THIRD EDITION

UMPHRED'S NEUROREHABILITATION

for the Physical Therapist Assistant

THIRD EDITION

UMPHRED'S NEUROREHABILITATION for the Physical Therapist Assistant

Editors

Rolando T. Lazaro, PT, PhD, DPT
Associate Professor
Department of Physical Therapy
Sacramento State University
Sacramento, California

Darcy A. Umphred, PT, PhD, FAPTA
Emeritus Professor
Retired Chair and Professor
Department of Physical Therapy
University of the Pacific
Stockton, California

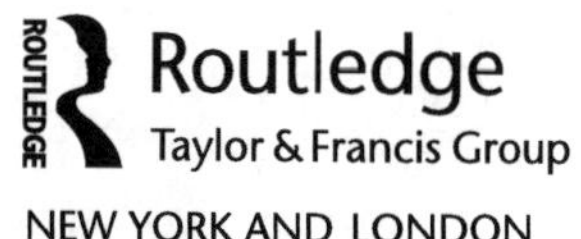

NEW YORK AND LONDON

Umphred's Neurorehabilitation for the Physical Therapist Assistant, Third Edition includes ancillary materials specifically available for faculty and clinician use. Please visit www.routledge.com/9781630915650 to obtain access.

First published 2021 by SLACK Incorporated

Published 2024 by Routledge
605 Third Avenue, New York, NY 10158

and by Routledge
4 Park Square, Milton Park, Abingdon, Oxon OX14 4RN

Routledge is an imprint of the Taylor & Francis Group, an informa business

Cover Artist: Katherine Christie

Library of Congress Cataloging-in-Publication Data

Names: Lazaro, Rolando T., 1965- editor. | Umphred, Darcy Ann, editor.
Title: Umphred's neurorehabilitation for the physical therapist assistant / editors, Rolando T. Lazaro, Darcy A. Umphred.
Other titles: Neurorehabilitation for the physical therapist assistant
Description: Third edition. | Thorofare, NJ : SLACK Incorporated, [2020] | Preceded by Neurorehabilitation for the physical therapist assistant / edited by Darcy A. Umphred, Rolando T. Lazaro. Second edition. [2014]. | Includes bibliographical references and index.
Identifiers: LCCN 2020012093 | ISBN 9781630915650 (paperback)
Subjects: MESH: Neurological Rehabilitation | Physical Therapist Assistants
Classification: LCC RC482 | NLM WL 140 | DDC 616.89/13--dc23
LC record available at https://lccn.loc.gov/2020012093

ISBN: 9781630915650 (pbk)
ISBN: 9781003525189 (ebk)

DOI: 10.4324/9781003525189

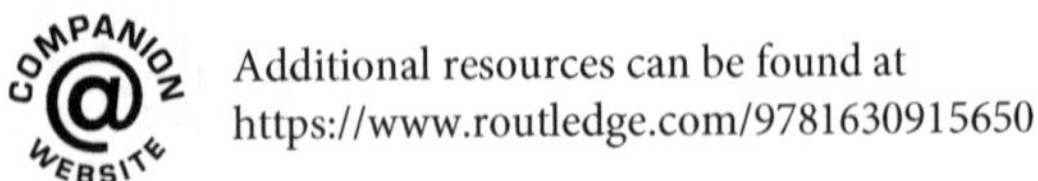

Additional resources can be found at
https://www.routledge.com/9781630915650

Dedication

The Third Edition of *Umphred's Neurorehabilitation for the Physical Therapist Assistant* is not only dedicated to all the professionals involved in its evolution, it is also dedicated to all the patients and family members that have taught us how they learn, what they value, what they want to relearn as far as movement function, and how they are best empowered to regain that function. Although the literature and ever-changing evidence creates maps to regaining function, the specific path within that map to success should be guided by the patient and the patient's motivation to retaining and continuing that learning. Once we as professionals see and listen to the voice of the patient, our clinical environment for both the clinician and patient become a wonderful world of learning for everyone.

—Darcy and Rolando

As in the first edition, I would also like to dedicate this edition to my immediate and extended family, whose support and encouragement has always given me energy to keep trying to provide to younger colleagues those materials that will help translate academic work into clinical competency. To my friends and colleagues who have deepened my belief in the empowerment of individuals to regain movement function in spite of body system problems, I truly thank all of you for your guidance in my evolution.

—Darcy

I dedicate this book to my mentors. Thank you for the support and encouragement, and for always believing in me. Most importantly, thank you for the friendship and love through the years. I honor your legacy by being the best mentor I could be to the next generation of physical therapy clinicians and educators.

—Rolando

Contents

Umphred's Neurorehabilitation for the Physical Therapist Assistant, Third Edition includes ancillary materials specifically available for faculty and clinician use. Please visit http:// www.routledge.com/9781630915650 to obtain access.

Acknowledgments

Dr. Lazaro and Dr. Umphred would like to thank all the authors in the Third Edition of *Umphred's Neurorehabilitation for the Physical Therapist Assistant* who have shown such a commitment to the profession of physical therapy and to the evolution of practice for the physical therapist assistant. As this Third Edition has an online video portion with actual video clips of both normal and problems in movement patterns, we would like to thank everyone who participated in this aspect of this edition. Also, thanks is expressed to everyone at SLACK Incorporated who has helped with this Third Edition in order to make it a visionary textbook for the physical therapist assistant and their faculty. We would especially like to thank Tony Schiavo, Joseph Lowery, Kayla Whittle, Mary Sasso, Nathan Quinn, and Allegra Tiver for their devoted time and energy at SLACK Incorporated and for making our jobs easier and without extreme stress.

About the Editors

Rolando T. Lazaro, PT, PhD, DPT is currently an Associate Professor at Sacramento State University in Sacramento, California. He graduated from Touro University with a PhD in Health Science, from Creighton University with a Postprofessional Doctor of Physical Therapy, from the University of the Pacific with an MS in Physical Therapy, and from the College of Allied Medical Professions, University of the Philippines Manila with a BS in Physical Therapy. Dr. Lazaro has authored research articles and chapters for a variety of textbooks. He became the primary editor of the Seventh Edition of Umphred's *Neurological Rehabilitation,* which was published in 2019. He is also coeditor of the Seventh Edition of Goodman and Snyder's *Differential Diagnosis for Physical Therapists* and Associate Editor of the Fourth Edition of Goodman and Fuller's *Pathology: Implications for the Physical Therapist.* Dr. Lazaro was awarded a Fulbright Senior Scholarship to the Philippines from June to November 2013. Previously, Dr. Lazaro was a professor at Samuel Merritt University in Oakland, California, and assistant professor at the University of the Pacific in Stockton, California. He was also a part-time physical therapist assistant faculty at the Professional Skills Institute in Concord, California.

Darcy A. Umphred, PT, PhD, FAPTA graduated from the University of Washington with a BS in Physical Therapy, from Boston University with an MS in Allied Health Education, and from Syracuse University with a PhD in Theories of Learning and Teacher Education in 1978. She has taught in both physical and occupational therapy programs throughout the United States since receiving her MS in 1970. At the time of her retirement, she was professor and chair of the Department of Physical Therapy at the University of the Pacific and played a major role in its evolution to granting a Doctorate of Physical Therapy to its graduates. After retirement, she was made an emeritus professor with all the honors that it brings. Throughout her professional career and throughout the world, she taught courses that combined theories of central nervous system function, movement science, evidence-based practice, and the unique qualities of the learning styles of the patient and clinicians into an integrated approach to analyzing individuals with central nervous system dysfunction creating functional movement problems. Her love of clinical practice and analyzing movement problems has driven her to question the "why's" behind patients' functional restrictions. Similarly, she has studied how our limbic, cognitive, and belief systems affect the interactions between the client and the therapist. She was the primary editor of the textbook *Neurological Rehabilitation,* for the first 6 editions between 1985 and 2012, which were translated into many different languages throughout the world. She has received numerous awards at the local, state, and national levels within the American Physical Therapy Association and was made a Catherine Worthingham Fellow in 2003. Her respect for the profession of physical therapy and the 2 educated clinicians—the physical therapist and the physical therapist assistant—has been demonstrated by her commitment to the responsibilities and services both professionals play in the delivery of physical therapy services throughout the world. It is her belief that physical therapy can and should play a unique role in the delivery of services for individuals with functional movement problems whether those problems arise from disease, pathology, or from everyday life experiences. Optimal quality of life is defined by each individual, and it is the therapist's role to help that person regain as much of that quality available. Thus, listening to the patients' voice—their beliefs, their true desires, and what will motivate each patient to retain and continue to learn—has become a major focus in her role as a patient and family advocate within the health care delivery system today.

Contributing Authors

Hazel Anderson, PT, DPT, cert. MDT (Chapter 17)
Assistant Professor
University of St. Augustine for Health Sciences
Austin, Texas

Fritzie Arce-McShane, PT, PhD (Chapter 4)
Research Assistant Professor
Department of Organismal Biology and Anatomy
University of Chicago
Chicago, Illinois

Rodiel Kirby Baloy, PT, DPT, EdS, MS (Chapter 8)
Adjunct Professor
Transitional Doctor of Physical Therapy Program
Department of Physical Therapy
The College of St. Scholastica
Duluth, Minnesota
Adjunct Faculty
Physical Therapist Assistant Program
Stanbridge University
Irvine, California

Ronald De Vera Barredo, PT, DPT, EdD, FAPTA (Chapter 16)
Dean and Professor
College of Health Sciences
Tennessee State University
Nashville, Tennessee

Kristen Barta, PT, PhD, DPT, NCS (Chapter 15)
Assistant Professor
University of St. Augustine for Health Sciences
Austin, Texas

Jan Black, PT, MSPT (Chapter 5)
Co-founder/Clinic Director
Neuroworx
Sandy, Utah

Amy Broekemeier, PT, DPT, COMT, PMA-CPT (Chapter 18)
Pinnacle Performance Owner
Doctor of Physical Therapy
Certified Manual Physical Therapist
Salt Lake City, Utah

Gordon U. Burton, OTR/L, PhD (Chapter 7)
Professor Emeritus
Past Chair and Professor
Department of Occupational Therapy
San Jose State University
San Jose, California

Elizabeth Ching, OTD, MEd, BSOT, OTR/L (Chapter 7)
Associate Professor
Department of Occupational Therapy
Samuel Merritt University
Oakland, California

Barbara H. Connolly, PT, DPT, EdD, C/NDT, FAPTA (Chapter 10)
Professor Emeritus
Department of Physical Therapy
University of Tennessee Health Science Center
Memphis, Tennessee

Kristine N. Corn, PT, MS, DPT (Chapter 9)
Owner and Clinician
Sierra Pediatrics
Roseville, California
Founder and Clinician
Ride To Walk: Therapeutic Horseback Riding
Granite Bay, California

Carol Davis, PT, DPT, EdD, FAPTA (Chapter 18)
Professor Emeritus
Department of Physical Therapy
University of Miami Miller School of Medicine
Coral Gables, Florida

Lauren Eberhardt, PT, DPT, NCS (Chapter 8)
Director
Physical Therapist Assistant Program
Stanbridge University
Irvine, California

Germaine Ferreira, PT, DPT, MSPT, BHMS (Chapters 15 and 17)
Assistant Professor
University of St. Augustine for Health Sciences
Austin, Texas

Lisa Ferrin, PTA, AS (Chapter 6)
Physical Therapist Assistant
Outpatient Rehabilitation
Methodist Hospital
Sacramento, California

Amanda A. Forster, PT, DPT, NCS (Chapter 14)
Senior Physical Therapist
Kaiser Permanente
San Jose, California

Patricia Harris, PT, MS (Chapter 6)
Professor, Retired
Physical Therapist Assistant Program
Sacramento City College
Sacramento, California

Brian Hickman, PT, DPT, NCS, GCS, CEEAA (Chapter 11)
Physical Therapist
Alameda Health System
Oakland, California

Bret Kennedy, PT, DPT, NCS (Chapter 11)
Adjunct Assistant Professor
Department of Physical Therapy
Samuel Merritt University
Oakland, California

Dennis Klima, PT, MS, PhD, DPT, GCS, NCS (Chapters 1 and 12)
Assistant Professor
Department of Physical Therapy
University of Maryland Eastern Shore
Princess Anne, Maryland

Tony Lema, PT, DPT (Chapter 11)
Physical Therapist
Alameda Health System
Oakland, California

Nelson Marquez, PT, EdD (Chapter 1)
Vice President
Institutional Effectiveness and Research
Webber International University
Babson Park, Florida

Becky S. McKnight, PT, MS (Chapter 13)
Program Coordinator
Physical Therapist Assistant Program
Ozarks Technical Community College
Springfield, Missouri

Esmerita Roceles Rotor, PT, PhD (Chapter 10)
Department of Physical Therapy
College of Allied Medical Professions
University of the Philippines
Manila, Philippines

Kelly Ryujin, PT, DPT (Chapter 11)
Adjunct Assistant Professor
Department of Physical Therapy
Samuel Merritt University
Oakland, California

Dale Scalise-Smith, PT, PhD (Chapter 3)
Vice President
Physical Therapy Academic Services
Orbis Education
Hinsdale, Massachusetts

Eunice Shen, PT, PhD, DPT, PCS (Chapter 10)
Rainwater Foundation
Monterey Park, California

James M. Smith, PT, DPT, MA (Chapter 13)
Professor of Physical Therapy
Utica College
Utica, New York

Irwin S. Thompson, PT, MPT, EdD (Chapter 6)
Assistant Professor
Department of Physical Therapy
California State University, Sacramento
Sacramento, California

Arvie Vitente, PT, DPT, MPH, GCS, CDP, CCI, PhD(c) (Chapter 19)
Academic Coordinator of Clinical Education
Assistant Professor
DPT Program
University of St. Augustine for Health Sciences
Miami, Florida

Amy Walters, PT, DPT, SCS, GCS (Chapter 17)
Assistant Professor
University of St. Augustine for Health Sciences
Austin, Texas

Preface

This Third Edition of *Umphred's Neurorehabilitation for the Physical Therapist Assistant* was written for student physical therapist assistants, physical therapist assistants in practice, and for faculty who teach neurorehabilitation within programs for physical therapist assistants. The area of neurorehabilitation has evolved from specific approaches designed by master clinicians from around the world to an environment where treatment interventions are supported by evidence along with experience in practice. Evidence-based practice is a process that considers the available documented evidence, the patient's values and desired outcomes, and the clinical judgment of the practitioner. Evidence-based practice generally leads to optimal outcomes but may not always answer clinical problem questions or clearly show the most efficient way to provide best practice. The physical therapist should not ask a physical therapist assistant to perform an intervention that has no evidence to support that it will lead to the desired outcomes of the plan of care. In the future, evidence that is true today may become simplistic or proven to be ineffective. New evidence can only evolve into new practice when both the physical therapist and physical therapist assistant recognize that the intervention approaches that they were taught are not working effectively for specific patients or not working at all with the general patient population, and new ideas whether discovered by the physical therapist or physical therapist assistant seem to positively change the outcomes of the plan of care.

This Third Edition widens the role of the physical therapist assistant and also the responsibility of that therapist in the evolution of intervention approaches that will best benefit the individual coming to physical therapy. Both editors have spent many years working in the area of neurorehabilitation as well as in the direct education of physical therapists who will be evaluating and setting up plans of care for individuals with movement dysfunctions arising from central nervous system (CNS) problems. The majority of the chapter authors in this book have been involved in the education of physical therapist assistants as well. Therefore, this book is specifically and purposely designed to be used by physical therapist assistants.

As physical therapy educators and clinicians, both editors understand the differences between disease/pathology and movement dysfunction. Thus, the medical model is only briefly introduced within this book. The major focus of this book is on approaches to gain or regain functional movement, and, in turn, quality of life of the individual coming to physical therapy. As therapists dealing with movement problems, both editors have clearly seen the potential of the human body to gain or regain function following a disease or pathology. Therapists do not correct the disease or damage to the CNS, but they do help in learning or relearning movement function lost to the individual coming to physical therapy. The plasticity of the CNS has now been shown in the literature as well as ways to learn or regain movement function and why those activities become best practice. Similarly, literature supports the concept that individual potential is dramatically improved when the person values the activities practiced and is actively engaged in the plan of care. For that reason, the physical therapist assistant's roles are not only to provide intervention or follow-up examinations, but also to be actively engaged in the interactions during those treatment sessions. As roles change so must the responsibility of the clinicians who either delegate or actively assume treatment of individuals under their care. The one specific concept that should be the foundation for neurorehabilitation is that there is potential in all of us to change and learn as long as we believe that change is possible. Empowering the patient to participate and actively engage in functional recovering will always be a key to success in physical therapy.

Introduction

The initial conceptualization of this book began well over 15 years ago and has evolved from both First and Second Editions into what is seen in this Third Edition. The role of the physical therapist assistant has enlarged and become a critical link in successful outcomes of many interventions provided to individuals with movement dysfunctions. This Third Edition has been written to help students and colleagues who are working with individuals with movement dysfunction arising from central nervous system (CNS) problems. As the depth and breadth of the role of the physical therapist assistant expands to include acute care, use of complex technology throughout the continuum of care, as well as treatment of long-term or chronic movement disorders, so must textbooks expand and incorporate those areas of practice. Physical therapist assistant texts must introduce, discuss, and explain both the interventions as well as examination tools that a physical therapist assistant might be asked to implement within the plan of care for individuals with CNS movement deficits. Those movement problems can arise at birth, in early childhood, adolescence, adulthood, or as one ages toward and into geriatrics. The initial chapters lay the foundation for discussion of interventions and follow-up examinations that a physical therapist assistant might be asked to perform throughout the plan of care. The model for physical therapist assistant practice as identified by the American Physical Therapy Association has been used as a guide to direct the physical therapist toward appropriate interventions and examination tools that might be delegated to the assistant. For that reason, intervention precedes examination because the physical therapist assistant will be asked to begin components of the plan of care designed by the physical therapist before being asked to perform selected examination procedures to generate information regarding the progress of a patient/client. As this model is different from the model used by physical therapists, the differentiation of those roles are identified throughout the book. The World Health Organization's International Classification of Functioning, Disability and Health has been adopted as the foundation for both the physical therapist and physical therapist assistant focus of care and now places the patient/client as the one who identifies value or quality to the various movement goals used in the plan of care. Patient participation is the key to success in any therapeutic environment and the link to long-term function.

The intervention chapters introduce and discuss common movement dysfunctions caused by CNS injury across the lifespan and the intervention approaches a physical therapist assistant might be asked to perform, as well as examination tools used to measure outcomes of those interventions. A discussion of the cardiopulmonary issues that might affect neurorehabilitation should help the physical therapist assistant understand how other body systems can affect movement dysfunctions and complicate the plan of care. The entire spectrum of care from birth through geriatrics is incorporated into this Third Edition, including the acute care settings through management of lifelong impairments and movement limitations. Similarly, a chapter on complementary approaches to intervention should help the reader understand when these alternative techniques can be used under supervision of the physical therapist, when a physical therapist assistant has obtained expertise in one of these approaches and how those clinical skills might be used as part of the plan of care.

A thorough study guide has been developed to help the learner identify critical issues within each chapter. Study guide questions posed for specific case studies are found both within the text as well as online. Also, the reader will find online specific video clips of individuals with movement problems discussed in the various chapters along with treatment approaches. Video clips of specific handling or movement techniques have been developed by the editors to help the learner see how normal movements can be facilitated by a therapist. These video clips of handling techniques should assist the physical therapist assistant in ways that he or she can empower his or her patients and clients to learn or regain motor control leading to greater function and, hopefully, a higher quality of life.

The evolution of this edition hopefully parallels the evolution of physical therapist assistant practice. As more and more delegation is given to the physical therapist assistant, continued education and potentially higher degrees will become a reality. This edition is a thoroughly written textbook regarding interventions and examination tools used by the physical therapist assistant when working with patients with CNS problems; it also has a visionary component introducing the importance of visual analysis of movement problems and highlights the need for the physical therapist assistant to develop visual recognition of specific problems found in the population of individuals with CNS deficits. This visual aspect of this textbook should help faculty introduce specific movement problems seen in this population with consistency.

In the end, physical therapy is all about providing excellent care to the patients and clients we serve. As editors, we are confident that this text will provide readers with excellent information that elevates their clinical practice and incorporates the patient's voice within all care environments.

Chapter 1

Introduction to Neurorehabilitation for the Physical Therapist Assistant

Darcy A. Umphred, PT, PhD, FAPTA; Rolando T. Lazaro, PT, PhD, DPT; Nelson Marquez, PT, EdD; and Dennis Klima, PT, MS, PhD, DPT, GCS, NCS

KEY WORDS Activity | Body structure and function | Patient/Client management | Health condition | International Classification of Functioning, Disability and Health | Neurorehabilitation | Personal and environmental factors | Physical therapist assistant

Chapter Objectives

- Discuss the International Classification of Functioning, Disability and Health (ICF) model and its implications on physical therapy management.
- Discuss the difference between the western medical model and the ICF model used by physical therapists and physical therapist assistants today.
- Discuss the factors involved when a physical therapist determines which tests, measures, and interventions are appropriate to be delegated to a physical therapist assistant.

The topic of neurological rehabilitation encompasses knowledge of the neurosciences, behavioral sciences, and social sciences. It requires an understanding of development across the lifespan and the pathologies or diseases relating to the nervous system. The causes and medical treatments for all known neurological pathologies or diseases fall within the domain of medical practice. While physical therapists and physical therapist assistants do not medically treat those diseases, an understanding of the pathologies is important in selecting the appropriate tests and measures establishing goal expectations and parameters for interventions, and considering limitations on motor control, motor learning, and neuroplasticity.

A patient may present to physical therapy with impairments or abnormalities in body structures and functions, and/or activity limitations, or problems with performance of functional activities. These limitations may have developed from a combination of nervous system pathology and the preexisting health status of the individual. Traditionally, neurological rehabilitation (or *neurorehabilitation*) is the process of regaining optimal function following the pathology or disease of the peripheral nervous system (PNS) and central nervous system (CNS). Generally, patients with these conditions are sent to physical therapy through a referral process from medical doctors and other health care professionals. The focus of this text will be on this scope of practice and the role of the physical therapist and physical therapist assistant when a referral has been made. Although the focus of this text is on neurorehabilitation following CNS insult, physical therapist assistants must also be aware of the role of physical therapy in wellness or pre-disease, as well as maintenance of motor function or quality of life of individuals following physical rehabilitation.

As many physical therapy clinics offer health promotion, wellness, and risk-reduction activities, individuals who previously had a CNS condition may come to those

Lazaro RT, Umphred DA, eds.
Umphred's Neurorehabilitation for the Physical Therapist Assistant, Third Edition (pp 1-11).

clinics without a referral source but with a prior medical diagnosis. Again, physical therapists and physical therapist assistants may be involved in examining and establishing treatment protocols to enhance the wellness, promote the health, and reduce the risk of developing other mobility limitations. Similarly, individuals may be placed in care facilities where a physical therapist and physical therapist assistant provide service to maintain mobility and optimize function. In those situations, the individual may first be evaluated by the physical therapist, who establishes a plan of care. Then, the physical therapist assistant may perform subsequent interventions and appropriate portions of reexaminations.

The physical therapist and physical therapist assistant must closely collaborate to ensure that optimal care is provided to the patient/client. Similarly, the physical therapist and physical therapist assistant must understand and appreciate the models both professionals learn and use when interacting with the patient. The model used by a physical therapist begins with examination, followed by drawing conclusions that lead to a physical therapy diagnosis, prognosis, and the plan of care. The model used by a physical therapist assistant begins with discussion by both the physical therapist and physical therapist assistant of the plan of care, followed by the physical therapist assistant interventions when appropriate, and follow-up examinations at established intervals or when changes in the patient's motor skills would indicate it is appropriate. These practice models are different, and for that reason, the intervention chapter precedes the chapter on examination when considering the physical therapist assistant's responsibilities within neurological rehabilitation.

In the clinical setting, differentiation of the roles of the physical therapist and physical therapist assistant may not be as clear, especially when physical therapists or physical therapist assistants start at the particular practice setting as novice practitioners. Following graduation from an educational program, these practitioners must commit to becoming lifelong learners. Most physical therapist assistants continue their learning through continuing education courses, in-service education, mentorship opportunities, formal academic degree programs, and certification or licensure in other areas of health care delivery. For this reason, a physical therapist may direct certain basic interventions and reassessments to a novice physical therapist assistant while delegating more complex interventions, reassessment of functional skills and more complex impairments, and a role in discharge planning to a more experienced physical therapist assistant. Similarly, novice physical therapists may not realize that an experienced physical therapist assistant could have advanced knowledge and skills and provide high-quality care to individuals with complex movement problems secondary to neurological pathologies. In both scenarios, it is critical that the physical therapist and physical therapist assistant closely communicate and collaborate to develop a plan of care that returns the patient to the highest level of physical function.

This chapter aims to present a conceptual understanding of the model of neurorehabilitation that is pertinent in current physical therapy practice. This outlines the foundation for learning the specific neurological clinical problems presented in subsequent chapters of this text. These specific clinical problems, crossing a lifespan of development, will also play a role in determining what should and should not be delegated. The physical therapist assistant must always remember that although a specific age population may be the focus of a pathology topic, many clinical problems can occur at any age. Obviously, those problems that occur in utero, at birth, or with a genetic link will set the stage for alternative paths to development. But these individuals who have neurological issues early in their lives can develop any of the other clinical problems discussed in this text along with additional movement problems that may arise because of aging and other life choices. For example, someone with an early medical diagnosis of cerebral palsy can later have a stroke, a spinal injury, or a head injury, or can develop some demyelinating disease as an adult. Similarly, the individual can develop repetitive strain problems from overuse or can stop moving, go into a disuse problem, or, through life choices, may become obese. Thus, those interventions presented within each of the clinical problem chapters are within the scope of a physical therapist assistant and might be delegated as part of the treatment plan for an individual on a physical therapist assistant's caseload.

Model of Neurorehabilitation: Introduction to the International Classification of Functioning, Disability and Health

Disablement Models of the Past (International Classification of Impairments, Disabilities, and Handicaps and Nagi Models)

Physical therapy, like many health professions throughout the world, analyzes and implements theoretical models to link the relationship between movement dysfunctions resulting from acute disease and pathology to explain how these movement problems can affect an individual's life. Therapists working with movement problems can often directly relate specific activity limitations to a pathology within the brain, but, just as frequently, many pathologies within the brain can lead to the same movement problem. As the profession of physical therapy moved from technique-based interventions to an evidence-based approach, it was natural to link our examinations and interventions to the pathology or disease that seemed to have caused those movement problems. For that reason, models that identi-

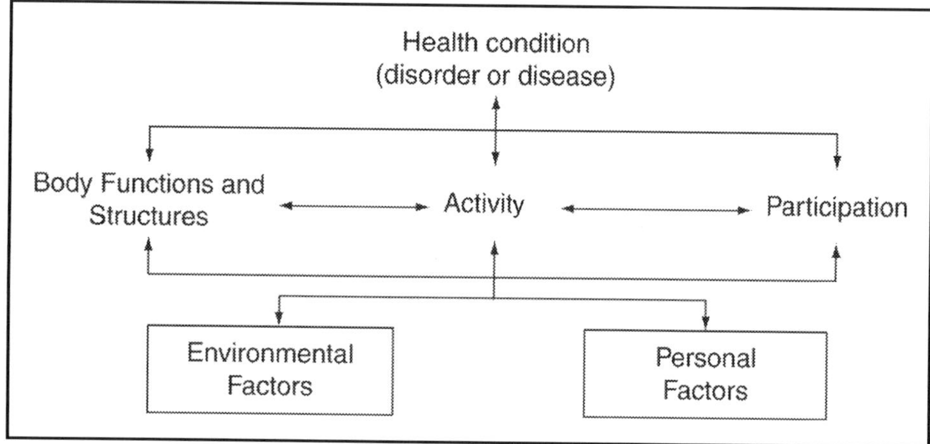

Figure 1-1. The International Classification of Functioning, Disability and Health model. (Reprinted with permission from World Health Organization. *Towards a Common Language for Functioning, Disability and Health*. Geneva, Switzerland: Author; 2002.)

fied the medical condition with the specific movement problems began to be developed and accepted by physical therapists. Two specific models were embraced in the 1980s and 1990s that clearly differentiated the disease or pathologies treated by medical doctors from the functional problems treated by physical therapists and physical therapist assistants. These 2 models, Nagi[1] and the International Classification of Impairments, Disabilities, and Handicaps (ICIDH),[2] basically followed a linear, sequential model in which a medical condition/disease or pathology lead to specific system impairments denoting body system or subsystem abnormalities. These impairments lead to functional limitations (Nagi) or disability (ICIDH), which describe what the person cannot do functionally, such as rolling, coming to standing, and reaching. These then lead to disability (Nagi) or handicaps (ICIDH), which are the person's perceived limitations in the ability to perform societal roles. Both models were based on a model of disablement and did not take into account the strengths of the patient that may assist in recovery and rehabilitation. The *Guide to Physical Therapist Practice* (the *Guide*) adopted the Nagi model in its first and second editions.[3]

Today's Enablement Model: The International Classification of Functioning, Disability and Health

In 2002, the World Health Organization introduced the ICF model.[4] This is a model of enablement, which takes into consideration the strengths of the patient/client, in addition to the patient's problems or limitations. This model identifies the complex, multidirectional, and integrated relationship among medical pathology, body systems, and movement, encompassing functions, functional activity, and participation in life. It also takes into account contextual factors, which could be personal, societal, and/or environmental considerations that may influence the person's path of rehabilitation, personal choices, and potential to return to optimal health and well-being. As such, the ICF subscribes to the biopsychosocial model of human functioning following a disease or illness.[4]

In the ICF model (Figure 1-1), the interaction between *health condition* and *contextual factors* forms the basis for disability and functioning. Also, in the model, human functioning is classified according to 3 levels: body or body part, the person as a whole, and the person in relation to the larger society.

Starting from the left, the diagram indicates the following aspects:

- *Body functions and structures* refers to the anatomical and physiological functioning of the human systems and subsystems.
- *Impairments* denotes problems in body structures and functions such as a CNS trauma or a fractured femur.
- *Activities* refers to the ability of a person to perform functional tasks such as rolling in bed, transferring to a chair, or walking.
- *Activity limitations* indicates problems with performance of functional activities, such as the inability to dress or walk in one's home.
- *Participation* involves choices and the ability of a person to be engaged in community situations such as going to a family gathering, shopping, or playing cards with friends. Problems with participation are termed *participation restrictions*, and the patient determines their value or worth as a way to participate in life.

A therapist could therefore assess each level of ICF functioning in relation to the presenting strengths and weaknesses at each level. Body functions and structures, activities, and participation highlight dimensions of functioning that are normal for the individual, while impairments, activity limitations, and participation restrictions are prob-

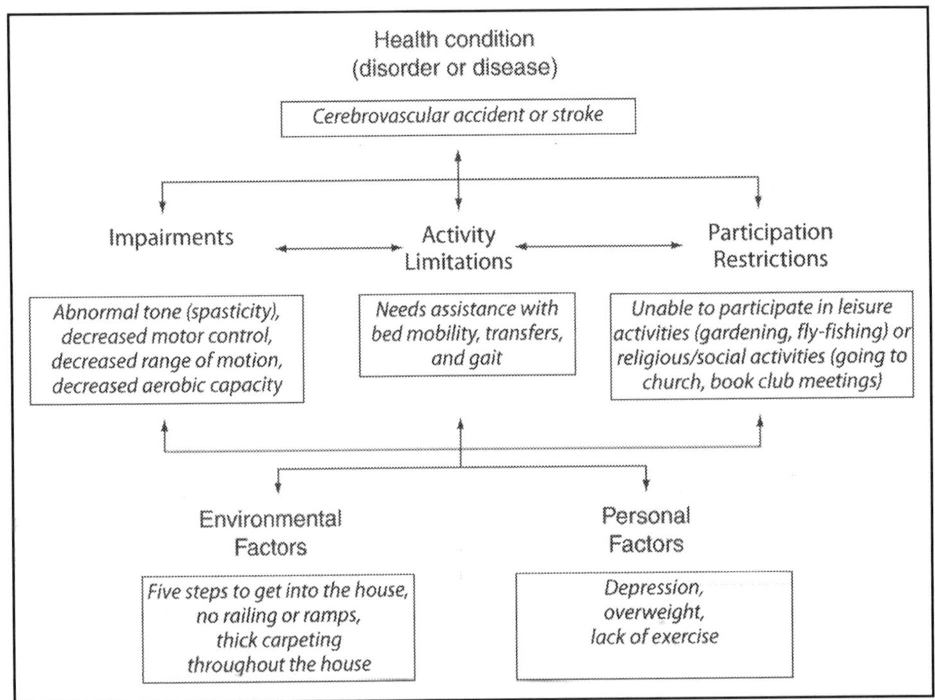

Figure 1-2. Application of the International Classification of Functioning, Disability and Health model to physical therapist and physical therapist assistant practice. The headings show the original model, and the italicized words and phrases in the boxes show how the model is applied to physical therapy practice.

lems that may be addressed by therapeutic interventions by a physical therapist or physical therapist assistant.

Moreover, contextual factors could also affect functioning. Environmental factors include the physical, social, and attitudinal attributes that may facilitate or hinder the return to optimal function. This return to function may also be facilitated or inhibited by personal factors or specific attributes of the individual.[4] This is why a therapist needs to be sensitive to what the patient values or wants to participate in and that determination is not made by the therapist.

Figure 1-2 provides an example of how the ICF model can be applied to physical therapy practice. Assume that the patient has a medical diagnosis of cerebrovascular accident or stroke (health condition/disorder or disease). This person may demonstrate activity limitations such as the need for assistance to perform bed mobility, transfers, and gait performance. The therapist must then hypothesize the possible impairments that may explain the noted activity limitations. The activity limitations may be due to impairments such as tone abnormalities, motor control problems, lack of range, decreased aerobic capacity, and possible cognitive deficits[4] or lack of motivation of the patient. Some of these limitations may be due to the stroke, while others may be due to other factors such as aging and physical activity levels. The patient or patient's family may also provide information about how the body structure/function and activity limitations impact the patient's ability to perform societal roles or participate in life (participation restrictions). Integrating personal and environmental factors will determine if such factors facilitate or hinder the rehabilitation process.

In 2008, the American Physical Therapy Association (APTA) joined international health care entities and the World Health Organization in endorsing the ICF model.[5] This model is now widely used in the national and international physical therapy communities; therefore, this model will be consistently used throughout this text. The third edition of the *Guide to Physical Therapist Practice* used this model when determining the components of the *Guide*.[6] Also, the reader can always find new and expanded information regarding the clinical applications of the ICF model through websites.[7,8]

This book will also consistently incorporate the terminology and definitions of terms used in the *Guide*,[6] published by the APTA. The intent of the *Guide* is to discuss the common features that describe the physical therapy management of selected patient/client conditions and diagnostic groups.

Central to the understanding of the *Guide*[6] is the understanding of the elements of patient/client management: examination, evaluation, diagnosis, prognosis, intervention, and outcomes (Figure 1-3). The following describes each element and the role of the physical therapist assistant.

Examination

A physical therapy examination includes obtaining a patient history, performing a systems review, and administering tests and measures to gather relevant data about the patient. Often the systems review and subsequent tests and measures are merged as the therapist proceeds through the examination. However, in a primary care practice setting, the physical therapist may elect to partition the systems review as a screen for potential red-flag conditions. The initial examination is comprehensive and leads to a diagnostic classification or identification of specific body systems, activity limitations, and participation restrictions that may benefit from physical therapy intervention. This process may also result in identification of problems that may require consultation with or referral to other health care providers.[6] The physical therapist conducts the initial examination. The physical therapist assistant may assist in collecting data as determined by the physical therapist. If the physical therapist assistant is asked to participate in this initial examination, then those data or results must be reported to the supervising physical therapist in an effort to generate an appropriate plan of care.

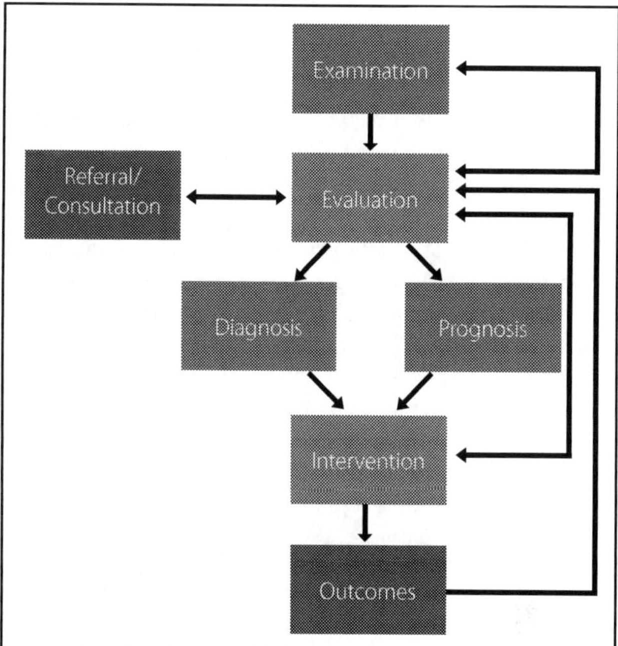

Figure 1-3. Elements of the Patient/Client Management Model. (Reprinted from http://guidetoptpractice.apta.org/, with permission of the American Physical Therapy Association. © 2019 American Physical Therapy Association. All rights reserved.)

Evaluation

This is a process in which the physical therapist makes clinical judgments based on data gathered during the examination. The evaluation facilitates the determination of the systems or subsystems that may explain the corresponding functional loss, as well as the severity of the patient's mobility profile. Through examination, the physical therapist also identifies possible problems that may require consultation with or referral to other providers. This element is beyond the scope of practice for the physical therapist assistant and is conducted by the supervising physical therapist. However, the physical therapist assistant may be present for the evaluation process.[6]

Diagnosis

The physical therapy diagnosis identifies the body structure/function and activity limitations that may contribute to the functional problem. The physical therapy diagnosis also articulates the possible participation restriction and activity limitations that the patient values or wants to return to after therapy. The physical therapy diagnosis may also contain a brief discussion of the contextual factors that affect function. It is a "process and the outcome of examination and evaluation"[6] and provides the basis for determining the patient/client prognosis and planning intervention strategies. For example, the physical therapist may formulate a diagnosis for a patient with a traumatic brain injury that describes altered cognition, hemiparesis, and limited gait performance impeding participation in employment and recreational activities.

The referring physician is responsible for the medical diagnosis that should identify the disease and/or pathology, and the supervising physical therapist determines the diagnosis of impairment, activity, and participation loss. Remember that the patient and family always determine participation activities. The determination of both types of diagnoses is beyond the scope of physical therapist assistant's practice. However, it is the responsibility of the physical therapist assistant to comprehend the meaning of the diagnosis and how it relates to intervention. It is the physical therapist's responsibility to communicate to the supervising physical therapist the changes in the patient/client's functional performance to allow the physical therapist to make the necessary changes in the treatment plan.[6] Although the roles and responsibilities of the physical therapist and physical therapist assistant will change, the relationship and responsibilities to communicate with each other will always remain a key to best practice.

Prognosis

The prognosis identifies the predicted optimal improvement in function and the time parameters needed to change the existing limitations into functional activities the patient will be able to perform.[6] Part of the prognosis will deal with specific body systems that require change before function can be expected. In addition, when establishing the prognosis, the physical therapist must consider the patient's health and nutritional status. Examples of those body system problems may be as simple as strengthening a specific muscle group or increasing general range of motion (ROM) in joints, or as complex as improving balance and postural control. Another part of the prognosis will deal with specific activities that the therapist, patient, and family have identified as needing improvement to regain optimal function. These activities may include having bed mobility, walking, climbing stairs, getting in and out of the shower, dressing, feeding, and getting in and out of the car. In some rehabilitation environments, specific activities of daily living tasks may be the responsibility of other professionals such as occupational therapists or occupational therapy assistants. Also, it is important to link therapy goals to those of the patient/family and what that individual wants and needs to do once they leave the rehabilitation environment. These are often considered participation activities and certainly may include golfing, fly fishing, going to religious services, shopping, or other activities that allow the individual to participate in life. As such, the patient and the family, not the therapist, should identify those activities.

The prognosis also includes the plan of care established by the physical therapist. The plan specifies the anticipated goals and expected outcomes, and the specific interventions to be used, including the timing and frequency. It includes both short-term and long-term goals. While the establishment of these goals is the responsibility of the physical therapist, the physical therapist assistant could provide input on the development of these goals and how they should be changed based on the patient's response to the interventions.

Regardless of the delegated responsibilities, the physical therapist assistant is always responsible for communicating any changes in the patient's response to the plan of care. The physical therapist assistant provides this input to allow the supervising physical therapist to modify the prognosis and the treatment plan as appropriate. The observed changes may be due to development of new problems that may require reexamination or referral to other professionals including the physician.

Intervention

This element of the Patient/Client Management Model involves the use of physical therapy procedures to achieve the patient goals. A reexamination may be conducted to determine any changes in the patient/client status, progress toward established goals, or the modification of the current plan of care.[6]

In the area of neurorehabilitation, common interventions delegated to physical therapist assistants include body structure/function training, such as strength training or ROM exercises, and activity training, such as task-specific exercises to improve bed mobility, sit-to-stand, walking, or sitting (see Chapter 5). Functional training will include interventions to facilitate the return to participation in work, community, and civic life. Additional domains include airway clearance techniques, assistive technology applications, and motor function training. Patient instruction, such as with a home exercise program, will be a common intervention the physical therapist assistant performs. The physical therapist assistant may assist in data collection to determine if the current plan of care is on track in meeting the established goals, or if the plan of care needs to be modified.

The depth and breadth of the physical therapist assistant scope of practice may change if the educational preparation for the physical therapist assistant moves from an associate to a baccalaureate degree. The roles of the physical therapist assistant may also be influenced by the acquisition of additional treatment skills through continuing education. The specific direction to the physical therapist assistant has to be based on the physical therapist assistant's abilities and the scope of practice identified within the respective state law. It is not clear how the roles of the physical therapist and physical therapist assistant will change, but both professionals must work closely together to provide the best care for the patient.

Outcomes

Physical therapy outcomes refer to the product of the patient/client management process and the impact of physical therapy care on the impairments, activities, and participation, as well as patient/client satisfaction following the physical therapy intervention.[6] The physical therapist assistant could participate in tracking outcomes by assisting in collecting objective and measurable data. Outcomes can, in turn, drive continuous quality improvement for the practice setting.

Physical Therapy Practice Areas

The *Guide* includes practice patterns that provide details on the possible examination, intervention, and prognostic indications given specific practice patterns. Following are 4 content (practice) areas under which these practice patterns are classified:

1. Musculoskeletal (muscles, joints, and bony structures)
2. Neuromuscular (sensory and motor peripheral nerves and CNS processing, including somatic and autonomic)
3. Cardiovascular and pulmonary (heart and lungs)
4. Integumentary (skin)

This text will focus on the clinical problems that develop within the area of neuromuscular practice, although any patients can develop movement problems that arise from other bodily system areas such as musculoskeletal, cardiovascular, pulmonary, integumentary, or endocrine. The reader must be aware that patients may have difficulty in more than one bodily system area, and the interactions may be significant. For example, a person with movement dysfunction following a neurological condition may also develop cardiopulmonary problems, or the person may already have a cardiopulmonary issue prior to the neurological insult (see Chapter 16). Both body systems must be considered when implementing appropriate physical therapy plans of care. (See Chapters 9, 10, 11, 12, 13, 14, 15 and 16 for additional information on these other systems interactions with observed movement problems of those patients.)

Although the *Guide*[6] identifies body system problems that physical therapists generally treat, additional systems can affect movement problems seen as part of the habilitation or rehabilitation of those individuals. Organ systems can play a critical role in the effectiveness of the physical therapy interventions. The gastrointestinal system plays a primary role in nutrition intake and elimination of waste. The hepatic and urinary systems play a vital role in filtering out chemical waste and excess fluid. The lymphatic system helps the vascular system with fluid elimination. Any body system can dramatically affect the cardiac, smooth, and striated muscles' metabolism and function.

Similarly, a dysfunction of the neuromuscular system can affect the function of other organ systems as well. For example, an individual may be referred to physical therapy with the medical diagnosis of early-stage Parkinson's disease. A patient may complain of constipation, which may be a result of decreased level of mobility, medication side effects, and rigidity of the trunk and the abdominal muscles. In this case, the patient may benefit from an increase in mobility and ambulation and interventions to decrease torso rigidity. The interventions may lead to an increased level of activity performance and participation and may also provide the added benefit of improvement of gastrointestinal function, leading to decreased complaints of constipation.

Role of the Physical Therapist and Physical Therapist Assistant

Although the licensing board of the state dictates the role of the physical therapist assistant within a clinical setting, the specific types of delegation fall under the responsibilities of the physical therapist and should directly relate to the needs of the patient. The physical therapist assistant is the physical therapist's assistant and should function within that scope of practice. The physical therapist will have ultimate responsibility for the physical therapy provided to the patient.

Theoretical Framework

The authors have developed a theoretical framework to assist the reader in understanding the role of the physical therapist assistant in working with patients/clients with neurological conditions. The theoretical framework is aligned with key components of the ICF model, the Patient/Client Management Model, and effective delegation principles (Figure 1-4).

Designated interventions for a patient recovering from neurological pathologies are directed at improving the patient's functional status through comprehensive interventions at both the activity and body systems and functions level. These interventions may simultaneously improve activity and participation (such as returning to leisure activities like golfing or fly fishing) or may be directed at resolving impairments that could ultimately improve activity and participation.

For example, if the patient's ultimate goal is to be able to return to fly fishing, the physical therapist assistant can work with the client in sitting or standing and having the client hold, or hold with assistance, a fishing rod placed in a large can stabilized with sand. As the activity is performed, the client will, by virtue of the task, be working on ROM, strength, balance, and postural control of the trunk, limbs, and shoulder girdle, all of which may need retraining after the neurological insult. In addition, the physical therapist assistant must employ effective strategies to address the cognitive, musculoskeletal, and neuromuscular needs of the patient while working on specific activities selected by the patient or family.

Delegation Strategies: Decision-Making Versus Doing

In the Patient/Client Management Model continuum, the physical therapist assistant will ultimately be delegated select reexamination procedures and interventions.[6] The determination of these interventions follows a thorough initial examination by the physical therapist. The physical therapist will summarize findings of the examination in the evaluation and will formulate a diagnosis and prognosis based on these findings. Designated interventions will then be indicated in the plan of care, and the physical therapist assistant will perform select intervention activities in conjunction with ongoing communication with the supervising physical therapist.

In 1971, within a few years of the development of the physical therapist assistant, Nancy Watts, PT, PhD, FAPTA, presented effective delegation strategies to our profession.[9] The physical therapist's responsibility for determination of the tasks that can be delegated to a physical therapist assistant, including interventions and reexaminations, is a complex issue. Watts proposed a decision-making method that includes analyzing the physical therapy tasks involved in the interventions under consideration to determine the degree to which it represents decision-making vs doing, and the degree to which the elements are separable. She suggested that both components interact, and both are necessary to quality care and best practice (Box 1-1).

The decision-making aspect of care requires evaluation and treatment planning skills. These skills require complex problem-solving, up-to-date knowledge of the science of physical therapy, and a sophisticated ability to analyze and synthesize information from various sources to rationally

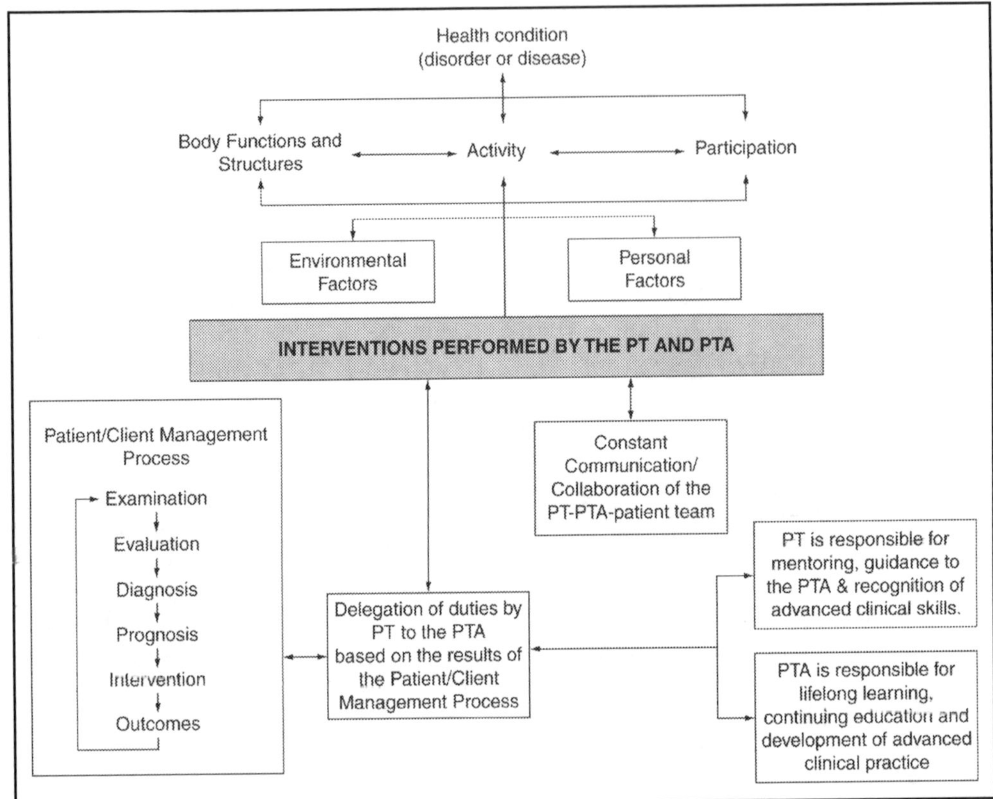

Figure 1-4. Theoretical framework for interventions provided by the physical therapist assistant. Abbreviations: PT; physical therapist, PTA; physical therapist assistant.

Box 1-1

Delegation Strategies: Decision-Making Versus Doing

1. Predictability of consequences: How uncertain is the situation? How confident can the decision-maker be in the predictions about the consequences of action?
2. Stability of the situation: How much and how quickly is change likely to occur in the factors on which decisions are made?
3. Observability of basic indicators: How difficult is it to elicit the phenomena on which decisions are based? How easy are these phenomena to perceive or observe?
4. Ambiguity of basic indicators: How difficult are the key phenomena to interpret? How easily might they be confused with other phenomena?
5. Criticality of results: How serious are the consequences of a poor choice of method?

choose the best alternative. To a large extent, these responsibilities fall into the physical therapist's scope of practice.

The doing aspect of care requires excellence in skill, the knowledge of therapeutic interventions, the capacity to recall correct treatment sequences, the artful manipulation of one's hands and body, and the ability to be sensitive to patient response moment-to-moment. Watts maintains that, in general, "decision-making skills involve dealing with data, while doing skills require dealing with people and things."[9] She also added that "the distinction drawn in this model between these 2 categories of skill should not be misconstrued as implying any hierarchy of importance nor any lack of interdependence between activities in the 2 realms."[9]

Watts also identifies 5 factors present in treatment that more adequately characterize the continuum that flows between deciding and doing:

1. Predictability of consequences: How uncertain is the situation? How confident can the decision-maker be in the predictions about the consequences of action?

   For example, a gait-training program for an individual with a sprained ankle with no other medical conditions is very different from a gait-training program for a person with a stroke, cardiac and pulmonary complications, uncontrolled diabetes, and a new orthotic device because of ankle weakness and instability.[9] The predictability of the probable consequences of gait-training decisions made for a patient with a sprained ankle seems more certain than those made for a person following a stroke with added complicating medical variables.

2. Stability of the situation: How much and how quickly is change likely to occur in the factors upon which decisions are made?

   For example, a mat exercise program for someone with a complete spinal cord injury (SCI) will remain relatively unchanged for a period of time compared with a mat program for an individual with an incomplete SCI. The person with the incomplete SCI may demonstrate significant functional improvement within a short period of time. However, considering the medical condition, a physical therapist assistant with accurate visual recognition skills and experience and additional education in SCI management may be delegated intervention strategies, but will be expected to report to the physical therapist any changes that might indicate an alteration in the plan of care.

3. Observability of basic indicators: How difficult is it to elicit the phenomena on which decisions are based? How easy are these phenomena to perceive or observe?

   For example, an obligatory reflex may be easy to elicit and observe, whereas a maximal voluntary contraction requires full patient participation and may be more difficult to elicit.[9] When adjustments in treatment are needed on a moment-to-moment basis, the intervention should remain with the physical therapist. As soon as those movements begin to stabilize and changes are easily recognized, then delegating to the physical therapist assistant is appropriate.

4. Ambiguity of basic indicators: How difficult are the key phenomena to interpret? How easily might they be confused with other phenomena?

   For example, possible signs indicating the possibility of a cerebrovascular accident would be more difficult to identify and interpret than determining whether a muscle substitution was used in a manual muscle test.[9] A physical therapist assistant can easily recognize muscle substitution and certainly an obvious stroke in transition, but noticing subtle changes that reflect worsening of a medical problem is the responsibility of the physical therapist, and a patient who may be that unstable should not be delegated.

5. Criticality of results: How serious are the consequences of a poor choice of method?

   For example, a wrong choice in a facilitation method that resulted in no response of the muscle would be of less consequence than the wrong choice in the amount of exercise without rest to be given to a patient with cardiac compromise.[9] If the intervention needs constant reexamination throughout the treatment, the physical therapist should not be asking the physical therapist assistant to make those decisions. On the other hand, a very skilled and experienced physical therapist assistant might be able to monitor a patient and recognize when the physical therapist is needed. Thus, the decision to delegate or retain control over the intervention should be made with serious consideration of the patient's needs and the stability of the vital organ systems of the patient.

These 5 determinants are present to varying degrees in all treatment situations. In deciding which interventions and reexaminations to delegate to the physical therapist assistant, the physical therapist must clearly differentiate between the deciding and doing aspects of the intervention and then, using the factors listed previously, determine the extent to which these 2 aspects of care can be separated. These components will guide a physical therapist regarding when to delegate select interventions for a client with CNS damage to a physical therapist assistant. Obviously, the experiences and continuing education of the physical therapist assistant may change how a physical therapist decides to delegate. The patient must always be the one constant factor, and the belief that "we do no harm and provide best practice" should be the guiding factor in that decision-making.

If the patient requires constant guarding and guidance to carry out a specific functional task, and the amount of guarding and guidance varies from moment-to-moment, delegation of that activity to a physical therapist assistant may be inappropriate. On the other hand, if the patient is able to run a motor program, such as moving from sit-to-stand, but needs guidance to stay within a parameter of range of limits of stability or balance, delegation of the intervention to a physical therapist assistant is appropriate. If the patient does not need guidance and only needs practice to overcome functional limitations, usually a family member or an aide can assist, and this may not be an appropriate use of the physical therapist assistant. Although many overlapping variables might determine when a physical therapist vs a physical therapist assistant should be responsible for the intervention, having time to provide a service should not be a reason. If the physical therapist assistant is being asked to treat someone because he or she has time and not because the physical therapist assistant is the best provider given the needs of the patient, then that delegation is inappropriate and is a misuse of the physical therapist assistant within a clinical setting.

Effective delegation strategies are enhanced by ongoing communication with the supervising physical therapist to optimize interventions performed by the physical therapist assistant to enhance the plan of care. If an intervention is delegated to a physical therapist assistant and the skill is outside of what the physical therapist assistant has learned, it is always appropriate for the physical therapist assistant to ask the physical therapist for help or guidance. If what was delegated seems to contradict what the physical therapist assistant has learned as contraindications, the physical therapist assistant should always ask the physical therapist for clarification before beginning treatment.

Career Development and Clinical Interaction Issues

Career development is important to every individual. Every person strives to perform work that provides a sense of satisfaction and purpose. In the case of a physical therapist assistant, career pathways have emerged with the advancement of the practice of physical therapy. It is, however, important to have a clear picture of the implications of these career pathways in relation to the ethical and legal aspects of practice.

Within the profession itself, the APTA initiated the physical therapist assistant Recognition of Advanced Proficiency. This is the equivalent of the clinical specialist certifications for physical therapists. This advanced proficiency designation recognizes physical therapist assistants who have furthered their careers beyond their entry-level preparation by achieving advanced skills through experience, leadership, and education.[10] This also recognizes the exceptional physical therapist/physical therapist assistant team collaboration that facilitates the provision of the best possible care to the patient/client. Currently, physical therapist assistants can obtain advanced proficiencies in the following areas: acute care, aquatic, cardiovascular/pulmonary, geriatric, integumentary, musculoskeletal, neuromuscular, oncology, and/or pediatric physical therapy. More information regarding Advanced Proficiency Pathways for the physical therapist assistant can be found on the APTA website.

The following clinical scenarios describe potential areas of conflict in the physical therapist/physical therapist assistant dynamic. The first pertains to the clinical interactions between a physical therapist and physical therapist assistant from a business model. One scenario that has developed is the physical therapist assistant owning a physical therapy practice that employs physical therapists and physical therapist assistants. Most state physical therapy licensing boards have identified the practice relationship of this business model. If the physical therapist assistant owns the practice, then *that individual cannot function as a physical therapist assistant within that setting*. The conflict of interest between the role of a boss to the physical therapist and being the assistant to the same individual is self-explanatory and legally controlled by most state regulations governing the practice of physical therapy.

Another role the physical therapist assistant may assume in a clinical setting is that of receiving certification or licensure in a complementary approach to patient management. Examples of these certifications or licensure include being a Feldenkrais practitioner, being a Rolfer, or training in craniosacral techniques (see Chapter 18). In these cases, the physical therapist assistant may develop intervention skills outside the skills of the physical therapist but complementary to providing intervention. Hopefully, open communication exists between the physical therapist and physical therapist assistant that encourages implementation of all interventions that can benefit the patient, but again, the physical therapist assistant must remember that the physical therapist is responsible for deciding which interventions are to be used and which interventions will be delegated to the physical therapist assistant.

The physical therapist assistant should always make the physical therapist aware of intervention strategies that may be helpful but are not already provided within the plan of care and never begin interventions without clarifying the intent with the physical therapist. If the physical therapist assistant is practicing as a complementary therapist independently of a physical therapy practice setting and outside the supervision of a physical therapist, then the physical therapist assistant must remember that he or she is not practicing as a physical therapist assistant, and that what is offered is not physical therapy and cannot be billed as such. Physical therapist assistants who have additional certification should also be aware of the legal and liability issues that may apply to them as licensed physical therapist assistants practicing in the complementary therapy arena. Discussion of these issues is beyond the scope of this text, but physical therapist assistants with complementary training must become familiar with the laws within the state in which they practice.

Future Roles

Physical therapy is a profession that has been evolving since its conception. The roles of the physical therapist and physical therapist assistant will change. Yet, the interactions should remain as 2 clinicians whose responsibility is to help guide patients toward functional recovery and a higher quality of life. As physical therapists develop more wellness clinics and risk-reduction programs, the roles of physical therapist assistants will enlarge in these practice areas as well. As the aging population copes with chronic diseases and the life-altering loss of functional skills, optimizing quality of life vs regaining function will become part of an ever-expanding scope of practice. As the population ages, maintaining independence will decrease individuals' care costs. The physical therapist assistant will continue to play an important role in that maintenance of functional skills in a cost-effective manner.

The role of the physical therapist assistant has the potential of enlarging with increased responsibilities for patient care. As these roles change, so will the educational requirements for entry-level practitioners, as seen in the move to an entry-level clinical doctorate for physical therapists. Physical therapist assistant educational requirements may change to require a baccalaureate degree. Physical therapist assistants of today may well be facing the same dilemma as physical therapists who graduated with bachelor's and master's degrees in the past. Younger graduates today may have a degree higher than the one a current practitioner has. This means only that the younger therapist, whether a physical therapist or a physical therapist assistant, may have new knowledge to teach the experienced clinician, just as the clinician has skills to teach the novice. The key to not being caught with limitations in practice parameters is to continue with one's learning no matter the degree received that opened the door to entry into this profession.

It is hoped that this text will provide a background to the physical therapist assistant that will not only help during study as a student but also provide insight and guidance once the student moves into an exciting practice arena as a physical therapist assistant.

References

1. Nagi S. *Disability Concepts Revisited: Implication for Prevention.* Washington, DC: National Academy Press; 1991.
2. World Health Organization. *International Classification of Impairments, Disabilities and Handicaps (ICIDH).* Geneva, Switzerland: Author; 2001.
3. *Guide to Physical Therapist Practice.* 2nd ed. Alexandria, VA: American Physical Therapy Association; 2001.
4. International Classification of Functioning, Disability and Health. World Health Organization. https://www.who.int/classifications/icf/en/. Accessed November 2, 2012.
5. American Physical Therapy Association. APTA Endorses World Health Organization ICF Model. http://www.apta.org/Media/Releases/APTA/2008/7/8/. Accessed November 2, 2012.
6. American Physical Therapy Association. Guide to Physical Therapist Practice 3.0. http://guidetoptpractice.apta.org/. Accessed August 1, 2018.
7. Sykes C. Health classifications 2: using the ICF in clinical practice. WCPT Keynotes. http://www.wcpt.org/sites/wcpt.org/files/files/KN-ICF-Clinical_practice.pdf. Accessed August 29, 2013.
8. Rauch A, Cieza A, Stucki G. How to apply the International Classification of Functioning, Disability and Health (ICF) for rehabilitation management in clinical practice. *Eur J Phys Rehabil Med.* 2008;44(3):329-342.
9. Watts NT. Task analysis and division of responsibility in physical therapy. *Phys Ther.* 1971;51(1):23-35. doi:10.1093/ptj/51.1.23
10. American Physical Therapy Association. PTA recognition of advanced proficiency. http://www.apta.org/ptarecognition/. Accessed August 1, 2018.

Chapter 2

Functional Neuroanatomy

Darcy A. Umphred, PT, PhD, FAPTA

KEY WORDS Brainstem | Cortical structures | Diencephalon | Gray and white matter | Neuron (dendrites, cell bodies, axons, and synaptic junctions) | Peripheral and central nervous system | Spinal cord

Chapter Objectives

- Comprehend the structure and function of the areas of the central nervous system (CNS).
- Comprehend the function of the peripheral nervous system and its importance in sensory awareness, processing, and, ultimately, motor function.
- Differentiate the areas of the CNS and where those areas are located in relation to each other.
- Identify the difference between sensory and motor processing and where that processing occurs.
- Discuss the difference between gray and white matter and the part of the neuron each represents.
- Describe the vascular system within the CNS and how important that is in brain health.

This chapter is not written to replace traditional functional neuroanatomy or neurophysiology textbooks[1,2] or courses, but rather as a review for the physical therapist assistant of the neuroanatomical structures and function of the human nervous system.[3,4,5] The analogies used within this chapter may seem at times simplistic, but are used to help the physical therapist assistant not only understand this system, but also develop communication skills with patients with nervous system impairments and their families. These analogies are designed to help patients and families comprehend the structure and function of the nervous system. For many people, the nervous system seems so complex and confusing that patients and family members feel overwhelmed and unable to comprehend the role that they play in helping to improve function.

If the analogy is made between the nervous system and a large car with all its components, it is the interactions of all the parts, and not necessarily each part itself, that produces the complex function. The driver of the car, as is the patient's nervous system, is the most important. When considering a car, the individual does not have to be able to name each aspect of the many components; the person just has to recognize when something is not functioning. When the air conditioning does not work, the driver takes the car to the mechanic. It may be determined that a hose is leaking, or the water pump failed, but not a problem in the air conditioning itself.

The nervous system is similar, and the result of its function is participation in life. Patients may have anatomically similar lesions that lead to different problems, while other patients may have different lesions that lead to similar problems. Whether an individual wants to pick up a cup of coffee but sees double, is unable to feel where the cup is located, or reaches for the cup and his hand or arm shakes too much to hold the cup, the result is loss of function. No matter the cause, functional impairments affect performance. Those individuals often feel they can no longer participate in activities they want, and their quality or control in life has changed. These individuals often get frustrated and show other emotional responses that can make the problem seem worse. An individual with nervous system problems temporarily or permanently comes to therapy to have someone help them correct these system problems.

Lazaro RT, Umphred DA, eds.
Umphred's Neurorehabilitation for the Physical Therapist Assistant, Third Edition (pp 13-36).

A patient may need to learn a new way to function to compensate for a loss, to relearn how to regain function through its original means, or to learn to perform the same function using different components. Like the mechanic with the car, the physical therapist needs to recognize the functional problems of the patient and how to correct them. The physical therapist does functional examinations to evaluate the problems and set up a plan of care. When the physical therapist delegates tasks to an assistant, both professionals need to understand the larger problem within the nervous system, understand how those problems affect the function of the entire system, and recognize when what is being practiced does not match the direction of the desired plan of care. Thus, understanding the basic principles of neuroanatomy, neurophysiology, and function is critical for a physical therapist assistant to practice effectively with clients with CNS dysfunction.

This chapter is designed to help the physical therapist assistant comprehend how all the parts of the nervous system fit together, what to recognize when a part is not functioning, and how to help the nervous system relearn once something affects its function.[4] As in a car, some parts are more critical than others. The physical therapist assistant should be able to recognize the behavioral structures, analyze how those behaviors affect patients, and recognize faults in patients' abilities to produce those behaviors. A wide variety of complications can lead to development of movement disorders. Such complications include birth trauma, genetic predisposition, traumatic injury, severe chemical interaction, structural degeneration over time, or a decision not to participate in movement that leads to abnormalities. Although it is the physical therapist's responsibility to recognize the specifics of those deviations from normal function, it is also the physical therapist assistant's responsibility to recognize changes from what the physical therapist has already evaluated and identified. If, after reading this chapter, physical therapist assistants have that overview, they can later pursue more inclusive and complex functional or complex neuroanatomy texts. Using this model may help the physical therapist assistant make more sense of knowledge, and help make learning more fun and challenging.

When looking at a person, one can see structures on the outside. In the head, one finds eyes, ears, a nose, a mouth, a tongue, skin, and hair. These structures send information or sensory input to central structures through what are called *cranial nerves* (CN). Information coming from the body from the skin, joints, and muscles are called *peripheral nerves.* Cranial and peripheral nerves carrying information toward the CNS are called *sensory nerves.* Nerves carrying information from the CNS to the peripheral systems are called *motor nerves.* The entire system is considered the *somatic nervous system.*

Another nervous system is called the *autonomic nervous system*, which receives input from and carries responses to the internal structures or organs such as the heart, lungs, stomach, intestines, kidneys, liver, and blood vessels. When talking about the skin and thermal regulation, some overlap exists between the somatic and autonomic nervous systems. These systems are certainly more complex and interactive and critical in life function, but that degree of complexity can become overwhelming to both the clinician and the patient or family.[6]

Peripheral Nervous System

The peripheral nervous system is made up of both sensory and motor nerves. These nerves are made up of a large number of fibers called neurons. The anatomy of the neuron will be discussed later in this section.

Sensory System

All information traveling from the periphery of the head and body toward the central system is considered sensory. Information coming in from one side of the body will communicate or synapse on another neuron and cross over to the opposite side of the CNS. This is critical, for the right side of the body is controlled by the left side of the nervous system, and vice versa. Every sensory nerve's role in body function is to inform the nervous system about environments outside and inside the human body. Information regarding pain, touch, joint positioning, temperature, and muscle contractions is considered somatic sensory input, while information coming from internal organs regarding pain, heart rate, respiration, blood pressure, and bowel and bladder filling is considered autonomic input.

These nerves are made up of hundreds or more smaller fibers called *neurons.* The neuron is made of receptors called *dendrites*, cell bodies or the brain of the neuron, and then an axon or the tract that carries the information onward (Figure 2-1). All cell bodies for the somatic sensory system are located within the dorsal root ganglia at the anterior part of the spinal column and considered part of the CNS. Their axons travel into the spinal cord and synapse on another neuron either at the cord level or above. Each neuron plays a role in the type and function it serves. Without this information, a body could not function, because it would have no idea how to protect itself or learn about and react to the external and internal environments. In Chapter 6, the reader will find further discussion of both somatic and cranial sensory systems and how to test for them in patients. When testing for patients' perception of that sensory information, the reader needs to know that at least 2, and often more, junctions or synapses are part of this transmission, and the information can be altered or changed at these junctions.[3] Thus, the concept of sensory perception is quite complex.

Motor System

Striated Motor

Information, or neurons traveling from the nervous system out to the head and body, will be considered *striated motor neurons* or lower motor neurons because they are the last neurons before exiting the nervous system. Striated motor neurons carry information or programs out to all striated muscles throughout the body. These programs run combinations of muscle interactions for an individual to control movements and activities that lead to independence and quality of life.

Some motor programs seem inherent or are learned in utero as reflexes, while others are learned through experiences throughout life. A small child must first learn to hold his head against gravity by developing core postural strength, then continue to integrate that strength to begin to roll over, be held and hold his body against gravity, come to sit, sit, come to stand, stand, walk, and run. Within the first few years, the child will learn to control bowel and bladder function using somatic motor control over both areas of the pelvic floor and distal sphincters. Simultaneously, a child will learn to make and listen to sound, and later talk in the parents' or caregivers' language, as well as control the use of the 2 eyes to focus on people and objects in the external world. The child similarly is learning to control his hands to manipulate toys and play. During this time the child will learn what he is feeling with what he is seeing. All this learning is going on simultaneously and sequentially within the nervous system.

Terms are often used for different degrees of motor function. Gross motor activities are considered when the movements are large and require multiple joints and combinations of muscle groups. Fine motor activities are defined as movements requiring precision and often occurring in a small range of motion such as prehension, manipulation of food, talking, and controlling the muscles of the eyes. As a child learns, gross and fine motor activities are integrated so the child can stand while brushing his teeth or talk, or listen at the dinner table without falling out of the chair. Progressing from daily living activities to complex play, and later to even more complex adult activities, demonstrates the complexity of this motor system. For the individual to learn to control and modify these motor behaviors, there is a need for sensory feedback to recognize error and change or modify all these complex programs (see Chapter 3).

Autonomic Motor

Autonomic motor neurons go to smooth muscle found in organ systems that include the stomach, intestines (bowel), kidneys, liver, vascular system (both arterial and venous), and vessels in the skin for temperature regulation and sweating. The regulation of this system varies from the regulation of the somatic system, but within the CNS, communication is again vital for survival.

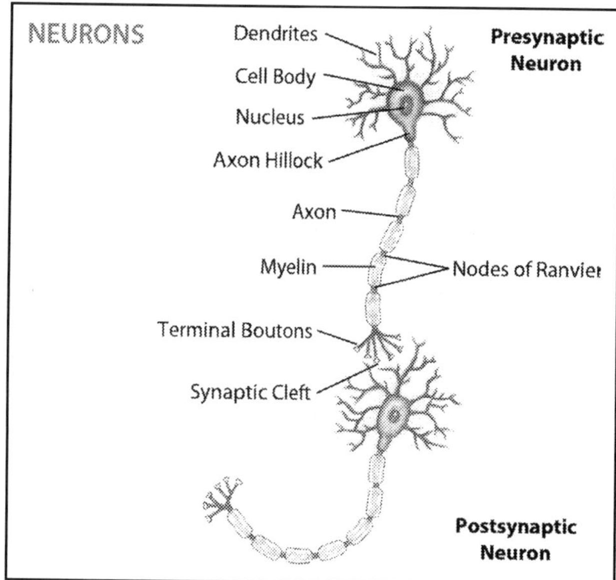

Figure 2-1. Neuron. (Reprinted with permission from Gutman SA. *Quick Reference Neuroscience for Rehabilitation Professionals*. 3rd ed. Thorofare, NJ: SLACK Incorporated; 2017.)

Interaction of Somatic and Autonomic Motor

Motor neurons carry information to the heart and lungs for those systems to function throughout life without the individual thinking about running them. The interaction between automatic breathing within the lung structure, and contraction of striated muscles of the diaphragm and the abdomen, again demonstrates the complexity of running the human body. Some of those nerves or bundles of neurons are somatic motor, while others are autonomic motor which obviously need to be coordinated by the central portion of the nervous system.

There are differences in the types and ways somatic motor and autonomic motor neurons disseminate the desired responses of the end organs or muscle fibers. The complexity of these differences cannot be seen in movement analysis, and therefore will not be included in this chapter.

Central Nervous System

Whether the neuron starts in the periphery going toward the CNS, is sent from the CNS going to the peripheral system, or is transmitted from one area to another within the central system, all neurons have 4 anatomical parts: dendrite, cell body, axon, and synaptic cleft.

All dendrites receive information, whether from peripheral receptors or from another neuron within the nervous system, and carry the information toward the cell body within the CNS. From the cell body, the information travels along the axon toward the end of the neuron to a junction called a *synapse* (Figure 2-1). At these synapses, the information is communicated to another neuron, straited mus-

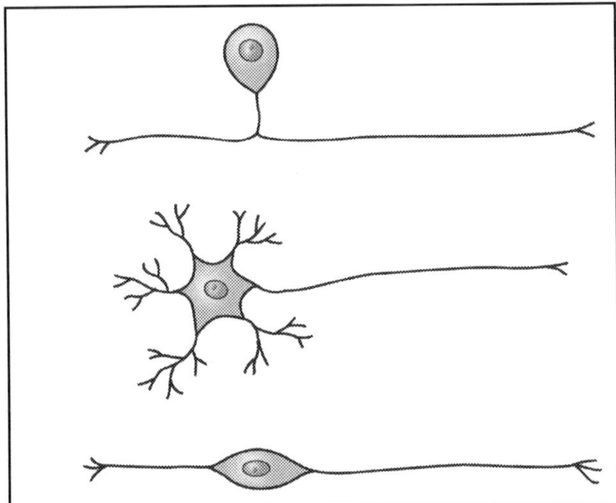

Figure 2-2. Morphologic cell types in the nervous system. (Reprinted with permission from Nolan MF. *Cram Session in Functional Neuroanatomy.* Thorofare, NJ: SLACK Incorporated; 2012.)

cle, or organ system. These axons can travel long distances within the nervous system, or can go very short distances and just synapse on a cell body near where they originated. Within the CNS, the axons can synapse on either dendrites or cell bodies. Those synaptic junctions use chemicals to transmit the information, and the dendrites and cell bodies are sensitive to the types of chemicals released. Neurons are the most diverse cell type in the human body, both in relation to size and anatomical structure, but they only have 3 functional shapes: bipolar, pseudo unipolar, and multipolar (Figure 2-2). Multipolar cells make up more than 99.9% of all cells in the CNS. When looking at Figure 2-1 the reader can see that a multipolar cell has many dendrites and a large cell body. With many synaptic junctions, the total information sent to the cell body gives rise to huge variance in what the cell body will communicate down its axon toward the synapse and next neuron.

No matter whether the axon is motor, sensory, or an interneuron within the CNS, it is surrounded by non-nervous system cells called *myelin* (see Figure 2-1). The thickness of the myelin determines the speed of conductivity of the information. Whether it is going to the brain as sensory, communicating between centers for associations, or descending from the brain as motor tracts, myelin plays a role, and is a critical anatomical component of the successful functioning of the entire nervous system. Damage to this myelin leads to conductivity problems and ultimately movement dysfunction. See Chapters 10, 14, and 15 for problems with demyelination and their ultimate effect on motor performance and functional movement.

It is difficult to provide a simple general overview of the CNS because of the many parts that work simultaneously as well as sequentially.[4] How all these clusters of cell bodies or nuclear masses are coordinated is the mystery of the overall function of the CNS. These anatomical structures will be discussed separately, and figures used to identify the relationships of structures will also be discussed.

The ultimate goal of the CNS is to take in and process all information from outside and within the human body, put meaning to that data, and decide how to control the body's response. Simultaneously, that information leads to higher-level cognitive thought processes. During the initial phases of a small child's life, the CNS is learning, and that learning will continue throughout life. The individual will learn to process sensory information, and then learn to respond to that input. The brain initially responds automatically to sensory inputs such as light touch or pain that causes a baby to withdraw, bladder or intestinal filling that causes emptying, or lack of food in the stomach that causes the baby to cry for food. These are for survival and are critical for the human infant. Very quickly, the child will learn to recognize faces and begin to respond to the environment.

This young nervous system will learn early in life to move against gravity; communicate with other members of our species; differentiate safe and dangerous environments; run motor programs without the need for input until the program is no longer effective; begin to use complex language; and process information for higher-level thought such as reading, doing math, writing, abstract thinking, running machinery, using computers, and other complex life tasks that can lead to success as an adult. As adults age, the brain will change, and cells will die, which causes the nervous system to adapt and make accommodations to remain functional. It is not until the brain reaches a critical level of insult that friends, family, or medical practitioners recognize changes in behavior or function that bring that individual to today's health care environment.

How all these systems communicate and process all this information simultaneously and sequentially is an amazing and complex interaction that has led to humans being considered the most complex animal on earth. How emotions and belief systems interact with the sensory and motor systems again becomes complex, and how they are expressed in our patient's actions will be discussed later in this chapter.

Anatomy of the Nervous System

The nervous system is made up of various areas (Figure 2-3). This chapter first deals with each of the gross anatomical structures, with brief discussions of what movement dysfunctions arise with specific structure damage.

Prior to discussion of specific anatomical parts of the nervous system, the physical therapist assistant needs to become familiar with 2 terms: gray matter and white matter.

Gray matter contains high concentrations of cell bodies, while white matter contains bundles of axons taking information from one area of the nervous system to another. The discussion of the anatomy will begin with the spinal system and progress to the highest centers, the cortices. Within the spinal system, the central structures are made up of gray matter and clusters of cell bodies with gray structures that radiate from the dorsal and toward ventral roots attached to the spinal cord. Sensory information enters the dorsal root and mostly synapses in the posterior areas of the cord, while motor cell bodies cluster in the anterior areas and send axons out to the periphery. Information or axons traveling up and down from higher centers are located at the front, lateral, and posterior aspects or outer aspects of the spinal cord, and are made up of white matter. That functional representation remains somewhat consistent as tracts ascend and descend through the lower areas of the brain, but when looking at the highest aspect of the brain, the cortex or gray matter is on the outside, and white matter is found internally holding tracts going in both directions. Most second-order neurons, or those having cell bodies originating and synapsing within the CNS, will cross over and travel up the other side. This keeps consistency to information coming from one side of the body going to the cortices on the other side for processing. Similarly, those axons that originate in higher centers will cross over at some time to the other side, going to motor neurons that leave the system. A large number of axons carry information between parts of the brain; these are referred to as *within* and *interhemispheric* tracts. Distinguishing between white and gray matter within the CNS is important for the physical therapist assistant when reading patient charts. When the chart says there is white matter involvement, the physical therapist assistant should recognize that axons or tracts have been affected or damaged, and those tracts have the possibility to regenerate. When the chart reads that gray matter is involved, the physical therapist assistant should quickly recognize that cell bodies have been affected and may not regenerate.

An important principle within the nervous system is that the right brain receives and controls information on the left side of the body and trunk, while the left brain deals with information on the right side of the body and trunk. For that reason, all incoming information (sensory) needs to cross somewhere between the spinal level and its ultimate destination to the brain on the other side. As these incoming tracts cross over at specific locations onto the next nuclear cluster of cells, whether dendrites or cell bodies, they will synapse. The first-order neurons or tracts initially travel up on the outside of the cord and then synapse on clusters of cell bodies, and then travel more medial or internally within the system. This is how the white matter, initially on the outside at the spinal level, changes to being on the inside, and then radiates to the gray matter or the cerebral cortices on the outside. The motor system needs to follow the same anatomic arrangements with axons originating in the cortices and crossing over before synapsing on the motor cell bodies of CNs (going to the face) or motor neurons (within the spinal cord) going out to the periphery.

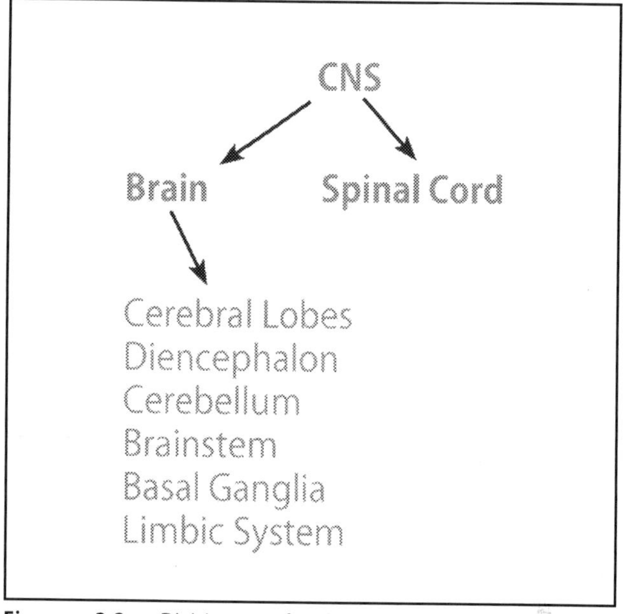

Figure 2-3. Divisions of the CNS. (Reprinted with permission from Gutman SA. *Quick Reference Neuroscience for Rehabilitation Professionals*. 3rd ed. Thorofare, NJ: SLACK Incorporated; 2017.)

Spinal System

The nervous system portion of the spinal system is found within the boney structure and called the *spinal cord*. The spinal cord enters the cranial vault at the base of the skull, and at that time, the remaining aspects of the nervous system is called the *brain*. The lowest part of the brain is called the *brainstem*, and the highest is the *cortex* or *cortical structures*.

The spinal system is the first system that receives information from the periphery and organ systems via the dorsal root ganglia that holds cell bodies for those neurons. The ventral root holds axons from spinal system motor neurons that leave the CNS going to both the somatic and autonomic motor systems (Figure 2-4). Peripheral nerves are labelled according to anatomical representation at the levels of the cord; when they are sensory or motor testing, they're referred to as *dermatomes* (see Chapter 6).

These spinal neurons are still made of neurons carrying specific information destined to the CNS or brain. Sensory information destined to higher centers will ascend in both posterior and lateral conduits or columns of axons going to higher centers. Some axons from the dorsal root will synapse on cell bodies within the spinal gray matter. This is where there are axons ascending, while others axons do not synapse and initially ascend and synapse in the next level, the brainstem. As soon as a synapse is made, the next order neurons are considered second-order neurons. Their axons continue their journey toward their final destination at higher centers within the brain.

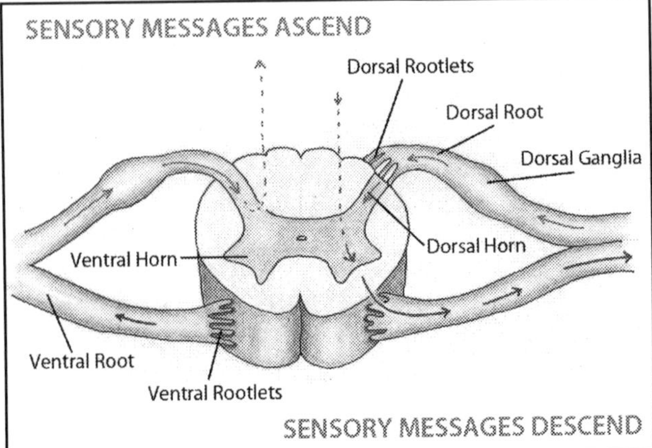

Figure 2-4. Dorsal root ganglia figure and ventral root showing both ascending (sensory) and descending (motor) activity at the spinal level. (Reprinted with permission from Gutman SA. *Quick Reference Neuroscience for Rehabilitation Professionals*. 3rd ed. Thorofare, NJ: SLACK Incorporated; 2017.)

Information from higher centers that carry the motor information or programs come down from higher centers or descend, cross over either in the brainstem or spinal cord, and synapse onto clusters of motor nuclei or gray matter on the opposite side within the anterior portion of the spinal cord. These spinal cord cells or neurons send axons out to the peripheral system via the ventral root, and are considered motor with their goal to control functional movement. Combinations of motor neurons from motor centers in the brain control and modify the spinal level and ultimately motor programs. Similarly, autonomic neurons descend upon the spinal system to send information out to regulate smooth muscle in organ systems. Within the spinal system, there are many interconnecting small neurons and synaptic connections onto dendrites and cell bodies of other neurons within the system that help regulate both input and output within this system. Refer to Box 2-1 as an example of the long chain neuronal loops.

The complexity of this system is amazing. Unfortunately, when this system is damaged, an individual can lose a tremendous amount of function, both in feeling from the periphery (sensory or input), as well as programming to run functional activities (motor or output). The specific areas that are affected in traumatic spinal injuries are discussed in Chapter 11. Figures 11-1, 11-2, and 11-3 deal with impairments within the spinal system and their ultimate effect on both sensory and motor function.

Box 2-1

Example of Patient Who Demonstrates How Long Chain Neuronal Loops Affect Motor Performance

A client had recurrent small strokes for more than 35 years. When she stood up, she developed horrible tonal patterns in her arm, and then one could see extreme extensor patterns in her leg, which limited her gait patterns. She had traveled the world receiving therapy from master clinicians as well as treatment from famous doctors. As a student, I was asked to do gait training after her next small stroke. I assumed she had received gait training from many masters, and thus I was not going to change her preexisting gait patterns. But if I could reduce the tone in her arm, she would be more presentable to society. This was one of her goals. So for the time I had remaining on my internship, I walked the patient from where I parked the wheelchair to the mat, and treated her arm with relaxation techniques. After therapy, I walked her back to the chair and considered that gait training. Within 2 weeks, I could get her arm to relax, and she could place the hand in her back pocket in external rotation. When she stood up and walked, she had no gait deviations at all and walked normally. I quickly determined that I had affected the long chain reflex loops within the spinal system, which led to her control over the spinal motor neurons and ultimately the movement of her leg. She called me a "good witch" because I never touched her leg, and she was "healed" from her perspective. She didn't want to comprehend my interpretation of what happened, which was okay, as long as I understood the interactions within the spinal system and recognized it was not magic.

Brainstem

The brainstem is an important relay system communicating input from the spinal system and CNs to other areas of the brain such as the cerebellum, the diencephalon, and ultimately the cortical structures. The brainstem often has neurons stop and synapse on clusters of cell bodies to communicate to the next-order neurons before they ascend.[3] At these synaptic junctions, input can be regulated in intensity and importance through small interneurons that modulate neurological signals locally. The brainstem can also be used to modify descending information carrying motor programs to control motor systems in the spinal cord that goes out to the body. The brainstem is also where CNs or neurons first enter the nervous system as cranial sensory input and synapse on CN nuclear masses. This information synapses on specific areas, and from there, second-order neurons relay to higher structures to communicate the information coming from the head and structures in the head. The only CN that does not transmit input via the brainstem is CN I, the carrying input regarding olfaction. That CN comes directly into the cranial vault at the front of the skull. CN II, the *optic nerve*, also enters the skull at the level of the eyes. Some axons then bifurcate, sending input to large nuclear masses in the upper brainstem, and other information goes directly to the diencephalon or thalamic structures. The complexity of the anatomy of these CNs does not affect the physical therapist assistant's ability to test for CN function. When problems arise with any CN, the physical therapist should communicate to the physical therapist assistant how those CNs affect function in the patient and how best to help the patient relearn or compensate for loss.

One specific nuclear mass or area found throughout the brainstem, the *reticular activating system*, is made up of many cell bodies and axons. This system helps regulate sleep and wake cycles, alert the nervous system to potential harm, and affect higher center concentration both with distraction as well as focus. It is also an important area for pain regulation.

The 3 major regional divisions in the brainstem—the *medulla*, *pons*, and *midbrain*—have a wide variety of functions:

- Medulla: The medulla, the lowest region of the brainstem, plays an important role in housing nuclear masses from sensory information from the spinal cord before the next neurons cross over the medulla and ascend to higher bundles of cell bodies to synapse again. Each cluster or group of cell bodies within the medulla can be regulated in intensity and importance by other nuclear masses coming from the peripheral system, other CNs as well as higher centers with the brain. Specifically, within the medulla, CN VIII (auditory/vestibular), CN IX (glossopharyngeal), CN X (vagus), and CN XI (accessory) have nuclear masses. The nuclear masses each have names, and whether the information is primarily sensory, or just motor, or both is specific to each CN. One important CN for the physical therapist assistant to comprehend is CN VIII, the *auditory/vestibular nerve*. Half of CN VIII carries sensory input regarding the vestibular system, and thus plays a key role in balance and awareness of head position in space. Some vestibular input goes directly to the cerebellum, while other axons synapse on large neuronal bodies regulating both ascending and descending vestibular information to the spinal system, to the motor nuclei going to the eyes in the midbrain, and to higher centers. The vestibular system not only plays a role in balance and postural tone, but also influences on all 3 cranial motor nerves controlling movement of the eyes. The vestibular nuclei also send a large number of second-order neurons to the reticular system to alert the person of danger such as a potential fall from rapid movement of the head in space. The complexity of the vestibular system can be seen in Figure 2-5, but it is not within the scope of this chapter to discuss all of these connections.[7,8] The medulla also plays a critical role in controlling breathing via CN X, which the physical therapist assistant should be monitoring throughout any treatment. Many problems can be found with lesions in the CNs, but that discussion is also outside the scope of this chapter.
- Pons: The pons is primarily a relay center. Axons from higher centers primarily from the front of the brain and from the basal ganglia (BG) descend onto cell bodies in the midbrain. Then those neurons send information to the cerebellum regarding desired movement programming.

  CNs enter and leave from nuclear bodies within the pons (Figure 2-6). CN V (trigeminal), CN VI (abducens), and CN VII (facial) have nuclear masses within the lower to mid-pons. Thus, input of sensory abilities on the face, head, inner oral cavity, and sensation of taste enter at this level, while motor neurons going out to the muscles for facial expression, eyelid closing, and jaw movement may be affected with pons involvement.

  A large number of descending neurons or white matter carry motor information that travels through the anterior or front of the pons to the spinal system. Sensory information from lower centers ascends through the pons on the lateral and posterior aspects.
- Midbrain: The midbrain is the highest division in the brainstem. The midbrain processes information carrying input from CN II (visual) and CN VIII (auditory) within nuclear masses or clusters of cell bodies called *colliculi*. The superior colliculi process visual information, while the inferior colliculi receive auditory input that entered at the medulla. Both areas send processed information to the next highest area, the *diencephalon*, specially the *thalamus*. The anterior portion of the midbrain houses many descending motor fibers or white matter from higher centers in the brain called *cerebral peduncles*.

  The midbrain is also a relay center for aspects of the reticular system, encompassing a portion of all aspects of the brainstem. Again, a large number of ascending sensory tracts travel through the midbrain. These ultimately will synapse on higher nuclear bodies above the midbrain, mainly the thalamus. CN III (oculomotor) and CN IV (trochlear) controlling eye muscles originate in motor nuclei or masses sending axons out to muscles of the eye (Figure 2-6).

In the brainstem, the reticular system plays a critical role in regulated attention, sleep cycles, and sensitivity to incoming information. The complexity of these interactions among neuronal bodies within the brainstem is fascinating and fun to study, but not necessarily critical for the physical therapist assistant to understand functionally (Figure 2-7). When this system is depressed, it can lead to consciousness problems or an inability to attend, but when it is excitable, it can lead to outbursts and hypersensitivity, especially to pain and light touch. The reticular system has the potential to trigger protective responses and, indirectly, motor behavior that is dangerous to both the patient and the clinician. Neurons on the way to the cortical structures often send collaterals or branches of the ascending axons into the reticular system, which can help alert the brain to important incoming information. Damage to the reticular formation within the pons can result in a condition called

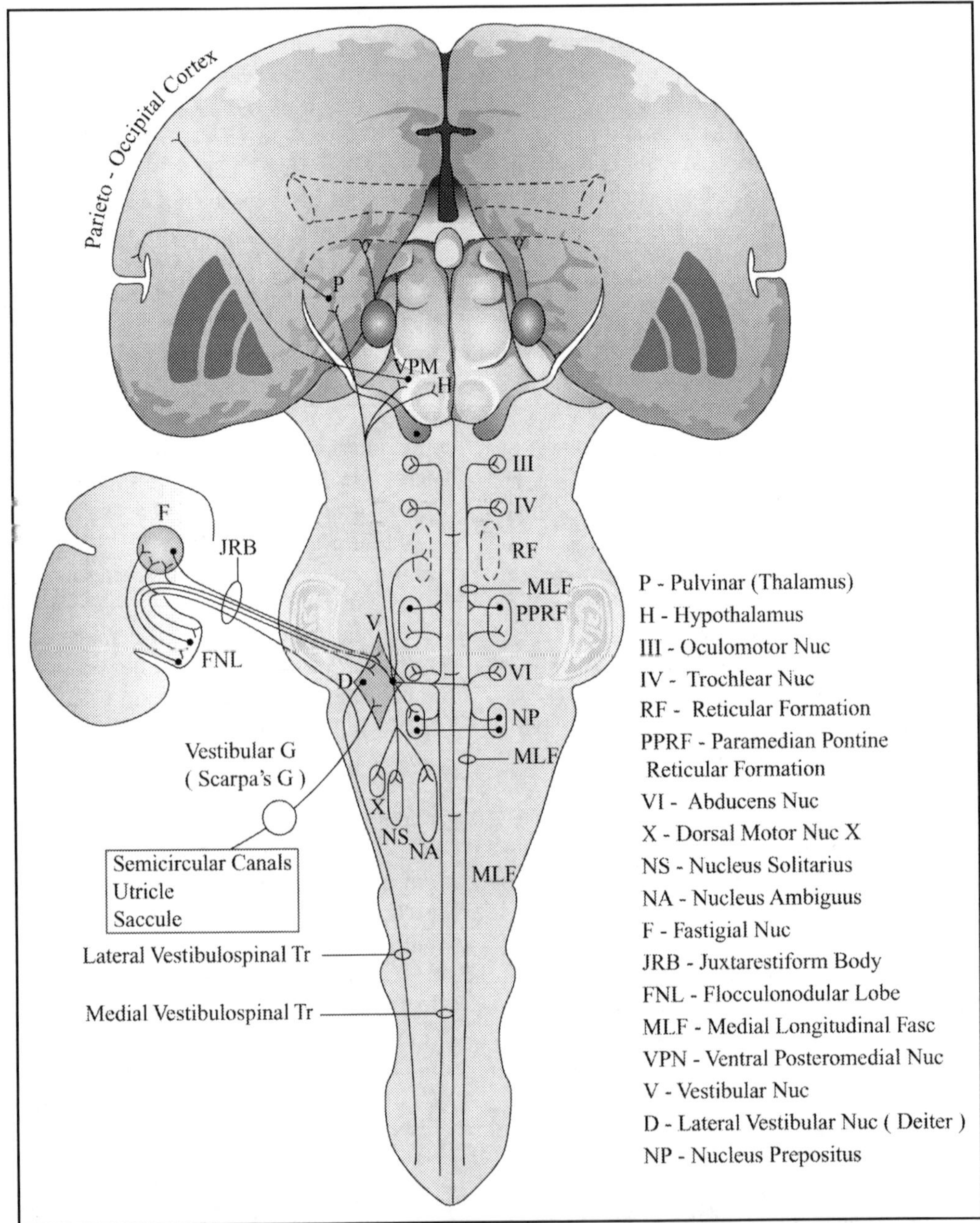

Figure 2-5. Schematic diagram of the afferent and efferent connections of the vestibular nuclei. (Reprinted with permission from Nolan MF. *Cram Session in Functional Neuroanatomy.* Thorofare, NJ: SLACK Incorporated; 2012.)

decerebrate rigidity which results in spastic extension of both the upper and lower extremities,[4] thus, showing the descending effect this system has on motor neurons in the spinal system.

Individuals with whiplash neck injury from auto accidents often have upper neck injuries. Those injuries often place traction on the brainstem causing involvement called neuronal shearing.[4] In this situation, white matter or axons ascending from the spinal system are pulled longitudinally and can shear or rip apart as they attach in the medulla. This situation can cause severe pain, headaches, and dizziness. Descending fibers can also be affected. Some of the movement problems will create tonal changes (both high and low tone) and balance impairments.

Again, these emphasize that brainstem damage can result in ascending tract involvement or sensory deficits and loss of descending fibers, causing motor deficits. Individuals with traumatic brain injury often show signs of brainstem involvement or damage, which can be seen on medical examination tools such as computed tomography scans, magnetic resonance imaging (MRI) scans, and positron-emission tomography studies. Discussion of these tools is not within the scope of this chapter, but information can be found online or in many other textbooks.[4,9]

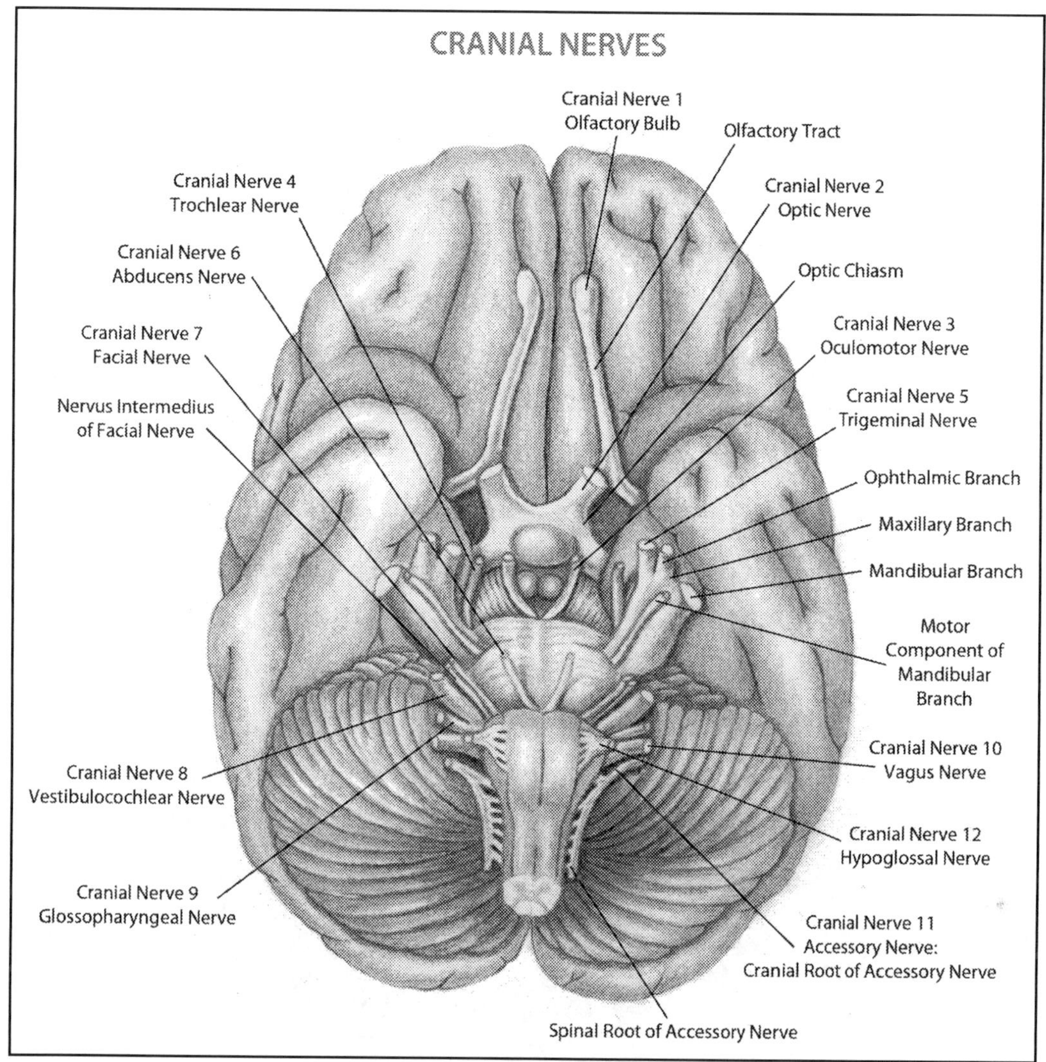

Figure 2-6. CNs entering and leaving various parts of the brainstem as well as higher centers. (Reprinted with permission from Gutman SA. *Quick Reference Neuroscience for Rehabilitation Professionals*. 3rd ed. Thorofare, NJ: SLACK Incorporated; 2017.)

The reader can refer to Chapter 12 for additional information on brainstem shearing and traumatic injury.

Cerebellum

The cerebellum plays a key role in balance, coordination of movement, and postural control. Its function is to automatically correct error in motor programs until the motor program no longer is effective. It uses primarily proprioceptive information from the head and body and sends that information back to modify muscle and joint activity. This structure compares the blueprint for a movement to the final product and makes the necessary adjustments. Higher centers will tell the cerebellum when a program needs to be changed. Its interactions with higher centers may also lead to spatial organization, memory, practice learning, and attention shifting.[3] This structure is found posterior to the brainstem and is connected to the brainstem through 3 large conduits, called *peduncles*, on each side: *inferior, middle,* and *superior.*

The inferior peduncles originate in the posterior/lateral medulla and carry both sensory and motor neurons primarily from the vestibular system. This sensory information comes directly from the ear as well as indirectly from the vestibular nuclei in the medulla. This information has not yet been projected to the opposite side of the body. The inferior portion of the cerebellum sends descending neurons back down this inferior peduncle to vestibular nuclei affecting the same side of the body. Important roles of these vestibular nuclei are to send descending fibers onto the motor nuclei in the spinal system to assist in postural tone, send ascending neurons onto the nuclear masses (CNs) that control eye movements, and send ascending fibers to higher centers in the brain.[7] These fibers going to higher centers will cross to go to the opposite side of the body for processing or interpretation. The relationship between

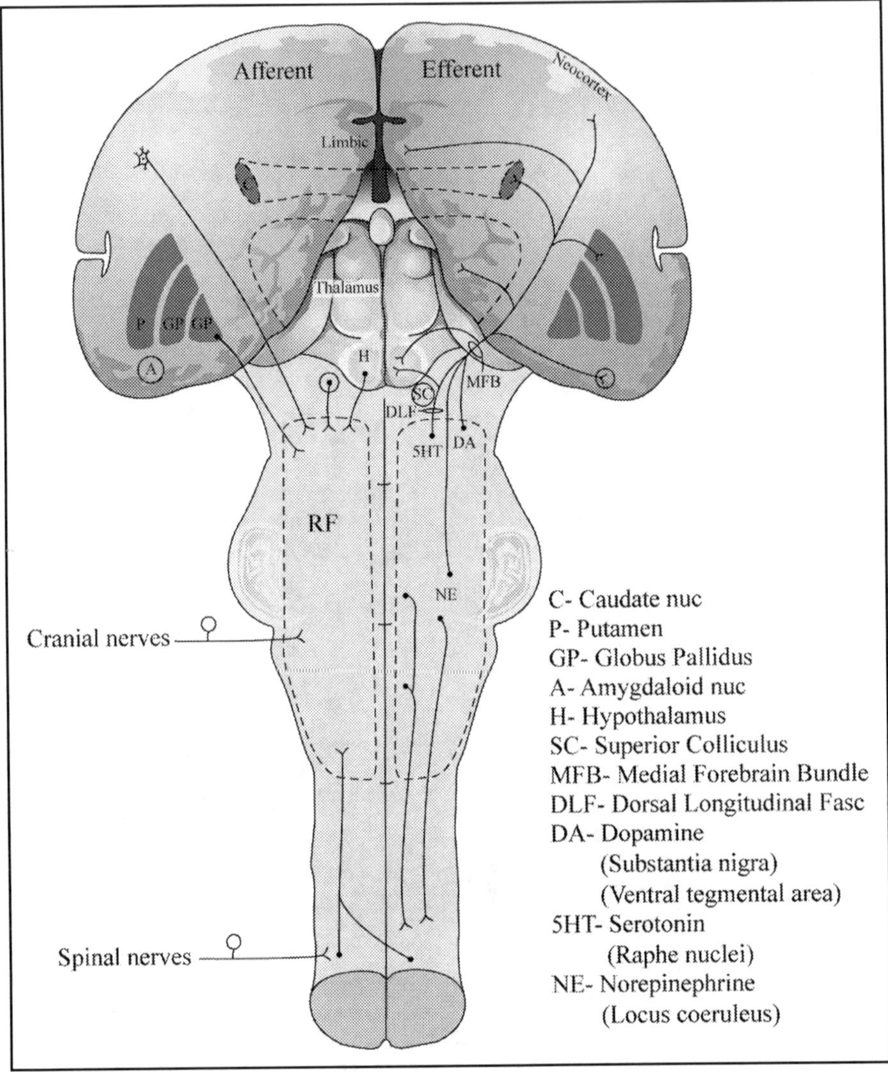

Figure 2-7. Afferent and efferent projections from brainstem reticular formation. (Reprinted with permission from Nolan MF. *Cram Session in Functional Neuroanatomy*. Thorofare, NJ: SLACK Incorporated; 2012.)

hearing (sound) from the other half of CN VIII and the control of the eyes is initially reflexive. It starts with hearing a sound on one side of the body, and in response, the eyes will reflexively turn or look toward the sound on that side. In time, the brain or higher centers will regulate this control from the opposite side and be able to separate eye movement from auditory and vestibular input.

The middle cerebellar peduncles at the pons level carry only input information that has crossed over from higher centers. This information is communicating to the cerebellum desired motor function and programming from higher centers. This information via the middle cerebellar peduncles radiates to large areas of the cerebellum and will condense and send integrated information back to the higher centers.

The superior peduncle originates in the cerebellum, enters at the midbrain level, and primarily carries information from the cerebellum that will ascend, cross over, and ascend to higher motor centers in the brain regarding motor programing. These superior peduncles are the primary way the cerebellum communicates with higher motor centers on the opposite side. The cerebellum plays a key role in regulating speed, trajectory, and force used to run any functional movement or motor program. Individuals with cerebellum damage often have problems with trajectory of movement.

During gait, these problems are referred to as *ataxia*. When observed in the trunk and upper extremities, these movements are referred to as *intentional tremors*, or tremors upon intentional movement. These problems can be seen when an individual is trying to reach a target. With cerebellum problems, the patient will often overshoot or undershoot. The more the intention is made to correct the problem, the more exaggeration one observes in the movement, thus the term *intentional tremors*. The person often tries to splint the most proximal joint to stabilize the movement patterns, but that will not lead to control over an integrated multi-joint movement pattern and obviously limits the individual's participation in functional control. Higher centers such as vision recognize the error and try to correct movement, but without cerebellar control, movement becomes very difficult.

The cerebellum also plays a key role in control over balance, axial control, and production of core strength. The cerebellum integrates information from higher centers, communicates that integration via the superior peduncle, and sends it back to the frontal lobes and indirectly to the BG. Damage in other areas of the brain can send incorrect information to the cerebellum via the middle cerebellar peduncles. This indirectly looks as if the cerebellum is involved or damaged when it is not. When regulation over the trunk or core muscles is involved, the physical therapist assistant could see excessive movement in the trunk when trying to run postural programs. The physical therapist should be able to differentiate motor problems in the cerebellum from those in the BG and frontal lobes. These higher centers are discussed in later sections. The physical therapist should help alert the physical therapist assistant to types of interventions that will help the person relearn motor control with movement problems originating from the cerebellum.

Diencephalon

These anatomical structures are above the brainstem and anterior to the cerebellum. Some anatomists believe 4 large gray matter structures make up the diencephalon: the *thalamus*, the *limbic system*, the *hypothalamus*, and the *BG*. Other anatomists place the BG and limbic structures in the *telencephalon*, or higher cortical areas. For this chapter, these 4 structures will be discussed. They play critical roles in the function of the nervous system. Some systems are involved in motor performance, relaying and controlling both input and output from higher centers, and integrating emotions with motor performance, while others are responsible for control over emotions and the ability to store and retrieve short-term and long-term memory.

- Thalamus: The thalamus is made up of a large number of nuclear masses with specific relay responsibilities. It is truly a relay center for all sensory information, although olfaction does project into the limbic structure before it gets to the thalamus.[4] All ascending sensory information from the periphery synapse will have crossed over and then synapse onto certain nuclear centers in the thalamus. Both CNs for vision (II) and hearing (VIII) have large relay centers called *geniculate bodies* at the posterior and lateral aspects of the thalamus where synapses are made and where new neurons are relayed to appropriate higher centers or lobes. Additional relay nuclear masses in the thalamus help communicate information from the emotional system (limbic) as well as to and from the cerebellum. Damage to the thalamus is catastrophic to a human and causes tremendous loss of function, because information from the body cannot be communicated to higher centers in the brain and then processed. When the thalamus is damaged at a young age, initial learning is very difficult. Relearning following injury to the thalamus is unavailable because feedback from peripheral receptors to change motor programs is not available. Damage to the geniculate bodies (CNs II and VIII) can lead to loss of sight or hearing.
- Limbic system: The limbic structure deals with emotions such as love, joy, fear, anger, rage, and depression, and directly impacts the rest of the nervous system, especially when strong feelings are present.[10] Anger can increase extensor tone, throw off balance, and cause a patient to possibly strike out. Depression can decrease all tone, especially core or trunk muscles, and make the patient feel weak and sleepy. The physical therapist assistant needs to learn to be sensitive to the emotional responses of the patient, because those responses affect functional movement. If a patient is angry and taught to do a transfer while angry, tone has been produced that won't necessarily be present when the individual tries to transfer when not angry. Trying to get a patient to be calm or relaxed and enjoy the interaction during any intervention will neutralize the emotional limbic system and allow the motor system to run without altering tone from the limbic system. Once the motor program is learned, reintroducing emotions such as anger, laughter, and sadness while still running the correct motor program will give the patient independence when participating in life and all the emotions that contribute to those interactions. Different emotions release different chemicals into synapses of neurons, and this ultimately affects the way a person thinks and responds. A feeling of safety is by far one of the most important emotions a patient needs to feel during interactions with the physical therapist assistant. One must remember that all of us have emotional feelings and biases, which can affect the way we interact with colleagues as well as with patients. That is, we all have a limbic system that affects our life and the way we respond to the world. As clinicians, we must also accept that we should not be putting those biases onto the patient. Setting a stage showing a patient that you are also human and have emotions allows the patient to share feelings and helps the physical therapist assistant determine if emotions are affecting motor performance and thus the plan of care.

The limbic structure has intimate communications with the reticular system in the brainstem, for it will alert the system to danger or safety. It can alter the sensitivity to incoming information by increasing the awareness of sensations, especially pain.

The limbic system plays a critical role in retention of new memory, retrieval of past memory, and communication with higher brain structures. This structure is extremely sensitive to alcohol and drugs and can be damaged with recurrent use of any of those substances. Many nuclear masses are within the limbic structures, and neuronal tracts go between them and radiate to higher centers, often through the thalamus.[3,4]

- Hypothalamus: The hypothalamus is a large nuclear mass that controls the autonomic nervous system and is often said to control flight, fight, fear, and reproduction. Similarly, this system plays a key role in autoregulation of the body's responses to the world and to illness by regulating body temperature and responses to diseases. When talking about regulation, remember that these structures are made up of neurons, and these neurons release chemicals that affect the neurons in the synapses and how information is passed on to other structures. The structure and function of the autonomic nervous system (both sympathetic and parasympathetic) are slightly different than the somatic sensory-motor system. The autonomic nervous system uses sensory information to drive the function of the autonomic motor systems going out to organs, blood vessels, and glands. Thus, it controls temperature, digestion, heart rate, respiration, metabolism, blood pressure, and balance of function of internal organs.[3]
- Basal nuclei or BG: These structures are critical aspects of the brain in regards to motor function. Some anatomists believe these nuclear structures are part of the cortical system or telencephalon, while others place them in the diencephalon. Whatever nomenclature is used, the BG are deep within the brain and have intricate connections among the structures as well as to both higher and to lower motor nuclei, which ultimately plays a role in motor programming of striated muscles.

  Part of the BG receives information from higher structures (primarily the frontal lobes), and sends information back to those lobes both directly and indirectly via the thalamus. In turn, that information is sent to the cerebellum, which in turn relays information back. These relay loops regulate stereotypic and automatic movements and control motor patterns or programs. Thus, they assist in higher center functional control over movement. The BG play a primary role in regulation and modification of the tonal characteristics seen in all movements. The sensory or receiving nuclei of the BG are called the *caudate* and *putnam*. The *globus pallidus* are nuclei that send efferent neurons back to the frontal lobe and are considered motor because they exit the BG (Figure 2-8). These nuclear structures are complex, and discussion of this complexity is not realistic in this overview. But it is important to understand that there are many interconnecting loops both within these nuclei and among nuclei within the BG. The BG also have relay loops into the upper brainstem. These nuclei are regulated by chemicals or neurotransmitters—primarily dopamine and acetylcholine—released at synaptic junctions. When any of these or adjacent nuclear masses begin to degenerate or lose cell bodies over time, then chemical imbalances, such as an imbalance due to a decrease in the chemical dopamine, cause specific motor impairments. For example, if the loop between the BG and a midbrain nuclear mass like the *substantia nigra which* relays information to and from the BG, degenerates, the resulting motor impairments leads to the movement dysfunction called Parkinson's disease. This disease creates tonal abnormality of proximal rigidity and distal non-intentional tremors found in the hands, tongue, and feet. Medication to replace the dopamine imbalance will often help alleviate the motor impairments for a substantial amount of time, but the degeneration of the BG will continue, and in time, the patient will lose functional control. This motor functional control problem for a patient may not cause any high-level thought processing difficulties. Colleagues and family often think that because the patient may be very slow in responding to a command, increasing their voice level will result in better understanding. In fact, to many patients, this is insulting and may increase tone due to an emotional reaction.[3]

BG also process emotional and cognitive information, which can affect areas within the BG.

Cortical Structures

The cerebrum, also called the *neocortex*, makes up the largest and most superficial division of the brain, and can be separated into 2 hemispheres. The 2 hemispheres are divided by indentations called the *longitudinal fissure*, which goes from the front to the back on the brain. Within each hemisphere, there are 4 cortical structures called *lobes*. Each lobe is separated by large fissures, each with a different name. Many smaller fissures are also located within each lobe. These indentations allow for more cellular mass within each lobe, as the fissures fold in and out down along the structure. These lobes are made up of a huge number of cell bodies, gray matter, with small dendrites that receive information, and often small axons that relay that information to other cells within these lobes. Longer axons relay to associating areas within each lobe, as well as to other lobes. Each lobe has 6 layers of cells, each with a slightly different function within the gray matter. Although the complexity of these layers of cells and how they interact and communicate are very important in brain function, it is not critical to analyze these interactions to understand the sensory-motor

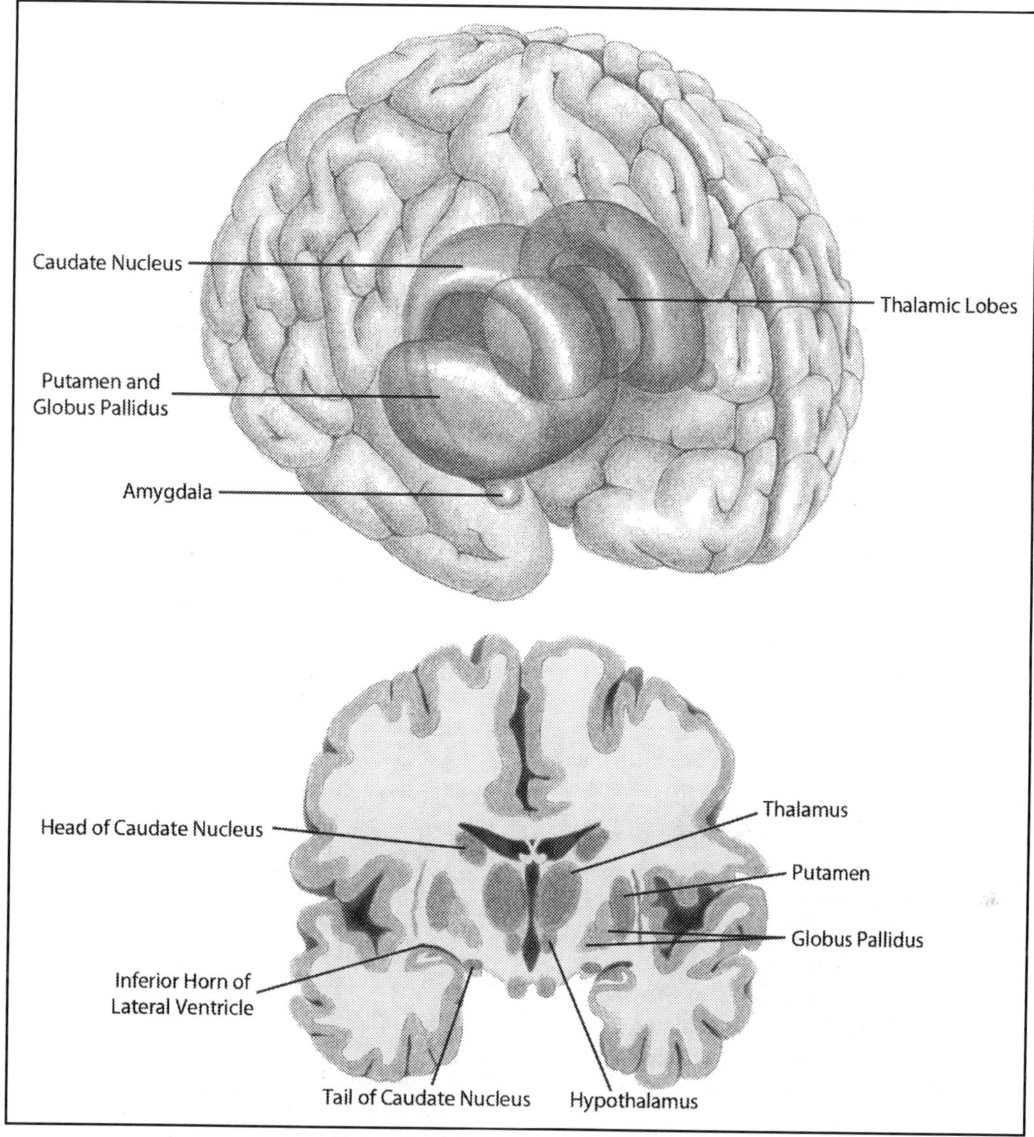

Figure 2-8. Basal nuclei or ganglia. (Reprinted with permission from Gutman SA. *Quick Reference Neuroscience for Rehabilitation Professionals*. 3rd ed. Thorofare, NJ: SLACK Incorporated; 2017.)

systems and how higher centers affect motor expression. All 4 lobes in each hemisphere are primarily made up of cell bodies, which are gray matter, while the longer axons, originating from these cell bodies in these lobes and used to communicate information between lobes and to lower structures, are white matter.[3,4,5]

Three lobes—*parietal*, *temporal*, and *occipital*—are located on each side and at the back of the brain, and primarily function to receive and process sensory information from both the head and body on the opposite side. The largest and fourth lobes are at the front of the brain directly behind the forehead and eyes, and they are called the *frontal lobes*. The frontal lobes integrate many aspects of brain function and are critical in sending descending motor neurons as the output system for motor control, and modifying the aspects of the head and body during motor function on the opposite side of the head and body. The frontal lobes have tremendous relay connections with the BG, limbic structures, and the cerebellum, as well as ultimate responsibility for controlling the muscles in the body and the face in all functional activities, no matter the complexity. Each lobe in the brain is discussed separately, although they are intricately interconnected via communications networks of interneurons.

- Parietal lobes: Also referred to as the *somatosensory* lobes. Information coming from the skin, muscles, and joints in the body enters the spinal system (some synapses in the cord and other fibers go directly to the medulla before the sensory input synapses). Whether the synapses are in the spinal cord or the medulla, they will cross over to the other side, be projected to the thalamus, synapse again, and then project onto

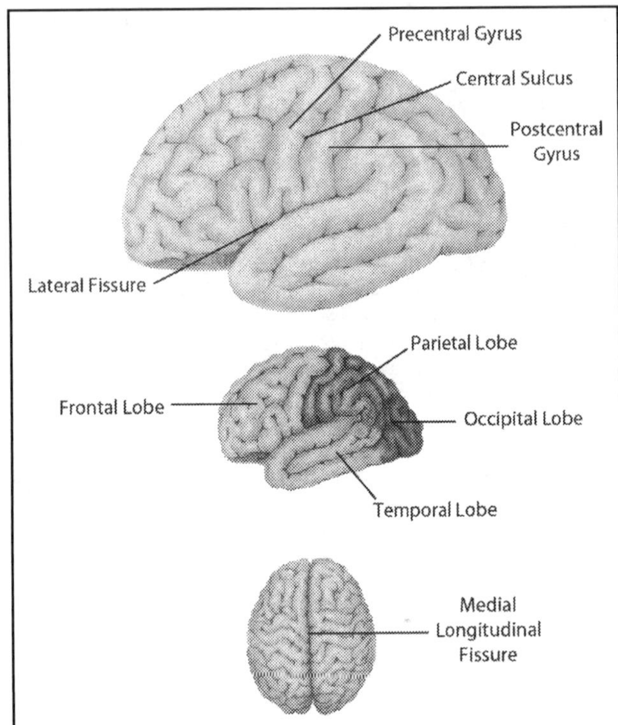

Figure 2-9. Cerebral lobes. (Reprinted with permission from Gutman SA. *Quick Reference Neuroscience for Rehabilitation Professionals.* 3rd ed. Thorofare, NJ: SLACK Incorporated; 2017.)

the primary somatosensory receiving areas of the parietal lobes. Information from the head carrying similar information synapses in CN nuclear masses in the brainstem, crosses over, projects to the thalamus, synapses again, and then projects to this lobe on the opposite side. That information, first processed as pure sensory information, includes touch; pressure; pain; joint position; stretch to muscles from the body, limbs, and the head; and vestibular information. Information from the peripheral body comes in at the spinal level, while information from the head comes in at the brainstem level via CNs (see Chapter 6). Once the primary sensory is projected onto the parietal lobes, it is represented according to the importance of that information and how the brain will use it. That is, the face and hands have higher representation, or more cell bodies, to process the information than representation given the calf or upper arm. All sensory input is processed multiple times in what is considered the association area within the lobe. That input is then projected to other areas of the brain, as well as posteriorly to other cell bodies for further integration and meaning. This information leads to an understanding of body image, body schema, and position in space both within and outside the body, and it leads to the sensory aspect of motor planning and spatial relationships. The projection of this information into the limbic structures leads to the integration of the emotional aspect of body image, and not just the physical size. This complex processed information will be integrated with other sensory lobes of the brain to link vision and auditory information, and is considered multimodal. These neurons are then relayed via long axons sent forward toward the frontal lobe to be integrated for higher-level thought as well as motor performance. The reader is encouraged to study more about these perceptual strategies as part of an analysis of the somatosensory system.[11]

- Temporal lobes, or auditory processing lobes: The temporal lobes are located at the level of the ear and receive sensory information from the auditory or hearing system from the ear or CN VIII. That information enters the brain at the lower brainstem, synapses in large nuclear masses, crosses over, projects upward, synapses again in the thalamus, and then radiates onto the primary auditory receiving areas of the temporal lobes. This lobe initially processes the auditory input in pure sounds or sensory input, and then integrates that information in associated areas into tones, frequencies, and meaning. The brain will identify those sounds and localize them as to their position in space to learn to identify meaning and importance. Sound is integrated with the limbic structures through cells projecting information leading to emotional interactions, which give the meanings of those sounds. Bombs blasting will lead to withdrawal and alert the CNS, while soft rhythmic sounds lead to relaxation. Similarly, the noise level and types of sounds can affect your patients' motor responses and attitudes toward the sessions. Similar to the parietal lobes, the information projecting onto the primary temporal areas will be integrated and sent posteriorly to other cell bodies and link other information regarding the auditory system and, in time, the somatosensory and visual cortices. Thus, the temporal lobes, when linked with the occipital lobe (Figure 2-9), are involved in verbal and visual memory, interpretation of emotional reactions of others, and the complexity of language development and learning. These lobes will be used as part of the communication system and integrated with the frontal lobes leading to language production and control over the larynx and tongue for speech.[12]
- Occipital lobes: These visual cortices are at the back of the skull. Neuroanatomy of CN II, or the optic nerve, is very complex. The reader is referred to additional references at the end of this chapter for an in-depth study of the complexity of this system. Part of the input tract crosses, and part stays on the same side, thus allowing all visual information from one side of the external world to cross over and go to the opposite occipital lobe. In this way, the brain can process all the information from one side of the external world onto the opposite side of the brain. The input from CN II sends neurons to the thalamus, synapses in the poste-

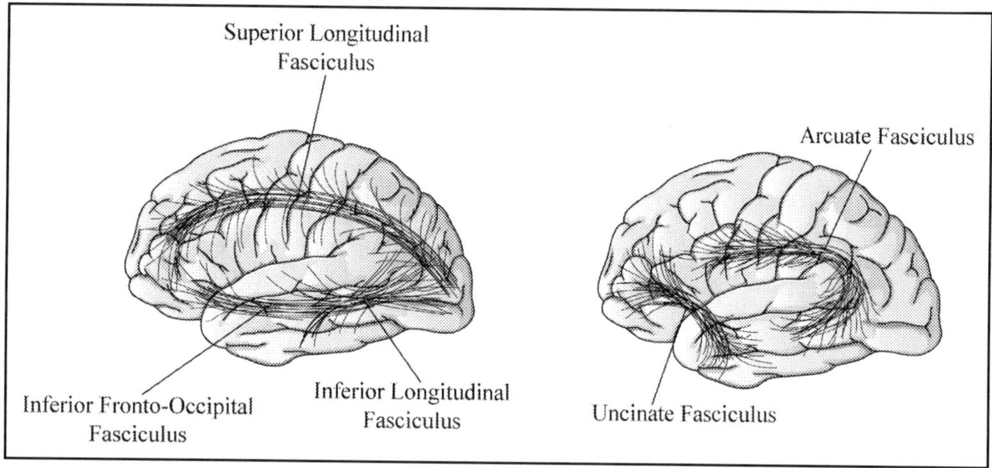

Figure 2-10. Schematic diagram of the major intra-hemispheric association bundles. (Reprinted with permission from Nolan MF. *Cram Session in Functional Neuroanatomy*. Thorofare, NJ: SLACK Incorporated; 2012.)

rior geniculate bodies, and then projects onto the primary visual receiving lobes. Simultaneously, the same input sends collateral neurons or axons radiating to the brainstem's large nuclear masses, which play a role in controlling the cranial neurons leaving the brainstem going to muscles controlling eye movements.

Information in the primary occipital receiving areas will be initially processed as pure visual information, and then sent to associated nuclear masses or other adjacent cells bodies for integration and processing. Information within the occipital lobe will make its way forward anteriorly and laterally to synapse on nuclear masses that associated information coming from the temporal and parietal lobes to integrate and associate multiple types of input for higher-level processing.[13] Hearing and localizing a sound to guide the eyes to look and process visual information are very complex neuromechanisms and one of the wonders of brain processing.

Information that has been processed and associated with other information from all 3 sensory cortical lobes is radiated via large bundles of white matter to the frontal lobes (Figure 2-10).

- Frontal lobes: Some refer to these lobes as the *motor cortex*, but they do play roles besides motor regulation. These lobes are the largest and are located at the front of the brain behind the forehead. The frontal lobes coordinate high-level behaviors such as motor skills, problem-solving, judgment, planning, and attention. The frontal lobes are also intricately connected to the limbic system and manage emotions and impulse control. Each frontal lobe has 4 distinct areas: the *prefrontal*, *premotor*, *supplementary motor*, and *primary motor*. Each area plays unique roles within the frontal lobes. The interactions or relay loops between the premotor and supplementary motor areas with the BG and with the cerebellum play a critical role in the development and modification of motor programs and control over all movements, whether it involves new learning, adjustments to old programs, or relearning functional movement (Figure 2-11). The primary motor area plays a role in fine motor control over movements of the hand, face, eyes, and tongue, as well as fine motor control over proximal joints when learning complex skilled movements such as pitching, throwing a baseball, or playing golf. Once motor plans are ready to be executed and sent to large masses of motor neurons in the brainstem and spinal systems, the motor tracts from the supplementary and primary motor tend to send that information directly without using additional synaptic junctions to modify the information. At that time, the motor programs will run through the interactions of the BG, cerebellum, and frontal lobes without the need for sensory feedback from those other cortices. These are considered *feedforward motor programs*. If the feedforward motor programs are accurate, they run effortlessly, but if the feedforward program does not match the sensory input, then the system becomes alert and needs to modify or change the existing program to match or readjust to the needs of the environment.

The complexity leading to the variance in control over movement depending upon the external environment is enormous and certainly changes as a child grows into an adult and then ages. For example, rising from sitting depends upon the individual's body size, both height and weight, as well as how far the seated structure is from the ground. A child first learns to come to stand off a small chair, while adults learn differently. Thus, the parameters for coming to stand are patient-dependent. As the child grows, those parameters change as does the height of the structures used in sitting. As an individual ages and power production decreases or diminishes, the environment for independent control will also change. If the problem is

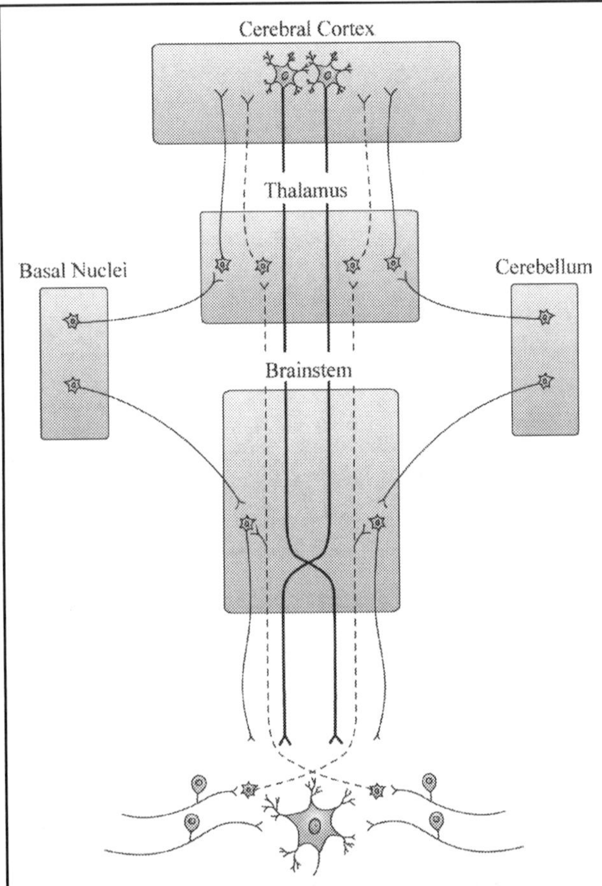

Figure 2-11. Schematic diagram illustrating segmental (afferent) and suprasegmental (brainstem and cerebral cortex) influences on lower motor neurons together with the 2 major influences (cerebellum and BG) on these cells. (Reprinted with permission from Nolan MF. *Cram Session in Functional Neuroanatomy.* Thorofare, NJ: SLACK Incorporated; 2012.)

weakness due to disease, trauma, or disuse, a riser can be placed on the chair to help the person come to stand. A raised toilet seat serves the same purpose. Whether a patient needs strengthening to be able to stand up independently, or needs to be introduced to an adaptive piece of equipment, should depend upon the evaluation, reevaluation following intervention, and the prognosis of the patient's recovery.

Ventricular System and Meninges

Now that the reader has an appreciation for the gross anatomy of the brain, a couple of additional areas need to be introduced.

The *ventricular system* is made up of a fluid substance that gives buoyancy to the brain and spinal system to protect them from forces placed upon those structures from the outside world. This system lays to the outside of the spinal system and brain itself, as well as having large reservoirs within the brain and brainstem (Figure 2-12). Understanding how fluid is transferred from the internal reservoirs to the fluid surrounding the outside is not relevant to the physical therapist assistant's understanding of brain function. What is important is comprehending that when transference of fluid is blocked within this system, the fluid can build up and damage the structures. The brain cannot accommodate the buildup of ventricular pressure, and the resultant damage can lead to pressure on the gray matter—whether it be cortical, brainstem, or spinal structures—and cause trauma and, at times, permanent brain damage. When the ventricles within the brain enlarge, the resultant condition is called *hydrocephaly.* In a child, when the boney plates of the head or skull have not yet closed, the boney structures of the skull itself can get bigger with ventricular enlargement, which causes additional problems. Today, the most common way to deal with this problem is for a neurosurgeon to place a shunt into the ventricles and allow the excess fluid to drain into the lower quadrant of the body. If a patient has a shunt, the physical therapist assistant needs to be aware of any change in normal interactions with the patient, or if the patient complains of severe headaches while under the care of the physical therapist assistant. These symptoms need to be reported to the physical therapist immediately to make sure the shunt has not plugged. Individuals with ventricular swelling problems can be hypersensitive to humidity, whether that be too humid or too dry. Patients with post-traumatic head trauma often complain of pressure changes in their head as the weather shifts back and forth. Again, dealing with these problems is outside the scope of the physical therapist assistant, but being sensitive to them and referring observations to professionals who can differentiate these issues is important.

The second structures are found in the skull and separate the fluid surrounding the brain from the skull bone itself. These structures are called *meninges* (Figure 2-13). The outer structure is similar to having a skull cap made up of strong connective tissue that allows the fluid to surround the brain and keep the brain buoyant and protected it from outside forces. The outside layer of meninges is called *dura mater.* The middle layer is the *arachnoid mater,* and protects the brain, similar to a sealant. Below the arachnoid is the *subarachnoid space,* which holds in the cerebral spinal fluid surrounding the brain. The lowest layer is called *pia,* and it is the deepest meningeal layer and specifically follows the indentations of the brain and the spinal cord. The anatomy of the meninges and the ventricular system is more complex than presented in this section, but the physical therapist assistant just needs to comprehend and be able to identify when behaviors change that might be caused by problems in the brain.

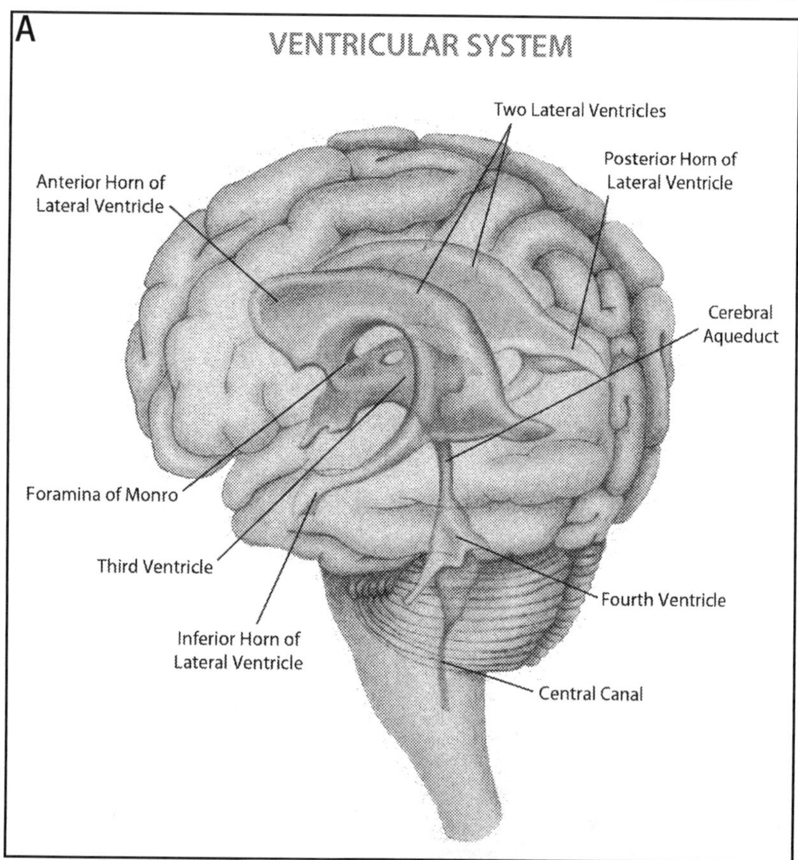

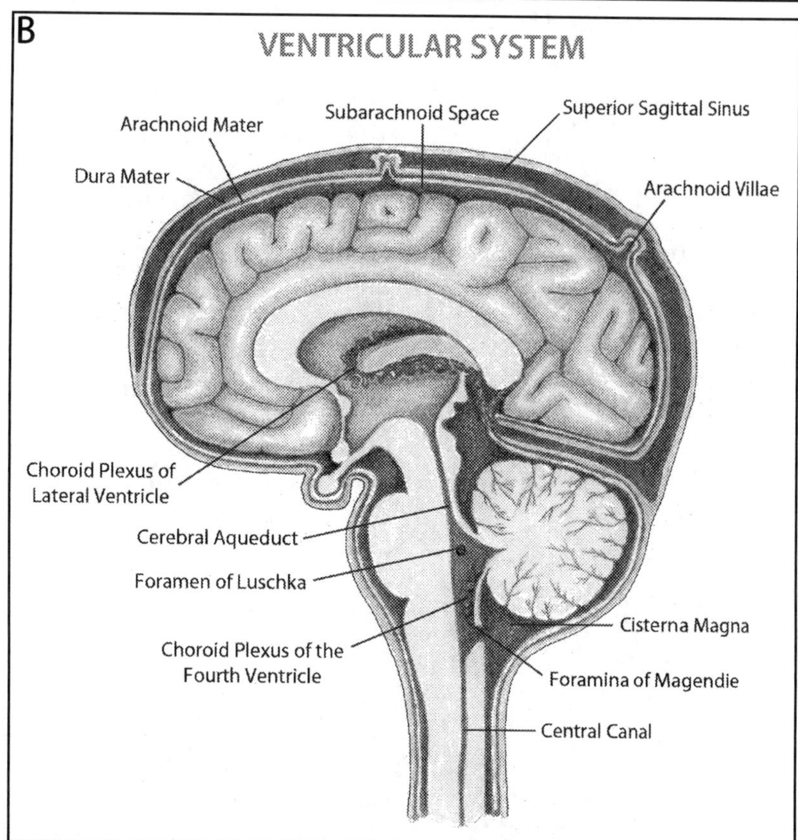

Figure 2-12. (A) Internal three-dimensional structures of the ventricular system. (B) Cross-sectional view of the entire ventricular and meningeal system. (Reprinted with permission from Gutman SA. *Quick Reference Neuroscience for Rehabilitation Professionals*. 3rd ed. Thorofare, NJ: SLACK Incorporated; 2017.)

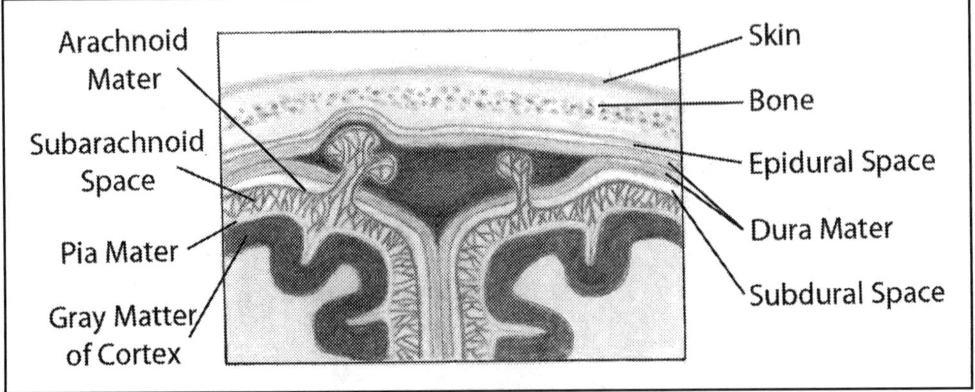

Figure 2-13. The meninges: dura mater, arachnoid mater, pia mater. (Reprinted with permission from Gutman SA. *Quick Reference Neuroscience for Rehabilitation Professionals*. 3rd ed. Thorofare, NJ: SLACK Incorporated; 2017.)

Circulatory System, or Blood Supply to the Nervous System

The second fluid structure that encompasses the nervous system is the circulatory system. Similar to what is found in the body and peripheral system, the spinal and brain nervous system has both arterial and venous circulation. The arterial system brings oxygen and food stuff to the spinal and brain neurons so those cells and the surrounding support structures can function and remain alive. The venous system drains the diminished blood once the oxygen and food stuffs have been removed and waste transferred.

The physical therapist assistant needs to have some comprehension of the arterial circulatory system of the brain. Two large anatomical arterial structures enter into the brain (Figure 2-14). These arteries come off the common carotid artery that leaves the heart, and branch into the 2 internal carotid arteries that enter the skull near the optic chiasm or the entrance of the optic nerve (CN II). These 2 branches provide most of the blood to the brain. A second arterial structure gives rise to the 2 vertebral arteries that form the descending spinal arteries that supply the medulla and spinal cord. The rest of the vertebral arteries give rise to arterial structures that supply blood to the remainder of the brainstem and the cerebellum.

The internal carotid arteries on each side of the skull create an arterial map called the *Circle of Willis*.[14] Within this map, one finds the common middle cerebral arteries on each side, with communicating arteries giving rise to both the anterior and posterior cerebral arteries. Both the anterior and posterior arteries have a communicating artery that joins those 2 arteries in both the back and front of the Circle of Willis. These circuits of interconnecting arteries on both sides of the brain allow blood to flow to all areas of both hemispheres of the brain, as well as interconnecting arteries from one side of the brain to the other, even if one of these arteries gets blocked or damaged. Each of these major arteries will branch into smaller and smaller arterial vessels to project the blood into all areas of the brain. Small veins begin deep in the brain within all the lobes and accompany the small arteries. The veins will enlarge as they collect more and more unoxygenated blood on their way back through the chiasm and into the descending vena cave to join other venous blood going to the heart and then to the lungs for reoxygenation.

The physical therapist assistant needs to be aware of problems that can arise in the circulatory system, leading to potential damage within the nervous system. A common term used to describe problems arising from this arterial system is a *stroke*, or *cardiovascular accident*.[4] It is called cardiovascular because the arteries originate from vessels from the heart or cardiac system, and it is the interaction of both the cardiac and ascending arterial vascular system that can cause strokes. When plaque or cholesterol builds up in the arteries leaving the heart, it can break loose from trauma or increased blood pressure. This plaque, once broken off, will float upward or toward the brain until the vessels begin to reduce inside, and the clot plugs the artery. Clot-buster drugs can dissolve this plaque and remove the symptoms of the stroke if caught early enough. Plaque can also lie down in the arteries within the brain and cause a stroke. Again, clot-buster drugs can eliminate or reduce the clinical symptoms. The plaque can be large and block larger arteries, or it can be small and only block off tiny arteries. The areas unable to receive oxygen can be permanently damaged if collateral circulation or removal of the clot cannot be made. As the circulatory system is in map form, certain arteries are more likely to have these floating clots enter into their branches. Thus, the most common is the middle cerebral artery on either side of the brain, which sends blood supply to areas more often affecting the upper extremity more severely than the lower extremity.

Clots are not the only cause of strokes within the brain. Some people have what are called *aneurysms* within the arterial systems. These aneurysms are weaknesses in the arterial vessels and usually found at junctions where arteries divide the arterial pressure is greatest. These aneurysms

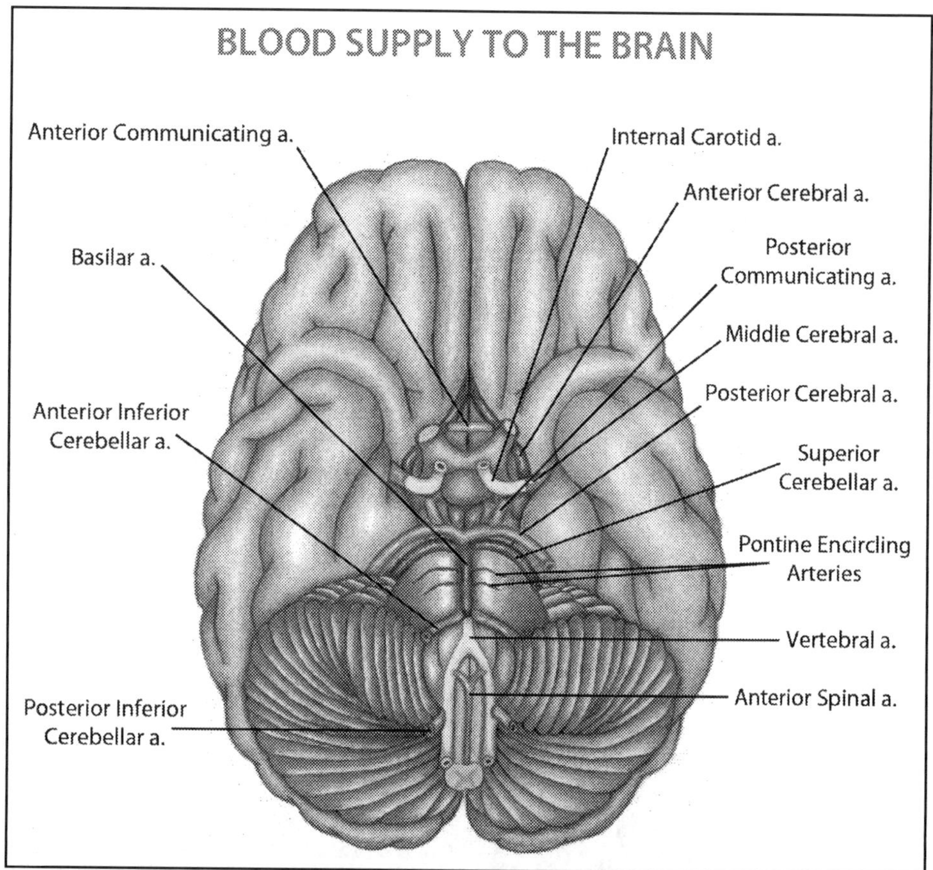

Figure 2-14. Blood supply for the brain. (Reprinted with permission from Gutman SA. *Quick Reference Neuroscience for Rehabilitation Professionals.* 3rd ed. Thorofare, NJ: SLACK Incorporated; 2017.)

begin to balloon out with blood until they can potentially burst, creating a bleed within the brain. The larger the aneurysm, the greater the danger for a catastrophic event that can lead to death. Arterial aneurysms are more frequently found in young adults[4] than in the elderly or older adult, where plaque formation and clots causing strokes are more frequent. Getting an individual medical care quickly is important, so the physician can differentiate whether the stroke is due to a clot or a bleed. Obviously, a clot-buster medication must never be given if the stroke is due to a bleed, because the clot buster medication will increase the bleeding (see Chapter 13).[4]

A third type of stroke is called a *transient ischemic attack,* often caused by vessels spasming within the brain or very small clots. Both causes of transient ischemic attacks often resolve within 24 hours without any permanent damage. If damage does exist, the brain will accommodate to the insult and often regain functional motor skills to get back to life.

Depending upon the size of the stroke and whether it is due to a blood clot or a bleed, functional loss of sensory processing, high-level thought, or motor function (both gross and fine of the hand and mouth) can be severe, and recovery takes time.

Clots and bleeds can also affect vessels sending blood to the spinal system and throughout the brainstem, cerebellum, and diencephalon. These are much less common. Bleeds following trauma to the nervous system can be found whether the trauma occurs in utero, at birth, as a child ages, as an adult, or as an elderly person. See Chapters 9 and 13 on both pediatric and adult clients with stroke for greater details on the human vascular system and related problems.

Gray and White Matter

The physical therapist assistant may read in the chart that a patient has gray or white matter damage following some insult to the nervous system. This is important, as the cortical areas are responsible for taking in data, processing it, and passing that on to be processed by other areas of the brain, whether that information is still within a specific lobe or communicated to other lobes for integration. For example, the *spinal thalamic* tract refers to the origin (spine) and destination within which the axon is going (thalamus). In this tract, the cell body originates at the spinal level, then its axon ascends, crosses over, and continues to the next synapse in the thalamus. Thus, it is an ascending tract and carries sensory information to the brain. If the tract is called *reticulospinal* or *corticospinal*, it means the tract originated either in the reticular system or in the cerebral cortex (usually frontal lobe). Both have axons that descend and synapse onto a spinal cord gray matter.

Discussion of all the sensory or motor tracts is beyond the scope of this chapter, but once the physical therapist assistant understands how to interpret the names of the tracts, it is easy to differentiate ascending afferent or sensory input tracts from descending motor tracts that ultimately will control the muscular system in the periphery. Many tracts originate in a cortex and project to another lobe. These tracts would be called *cortico-cortico* tracts. There are many tract systems whose purpose is to communicate information within and between lobes to do higher-order processing. Information from sensory lobes needs to be projected to the frontal lobe before motor planning. This sensory aspect of what will eventually be a motor plan has to be formulated. Information from the frontal lobes needs to be communicated to the BG and to the cerebellum, which will then communicate processed information back to the frontal lobes.

The brain obviously is a complex neuro-network, from reception of raw sensory data, to complex processing of that data for perception, to communication and integration of other sensory systems for higher-level thought. Similarly, formulating and controlling motor programming is very complex and involves many centers in the brain.

A child begins to process all sensory input even in utero, and certainly is forced to process input as soon as the first breath is taken, then continues to learn and modify input with appropriate motor responses throughout life.

Discussion of the names and functions of the large nuclear masses found within the spinal, brainstem, diencephalon, cerebellum, and cortical structures did not include presentation of large bundles of white matter carrying information back and forth among these neuronal cell body structures. There is more than one name for these bundles of axons; they are referred to as *tracts*, *callosa*, *peduncles*, *fornices*, *fasciculi*, and *capsules*. They all are made up of axons going toward or away from some area of the brain. Axons from one side of the cortex need to cross over to the other side the brain and use a large white matter area called the *corpus callosum*. Descending and ascending axons from the thalamus to and from the cortices within the brain go through an area called the *internal capsule*. Many descending axons from the frontal lobes keep descending through the internal capsule. Going by the thalamus, they enter into the cerebral peduncles in the anterior portion of the midbrain. Some of these axons are descending onto nuclear masses in the brainstem, some are going to the cerebellum, while still others go as far as the spinal cord, carrying motor information from higher centers. Axons from the frontal lobes to the spine are called *corticospinal* because they start in the cortex and synapse on motor nuclei in the anterior portion of spinal system before the next-order neuron's axons travel out to the peripheral system and run what are called *motor programs*. These axons ultimately drive functional movements the physical therapist assistant observes and examines.

Similarly, ascending and descending fibers are part of the autonomic nervous system. Their structure is slightly different, but ultimately the nervous system controls the human body and all the organ systems (Figure 2-15). Discussion of the complexity of the parasympathetic and sympathetic nervous system is not within the scope of this chapter.

Conclusion

The chapter began with the use of an analogy showing how a car with all its parts might be equated to the CNS. When looking at the parts of a car, you have a person driving, a steering wheel, gear shifts, the brake, an accelerator, and then everything under the hood. Under that hood, one finds an engine, a fuel pump, a battery, spark plugs, a radiator, a pump and fluid container for window cleaner, and all sorts of connecting wires that go from one part to the other. Now, how do we equate all these parts to the nervous system?

If we start at the cortical structures, the visual cortex needs to recognize all the parts of the car and their meaning. The parietal lobe needs to recognize the tactile touch when holding the steering wheel, turning it as needed, turning the key switch, or pressing the button to turn on the engine. The limbic lobe drives the desire to do these things. The temporal lobe needs to recognize the sound of the motor when it is on and if it sounds correct. All this information needs to be sent to the frontal lobe to plan which gear to put the car in and the amount of pressure needed on the gas pedal to move the car. The force placed on the gas pedal or on the brake will be set up by the interaction of the BG and the cerebellum. The BG and cerebellum need to recognize which gear to use, and the force and speed needed to move the car in the direction desired, which will direct the engine how to perform. At times, additional assistance is needed, such as turning on the windshield wipers when it is raining, turning on a blinker light, or turning the steering wheel to direct the car.

This is all done through an electrical system similar to the neuron network, which required first a starting point with an electrical charge similar to the dendrites and cell bodies. The electrical charge then travels to a receiving site where the next system responds whether that system is a large nuclear mass of new cell bodies in the brain or another system in the car. These next systems, whether a system in the CNS or a system in the car, help the entire system to function. Now, when any one system in the car (eg, engine, radiator, battery, steering system, or brakes) or the CNS (eg, stroke, head or spinal trauma, birth injury, or degeneration) has a problem, we have to go to someone who can analyze what is damaged and why. No matter if it is an automobile or the CNS, when something breaks

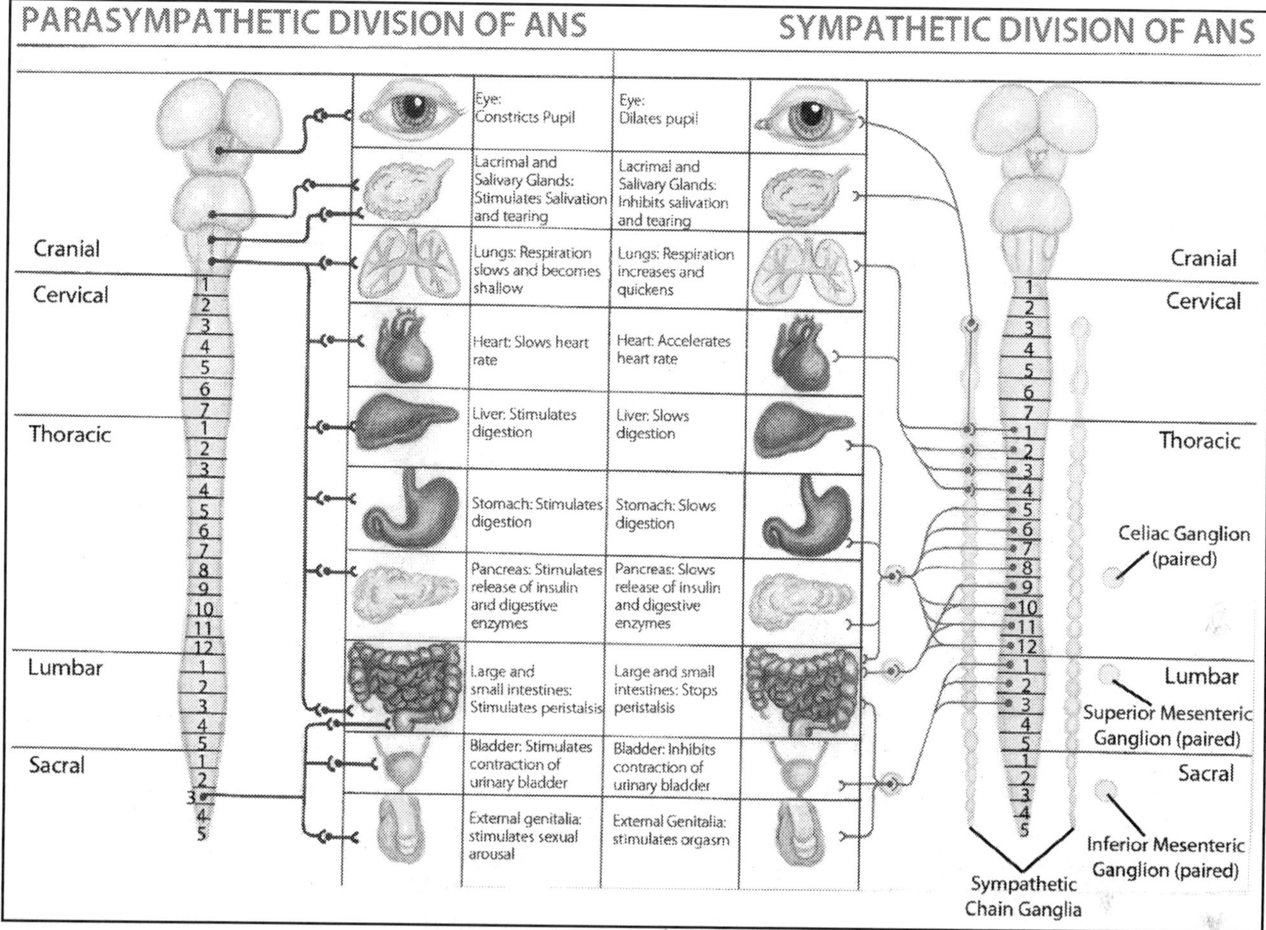

Figure 2-15. The autonomic nervous system. (Reprinted with permission from Gutman SA. *Quick Reference Neuroscience for Rehabilitation Professionals*. 3rd ed. Thorofare, NJ: SLACK Incorporated; 2017.)

down, the system becomes dysfunctional. A mechanic will diagnosis the problem in the car and hopefully be able to repair it or replace a part, or eventually the system will fail. Fortunately, the brain has many more parts and mechanisms that can relearn (motor learning), substitute for damaged cells (functional recovery), or even in time have other parts function as replacements for damaged areas (neuroplasticity). Each system in the brain serves an important function and as an individual ages, these systems learn new ways of responding to the external world, whether that be a motor function, a cognitive thought process, or an emotional interaction. The CNS is much more pliable than a car and able to adapt to system problems, which is why the physical therapist assistant's role in empowering a patient to regain functional control over the motor system is critical in the patient regaining the quality of life desired.

Pearls of Application to Function

1. When the chart or associated test such as an MRI reads:
   a. "A bleed in the internal capsule area," the reader should be able to identify that some sensory fibers or axons from the thalamus would be involved and sensory testing would be appropriate. Similarly, motor tracts going from the frontal lobes to the brainstem CNs and spinal system may be affected, and thus functional testing is appropriate (see Chapter 6).
   b. "Trauma to the frontal lobe," information going back and forth to the BG and the cerebellum can be affected. Patients will demonstrate specific motor programming problems. Understanding what each system does will help the physical therapist assistant recognize those movement problems.
   c. "A bleed in the brainstem," this can potentially involve the area of the descending fibers in the front of the brainstem (cerebral peduncles) going to motor nuclei in the spinal system, or fibers going to cranial motor nerves. Obvious motor programming problems can result with brainstem involvement and involved movement in the face. Motor control over CNs controlling muscles in the face, tongue, and throat can be tested. Tracts going to vestibular nuclei affecting balance and postural core strength can also be affected and should lead to balance and proximal postural test-

ing. Brainstem deficits certainly can alter the way a person moves in functional activities.

d. "Arterial clot affecting association areas of the brain," this suggests sensory cortices such as parietal, temporal, and occipital involvement. The resulting problems can affect perception and can include sensory awareness, sensory processing, communication between lobes, and control over descending fibers that lead to motor control.

e. "A tumor in specific areas of the brain," the physical therapist assistant should ask the physical therapist what cognitive, emotional (affective), and motor involvement the placement of that tumor might affect.

f. "The patient has a degenerative disease process," the physical therapist assistant should ask the physical therapist whether the degeneration is causing death of the cells themselves, is a problems with chemical transmission between cells such as a dopamine imbalance within the BG, or is a demyelination of the sheath that surrounds the axons, thus changing conduction of the information going to or from the brain. Each degenerative problem creates different movement prognoses and thus should affect the plan of care. It is the physical therapist's responsibility to communicate and differentiate for the physical therapist assistant which type of degenerative disease process is occurring and the type of sensory-motor processing will be affected.

g. "Involvement in the descending portion or anterior portion of the brainstem," those descending fibers carry motor information, and thus motor programming will be affected at the spinal level, as well as in fibers going to the cerebellum. The physical therapist assistant may be told that motor function is lost, but must remember that only about 30% of the fibers are seen in the MRI, so if the patient demonstrates functional movement when the demand of that movement is reduced, then fibers are still functioning and potential present.

h. "Damage to specific areas of the spinal system," the reader should refer to Chapter 11 and be able to understand what types of motor and sensory involvement might be affected, and how that will change motor performance and functional activities.

2. Differentiation among tumor, clots, bleeds, trauma, or developmental problems: Given the type of trauma to the CNS, recovery can be very different.

   a. Any tumor, whether malignant or not, will take up space in the CNS. Spinal tumors, whether treatable or not, are extremely painful due to the extreme limitation of space for the tumor to grow within the boney structure of the spinal system. Cranial tumors can often grow into the size of lemon, orange, or grapefruit without any pain, but they may show subtle signs of paralysis on one side similar to a stroke. This is why a physical therapist always needs to do medical screening before developing a plan of care. Often non-malignant cranial tumors are operable, and following surgery, the individuals will return to normal function, although initially they may show signs of weakness or movement dysfunction on the opposite side from the tumor. The physical therapist assistant may be treating a problem of pain in the back when the patient subtly develops weakness on one side of the body. This new problem should alert the physical therapist assistant that it is appropriate to ask the physical therapist to retest for a slow progressive problem within the brain, such as a stroke or tumor.

   b. Individuals with vascular insults, whether a bleed or a clot, may regain normal function depending upon the sight and degree of the insult. The individual may need to take intensive therapy with repetitive practice to regain function (see Chapter 13).

   c. Individuals with traumatic brain injury may have lesions anywhere in the CNS depending upon the initial impact and the contra-coup injury as a result of movement of the brain. Generally, the MRI will pick up this damage, but it may take additional MRIs to clearly identify the extent of the damage which will affect the ultimate plan of care (see Chapter 11).

3. Differentiation between the age of the patient and the type of insult: Individuals who have birth or pre-birth injuries have never had an opportunity to normally develop the CNS or learn. It may take an optimal environment to help the child learn sensory processing, perceptual concepts such as reading and math skills, and motor function (see Chapters 9 and 10). These sensory and motor problems differ from those of older children or adults because these populations have already learned perceptual processing and movement programs. New learning and relearning are different. New learning takes much more time and opportunity to practice, whether it be higher-level learning or motor programming. Relearning or substitution will not take the same amount of practice, while development of neuroplasticity within the brain takes a very long period of time (see Chapter 4).

4. The limbic system, within the diencephalon, deals with emotions and memory. One progressive emotional reaction within the limbic system is called the *F2ARV continuum*. F2ARV stands for fear/frustration, anger, rage, and violence. This continuum is driven by

chemistry within the limbic system, and starts with the emotions of fear and frustration. If the chemical or emotional reaction is not suppressed by higher cortical centers, an individual will often demonstrate anger. If the chemistry continues to amplify, internal chaos or rage can follow. If emotional control at this point is not regained, violence can occur. In some women, instead of violence, total emotional withdrawal from the environment is seen. The physical therapist assistant must be aware that some patients through life experiences can go down this continuum quickly and physically strike out at the therapist. Individuals with traumatic brain injury may come from an environment where violence is common, and violence may have led to the brain injury (see Chapters 7 and 12). It is much easier to create an environment that the patient enjoys, and is able to laugh and be relaxed, compared to an environment where the patient feels failure, which usually leads to frustration. Patients in early phases of brain injury may be confused, disoriented, and frustrated so it is the physical therapist assistant's responsibility to help the patient feel safe (see Chapter 8). Both physical and emotional pain can also trigger this continuum as a protective response. The physical therapist assistant must be sensitive to the emotional level of the patient to recognize when the patient is getting frustrated and angry. Most clinicians likely recall they preferred enjoying the learning vs feeling failure and frustration within the environment. Teaching slow deep breathing exercises or diaphragmatic breathing often relaxes the patient, lowers blood pressure, and helps avoid anyone going down this continuum. Changes to the specific activity can also redirect the patient's emotions and help stop the frustration. Pointing out the frustration or fear may also help the patient regain emotional control, thus empowering the patient to take control of the internal environment.

Acknowledgement

I would like to thank Davis Reina-Guerra for the time and energy he put forth in reading and making recommendations to enhance the reader's comprehension of the complex topics presented within this chapter.

References

1. Mancall EL, Brock DG, Standring S, Crossman A. *Gray's Clinical Neuroanatomy*. Philadelphia, PA: Elsevier Saunders; 2012.
2. Martini FH, Tallitsch RB, Nath JL. *Human Anatomy*. 9th ed. Glenview, IL: Pearson Education; 2017.
3. Gutman SA. *Quick Reference Neuroscience for Rehabilitation Professionals*. 3rd ed. Thorofare, NJ: SLACK Incorporated; 2017.
4. Kandel ER, Schwatz JH, Jennell TM, Siegelbaum SA, Hudspeth AJ. *Principles of Neural Science*. 5th ed. New York, NY: McGraw-Hill; 2013.
5. Nolan MF. *Cram Session in Functional Neuroanatomy*. Thorofare, NJ: SLACK Incorporated; 2012.
6. Loewy AD, Ratcliff G, Nathan PW, Haines DE, Matthews PBC, Noback CR. Human nervous system. Encyclopædia Britannica. https://www.britannica.com/science/human-nervous-system. Published June 14, 2019. Accessed July 17, 2019.
7. Herdman, SJ, Herdman S, Clendaniel RJ. *Vestibular Rehabilitation (Contemporary Perspectives in Rehabilitation)*. 4th ed. Philadelphia, PA: FA Davis; 2020.
8. Kingma H, van de Berg R. Anatomy, physiology, and physics of the peripheral vestibular system. *Handb Clin Neurol*. 2016;137:1-16. doi:10.1016/B978-0-444-63437-5.00001-7
9. Jang SH, Kwon YH. A review of traumatic axonal injury following whiplash injury as demonstrated by diffusion tensor tractography. *Front Neurol*. 2018;9:57. doi:10.3389/fneur.2018.00057
10. Thompson MH, Umphred DA. The limbic network: influence over motor control, memory, and learning. In: Lazaro RT, Reina-Guerra SG, Quiben M, eds. *Umphred's Neurological Rehabilitation*. 7th ed. St. Louis, MO: Elsevier; 2019.
11. Miller LJ, Anzalone ME, Lane SJ, Cermak SA, Osten ET. Concept evolution in sensory integration: a proposed nosology for diagnosis. *Am J Occup Ther*. 2007;61(2):135-140. doi:10.5014/ajot.61.2.135
12. Moller AR. *Hearing, Anatomy, Physiology and Disorders of the Auditory System*. 3rd ed. San Diego, CA: Plural; 2012.
13. Remington LA. *Clinical Anatomy and Physiology of the Visual System*. 3rd ed. St. Louis, MO: Butterworth-Heinemann; 2012.
14. Gupta G, Mahtabfar A, Meleis A. Circle of Willis Anatomy. Medscape. https://emedicine.medscape.com. Accessed July 16, 2019.

Recommended Readings

Cortical Lobe Activities

Bronstein AM. A conceptual model of the visual control of posture. *Prog Brain Res*. 2019;248:285-302. doi:10.1016/bs.pbr.2019.04.023

Fiori F, Chiappini E, Avenanti A. Enhanced action performance following TMS manipulation of associative plasticity in ventral premotor-motor pathway. *Neuroimage*. 2018;183:847-858. doi:10.1016/j.neuroimage.2018.09.002

Harmon-Jones E, Gable PA. On the role of asymmetric frontal cortical activity in approach and withdrawal motivation: an updated review of the evidence. *Psychophysiology*. 2018;55(1):e12879. doi:10.1111/psyp.12879

Lebon F, Horn U, Domin M, Lotze M. Motor imagery training: kinesthetic imagery strategy and inferior parietal fMRI activation. *Hum Brain Mapp*. 2018;39(4):1805-1813. doi:10.1002/hbm.23956

Rice P, Stocco A. The role of dorsal premotor cortex in resolving abstract motor rules: converging evidence from transcranial magnetic stimulation and cognitive modeling. *Top Cogn Sci*. 2019;11(1):240-260. doi:10.1111/tops.12408

Savelov AA, Shtark MB, Kozlova LI, et al. Dynamics of interactions between cerebral networks derived from fMRI data and motor rehabilitation during strokes. *Bull Exp Biol Med.* 2019;166(3):399-403. doi:10.1007/s10517-019-04359-6

Brainstem Function

Kragel PA, Bianciardi M, Hartley L, et al. Functional involvement of human periaqueductal gray and other midbrain nuclei in cognitive control. *J Neurosci.* 2019;39(31):6180-6189. doi:10.1523/JNEUROSCI.2043-18.2019

Poretti A, Boltshauser E, Huisman TA. Cerebellar and brainstem malformations. *Neuroimaging Clin N Am.* 2016;26(3):341-357. doi:10.1016/j.nic.2016.03.005

Perception and Learning

Bundy A, Lane SJ, Murray EA. *Sensory Integration: Theory and Practice.* 2nd ed. Philadelphia, PA: FA Davis; 2003.

Carr J, Shepherd R. *Movement Science: Foundations for Physical Therapy in Rehabilitation.* 2nd ed. Gaithersburg, MD: Aspen; 2000.

Merzenich M. *Soft-Wired: How the New Science of Brain Plasticity Can Change Your Life.* San Francisco, CA: Parnassus; 2013.

Pessoa L. *The Cognitive-Emotional Brain: From Interactions to Integration.* Cambridge, MA: The MIT Press; 2013. doi:10.7551/mitpress/9780262019569.001.0001

Rizzo M, Anderson SW, Fritzsch B. *The Wiley Handbook on the Aging Mind and Brain.* Hoboken, NJ: John Wiley & Sons; 2018. doi:10.1002/9781118772034

Chapter 3

Normal Movement Development Across the Lifespan

Dale Scalise-Smith, PT, PhD

KEY WORDS Cognition | Development | Dynamic systems theory | Innate motor behaviors | Locomotion | Motor development | Osteoporosis

Chapter Objectives

- Recognize the interaction among multiple systems in performance of motor behaviors.
- Explain motor behaviors and changes that occur across the lifespan, and the variability of motor performance among individuals.
- Examine the impact of health and fitness (physical activity) sustained over the lifespan on motor skill performance.
- Discuss the impact of age and age-related changes in exercise and training programs.
- Recognize that movement analysis is based on the central nervous system's (CNS) ability to run programs, adapt, and learn those programs to meet the functional demands of the individual.

Effective practitioners recognize the interactional processes that lead to changes in motor development across the lifespan. The human motor system is comprised of more than 700 muscles and the nerves that supply them. Motor behaviors require coordinated efforts among these and other bodily systems to produce movements. Motor behavior, the study of how movement is learned and controlled and changes with increasing age, is divided into subdisciplines: motor control, motor development, and motor learning (see Chapter 4).[1]

This chapter provides an overview of motor development to help the reader recognize typical and atypical changes in motor behaviors across the lifespan, appreciate factors that influence motor development, and apply knowledge of motor development, and associated mechanisms of change, to intervention strategies.

Until the late 1960s, research in motor development focused on infants and children. In the 1970s, developmentalists came to realize that changes in motor behaviors did not end in adolescence, but rather were dynamic processes with changes occurring through older adulthood. Thus, models of motor development have expanded to include changes that occur throughout the lifespan. Consequently, lifespan motor development now examines movement from early infancy through older adulthood. Motor development, a subdiscipline of motor behavior, is characterized by acquisition of motor skills during infancy (birth to 1 year) and childhood (1 to 10 years), followed by a period of stability from adolescence (10 to 19 years) through early and middle adulthood (20 to 59 years), and finally, a decline in execution of movements during late adulthood (60 years to death).

Lifespan motor development reflects motor behaviors observed from the prenatal period through older adulthood. The acquisition, control, and retention of motor skills is not confined to any specific part of the lifespan. During early infancy, acquisition of postural control and grasp-

Lazaro RT, Umphred DA, eds.
Umphred's Neurorehabilitation for the Physical Therapist Assistant, Third Edition (pp 37-59).

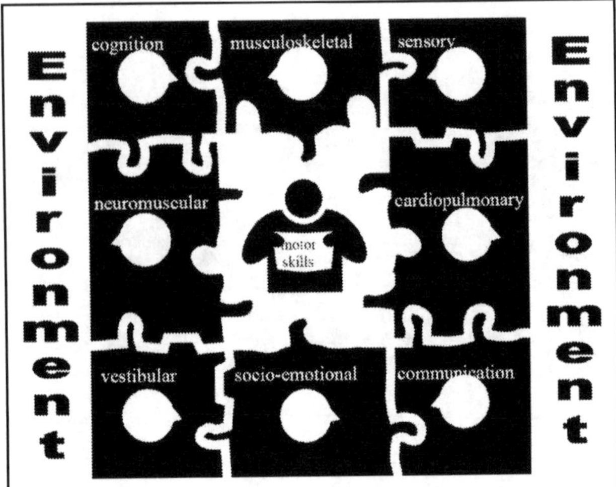

Figure 3-1. Interaction between intrinsic and extrinsic factors.

ing are primary foci. Later in infancy, mobility and object manipulation become primary objectives. During childhood, the skills acquired earlier are refined and coalesce to produce complex motor behaviors. Throughout adolescence and adulthood, opportunities to practice motor behaviors in different environmental contexts expand, and motor skills mature. As individuals grow older, successful aging is the ability to control motor skills without decline. Whether this decline is due to aging, lifestyle choices, disease or a combination of these factors is open to debate. Within this context of motor development, the impact of internal and external factors on motor skill acquisition will be considered both individually and collectively.

Theories of Development

Development is defined as *the changes that occur in one's life from conception to death.*[2] Development is described as a dynamic process focused on the individual adapting movements to physical changes in the system throughout the lifespan.[3] Changes in human behavior—including cognitive, motor, language, social-emotional, and physical characteristics—result from aging, lifestyle choices, experiences, genetics, and their interactive effects.

Early studies of motor development were based on maturational models of CNS organization.[4,5] These studies provided elegant descriptions of posture acquisition and a timeline for skill development. Most research development has focused on the emergence of cognitive and affective behaviors, and neglected the processes and mechanisms involved in learning motor tasks.[6] Development was thought to occur in a fixed sequence, and behaviors observed were a direct reflection of the maturation of intrinsic mechanisms.[7]

This traditional model of development relied on motor milestones to evaluate ability levels in infants and children. While motor milestones provided an assessment of actual motor skills a child performed, they failed to provide information about the process of attaining motor skills.

Researchers have proposed theories on motor development that emphasize the forces behind behavioral changes. Some scientists[4,5] theorized that developmental changes arise from internal factors (eg, genetics and/or maturation), while others associated changes with external variables (eg, environmental, experience, and/or learning).[8,9] While sufficient evidence exists to support the idea that some predetermined processes occur at relatively similar points in development, not all motor behaviors emerge at the same biological, chronological, or psychological age in every individual. The traditional theories on development and maturation fail to adequately address the variation inherent in human motor development. Successful acquisition of motor skills may be directly related to the individual's need to solve a problem within the context of the environment.

Researchers who have focused on developing new models for motor skill acquisition in infants and young children include Heriza, Thelan, and Zelazo et al.[10-12] Rather than using traditional methods to measure changes in motor development and assess the outcomes, these researchers examined the process of motor skill acquisition.[13,14] These contemporary developmentalists support an interactive model of motor development in which both intrinsic and extrinsic variables impact the development and acquisition of motor skills (Figure 3-1). The primary foundation for this model is *dynamic systems theory.*

Dynamic systems theory states that an individual uses all possible strategies to accomplish a task, and as physiological systems are modified, the motor behavior changes.[15] Systems theorists purport that modifications in motor behaviors are the result of dynamic interactions between and among the musculoskeletal, neuromuscular, cardiovascular and pulmonary, and cognitive systems. Communicative and social-emotional aspects are equally considered. Interactive, multidimensional systems are susceptible to changes in organizational and behavioral capabilities as one ages.[16] As an individual acquires a skill, the organization of the behavior may change, thereby allowing the person to identify the most efficient strategy for effective functioning.

It is clear that a small change in any subsystem may result in a change in a motor behavior. For example, Thelan examined stepping in infants 8 weeks old.[15] During the baseline phase of this study, the infants' feet were placed on a treadmill with trunk support in an upright position. When the treadmill was turned on, the infants stepped. Immediately afterward, weights were applied to each leg, and the infants were again placed on the treadmill. The treadmill was turned on, but no infant stepped. The author concluded that small changes in one subsystem—in this case, the musculoskeletal system—resulted in a change in the whole behavior: stepping. This evidence supported the premise that modifying one aspect of a multicomponent system, especially during a critical period, results in a change in behavior.

As one ages, organizational changes of bodily systems increase the complexity of the collective system, allowing for greater adaptability and more efficient functioning. Scott defined periods of rapid differentiation or change during development when an organism is most easily altered or modified as *critical periods*.[16] These periods are when physiological systems are most vulnerable and may be positively or negatively affected by intrinsic as well as extrinsic factors acting on the system.[17] Thelan and Smith[17] acknowledge that, while behaviors appear in a fairly typical temporal sequence, individuals exhibit delayed or accelerated timing with different environmental contexts. These periods occur at different times for different systems throughout the body.

Understanding systems theory and the concept of critical periods is crucial to all aspects of motor development. These theories illustrate the complexity of development and the difficulty in identifying the variables that influence performance of motor behaviors across the lifespan, and in identifying the most effective treatments to use when a motor skill is compromised.

Age and Aging

Just as changes in intrinsic and extrinsic systems affect movement early in development, aging also affects motor performance. Age is defined in terms of chronological age and biological age.[18] Chronological age is the period of time that a person has been alive expressed in years and months. In infants, it is measured in days, weeks, or months, while in adults, it is expressed in terms of years.

Unlike chronological age, biological age is not measured according to the calendar. Instead, biological age measures functional age in body systems in relation to chronological age.[19] For example, an individual who competes in marathons may have biologically younger cardiovascular and pulmonary systems than same-age peers who are not runners. As another example, a female may go through menopause prematurely. A postmenopausal woman experiences a decrease in estrogen levels that, in turn, negatively affects bone strength as measured by bone density. This woman has less-dense bones than her same-age peers who will experience menopause later. While no consistent method has been established for measuring biological age, general agreement is that a wide variability of biological aging exists among individuals. More recently, researchers have examined biomarkers examining risk for age-related diseases.[20] They suggested that measuring biomarkers in early adulthood may provide information on predicting disease up to 2 decades before the disease emerges.

"Aging refers to the time-sequential deterioration that occurs in most animals including weakness, increased susceptibility to disease and adverse environmental conditions, loss of mobility and agility, and age-related physiological changes."[21] Factors associated with aging are characterized as *age-dependent* or *age-related*.

Age-dependent behaviors are physiological changes that affect tissues, organ systems, and functions that, cumulatively, can affect activity and participation levels of older adults. Age-related behaviors are observed in many people but may be accelerated or decelerated in individuals of the same chronological age.

One reason why behaviors may be designated as age-related rather than age-dependent is that individuals of the same chronological age are not necessarily the same biological age. From a genetic perspective, structural and functional changes in general are thought to be a consequence of aging and are, therefore, predictable and consistent across physiological systems. Affecting the genetic potential for longevity are the strong effects of environmental factors (eg, toxins, radiation, and oxygen-free radicals), acute temperature extremes and mobility barriers.[22] Consequently, using biological age rather than chronological age may be a more accurate reflection of changes in a biological system.

Researchers are unsure how much of the decline in motor behaviors in older adults is due to a decline in physiological systems or to decreased practice and/or conditioning.[23] Rowe and Kahn found that "with advancing age, the relative contribution of genetic factors decreases and the nongenetic factors increases."[23] Nongenetic risk factors can be identified through screening and addressed through clinical intervention and patient education. Lifestyle choices, including nutrition, physical activity, and other health habits, as well as behavioral and social factors, have a potent effect on aging processes. Researchers reported that well-being later in life is affected by lifestyle established earlier in life.[20,24,25] This suggests that interventions focused on positively influencing aging are important to preventive care, earlier in life, with the goal of improving successful aging and reducing sequelae associated with disease or injury.

Physiological Changes in Body Systems Across the Lifespan

Following dynamic systems theory, researchers and clinicians examining motor behaviors across the lifespan acknowledge that many biological systems involved in the execution of motor skills and their associated behaviors undergo physiological changes as a consequence of aging. Using a dynamic systems theory approach to lifespan development may explain how seemingly small changes in one system can affect an individual's functional abilities.

Musculoskeletal System

The musculoskeletal system is composed of muscles, bones, cartilage, tendons, fascia, and ligaments. The roles of the musculoskeletal system are to provide a structural framework for the body to move and to protect internal organs.

Development of the muscular system initiates in utero and continues into young adulthood as a direct result of growth in the number and size of the fibers. Differentiation and development of the fibers is first observed during the fifth and eighth weeks of fetal life.[26] Evidence of rapid differentiation in the musculoskeletal system translates to discernible, complex movements early in prenatal life.

Muscle tissue reportedly grows at a rate 2 times faster than bones between the ages of 5 months to 3 years.[27] Throughout development of the musculoskeletal system, changes occur in muscle length, width, and girth, but the overall outward appearance remains unchanged. There is considerable variation in this growth. The structural and functional capabilities of an infant's muscular system differ from those of an adult. One example of a structural difference between the infant and adult is in muscle fiber type. Compared with adults, a high prevalence of Type I muscle fibers is present in infant muscles that contain both Type I and Type II fibers. Functionally, the infants' predominance of Type I fibers results in a predominance of postural motor behaviors that rely on slow-twitch fibers, whereas adults are able use both muscle fiber types to produce ballistic movements and postural activities.

Differences exist in the temporal differentiation of muscular changes of same-age males and females. Males exhibit rapid increase in the number of muscle fibers during 2 periods: from birth to 2 years, and again between 10 and 16 years.[28] Females experience a longer and more gradual increase in fiber size between 3.5 to 10 years. In addition, during adolescence, males experience an overall fiber size increase of 14-fold, compared with a 10-fold increase in females. While muscle fiber development continues into middle adulthood, the pace of fiber development is slower in both males and females as they age. Age-related changes in the musculoskeletal system include decreased fiber size, muscle fiber recruitment, and quantity of fast-twitch fibers.[29] By age 50, muscle mass begins to decrease and continues to deteriorate through the eighth decade of life.[30,31] Similarly, muscle performance continues to decline beyond age 80.[32]

Strength and flexibility are 2 areas of the muscular system central to an individual's level of activity and participation. *Strength* is defined as the ability of a muscle to generate force against a specific resistance or produce torque at a joint.[33] *Flexibility* is the ability to bend. Strength increases because of higher levels of resistance applied gradually during a muscular contraction. Changes in the cross-sectional area of muscles directly influence the force production of a given muscle. As the cross-sectional area of the muscle fibers hypertrophy, the ability to produce force increases. Conversely, as the cross-section of muscles diminishes, the ability to produce force decreases.

Sarcopenia, the age-related loss of muscle mass, results in a loss of strength and power with decreased functional independence.[34] As an individual ages, the number and size of the muscle fibers decrease, resulting in a reduction in strength.[22] Although all muscles experience a reduction in strength as a consequence of age, the impact is greater on the lower rather than upper extremities.[25,32]

While strength is critical to musculoskeletal function, flexibility is equally as important. Flexibility incorporates joint motion and the extensibility of the tissues that cross the joint.[33] Flexibility changes across the lifespan and is directly related to the amount, frequency, and variability of motor activity in which the individual participates.[9] Early in postnatal life, infants exhibit limited flexibility due to the environmental constraints of the uterine environment. As the infant ages, flexibility increases in direct relation to increased joint play and extensibility of surrounding tissues. Flexibility increases in males and females through early childhood. By age 10 for boys and age 12 for girls, flexibility begins to decrease. However, this may not be true of athletes, dancers, and other individuals involved in activities that incorporate flexibility training. While strength and flexibility changes appear to be age-dependent, it may be more likely that it is age-related.[29] Regularly performing motor activities (exercise) directed toward improving strength and/or flexibility can reverse the effects of inactivity for most individuals, even those older than 90 years.[35] While it may take longer for older individuals to regain strength and/or flexibility than young adults or children, musculoskeletal tissue is modifiable. Modifying strength and flexibility in an older adult requires that other systems are capable of modifying performance levels to meet the increased needs of the musculoskeletal system.

Current research supports the premise that changes in the muscular system are more likely age-related and attributable to sedentary lifestyle, nutritional intake, excess weight, smoking, and alcohol intake which pose a greater threat to motor performance and function.[29,32] Thus, keeping physically active across the lifespan may be key to maintaining functional independence and may positively affect (decelerate) age-related changes.

Today, one cannot discuss the muscle system without incorporating the importance of the fascial system that infusions all identified bodily structures. It is made up of one dynamic matrix that is seen throughout the body and stretches and moves without restrictions in the normal healthy activity. Most colleagues think of the fascial system in relation to the muscle structures, but it encompasses the entire body. In normal growth and development, the fascial will expand along with the bone and muscle tissues as an individual matures, and can develop restrictions along with the muscles when mobility becomes limited. Physical therapists and physical therapist assistants generally consider this fascial system in relation to muscle function, and thus consider its effect on movement following trauma such as whiplash, falls, surgery, or repetitive strain, or due to poor posture or inactivity no matter the specific age of the individual.[36] As the fascial matrix is part of the entire body, restrictions can certainly develop in the abdominal and chest cavities without the direct relationship to muscle function. When considering normal development and movement across the lifespan, this fascial system is dynamic and a critical part of normal function.

The skeletal system, similar to the muscle fascial system, experiences phases of growth, stability, and degeneration. The skeletal system of infants and children is immature; bones are flexible and porous, with a strong periosteum.[37] Movement plays a key role as a "modeling force" in joint formation beginning in the prenatal period and continuing into postnatal development.[38] Early in prenatal development, the acetabulum is deep and surrounding the femoral head, whereas during prenatal development, the rate of growth in the femoral head is greater than the socket, and thus, by birth, the hip is the most unstable joint. Developmental changes of the acetabular socket may be attributed to fetal growth within a restricted uterine environment. These changes may in turn facilitate the infant's ability to successfully pass through the vaginal canal during birth.[38]

A primary difference between the child's and adult's skeletal system is the presence of the growth plate complex in children. Ossification centers appear from birth through skeletal maturity.[39] While primary ossification occurs in utero, secondary ossification is not complete until the individual reaches skeletal maturity, usually by age 14 in females and age 16 in males.

Even after bone length is complete, bones continue to grow on the surface. This is termed *appositional growth* and continues throughout most of life. During childhood and adolescence, new bone growth exceeds bone reabsorption and bone density increases. Until age 30, bone density increases in most individuals, and bone growth and reabsorption remain stable through middle adulthood. Later in adulthood, reabsorption exceeds new bone growth, and bone density declines.[29]

Women exhibit more loss of bone mass than men. Decreased bone density in women is generally attributed to differences in the type and level of hormones present. While the difference is most significant during menopause, premenopausal women still lose bone density at a higher rate than their male peers.[35]

Osteopenia is the presence of a less-than-normal amount of bone and, if left untreated, can lead to osteoporosis. Progressive loss of bone density, observed into older adulthood, is commonly identified as osteoporosis. Osteoporosis is more common in women, and it is estimated that up to 50% of postmenopausal women are at-risk for osteoporosis, and subsequent fractures and postural changes in older adults.[31,35]

Overall, many of the changes in the musculoskeletal system relate to demands placed on the system. The extrinsic and intrinsic forces imposed on musculoskeletal systems of typically and atypically developing children may contribute to functional and structural differences in their musculoskeletal systems. Similarly, accelerated or decelerated age-related changes in the older adult may be the direct result of the individual's activity level and other lifestyle choices.[40]

As an integral part of intervention, education is central to the patient/client recognizing the significance and long-term benefits of an active lifestyle. While all systems contribute to and are affected by one's lifestyle, the cardiovascular and pulmonary systems play an important role.

Cardiovascular and Pulmonary Systems

The cardiovascular and pulmonary systems comprise the heart, lungs, and associated vascular complex. The cardiovascular system is responsible for pumping blood through the pulmonary, coronary, cerebral, and systemic circulation for the purposes of perfusing tissues with oxygen and nutrients and removing waste products. The pulmonary system is responsible for oxygen transport and gas exchange.

The symbiotic relationship between the cardiovascular and pulmonary systems means that small changes in one system can significantly affect both systems and, by extension, all other systems. In addition, other internal and external factors are important to maintaining physiological stability.

Changes within the cardiovascular and pulmonary systems directly affect an organism's growth and development. With aging comes a change in the cardiovascular and pulmonary systems' ability to adapt the intrinsic and extrinsic factors that contribute to the functioning of the system.

Regardless of the age of the individual, therapeutic interventions directed toward prevention and wellness are critical to continuing to function, performing activities, and participating as an active member of a community.

From 3 to 8 weeks of prenatal life, all the cardiac structures are formed.[41] All other structures of the cardiovascular system are fully developed and functional shortly after birth. At birth, the left and right ventricles are of similar size, but by 2 months, the muscle wall of the left ventricle is thicker than the right ventricle. The significance of the difference in thickness between the muscular wall of the left and right ventricles is related to function. The left ventricle is responsible for pumping blood to the whole body, while the right ventricle is responsible for pumping blood only to the lungs.

Structurally, the heart doubles by an infant's first birthday and increases its size 4-fold by age 5. Much of the changes associated with cardiac growth occur during childhood. As the size of the heart increases, the heartbeat decreases, and blood pressure (BP) increases.[42] Heart rate in a newborn is generally 120 to 140 beats per minute (bpm), 80 bpm by age 6, and 70 bpm by age 10. *Systolic BP*, defined as maximal pressure on the artery during left ventricular contraction or systole, increases from 40 to 75 mm Hg in the newborn, to 95 mm Hg by age 5.[43] BP continues to rise into adolescence. The capacity to maintain exercise for longer periods and at greater intensities increases throughout early childhood. Children as young as 5 years old who have not had opportunities for adequate aerobic exercise and nutritional intake may show signs of or be at-risk for cardiovascular disease.[44]

Development of the pulmonary system occurs during later prenatal and postnatal life.[45] The weight of the lungs triples by age 1. As the size of the lungs continues to grow, the capacity and efficiency of the lungs increase and respiratory rate decreases. The vital capacity of a 5-year-old is one-fifth that of an adult, but this is not usually a limiting factor during exercise. Overall, aerobic capacity increases during childhood and is slightly higher in males than in females. The work capacity of children increases most dramatically from age 6 to 12.[42] Peak oxygen consumption is achieved early in adulthood and changes in direct relation to activity levels.

As activity decreases in older adulthood, so do the structural and functional capacities of the cardiovascular and pulmonary systems. Many of these changes are the direct result of decreased elasticity of the tissues, decreased efficiency of the structures, and decreased ability to increase workload.[46] Functional changes include a decrease in the maximum heart rate from more than 200 bpm through young adulthood to 170 bpm by age 65. Older adults have fewer elastic vessels, and resistance to blood volume increases. Consequently, older adults reach peak cardiac output at lower levels than younger individuals do. These cardiovascular changes may be compounded by sedentary lifestyle, and the result may be decreased capacity to perform activities that raise metabolic demands.[47] However, some of these normal aging responses can be modified through lifestyle choices including exercise and nutrition.

Throughout life, performance of motor activities and activities of daily living depends highly on the integrity of an individual's cardiopulmonary and cardiovascular systems. Introduction of aerobic activities during early childhood has implications for improved health and wellness across the lifespan. While aging affects the performance and efficiency of the cardiopulmonary and cardiovascular systems, aerobic exercise can improve the capacity and efficiency of the cardiovascular and pulmonary systems.[35] All of these changes in the cardiovascular and pulmonary systems have a significant impact on other systems and consequently on overall body function. Information from the cardiovascular and pulmonary systems (eg, BP and oxygen saturation rates) is communicated through the nervous system. The nervous system, in turn, regulates responses of the cardiovascular and pulmonary systems through the autonomic nervous system.

Neurological System

The nervous system is composed of the CNS and peripheral nervous system. The CNS includes the brain and spinal cord and directs all bodily functions. The peripheral nervous system includes both the autonomic and somatic nerves and is responsible for transporting impulses to and from the CNS.[48]

Development of the CNS occurs as an integration of intrinsic and extrinsic variables and environmental and genetic influences. The most critical and vulnerable period in CNS development is the first year of postnatal life, when the infant's brain develops from one-fourth to one-half the size of the adult brain. Much of the growth during this period is related to increases in the number of glial cells, in myelin in the brain, and in the size of neurons. During this period, the cerebral cortex undergoes rapid growth. These structural changes observed in the brain are directly related to motor behaviors and cognitive development observed during the first few years of life. Growth in the CNS slows after 2 years old, but it continues into adulthood. As the nervous system matures, the complexity of the gross and fine motor skills and cognitive processes increases. By adolescence, the brain has reached adult size, but myelination and differentiation continue into adulthood.

While the CNS, much like other bodily systems, has the capacity to compensate for some age-related changes, the extent of the compensation depends on the task and "practice" over time. Repetition of motor activities may stimulate activation of new growth in dendrites located proximal to neurons previously lost. Activation of new pathways may or may not result in improved functional ability (see Chapter 4, specifically Motor Control, Motor Learning, and Neuroplasticity).

Neuromuscular systems of the older adult may be limited in the capacity to reorganize muscle synergies and produce variability in functional responses.[49] Decline of the nervous system generally begins after age 30 and is characterized by loss of nerve fibers, axonal atrophy, number of neurons, and decreased brain weight. This loss is especially true if the individual leads a sedentary lifestyle accompanied by poor dietary and consumption habits.[50-52] Loss of neurons in the centers controlling sensory information, long-term memory, abstract reasoning, and coordination of sensorimotor information negatively affect function. For some individuals, this may not have significant implications. For others, CNS changes have serious implications. Alterations in the CNS may play a role in mobility, postural instability, and impaired sensation, and these changes can result in falls.[53] Implicit in performance of many functional activities is cognition. If changes in cognition coexist with changes in other systems, it may be difficult to accurately interpret the underlying causes.

Cognitive System

Cognition may be defined as awareness, perception, reasoning, and judgment.[54] The cognitive system uses the 5 senses (ie, sight, smell, sound, touch, and taste) to process, interpret, store, and retrieve information. Existing theories support the premise that sensory information is integrated and stored to allow for interpretation, storage, and retrieval.[54] Cognition is directly related to problem-solving and information-processing. Often, cognition is not measured directly, but, rather, is inferred.

One of the most important skills that infants learn early in life is to differentiate familiar and unfamiliar people. The infant's ability to act on the environment improves as comprehension of cause-effect improves. Early in development, infants and young children are unable to recognize relevant cues when processing information and cannot chunk information for storage. Consequently, infants and young children may not use or interpret the information as efficiently as older children. An example may be a parent giving instructions to a young child. If the young child is given more than one instruction, the child may be delayed in processing, or may not accurately process the information. As a result, the child may produce an inaccurate response.

During childhood, higher-level cognitive processing skills emerge as skills such as the ability to accurately identify relevant cues, filter irrelevant information, and process information faster. Optimal higher-level processing begins in adolescence and continues into adulthood.

While cognitive processing has shown to deteriorate in older adults, the degree or rate of deterioration is highly variable.[25,55] As an individual ages, information is processed more slowly, and the time necessary to perform motor skills increases.[56] Other motor tasks may be altered because of processing time. One example is driving a motor vehicle. Delayed processing in individuals older than 70 years old may significantly delay execution of the task and pose a danger to the driver, passengers, pedestrians, and individuals driving other vehicles. While driving may be a long-standing activity of an older adult, changes in cognitive or motor abilities may impact the individual's capacity to safely operate a motor vehicle.

Additionally, while the time necessary to perform a task may increase, older adults are able to learn new and execute existing tasks without incident.[25] Finally, whether learning new skills or performing existing ones, participating in mentally and physically stimulating activities is thought to prevent or slow cognitive decline in older adults.[22,57] There is current evidence that although these changes usually occur as a person ages, maintaining physical activities through exercise can reduce if not reverse some of the cognitive changes that we once thought were an immutable part of aging.[58-60] Thus, both the physical therapist and the physical therapist assistant need to encourage all patients, no matter their age, to identify a physical activity they enjoy and then maintain a level of exercise within that or another activity throughout their lifetime. The best way to maintain cognitive and physical health is through physical exercise. Activities such as yoga and tai chi allow for group interaction while maintaining physical and cognitive health.[61] Refer to Chapter 18 for additional ideas regarding complementary therapies.

Throughout life, growth and development of many body systems play an important role in the acquisition and performance of motor skills. The interactive and interdependent nature of systems supports the idea that changes in one system can affect, positively or negatively, performance of motor behaviors. This also supports the concept that maintenance of one system may help improve all other systems. The consistent behavior that seems to have a positive effect on all systems as one ages is physical exercise.[60]

Motor Development

"Motor development is the study of changes in human motor behavior over the lifespan, the processes that underlie these changes, and the factors that affect them."[62] Haywood referred to motor development as the gradual process of refining skills and integrating biomechanical principles of movement so that the result is a motor behavior that is consistent and efficient.[9] Efficiency is attained through practice of a behavior to reduce intra-individual variability and improve stability of performance.

Traditional developmental researchers regarded infants as passive beings who were acted on (stimulated) by external forces in the environment, more often reactive to external stimuli than actively producing purposeful movements. Infants were thought to produce responses that were stereotypic in nature and referred to as primitive and postural reflexes.

Contemporary research refutes the premise that infants are passive beings. Rather, infants are seen as competent beings capable of complex interactive behaviors beginning at birth.[63,64] One example of the infant's ability to produce purposeful interactions at birth is observed when infants turns their head toward their mother's voice.

Primitive reflexes represent an example of infant behaviors that classify infants as passive beings. These reflexes, now referred to as *innate motor behaviors*, are based on traditional models of CNS organization and motor development theories. More recently, researchers have produced evidence that these behaviors are not solely dependent on the CNS, but rather are the result of interactions and interdependence of intrinsic and extrinsic factors.[65] One example of an innate motor behavior is sucking. An infant will generally suck if a stimulus is placed strategically in the infant's mouth. However, the stimulus may not produce a similar response if an infant has recently been fed and is sated. Innate motor behaviors, present at birth, are modifiable and represent functional behaviors observed in very young infants.

The extensive literature on motor development indicates that not all individuals acquire the same motor skills at the same chronological age, nor will every individual exhibit motor behaviors in a fixed sequence of activities.[7,64] Additionally, while most children acquire skills in a somewhat fixed order, the sequence in which motor behaviors emerge may also vary and does not affect functional independence later in life.

Changes in motor performance, measured both qualitatively and quantitatively, are evident throughout life. These changes are not thought to be purely age-dependent, but rather age-related. Practice of skills through repetition improves motor performance. Similarly, decreased frequency in performing activities, as individuals age, may be the factor that most contributes to a decline in motor skills. Acquisition of motor skills is multifactorial, interweaving maturation of systems and experience. Declines in motor skills may be attributable to changes that occur as part of the aging process. Equally as important are the frequency and level of activity and participation of the individual.[66] Changes in these behaviors do not occur at exactly the same time for any 2 individuals.

Aging is a process seen in all species on Earth, and it varies within and among individuals. This variability depends on intrinsic factors, such as maturation of physiological systems, and extrinsic factors, such as environment and lifestyle including nutrition and physical activity. Motor development, seen as changes in motor behaviors, can be recognized across the lifespan (Table 3-1).

Prenatal (0 to 40 Weeks' Gestation)

Motor behaviors appear early in prenatal life. Technological advances enable health providers and family members to observe fetal movements such as reaching, grasping, thumb-sucking, and kicking. These complex behaviors lend evidence to the theory that at birth, infants are competent beings. Postnatally, the extrauterine environment is quite different for the newborn infant. Behaviors observed in utero, through ultrasound, may not be observed immediately after birth, as the newborn must adapt to this new environment and modify movements given the new forces imposed by gravity. Consequently, the newborn must learn to perform these tasks under new environmental constraints.

Infancy (Birth to 12 Months)

Emergence of motor behaviors is more rapid during the first year of life than at any other time. At birth, the infant is an interactive, competent organism capable of purposeful movements. Brazelton reported that, even at birth, infants turn toward the sound of their mother's voice (Figure 3-2) and visually focus on and track objects 8 to 12 inches from their faces.[63]

Taking into consideration the abilities and interactions of which a newborn is capable, behaviors previously referred to as reflexive movements are more likely functional motor behaviors that infants are capable of modifying. Motor skills emerge out of the infant's need to interact and solve problems within the new environment. As the repertoire of behaviors increases, the infant integrates feedback to refine behaviors and adapt to intrinsic growth or environmental parameters.[59]

During the first 3 months of life, infant motor behaviors focus on acquisition of head control (Figures 3-3A and B) in all planes of movement. Gaining head control enables the infant to visually track people and objects and coordinate eye-hand activities during reaching activities. Manipulative skills acquired during this period include reaching for objects held 6 to 8 inches away, and grasping an object placed in the infant's hand. Initially, both grasping and reaching are inefficient, but with practice, efficiency and accuracy improve.

By age 3 to 4 months, the infant achieves head control in the upright position, and eye-hand coordination is first observed (Figure 3-4). Reaching requires integration of information from the sensory, motor, and cognitive systems. Early reaching activities allow the infant to gather information about depth perception and use this in improving the accuracy of reaching activities. As infants learn to vary the force and distance, their success in attaining the object improves.

When in the prone position, infants prop on their elbows and are able to roll. These motor behaviors represent the emergence of postural programming integrated with the power and range to maintain gravitational demand during upright holding and movement patterns.

At age 4 to 6 months, infants begin to maintain an upright posture during supported sitting and, soon after, begin to prop sit and then sit independently (Figure 3-5). Sitting is a functional behavior and serves as a prerequisite for performance of activities of daily living as well as higher-level activities related to work, school, and play. As infants' independent sitting improves, so does their perspective of the world. These motor behaviors not only require postural programming, but now integrate balance strategies as well. Manipulative skills that emerge from 4 to 6 months include retrieving objects if placed within reach, holding 2 objects (one in each hand), using 2 hands to hold an object (bottle), and holding a toy in one hand while retrieving another toy with the free hand.

During the second half of year 1, the primary focus is on mobility, as seen in rolling, belly crawling (Figure 3-6), creeping on all fours, cruising, and independent ambulation. Balance and posture (Figure 3-7), as part of mobility tasks, incorporate sensory input and motor actions, including visual, vestibular, and somatosensory systems.

Infants use visual input to modulate reaching and grasping to accurately retrieve objects as manipulative skills by age 8 months (Figure 3-8). By age 9 months, an infant can grasp a spoon and bang it on the highchair tray but is not yet able to feed himself with the spoon (Figure 3-9). These patterns illustrate the development of trunk and axial posture and mobility control, but the child still needs to link the fine motor and cortico-spinal systems to accomplish intentional fine motor activities.

Table 3-1

Motor Development

Age	*Prone*	*Supine*	*Sitting*	*Locomotion*	*Hand*
0 to 1 months	Lifts head. Turns to side.	Turns head side-to-side. Tracks objects. Prefers head to one side.	Holds head upright 1 to 2 seconds. Is slumped in supported sitting.	Makes crawling movements.	Has jerky arm movements.
2 to 3 months	Lifts head to 90 degrees. Elevates chest. Is weight-bearing on arms. May begin rolling.	Engages in hand-to-foot play.	When upright, head bobs. Head lags in pull to sit. Requires support to sit. Has rounded back.	Pivots 30 degrees prone.	Briefly holds toy placed in hand. Brings hand to mouth. Bats at bright objects. Brings hands to midline.
4 to 6 months	Reaches in prone. Pushes up onto extended arms.	Begins rolling supine to side-lying.	Moves from propped to independent sitting (Figure 3-5).	Pivots in prone.	Retrieves object within reach. Holds 2 objects. Holds object with 2 hands. Brings toy to mouth.
7 to 10 months	Rocks on hands and knees. Moves into sitting.	Lifts head as in sit-up.	Moves from sitting to prone or quadruped. Rotates in sitting to retrieve object.	Moves forward on belly. Pushes up to hands and knees. Pulls to standing. Briefly stands independently.	Progresses from radial grasp to inferior to lateral pattern. Spontaneously releases objects.
11 to 12 months	Moves from prone to standing (Figure 3-7).		Side-sits.	Walks with one hand held. Stands alone. Moves stand-to-sit.	Begins to use objects as tools.
13 to 14 months	Moves to standing using half-kneel.			Walks without support. Stoops to retrieve objects, regains standing. Walks backward. Assists with feeding.	Holds 2 cubes in same hand. Grasps with thumb and first 2 fingers. Pats pictures in book.
15 to 18 months	Creeps up stairs. Walks up stairs with support.			Carries objects while walking. Walks sideways. Runs immaturely.	Builds 3-cube tower. Propels ball. Pokes with finger.
19 to 22 months				Stoops and retrieves objects (Figure 3-11). Ascends stairs with step-to pattern.	Builds 5- to 6-cube tower.
24 months				Kicks ball. Throws ball forward. Jumps off low step.	
30 months				One foot leads jumping off step. Climbs on tricycle.	Builds 8-cube tower. Imitates circular and horizontal strokes with crayon.

(continued)

Table 3-1 (continued)

Motor Development

Age	Prone	Supine	Sitting	Locomotion	Hand
3 to 3.5 years				Propels self on tricycle. Balances one foot momentarily. Reciprocates arms in running. Is independent on tricycle activities. Balances one foot >3 seconds.	Builds 9-cube tower. Unbuttons and buttons. Attempts cutting. Dominant hand emerging. Builds bridge with blocks. Strings large beads.
4 to 4.5 years				Hops 2 to 3 times. Walks on tiptoes. Runs with arm swing. Catches large ball. Throws ball 8 to 12 inches. Jumps both feet 2 to 3 inches.	Has tripod pencil grasp. Attempts to trace line. Establishes hand preference. Places raisins in jar. Cuts shapes from paper.
5 to 8 years				Jumps forward and sideways. Jumps over 6- to 8-inch object. Skips, gallops, bounces large ball, and jumps.	Draws letters, shapes, and numbers. Places small pegs in pegboard. Prints well. Buttons small buttons.
9 to 12 years				Displays mature patterns in running, jumping, and throwing.	Develops handwriting. Learns to draw.

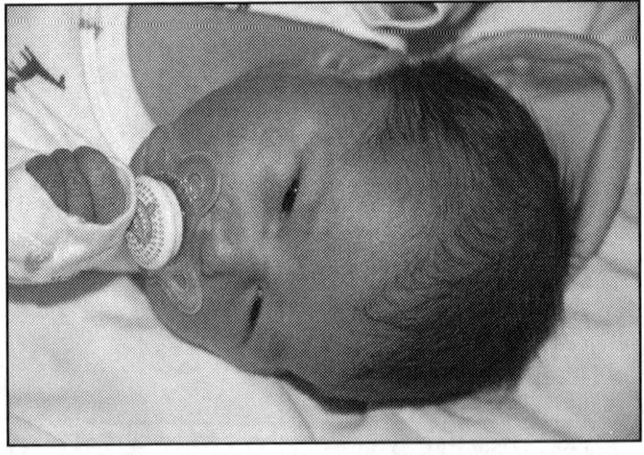

Figure 3-2. Newborn with head turned to mother's voice.

Early Childhood (1 to 5 Years)

While the first year of life is described as a period of motor skills development, the second year of life is when skills are refined, and higher-level motor function emerges. As infants develop independence in ambulation, they exhibit wide-based gait patterns with little rotation of the pelvis and little reciprocal movement of the upper extremities. While upright, infants begin to independently move sideways and backward in addition to moving forward. This allows them to maintain their center of gravity within a given base of support, as well as gaining lateral hip control. Manipulative skills observed during this period include banging 2 blocks together; retrieving small objects using a rake, finger-thumb, or pincer grasp; and placing objects into a container.[67]

As independent ambulation matures, dynamic balance in an upright bipedal posture evolves, allowing for new adventures and environmental exploration (Figures 3-10 and 3-11). With new opportunities come motor challenges and the emergence of new motor behaviors, including running, climbing, and jumping. Toddlers find particular pleasure in throwing (Figure 3-12), kicking, and catching balls. Additionally, toddlers begin to propel themselves on ride-on toys (Figure 3-13). The focus on this period for toddlers is independence.

Fine motor skills emerging during this period include eating with a utensil, usually a spoon, with fewer spills than before. Additionally, infants build small block towers, color with crayons, button large buttons, turn doorknobs, and open and close small jars. Integration of fine motor skills with cognitive spatial abilities and the desire to move is predicated on the emergence of postural control.[68]

Preschool-age children exhibit a mature gait pattern and ambulate using a narrow base of support, reciprocal arm swing, and a heel-to-toe gait pattern. Children mimic a true run but continue to have difficulty starting and stopping efficiently. In addition, receipt and propulsion of balls of all shapes and sizes improve qualitatively. By age 3, children

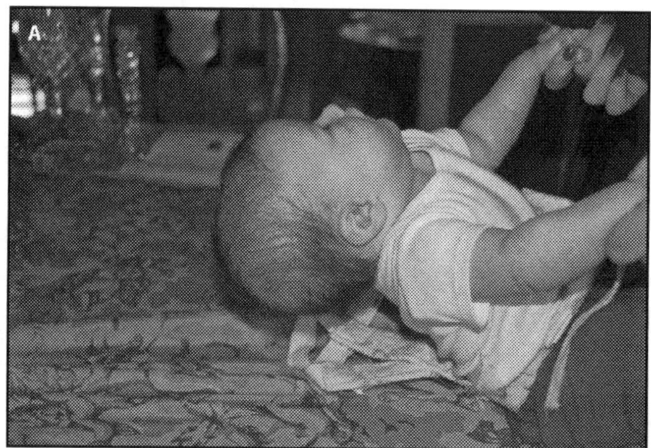

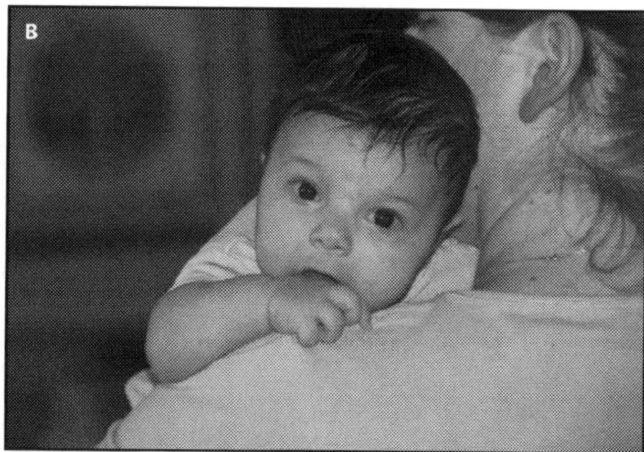

Figure 3-3. (A) Pulling to sit with head lag. (B) Head control in upright.

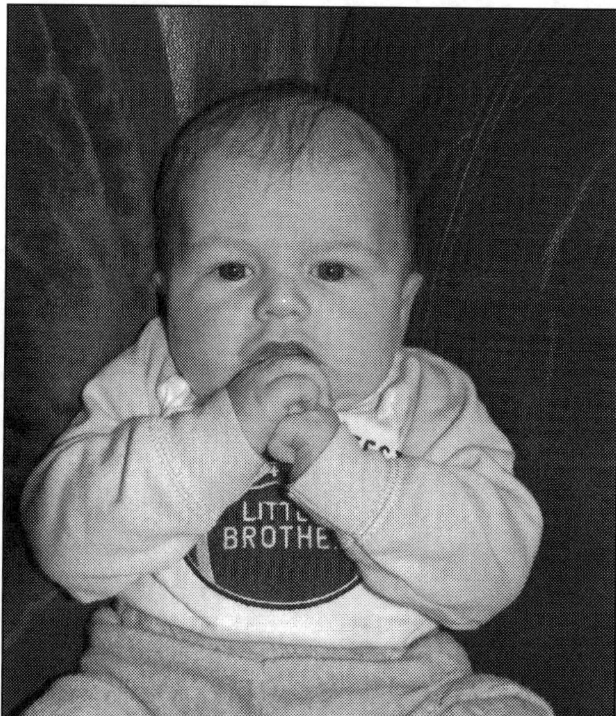

Figure 3-4. Hands in midline with binocular control of the eyes.

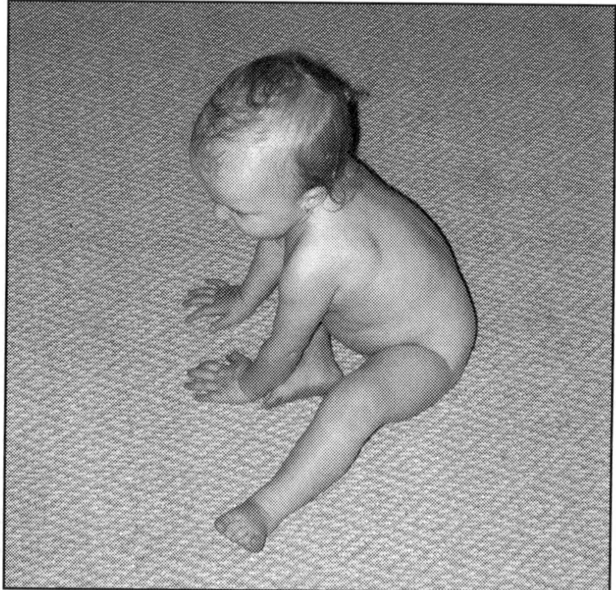

Figure 3-5. Prop sitting.

pedal a tricycle and ascends stairs, most using alternating feet, and by age 4, most children descend stairs alternately.

Fine motor behaviors emerge from environmental demands the child encounters in preschool and day care centers and other activities. Examples of the many fine motor skills observed during this period include cutting with scissors, copying circles or crosses, and matching colors, and some children demonstrate hand preference. These specific skills reflect the child's innate ability, environmental demands, repetition, and motivation to succeed.

Childhood (5 to 10 Years)

School-age children, from age 5 to 8, experience rapid increases in muscle growth that account for much of the weight gained during this period. Girls continue to be physically more mature than boys. Children at this age are extremely flexible, predominantly because muscle and ligamentous structures are not firmly attached to bones. Throughout development, acquisition of motor skills is directly related to practice and demand. A child who skis 6 months out of the year is developing different programs from a child who surfs daily.

Skills that emerge during this period include galloping, hopping on one foot for up to 10 hops (eg, hopscotch), jumping rope, kicking a ball with improved control (eg, soccer), and bouncing a large ball (eg, basketball). Mobility, balance, and fine motor skills improve dramatically. Girls and boys exhibit similar abilities in speed up to age 7, but by age 8, boys begin to outperform girls.

Qualitative changes are observed in coordination, balance, speed, and strength while performing previously acquired skills. These qualitative improvements of motor skills may be due to children's limbs growing faster than

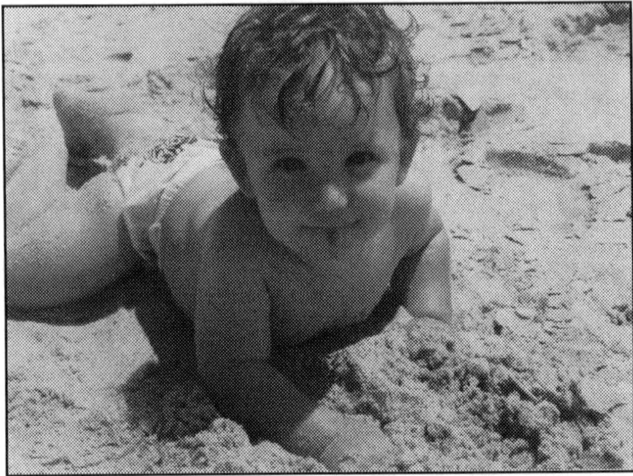

Figure 3-6. Belly crawling.

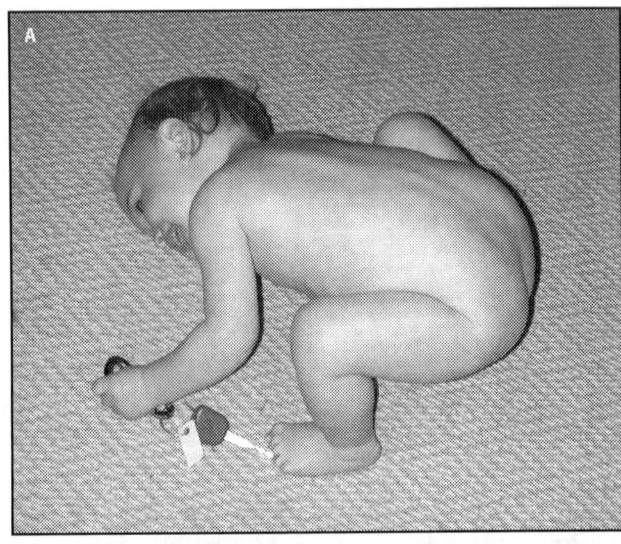

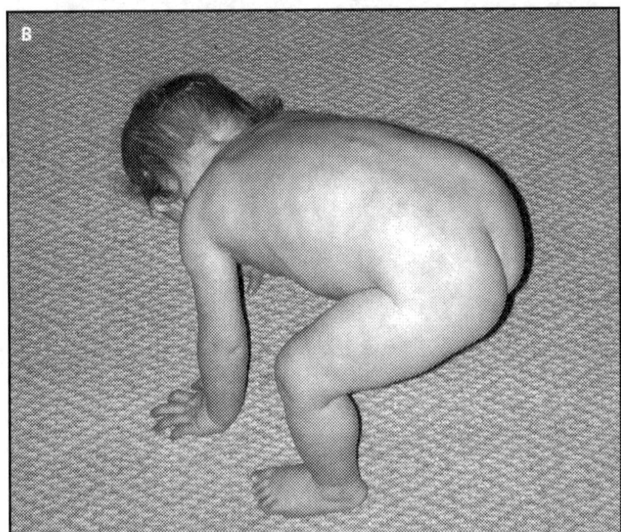

Figure 3-7. (A) and (B) Transition from sitting into standing.

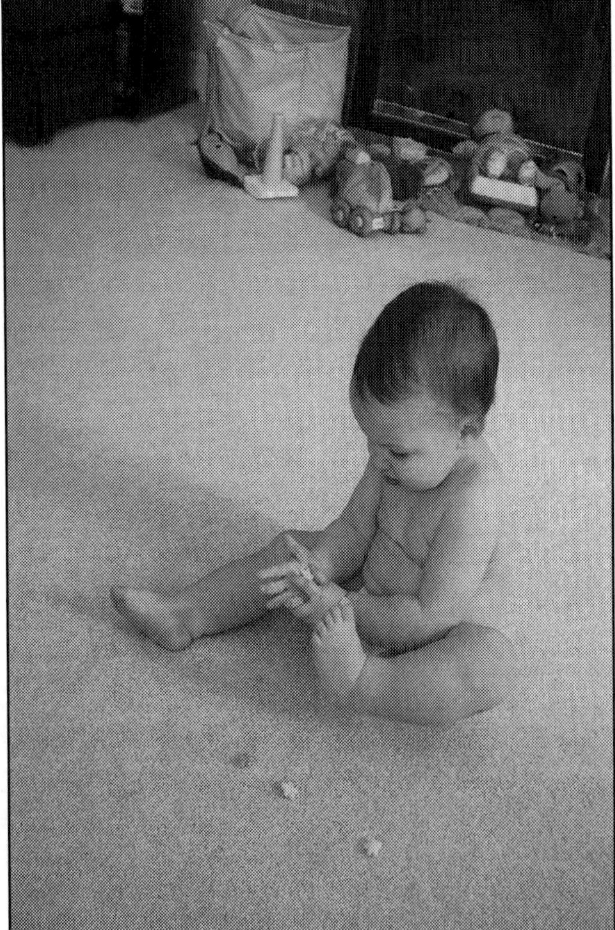

Figure 3-8. Developing prehension.

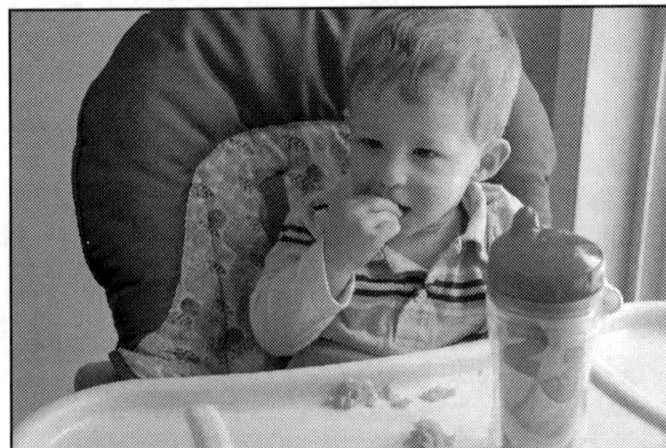

Figure 3-9. Finger feeding.

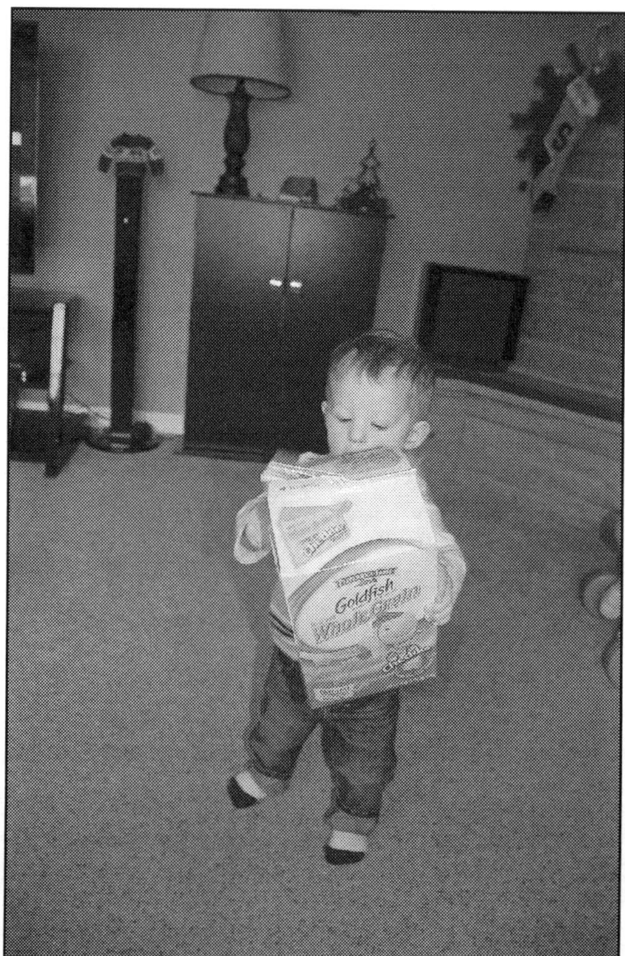

Figure 3-10. Walking holding an object.

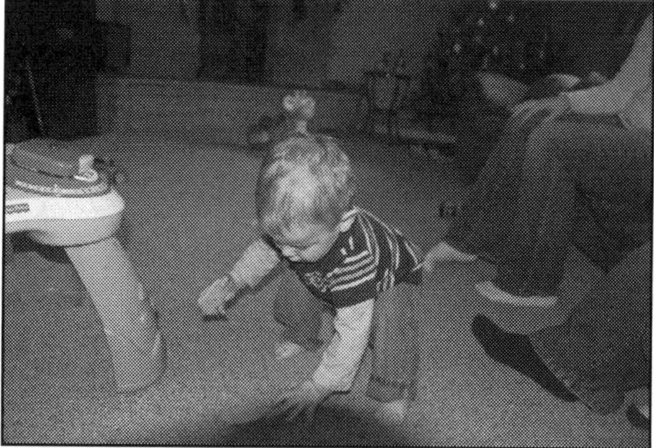

Figure 3-11. Squatting in play to retrieve an object.

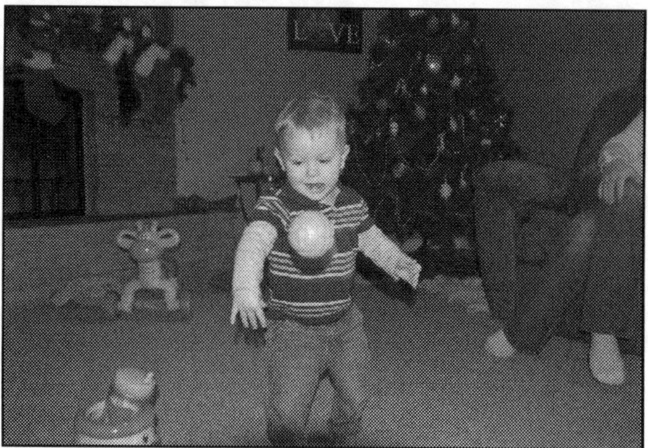

Figure 3-12. Throwing a ball.

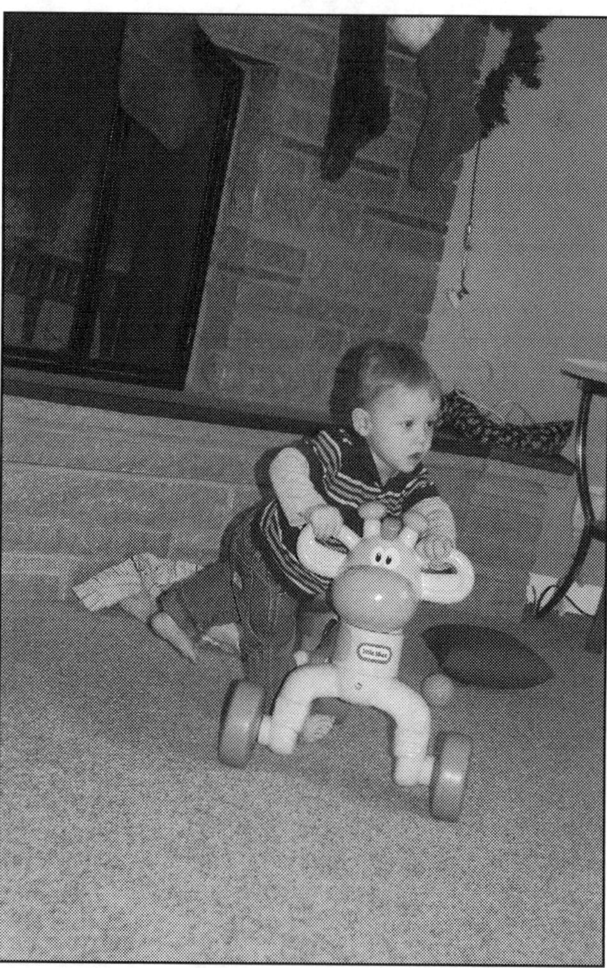

Figure 3-13. Mounting a riding toy.

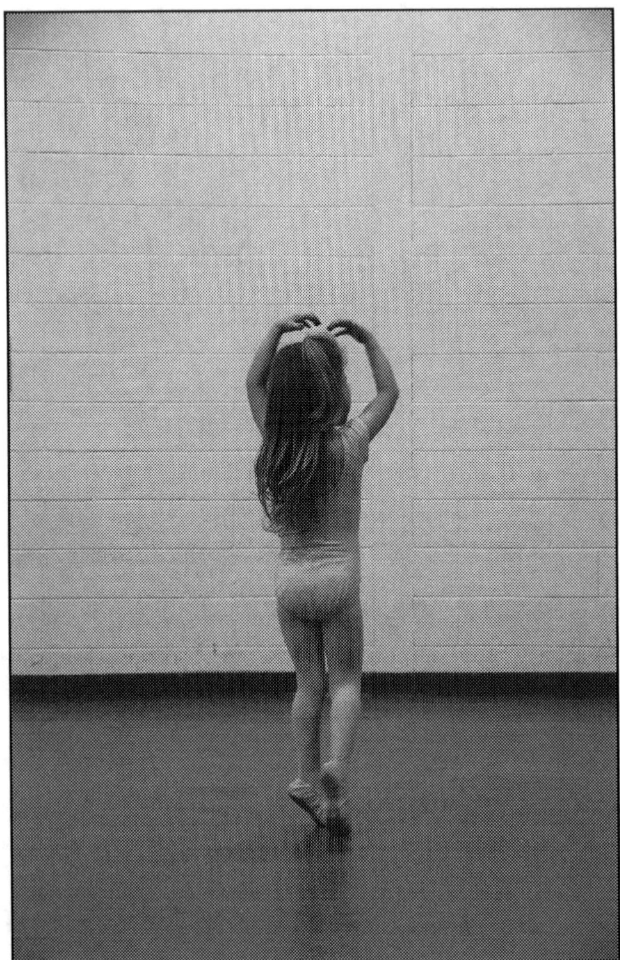

Figure 3-14. Early ballet training: tiptoes.

the trunk. Consequently, they exhibit better leverage. Existing motor skills become more refined, more controlled, more efficient, and more complex.[69] Motor skills have a strong influence in social domains, as boys and girls begin to perform in organized sports teams in school and the community (Figure 3-14). Competition within sports becomes a powerful force in motivating children to practice motor skills or directing children away from organized sports. Children with poorly developed motor skills, due either to genetics or opportunity, may be excluded from team activities and experience social isolation.[61]

Between age 5 and 8, manipulative skills increase exponentially. Hand preference is confirmed by this age. Children acquire and practice many manipulative and fine motor skills as part of their academic experience. Manipulative skills that improve dramatically include dressing oneself, particularly buttoning and unbuttoning clothing items; building with blocks; coloring with crayons; and handwriting and printing. As children move toward preadolescence from age 9 to 12, manipulative skills improve qualitatively. Children now progress to cursive handwriting and more complex drawings. Children in industrialized countries today are often exposed to computer-based programs, whether on a large home computer, hand-held mechanism such as an iPad, or devices in school. These academic and entertainment games have the potential of helping the child develop fine motor skills bilaterally depending upon the amount of repetition. These fine motor computer skills are becoming part of the academic curriculum and a substitute for past handwriting activities. How this will affect motor learning and fine motor development during childhood will be determined as these children mature into adulthood and progress into older age.[70]

Adolescence (11 to 19 Years)

In early adolescence, motor skills are refined and, for most individuals, considered mature. Balance skills, coordination, eye-hand coordination, and endurance may plateau. Exceptions may be elite athletes who continue to improve motor skills into adulthood (Figure 3-15).

Motor skills continue to develop until age 12. By then, individuals have achieved 90% of the mobility and the reaction times of adults. While most motor skills are acquired throughout childhood, proficiency continues into adolescence consistent with musculoskeletal growth, leading to increased strength, endurance, and coordination. Previously acquired skills, such as running, jumping, and throwing, progress quantitatively with respect to speed, distance, accuracy, and power (Figure 3-16). In adolescence, motor performance during competitive sports requires that basic skills are integrated and performed in more dynamic environments. During this period, children who may be genetically predisposed to performing high-level motor activities stand apart from their peers, as do children who are less competent in motor abilities. Always remember that practice and motivation to succeed also play a significant role in performance outcome. Similarly, environmental restraints also influence motor behavior. For example, a child who has the genetic predisposition for downhill skiing but lives in a warm climate may never ski and, thus, never actualize that ability.

By adolescence, manipulative skills are complex and resemble skills observed in adults. Greater dexterity of the fingers for more complex tasks—including art, sewing, crafts, knitting, and musical performance—enables adolescents to perform these motor tasks with greater precision and proficiency. How motor development skill might change as adolescents and adults become more sedentary through watching television and playing videogames is for future research to determine. It certainly has been shown that inactivity plays a primary role in the development of obesity in children.[71] Inactivity, as well as as tobacco smoking, poor nutrition, and harmful alcohol consumption, has also been identified as a risk behavior for adults.[72,73]

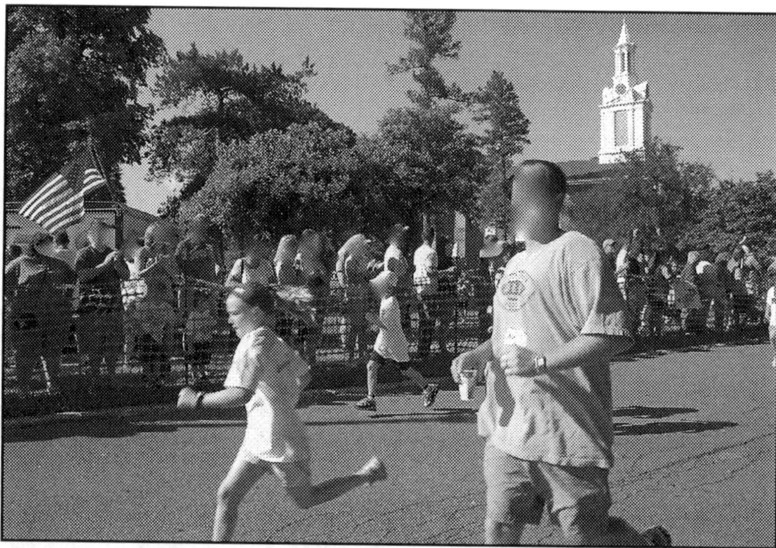

Figure 3-15. Running with a mature gait pattern.

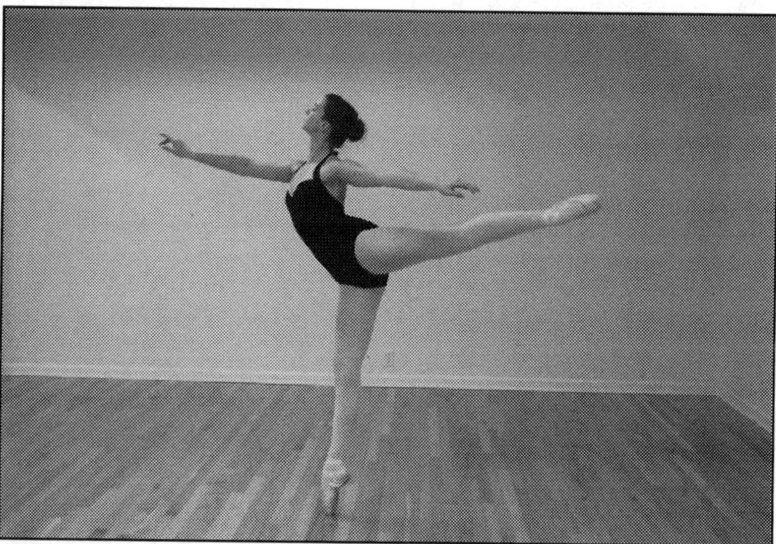

Figure 3-16. Advanced skill, ballet: young adult.

Adulthood (20 to 39 Years)

Motor performance is relatively stable in adulthood and directed at either leisure activities or high-level athletic competition. Exercise is probably one of the most easily modifiable behaviors affecting an individual's health and wellness. Adults exercise to remain physically fit and to decrease the risk of degenerative diseases. For those who do not routinely exercise, obesity and associated syndromes emerge as primary health problems. For the many young adults who integrate fitness training as part of their leisure activities, fitness continues as a way of life. Maintaining a healthy lifestyle can have positive benefits into older adulthood, reducing or slowing degenerative disease processes.

The peak of muscular strength occurs between age 25 and 30 in both males and females. After that period, muscle strength decreases as a result of reduction in the number and size of the muscle fibers.[68] Loss is related to genetic factors, nutritional intake, exercise regimen, and daily activities. Recent research findings suggested that it may be possible to quantify aging changes in young adults. Recognizing biomarkers and measuring changes in early adulthood, prior to emergence of clinical signs and symptoms emerge, may provide opportunities to modify lifestyle choices and prevent or reduce diseases. Employing preventative measures may lessen the impact of the disease, improve the quality of life, and reduce the financial impact on the client, family, and health systems.[20]

Middle Adulthood (40 to 59 Years)

Aging is associated with changes in the neuromuscular, musculoskeletal, and cardiovascular and pulmonary systems. Changes in these systems can greatly affect motor performance, although the degree of the impact is indi-

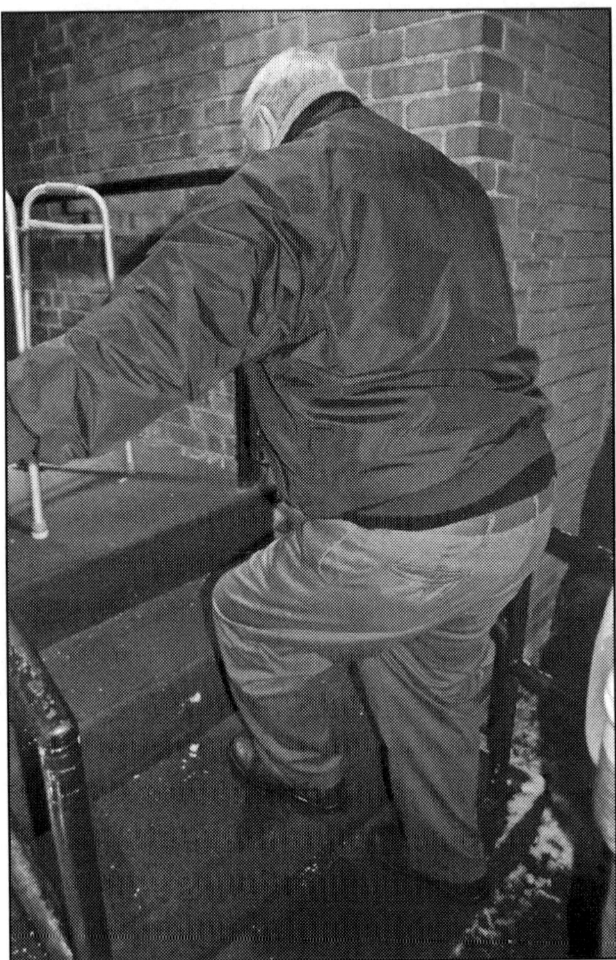

Figure 3-17. Older adult ascending stairs holding the rail.

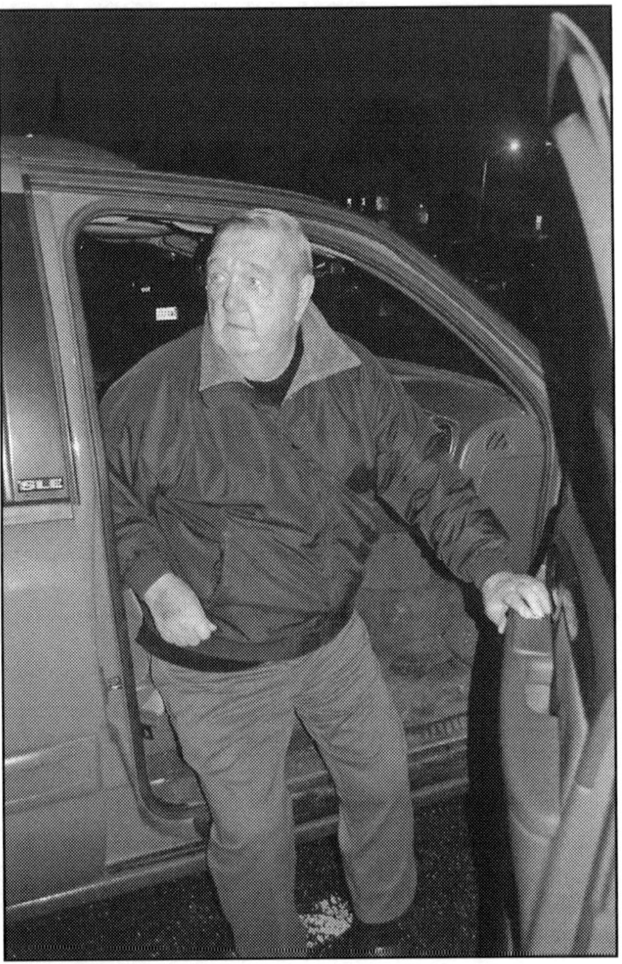

Figure 3-18. Older adult transitioning to sitting in a car.

vidually specific. Muscle mass and strength peaks in the third decade and then begins to decline through the seventh decade.[50] Mechanisms to counter muscle atrophy and assist in muscle strengthening include exercise regimens that emphasize aerobic and strengthening activities. The evaluative findings support the idea that for individuals with a highly active lifestyle, biological aging of the cardiovascular and musculoskeletal systems is slowed, likely attributed to the physical activity. The research supports the premise that lifestyle can positively impact aging. Similarly when high-level physical activity is reduced or removed, the decline in systems followed, and is seen in individuals with a more sedentary lifestyle. The following case study lends evidence that increased physical activity early in adulthood may have a profound impact in later adulthood, and that if the level of physical activity declines, the likelihood is that other systems will follow a similar decline. But, once that decline has occurred, the potential to regain system health is always possible as long as the individual is motivated and engages in physically activity of daily activities such as walking, group exercises, or group classes such as yoga or tai chi.

Older Adulthood (60 Years and Older)

Most older adults function reasonably well until an acute illness, a traumatic event such as a fall, or a compounding of small incidents results in an alteration of a motor skill or associated skills[34] (Figures 3-17 through 3-19).

While some effects are age-associated and may be reduced with regular exercise and increased motor activity, not all are modifiable. Timing appears to affect performance of motor skills. As individuals age, they appear less able to modulate timing of muscles during contraction and relaxation phases. The outcome is that motor skills are performed more slowly, and agonist-antagonist movement is more poorly coordinated than earlier in adulthood. A consequence of these changes may be that while older adults are able to produce adequate force to counteract a perturbation, delay in response time may alter the outcome and result in a step strategy.[34] Mackey and Robinovitch reported that deficits in strength and speed are directly related to poorer outcomes when balance is perturbed in older adults.[74] Besides being less efficient in movement production, variability in performance of motor skills increases. These age-related changes have serious implications for older adults because these changes put them at increased risk for falls.

Thirty percent of individuals over age 65 experience at least one fall each year.[75] Factors thought to be associated with falls include slower muscle activation, sensory deficits associated with impaired balance, muscle weakness, and medication.[34,76] The risks associated with falls increase with age and the number of associated risk factors. The most significant intrinsic alterations in the older adult with implications for performance of motor skills occur when functions of the neuromuscular, musculoskeletal, cardiovascular, pulmonary, and sensory systems deteriorate.

Jette and colleagues examined manipulative skills in older adults.[77] They found that changes in hand function associated with muscle weakness and decreased range of motion negatively affected activities of daily living performance.

Age-related changes may be attributed to compensations in the neural mechanisms in response to changes between and within the different systems involved in motor skill performance.[50] The integrated effects may include slowing in movement production and increased activation of agonist-antagonist muscle groups. An example of agonist-antagonist activation is during dynamic balance activities.[78] After age 70, most individuals are said to incur losses in muscle strength of up to 30% over the next 10 years. Overall, the loss of muscle strength through adulthood may be as much as 40% to 50% by the time an individual reaches age 80.[35] Again, the percentage correlates with the demand by the individual for repetition of the movements and daily physical activity level. Additionally, performing dual-task activities or conducting higher-level cognitive activities concurrent with a motor task has been shown to lead to delayed and altered balance responses in older adults. One thought is that executive functioning also declines with age.[79] Evidence supports the premise that decline in some systems leads to deterioration in motor behaviors. However, individual lifestyle choices, including playing tennis or pickleball, golfing, running, downhill skiing, or any physical activity that challenges aerobic activities, endurance, strength and balance may slow the percentage of loss and decline in successful performance of motor behaviors. Staying active may be one of the most critical aspect of maintaining functional independence and thus quality of life as one ages. The physical therapist assistant should identify activities the older adult client enjoyed prior to a change or decline in motor abilities and use technology such as the Wii (Nintendo) system to allow the individual to successfully engage in motor activities—such as bowling, skiing, and golfing—in a safe and supportive environment. As the older individual is able to execute the task in a supportive environment, the opportunity to participate in these real-life leisure activities may occur and provide additional social interactions.

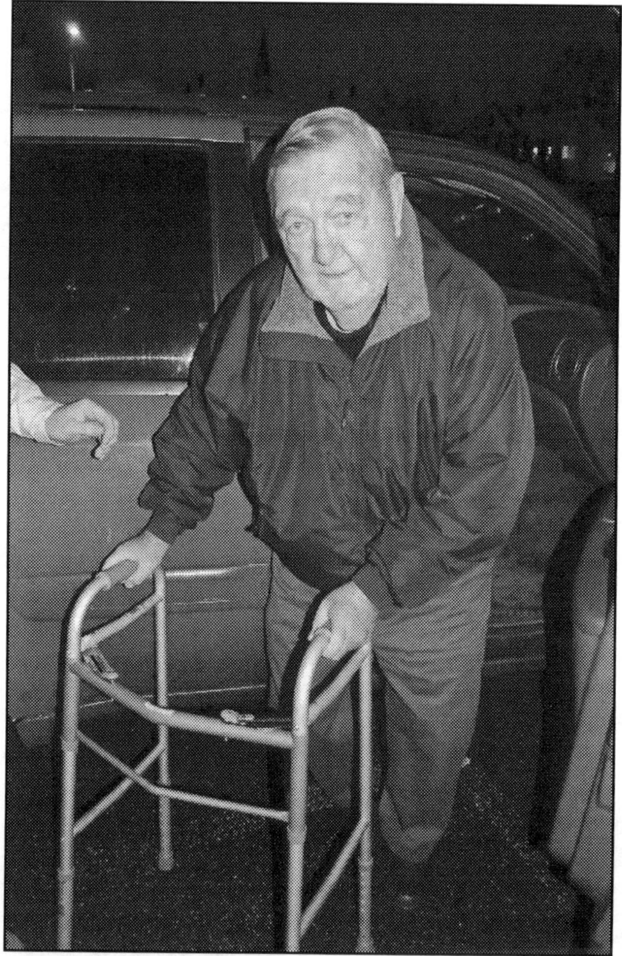

Figure 3-19. Older adult walking with a walker.

Promoting Motor Skill Development in a Therapeutic Environment

The relationship among physical therapist, physical therapist assistant, and patient/client is key to promoting a therapeutic environment focused on the individual client's needs, what motivates the client to move, and improving functional abilities. Regular communication and interaction foster an environment that is interactive and maximizes the skills, knowledge, and abilities of both the physical therapist and physical therapist assistant. Respecting the unique contributions each team member brings fosters a collaborative environment and is central to implementing a care plan designed to maximize the patient/client outcome.

Motor skill acquisition, refinement, and retention evolve from the individual's need and desire to interact in the environment. Through skill acquisition, the individual learns to meet the environmental demands contributing to function, activity, and participation in work, play, and leisure activities. Before intervening with clients or patients, clinicians must recognize motor behaviors that typically occur from infancy to older adulthood, and factors that affect the performance of these behaviors. A comprehensive approach that considers the individual is the optimal strategy for intervention. An interactive process among the physical therapist, physical therapist assistant, patient/client and family provides perspectives from multiple sources and promotes best practice by integrating the combined perspectives and unique contributions of health care practitioners, the patient, and family. Interventions are directed toward motor learning and organized around activities that challenge individuals, motivate them to practice tasks, and have been identified as leading to goals of the patient. Activities must be functional and appropriate to age and participation level. Movement and activity should be the emphasis of the program. Practice is critical to acquisition and refinement of motor skills (see Chapter 4).

The dilemma is that with practice comes repetition and boredom, and this may lead to decreased motivation. It is critical to vary tasks by frequently altering the environmental context to keep a child's or an adult's interest while practicing and refining a task. By setting up an environment that the patient knows will lead to reaching goals will motivate the patient to practice, whether physically or mentally, when not in therapy. Initially, the professional provides feedback to the individual about results and performance. The goal is for the individual to develop the ability to detect and correct errors in movement without the clinician present. Visual feedback in the form of mirrors and recordings can provide information about motor performance. If patients have visual/perceptional deficits, sometimes the use of a mirror has the potential to hinder or confuse them. Although the physical therapist should determine whether these perceptual problems exist, if the physical therapist assistant tried a mirror as part of the intervention, make sure the patient shows improvement and not confusion. Auditory feedback may be provided through verbal feedback or auditory switches.

The individual's desire to successfully perform a task and participate in activities may be the motivation needed for achieving the desired goal or outcome. Strategies that incorporate the target motor skills into the patient's daily life and encourage physical fitness as a lifelong activity to promote health and wellness of the body and spirit are important to prevention and wellness across the lifespan. During each therapeutic session, seeking client feedback on activity performance and participation emphasizes the valuable role and contribution the client contributes to achieving his or her desired outcomes. One strategy that the physical therapist assistant might employ is using music to facilitate client movement and participation in activities. Music might be used to facilitate the sequenced activities to integrate motor sequencing and cognitive skills. Devising simple movement sequences, choreographed to music with opportunities for expressive free movements, provides opportunities for the client to actively contribute to therapeutic sessions. As the client begins to attempt motor skills and participation increases, additional choreographed activities are integrated. Make sure the music selected is something the patient enjoys and relates to, and not just music the therapist enjoys. All types of music can be incorporated as part of a therapeutic activity, but the music preferred by the patient will be a higher motivator than sounds only appreciated by the clinician.

Physical therapist assistants can reinforce the concept of "use it or lose it" as it relates to all CNS function, including cognition and motor skills. Many computer programs and games provide leisure opportunities in addition to challenging the individual's cognitive and/or motor skills.[22] Playing Sudoku, computer games, or any activity that challenges the client's thinking ability will help with cognitive abilities. Promoting motoric activities through gaming also provides an opportunity to engage in activities focused on prevention and wellness activities designed to positively impact multiple systems. Another example is the Wii. This system allows the individual to successfully engage in preferred motor activities (eg, bowling, golf, tennis, basketball, and cycling) in a safe and supportive environment. As the client is able to execute the task in the health care setting, the opportunity to participate in these real-life leisure activities may occur and provide additional social interactions. The use of virtual reality can also motivate a patient to engage in the therapeutic environment. For example, practicing shopping using virtual reality can motivate the individual to guide the cart, turn toward objects, and reach for targets while walking on a treadmill. These activities encourage the patient to return to similar activities once leaving the therapeutic environment.[80,81]

Play as Therapy

Children perceive play time as an opportunity to engage in an enjoyable activity of their own choosing without any specific goal. Adults perceive play as a child-directed activity used to achieve a desired outcome. When involving movement, children and adults use play as a social context to promote acquisition and retention of motor skills. As infants and children grow, techniques for using play must be modified consistently with the children's cognitive and motor skill performance and social skills. While some genetic differences exist in play preferences between males and females, gender-neutral activities should be encouraged during therapeutic play sessions. Given that children see practice, the primary strategy for acquisition and retention of motor skills, as the opportunity to achieve the desired goal, they are excited to repeatedly practice activities. Directing the activities to the developmental ability and interest of the child motivates the child to practice motor skills by varying the task and the environment. Play positively reinforces development of motor skills in a noncompetitive environment.

Older children and adults may require different strategies that challenge affective, sensory, and cognitive systems to practice motor skills. Engaging the client in selecting age-consistent activities validates the client's role and responsibility and promotes investment in achieving the desired goals. In reality, adults usually enjoy playing as well. It is important that the tasks not be considered childlike or beyond a person's potential for success, but games can increase in difficulty if the adult shows improvement in the specific task. Games such as Sudoku and word puzzles are also available using technology and can be challenging, and successful experiences are good motivators to keep practicing. Computer games that challenge motor skill can also be fun for adults no matter their age, and can be incorporated into daily activities that are enjoyable as well as repetitive to encourage positive change in all biophysical, social, and cognitive domains.

At times, adults' goals in relation to functional movement may seem far beyond the level of function of the patient. For example, if an individual following a stroke has severe weakness in his right upper extremity as well as poor postural stability and balance in the trunk, and the patient's goal is to go deep sea fishing, the goal and the function seem incompatible. But, if the clinician can create an environment that simulates fishing, the patient should be more motivated to practice. Creating that optimal environment that motivates the patient while meeting both the therapist's and the patient's goals can be a challenge. Given the patient's goal of deep sea fishing, the patient can sit on the table mat, feet on the floor, with a therapeutic ball that keeps his arm abducted at 90 degrees, allowing for movement at the shoulder. A fishing rod can be planted into a large can full of sand to limit movement in front of the patient. The hand can be placed in a glove that can be attached with Velcro (Velcro) to the rod, then the patient can practice small movement of his right shoulder while automatically pulling in postural stability in an upright posture, which simulates fishing. As his posture and shoulder function improve, range of motion of the rod's movement can be increased. The activity will be working on trunk and shoulder stabilization, but in a functional pattern that reminds the patient of deep-sea fishing, thus working toward his stated goal. In this example, the patient is actually playing in therapy and hopefully engaged in his future.

Conclusion

Development of motor skills occurs out of a need to solve specific motor problems in the environment. Effective practitioners work cooperatively with patients or clients to identify motor problems and develop strategies that solve the problems and promote functional interaction in the environment. While genetic and environmental factors play a role in acquiring motor skills, the relative importance of these factors changes across the lifespan. During early acquisition of motor behaviors, genetics plays a greater role. Later, lifestyle factors are stronger.

Systems theory provides a model for why individuals exhibit motor skills at different biological ages and why the quality of motor behavior varies.[82] It is the physical therapist's responsibility to examine the influence of sensory, musculoskeletal, neuromuscular, vestibular, cognitive, and psychological systems on motor development to provide an understanding of how different systems exert influence at different points in development. Together, the physical therapist and physical therapist assistant select interventions that are designed to maximize patient outcomes and that are within the scope and abilities of the physical therapist assistant.

The human organism is complex and is composed of interactive and interdependent systems. The underlying theoretical constructs of systems theory may more fully explain development than traditional theories. Human systems function not in a unidirectional fashion, but collaboratively across the lifespan. Just as not all individuals exhibit motor behaviors such as sitting, creeping, or walking at the same time, not all individuals lose their ability to perform certain tasks (eg, driving a car or independently performing personal care) at the same biological, chronological, or even psychological age.

No one theory explains the development of complex motor behaviors completely, and none encompass the essence of inter- and intra-individual variability in aging. Aspects of theories provide evidence that an integrative perspective may be a more accurate reflection of aging. Lifestyle choices, including diet, physical activity, health habits, and behavioral and social factors, play a significant role on aging processes.

An integrated approach to intervention addresses the complex nature of motor behaviors observed throughout life. All systems discussed here play significant roles in the acquisition, refinement, and retention of motor behaviors. Careful consideration of each system individually and the interactive effects among systems is important to understanding motor behaviors. Remember, if a child, adult, or elderly individual repeatedly practices a stereotypic movement limited in function, that will become the program the individual uses. Thus, intervention can limit as well as expand the functional skills and abilities of the patient/client.

As physical therapists and physical therapist assistants specialize in movement function, understanding that movement development across the lifespan is very important as part of their basic knowledge. The profession of physical therapy is in the beginning phase of identifying exactly how to define and categorize the movement system and its changes across the lifespan to more clearly identify physical therapy movement diagnoses.[83] This movement system interacts with human bodily systems such as the cardiac, pulmonary, integumentary, neurologic, musculoskeletal, and endocrine systems. Thus, when discussing normal movement across the lifespan, one also needs to include individual differences in patients and their life environments that impact or influence their specific limitations. Diagnosing movement problems first begins with understanding and visually recognizing normal human movements and how they progress, how they add to one another to build or develop more complex movement patterns, what happens to that movement when a bodily system becomes negatively affected by trauma or disease, and how that all changes the way one moves. Having a clear appreciation of what is needed for an individual to perform any complex movement will be the physical therapist's responsibility as part of a diagnostic process, but it will often be the physical therapist assistant who will carry out the interventions that will lead the individual back to function. When a physical therapist assistant understands and can clearly identify what subcomponents of normal movement have affected a patient's functional movements, the physical therapist assistant will be more prepared to engage in correcting those functional movement patterns or substituting with something like an assistive device.

Case Study

This case study reinforces the hypothesis that exercise is important throughout one's lifespan for disease prevention as well as maintenance of a preferred quality of life. Exercise may help prevent disease progression even when pathology is present.

DB, a physical therapist, was an active adult engaged in playing tennis, downhill skiing, hiking in the mountains, scuba diving, and other physical activities with her family. At age 29, she was hospitalized with a thrombophlebitis and placed on blood thinners for a year. At age 30, she had her first child, and at age 35 her second, without any identifiable problems. At age 37, she began to study Taekwondo (TKD). She engaged regularly in TKD, obtaining a fourth degree black belt as well as qualifications as a certified instructor. While still very involved in TKD as her form of exercise, at age 45, a baseline bone scan was performed. Her bone density was 4 standard deviations above the norm for her age, thus suggesting very dense and healthy bones, possibly due to her physical activity level. Two years later, she was referred for a cardiology consult because she had thrown some pulmonary embolisms, and her primary care physician was concerned about cardiac disease.

The cardiac nurse was concerned as she took DB's heart rate and BP, because she felt that she did not hear normal cardiac sound for a woman of her age. The cardiologist listened, smiled, and told the nurse the heart sounds were like the heart of a 20-year-old competitive athlete. He said her heart had been enlarged due to demand from an obviously high physical activity level. He reported hearing a slow filling rate similar to a very healthy heart, with a strong contraction and slower beat of that heart than normally heard in a similar-aged woman.

At age 53, she had severe venous clotting problems that were determined to be genetic. The hematologist conducted a contrast study of her lower limbs and abdomen. The magnetic resonance imaging department called and asked her to come back the next day because something was wrong with the machine. She returned for another study, and the radiologist called with the second results, which were the same as the first. DB was told that she had developed what looked like a new venous return system from her legs, most likely due to the demands she placed on her legs during exercise. One highly respected radiologist who was asked to review the studies said DB had recantalized the cardinal vein from utero, which he had never seen except in autopsy. He also mentioned that a question regarding this possibility was always placed on the advanced specialist exam for radiologists.

DB was unaware of all of these changes in her body systems as they were occurring. Her body seemed to have adapted to the demands placed upon it. In the future, research may show that many systems in the body have plasticity. DB had continued to be very involved in a highly demanding form of martial arts until her doctors told her she had to stop. The doctors felt the medication she needed to take to prevent blood clots had the high potential of causing bleeding, especially if she ever fell. Thus, downhill skiing, martial arts, and scuba diving activities were all contraindicated.

A few years after stopping TKD at age 58, and after being placed on a heparin medication twice a day via injections, she spontaneously fractured her T12 vertebrae. Her hematologist ordered another bone density study. At that time her bone density was more than 4 standard deviations below her age norm. The causation, according to the hematologist, was due to the medication's effect on her bones. The medication had saved her life, but it had its side effects. Thus, over the previous 13 years, from her first to her second bone density study, she had dropped more than 8 standard deviations, which is a huge drop in density.

As a physical therapist, DB was acutely aware that exercise allowed her to remain engaged in life, and that to continue that quality, she needed to always be physically active no matter her age. Since her first spinal fracture, she has had 5 additional back fractures. She has had multiple pulmonary embolisms, venous clotting events, and life-threatening bleeds. If life forced her to stop moving, she has always been motivated to get up and move as soon as her body was capable of engaging in activities. The medical system has told her husband more than 10 times in the last 20 years that she would not survive the current medical event. Medical literature and research say that no one survives a thrombitic storm, and yet her body has done that 10 or more recorded times. She does have pain due to the chronic clots in large vessels in her legs and groin as well as the spinal compressions due to all the back fractures, but she has learned to reduce that pain through activity. At present she participates in yoga 3 times a week, and often engages in her own program at home. She walks and hikes when in the mountains, and knows that exercise is the one element that will keep her engaged in life.

References

1. Fairbrother JT. *Fundamentals of Motor Behavior.* Champaign, IL: Human Kinetics; 2010.
2. Short-DeGraf M. *Human Development.* New York, NY: John Wiley; 1988.
3. Jenkins SPR. *The Essential Guide to Kinesiology, Sport and Exercise Science.* Essex, UK: Multi-Science Publishing Co, Ltd; 2005. *Sports Science Handbook*; vol 2.
4. Gesell A. *The First Five Years of Life.* New York, NY: Harper & Brothers Publishers; 1940.
5. McGraw MB. *Neuromuscular Maturation of the Human Infant.* 2nd ed. New York, NY: Hafner; 1943.
6. Singer RN. The readiness to learn skills necessary for participation in sport. In: Magill RA, Ash MJ, Smoll FL, eds. *Children in Sport: A Contemporary Anthology.* Champaign, IL: Human Kinetics; 1978.
7. Smith LB, Thelan E. *A Dynamic Systems Approach to Development.* Cambridge, MA: The MIT Press; 1993.
8. Gibson JJ. *The Ecological Approach to Visual Perception.* Boston, MA: Houghton Mifflin; 1979.
9. Haywood KM. *Lifespan Motor Development.* Champaign, IL: Human Kinetics; 1986.
10. Heriza CB. Motor development: traditional and contemporary theories. In: Lister MJ, ed. *Contemporary Management of Motor Control Problems.* Alexandria, VA: Foundation for Physical Therapy; 1991.
11. Thelen E. Developmental origins of motor coordination: leg movements in human infants. *Dev Psychobiol.* 1985;18(1):1-22. doi:10.1002/dev.420180102
12. Zelazo PR, Weiss MJ, Leonard EL. The development of unaided walking: the acquisition of higher order control. In: Zelazo PR, Barr R, eds. *Challenges to Developmental Paradigms: Implications for Theory Assessment.* Hillsdale, NJ: Erlbaum Associates Inc; 1976.
13. Bradley NS. Animal models offer the opportunity to acquire a new perspective on motor development. *Phys Ther.* 1990;70(12):776-787. doi:10.1093/ptj/70.12.776
14. Thelan E. The role of motor development in developmental psychology: a view of the past and an agenda for the future. In: Lockman J, Hazen N, eds. *Action in Social Context: Perspectives in Early Development.* New York, NY: Plenum; 1990.
15. Thelan E. The (re)discovery of motor development: learning new things from an old field. *Dev Psychol.* 1989;25(6):946-949. doi:10.1037/0012-1649.25.6.946
16. Scott JP. Critical periods in organizational processes. In: Faulkner F, Tanner JM, eds. *Human Growth.* New York, NY: Plenum Press; 1986:181-196. doi:10.1007/978-1-4613-2101-9_10
17. Thelan E, Smith LB. *A Dynamic Systems Approach to the Development of Cognition and Action.* Cambridge, MA: The MIT Press; 1994.
18. Chodzko-Zajko WJ. Biological theories of aging: implications for functional performance. In: Bonder BR, Wagner MB, eds. *Functional Performance in Older Adults.* 2nd ed. Philadelphia, PA: FA Davis; 2001:28-41.
19. Karasik D, Hannan MT, Cupples LA, Felson DT, Kiel DP. Genetic contribution to biological aging: the Framingham Study. *J Gerontol A Biol Sci Med Sci.* 2004;59(3):218-226. doi:10.1093/gerona/59.3.B218
20. Belsky DW, Caspi A, Houts R, et al. Quantification of biological aging in young adults. *Proc Natl Acad Sci USA.* 2015;112(30):E4104-E4110. doi:10.1073/pnas.1506264112
21. Bengtson VL, Putney NM, Johnson ML. The problem of theory in gerontology today. In: Johnson ML, ed. *Cambridge Handbook of Age and Aging.* Cambridge, MA: Cambridge University Press; 2005:9. doi:10.1017/CBO9780511610714.003
22. Anton SD, Woods AJ, Ashizawa T, et al. Successful aging: advancing the science of physical independence in older adults. *Ageing Res Rev.* 2015;24(Pt B):304-327. doi:10.1016/j.arr.2015.09.005
23. Rowe JW, Kahn RL. Successful aging. *Gerontologist.* 1997;37(4):433-440. doi:10.1093/geront/37.4.433
24. Kaplan MS, Huguet N, Orpana H, Feeny D, McFarland BH, Ross N. Prevalence and factors associated with thriving in older adulthood: a 10-year population-based study. *J Gerontol A Biol Sci Med Sci.* 2008;63(10):1097-1104. doi:10.1093/gerona/63.10.1097
25. King M, Lipsky MS. Clinical implications of aging. *Dis Mon.* 2015;61(11):467-474. doi:10.1016/j.disamonth.2015.09.006
26. Sadler TW. *Langeman's Medical Embryology.* Baltimore, MD: Williams & Wilkins; 1984.
27. Ashburn SS. Biophysical development during infancy. In: Schuster CS, Ashburn SS, eds. *The Process of Human Development: A Holistic Life-Span Approach.* Philadelphia, PA: Lippincott; 1992:118-140.
28. Wilder PA. Muscle development and function. In: Cech D, Martin S, eds. *Functional Movement Development Across the Lifespan.* Philadelphia, PA: Saunders; 1995:137-157.
29. Lieber RL. *Skeletal Muscle Structure, Function, and Plasticity: The Physiological Basis of Rehabilitation.* Philadelphia, PA: Lippincott Williams & Wilkins; 2002.
30. Thompson LV. Age-related muscle dysfunction. *Exp Gerontol.* 2009;44(1-2):106-111. doi:10.1016/j.exger.2008.05.003
31. Distefano G, Goodpaster BH. Effects of exercise and aging on skeletal muscle. *Cold Spring Harb Perspect Med.* 2018;8(3):a029785. doi:10.1101/cshperspect.a029785
32. Hunter SK, Pereira HM, Keenan KG. The aging neuromuscular system and motor performance. *J Appl Physiol (1985).* 2016;121(4):982-995. doi:10.1152/japplphysiol.00475.2016
33. Dutton M. *Orthopedic Examination, Evaluation, and Intervention.* 3rd ed. New York, NY: McGraw-Hill; 2012.
34. Sturnieks DL, Menant J, Vanrenterghem J, Delbaere K, Fitzpatrick RC, Lord SR. Sensorimotor and neuropsychological correlates of force perturbations that induce stepping in older adults. *Gait Posture.* 2012;36(3):356-360. doi:10.1016/j.gaitpost.2012.03.007
35. Brown MB. The physiology of age-related and lifestyle-related decline. In: Guccionne AA, Wong RA, Avers D, eds. *Geriatric Physical Therapy.* 3rd ed. St. Louis, MO: Elsevier; 2012. doi:10.1016/B978-0-323-02948-3.00012-2
36. Davis CM. Fascia and the Extracellular Matrix: Latest Science Discoveries That Forecast the Importance of This Tissue to Health and Healing. In: Davis CM, ed. *Integrative Therapies in Rehabilitation.* 4th ed. Thorofare, NJ: SLACK Incorporated; 2017.
37. Carroll KL. Alterations of musculoskeletal function in children. In: McCance KL, Huether SE, eds. *Pathophysiology: The Biologic Basis for Disease in Adults and Children.* 6th ed. Maryland Heights, MO: Mosby; 2010:1618-1643.

38. Walker JM. Musculoskeletal development: a review. *Phys Ther.* 1991;71(12):878-889. doi:10.1093/ptj/71.12.878
39. Sullivan JA. Introduction to the musculoskeletal system. In: Sullivan JA, Anderson SJ, eds. *Care of the Young Athlete.* Rosemont, IL: American Academy of Orthopedic Surgeons and American Academy of Pediatrics; 2000:242-258.
40. Willardson JM, Tudor-Locke C. Survival of the strongest: a brief review examining the association between muscular fitness and mortality. *Strength Condit J.* 2005;27(3):80-85. doi:10.1519/00126548-200506000-00017
41. Larsen WJ. *Human Embryology.* Singapore: Churchill Livingstone; 1993.
42. Stout J. Physical fitness during childhood and adolescence. In: Campbell S, ed. *Physical Therapy for Children.* 2nd ed. Philadelphia, PA: Saunders; 2000:141-169.
43. Jarvis C. *Physical Examination and Health Assessment.* St. Louis, MO: Saunders; 2004.
44. Overbay JD, Purath J. Self-concept and health status in elementary-school-aged children. *Issues Compr Pediatr Nurs.* 1997;20(2):89-101. doi:10.3109/01460869709026880
45. Kelly MK. Physical therapy associated with respiratory failure in the neonate. In: DeTurk WE, Cahalin LP, eds. *Cardiovascular and Pulmonary Physical Therapy: An Evidence-Based Approach.* New York, NY: McGraw-Hill; 2004.
46. Jakovljevic DG. Physical activity and cardiovascular aging: physiological and molecular insights. *Exp Gerontol.* 2018;109:67-74. doi:10.1016/j.exger.2017.05.016
47. Lange-Maia BS, Strotmeyer ES, Harris TB, et al; Health, Aging, and Body Composition Study. Physical activity and change in long distance corridor walk performance in the health, aging, and body composition study. *J Am Geriatr Soc.* 2015;63(7):1348-1354. doi:10.1111/jgs.13487
48. Kandel ER, Schwartz JH, Jessel TM. *Principles of Neural Science.* 4th ed. New York, NY: McGraw-Hill; 2000.
49. Sleimen-Malkoun R, Temprado JJ, Hong SL. Aging induced loss of complexity and dedifferentiation: consequences for coordination dynamics within and between brain, muscular and behavioral levels. *Front Aging Neurosci.* 2014;6(140):140. doi:10.3389/fnagi.2014.00140
50. Greenlee H, Strizich G, Lovasi GS, et al. Concordance with prevention guidelines and subsequent cancer, cardiovascular disease, and mortality: a longitudinal study of older adults. *Am J Epidemiol.* 2017;186(10):1168-1179. doi:10.1093/aje/kwx150
51. Palmer VJ, Gray CM, Fitzsimons CF, et al; Seniors USP Team. What do older people do when sitting and why? Implications for decreasing sedentary behavior. *Gerontologist.* 2019;59(4):686-697.
52. Stringhini S, Carmeli C, Jokela M, et al; LIFEPATH Consortium. Socioeconomic status, non-communicable disease risk factors, and walking speed in older adults: multi-cohort population based study. *BMJ.* 2018;360:k1046. doi:10.1136/bmj.k1046
53. Ferrucci L, Cooper R, Shardell M, Simonsick EM, Schrack JA, Kuh D. Age-related change in mobility: perspectives from life course epidemiology and geroscience. *J Gerontol A Biol Sci Med Sci.* 2016;71(9):1184-1194. doi:10.1093/gerona/glw043
54. Papalia DE, Olds SW, Feldman R. *Human Development.* 11th ed. New York, NY: McGraw-Hill; 2008.
55. Ballesteros S, Mayas J, Reales JM. Cognitive function in normal aging and in older adults with mild cognitive impairment. *Psicothema.* 2013;25(1):18-24.
56. Eggenberger P, Schumacher V, Angst M, Theill N, de Bruin ED. Does multicomponent physical exercise with simultaneous cognitive training boost cognitive performance in older adults? A 6-month randomized controlled trial with a 1-year follow-up. *Clin Interv Aging.* 2015;10:1335-1349.
57. Avers D, Williams A. Cognition in the aging adult. In: Guccionne AA, Wong RA, Avers D, eds. *Geriatric Physical Therapy.* 3rd ed. St. Louis, MO: Elsevier; 2012. doi:10.1016/B978-0-323-02948-3.00017-1
58. Boa Sorte Silva NC, Gregory MA, Gill DP, McGowan CL, Petrella RJ. The impact of blood pressure dipping status on cognition, mobility, and cardiovascular health in older adults following an exercise program. *Gerontol Geriatr Med.* 2018;4:2333721418770333. doi:10.1177/2333721418770333
59. Chu CH, Chen AG, Hung TM, Wang CC, Chang YK. Exercise and fitness modulate cognitive function in older adults. *Psychol Aging.* 2015;30(4):842-848. doi:10.1037/pag0000047
60. Langoni CDS, Resende TL, Barcellos AB, et al. Effect of exercise on cognition, conditioning, muscle endurance, and balance in older adults with mild cognitive impairment: a randomized controlled trial. *J Geriatr Phys Ther.* 2019;42(2):E15-E22. doi:10.1519/JPT.0000000000000191
61. Pan Z, Su X, Fang Q, et al. The effects of tai chi intervention on healthy elderly by means of neuroimaging and EEG: a systematic review. *Front Aging Neurosci.* 2018;10:110. doi:10.3389/fnagi.2018.00110
62. Payne VG, Isaacs LD. *Human Motor Development: A Lifespan Approach.* 7th ed. New York, NY: McGraw-Hill; 2008.
63. Brazelton TB. *Neonatal Behavioral Assessment Scale.* London, England: Blackwell Scientific Publications Ltd; 1984.
64. VanSant AF. Motor control, motor learning and motor development. In: Montgomery PC, Connolly BH, eds. *Clinical Applications for Motor Control.* Thorofare, NJ: SLACK Incorporated; 2003:26-50.
65. Shumway-Cook A, Woollacott MH. *Motor Control: Theory and Practical Applications.* Philadelphia, PA: Lippincott Williams & Wilkins; 2001.
66. Fischer KW. Relationship between brain and cognitive development. *Child Dev.* 1997;68:623-632.
67. Bertenthal BI. Origins and early development of perception, action, and representation. *Annu Rev Psychol.* 1996;47(1):431-459. doi:10.1146/annurev.psych.47.1.431
68. Ashburn SS. Biophysical development during early adulthood. In: Schuster CS, Ashburn SS, eds. *The Process of Human Development: A Holistic Life-Span Approach.* Philadelphia, PA: Lippincott; 1992:556-577.
69. Owens KB. *Child and Adolescent Development: An Integrated Approach.* Belmont, CA: Wadsworth; 2002.
70. Baranowski T, Blumberg F, Buday R, et al. Games for health for children-current status and needed research. *Games Health J.* 2016;5(1):1-12. doi:10.1089/g4h.2015.0026
71. Kenney EL, Gortmaker SL. United States adolescents' television, computer, videogame, smartphone, and tablet use: associations with sugary drinks, sleep, physical activity, and obesity. *J Pediatr.* 2017;182:144-149. doi:10.1016/j.jpeds.2016.11.015

72. Fehily C, Bartlem K, Wiggers J, et al. Systematic review of interventions to increase the provision of care for chronic disease risk behaviours in mental health settings: review protocol. *Syst Rev.* 2018;7(1):67. doi:10.1186/s13643-018-0735-4
73. Weisman A, Fazli GS, Johns A, Booth GL. Evolving trends in the epidemiology, risk factors, and prevention of type 2 diabetes: a review. *Can J Cardiol.* 2018;34(5):552-564. doi:10.1016/j.cjca.2018.03.002
74. Mackey DC, Robinovitch SN. Mechanisms underlying age-related differences in ability to recover balance with the ankle strategy. *Gait Posture.* 2006;23(1):59-68. doi:10.1016/j.gaitpost.2004.11.009
75. Tinetti ME, Baker DI, McAvay G, et al. A multifactorial intervention to reduce the risk of falling among elderly people living in the community. *N Engl J Med.* 1994;331(13):821-827. doi:10.1056/NEJM199409293311301
76. Woollacott MH, Shumway-Cook A, Nashner LM. Aging and posture control: changes in sensory organization and muscular coordination. *Int J Aging Hum Dev.* 1986;23(2):97-114. doi:10.2190/VXN3-N3RT-54JB-X16X
77. Jette AM, Branch LG, Berlin J. Musculoskeletal impairments and physical disablement among the aged. *J Gerontol.* 1990;45(6):M203-M208. doi:10.1093/geronj/45.6.M203
78. Benjuya N, Melzer I, Kaplanski J. Aging-induced shifts from a reliance on sensory input to muscle cocontraction during balanced standing. *J Gerontol A Biol Sci Med Sci.* 2004;59(2):166-171. doi:10.1093/gerona/59.2.M166
79. Inzitari M, Baldereschi M, Di Carlo A, et al; ILSA Working Group. Impaired attention predicts motor performance decline in older community-dwellers with normal baseline mobility: results from the Italian Longitudinal Study on Aging (ILSA). *J Gerontol A Biol Sci Med Sci.* 2007;62(8):837-843. doi:10.1093/gerona/62.8.837
80. Aida J, Chau B, Dunn J. Immersive virtual reality in traumatic brain injury rehabilitation: A literature review. *NeuroRehabilitation.* 2018;42(4):441-448. doi:10.3233/NRE-172361
81. Cano Porras D, Siemonsma P, Inzelberg R, Zeilig G, Plotnik M. Advantages of virtual reality in the rehabilitation of balance and gait: systematic review. *Neurology.* 2018;90(22):1017-1025. doi:10.1212/WNL.0000000000005603
82. Adolph KE. Babies' steps make giant strides toward a science of development. *Infant Behav Dev.* 2002;25(1):86-90. doi:10.1016/S0163-6383(02)00106-6
83. The American Physical Therapy Association. Physical Therapist Practice and the Movement System. https://www.apta.org/MovementSystem/WhitePaper/. Accessed July 8, 2018.

Chapter 4

Motor Control, Motor Learning, and Neuroplasticity

Darcy A. Umphred, PT, PhD, FAPTA and Fritzie Arce-McShane, PT, PhD

KEY WORDS Extrinsic feedback | Intrinsic feedback | Limbic impact on motor system | Motor control | Motor learning | Neuromechanisms | Neuroplasticity | Practice context | Practice schedule | Stages of motor learning

Chapter Objectives

- Identify the differences among motor learning, motor control, and neuroplasticity.
- Differentiate between practice context and practice schedule.
- Discuss the stages of motor learning and their implications on the intensity of practice and the degree of external feedback.
- Discuss the differences between external and internal feedback, and identify which feedback schedule is appropriate for a patient's stage of motor learning.
- Conceptually differentiate between a cognitively run movement and an automatic/feedforward motor program controlled by the central nervous system (CNS).
- Discuss the difference between new motor learning, as seen in a child, with and without CNS damage, and relearning of movement patterns, as seen in a patient with CNS dysfunction and prior motor learning.
- Explain current theories of neuroplasticity and the critical elements that are needed to encourage motor control and motor learning.
- Identify the interactions among sensory processing, motor learning, and sensory input that can be used to retrain the motor system.
- Discuss the impact of the limbic system on motor learning and motor control.
- Understand the concept of priming the nervous system to learn.

Introduction

Motor control, motor learning, and neuroplasticity are 3 areas of interest to the physical therapist and physical therapist assistant when working with patients of various ages diagnosed with disease or trauma to the CNS and, as a result, have movement problems. New advances in research in the areas of neurophysiology, theories of motor control and learning, and adaptation of the nervous system following injury (termed *neuroplasticity*) are significantly affecting physical therapy management.[1-11] Although the specific rationale for each component of an intervention design is the responsibility of the physical therapist, a general understanding of the theory within these 3 areas and their relationship to treatment and reexamination should enhance the physical therapist assistant's knowledge and understanding for why specific interventions for a particular patient may or may not be delegated. In addition, similarly, explanations can be provided to justify why certain practice environments need to be the responsibility of a caregiver or family member. Lastly, knowledge of

Lazaro RT, Umphred DA, eds.
Umphred's Neurorehabilitation for the Physical Therapist Assistant, Third Edition (pp 61-82).

Table 4-1

Summary of Motor Control, Motor Learning, and Neuroplasticity Concepts and Implications for the Physical Therapist Assistant

	Control Function	***Neuromechanism and Implications for the Physical Therapist Assistant***
Motor Control	Using existing synaptic connections and existing programming.	Neurotransmitters: 10th to 100th of milliseconds to respond. Neuropeptides: Hour or days for transmission to synapse; response can be hours, days, months, or lifetimes (in the case of certain drugs). Thus, the physical therapist assistant needs to give time to the patient once asked to perform before another instruction is given. The physical therapist assistant uses prior learning to regain motor control.
Motor Learning	Modification of existing motor programs and synaptic firing patterns.	Repetition of practice of new motor program takes days, weeks, or months, and needs continual practice to ensure permanent learning. Practice must continue from site to site as patient's skills improve. Variation of practice within the program is critical for adaptability. Physical therapist/physical therapist assistant must first establish motor control before new learning can occur.
Neuroplasticity	Modification of surviving cellular structure to reform primary function, assume a different function, and enhance neuroplasticity.	Based on environmental demands placed on the organism and potential for the organism to regain control of sensory processing and motor programming. Repetition of practice takes weeks, months, or years, and continual environmental demands. Internal motivation to regain function is paramount to this type of neurofunction. Thus, never say "never," because the "never" is up to the patient's internal motivation and potential.

neuroplasticity principles can assist the physical therapist assistant in selecting the appropriate intensity of treatment, saliency of the activity itself, need for a home program, and importance of patient adherence and maintaining an exercise program once discharged. Table 4-1 identifies the differences among these 3 conceptual areas of CNS function, as well as the time parameters needed for the CNS to control, learn, and adapt to the motor requirements of the environment.

Theories within the areas of motor control, motor learning, and neuroplasticity will be introduced in this chapter. For theories of development and how they affect stages of learning, see Chapter 3. Before discussing how theories might guide intervention and reexamination decisions, a clear definition of each topic and the specific role it plays in activity and functional movement will be introduced. Once each topic has been discussed, the interaction of these theories will be presented through case examples as possible explanations for treatment sequences, reexamination, and required intervention changes. For specific intervention techniques appropriate to the physical therapist assistant, see Chapter 5. As the responsibility of the physical therapist assistant enlarges and both the reexaminations and treatment protocols are falling under the physical therapist assistant's scope of practice, clinicians need to be able to identify signs of new motor control problems as well as progressions in motor learning when working with individuals with movement problems associated with CNS changes. The goal of this chapter is the discussion of theory and its application to the practice of physical therapy, and specifically to those concepts within the practice of the physical therapist assistant.

The roles of the physical therapist and physical therapist assistant are directly linked to interventions that improve performance of functional activities, thus improving a person's quality of life. These activity limitations can often be linked to disease, pathology, trauma, or preexisting life experiences that affect a specific system and its interactions with the functions of the cardiopulmonary, integumentary, musculoskeletal, and neuromuscular systems. Regardless of the specific system involvement, the individual's ability to manage movement in functional activities (motor control), capacity to learn new movement options (motor learning), and capability to regain motor function following direct or indirect CNS insult (neuroplasticity) is regulated by the individual's existing potential and by the environment created for learning. Although this chapter will focus on individuals who have movement deficits associated with CNS problems, physical therapists and physical therapist assistants need to remember that the theories presented relate to motor output controlled by the nervous system and those functional movement problems seen in any one individual, despite what the identified medical problems or diseases may be.

This chapter's organizational structure begins with a historical perspective, and then proceeds to current theories of motor control, motor learning, and neuroplasticity. This order was selected to help the reader understand how treatment philosophies have evolved, and to emphasize theory in the order consistent with CNS processing. An individual will need to learn a behavioral sequence or motor program before gaining the ability to control that motor pattern or behavior. Most motor learning uses sensory input initially to give the nervous system needed information that will be used to facilitate motor learning and to gain control over that movement. Sensory input is also needed when changes in programming are necessary. Thus, it is very important not to totally separate the concepts of sensory input from motor learning and motor control. Although the literature cannot substantiate which or how much sensory input is needed for specific motor learning, it continually identifies that sensory input is a key element to motor learning and neuroplasticity.[12-14] Sensory input is considered a primary component to priming the nervous system to learn, and there is more evidence that somatosensory neurons are active during all movement.[15,16] Some motor learning occurs in utero and is often called *reflexive* or *preexisting* motor programs. In a 6-month gestational-aged infant born premature, the heart muscle and most autonomic smooth muscle control have already been established; however, the skeletal muscle tone characteristics observed will be hypotonic with no muscle control evident. These types of observations help therapists understand that motor learning begins very early in the development of a fetus, because between 6 and 9 months of gestation, a fetus will develop a substantial amount of tone. The newborn comes into the world in a dominant flexor tone pattern, but has already spent a lot of time extending the limbs, as can be identified by the pregnant mother. Motor learning will continue throughout life as long as the environment asks for change and the CNS has the pliability and desire to retain control over functional movements. As individuals grow during childhood; move into adolescence and adulthood selecting specific activities of daily living (ADL) or recreational sports they enjoy or are required to perform; and progress into aging with structural changes within their frames or system deficits such as heart conditions, circulatory problems, or respiratory function, motor control will need to adapt for them to maintain control over their life's environment. The role of a therapist, whether a physical therapist or a physical therapist assistant, is to help individuals learn initially to maintain or regain control over those functional movements. The ultimate goal of therapy is to provide and enhance an individual's opportunity to control those valued movement patterns, which in turn enhances the person's respective quality of life and motivation to move. The concept of "use it or lose it" is applicable from birth to death. A child is motivated to use inherent programs to initiate early motor movement, and that motivation will drive that child throughout life. If, as the person ages, there is no motivation to move, and the person stops engaging in life activities, motor function will deteriorate.[17,18] Thus, when working with adults and especially the elderly, determining what motivates that individual to move is much more important than predetermining what functional activity you as a clinician will work on with that individual during treatment. Thus, it is crucial to have the participant or patient become an active participant in determining what functional activities should be selected as part of the functional training.[17-19] Stress perceived by the individual also affects performance,[20] and thus keeping the patient relaxed and motivated while reducing stress during performance of a functional task should also drive learning and, in time, neuroplasticity. The terms *motivation*, *drive*, and *stress* are all derived from structures known as the *limbic system*. This system places a key role in driving motor learning, control, and neuroplasticity.

Historical Perspectives

Existing theories on motor control and learning have shaped the science and practice of rehabilitation medicine. Since regaining movement function through therapeutic exercise has been a central theme for the field of physical therapy, the decision of how best to regain or learn motor skill in various functional activities was based on master clinicians' understanding and observations of movement to guide their clinical decision. Then those masters tried to base their approximations on the best science theory of the time, or the available evidence. Motor control models and their corresponding neurological rehabilitation models have evolved through the years. The motor control models attempt to answer 2 basic questions: "What are the control parameters?" and "What are the underlying processes involved in the generation of movement?" The neurorehabilitation models, on the other hand, incorporate the evaluation and treatment intervention that respond to the principles of the motor control model they adhere to, but are also based on the functional outcomes of the patient.

In the first half of the 20th century, exercises were based on theories of reinforcement, existing muscle physiology, and practice schedules related to maximal and submaximal strength of existing muscles. In the mid-20th century, treatment techniques in the area of neurorehabilitation began to be explained using theories of neurophysiology, neuroanatomy, and childhood development. The accepted neurophysiology was based on research conducted by the physiologist Sherrington.[21] The theory was based on the assumption that functional movement was under rigid hierarchical control within the nervous system. It was during this era that treatment approaches, such as proprioceptive neuromuscular facilitation,[22] as well as those developed by Bobath,[23] Rood,[24] Ayres,[25] Johnstone,[26] and Brunnstrom,[27] were established. The therapists who developed these approaches had one thing in common: they were movement specialists and based their theories and approaches on movement analysis. These individuals successfully created environments within which patients learned or regained motor function. Thus, these early approaches were based on clinical observation of movement, and not science. But, they did try to explain their treatment protocols using scientific theories of that time. Unfortunately, that early research was proven wrong, and our understanding of motor control, motor learning, and neuroplasticity has evolved. But the movements observed by therapists during that time are often movements observed by therapists today. Theories will change as new research opens new avenues of science analysis, but keen *visual observations of functional movements* and limitations will always remain a critical skill for the physical therapist and physical therapist assistant as movement specialists. Many of the previously mentioned approaches are still used and retain similar treatment applications and interventions; however, the treatment rationale for each of the approaches uses more current research and evidence to explain its validity. In the 1970s and 1980s, some therapists[28,29] were teaching integrated approaches based on a systems model and functional training vs a more traditional Sherringtonian/hierarchical[30] sequential model. Once physiologists and neuroanatomists began to analyze movement while the animals were awake, they realized that the Sherrington model was not as accurate as Bernstein's model[14,15] presented decades before. Since the latter part of the 20th century, therapists have changed the model used for CNS control and learning, although the movement analysis may still have similar commonalities. All bodily systems influence how the CNS controls movement, and that ultimate control may be generated using a dynamic multiple systems interactions model,[31,32] or in a dynamic hierarchical fashion[33,34] in a top-down model.[35] The complexity of the human body and the motor control needed to maintain functional control over striated and smooth muscle during normal activities cannot be denied. Yet, only within the past 20 years has the concept of neuroplasticity evolved and begun to play a critical role in decision-making regarding how a patient should be evaluated and which interventions might best lead to optimal functional outcomes following CNS injury, whether that injury occurred in utero, early childhood, adolescence, or adulthood.[36] The complexity and variety of variables that influence motor learning and neuroplasticity and create motor control have not been identified using traditional controlled research models. Some investigators are trying to look at multiple variables and the mechanisms that create change in motor performance and that should drive intervention.[37] The answers to all effective interventions from the best to the least have yet to be determined. These interventions will change as future research is reported. Thus, the literature can only guide the therapist toward best practice or parameters of care, while each patient needs to guide the specifics and show what motivates that specific CNS to change (Box 4-1).

Motor Control

Motor control is the study of how the CNS regulates the musculoskeletal system and the environment in the generation of movements for the attainment of specific task goals. In motor control, 3 elements are crucial. It involves a neural circuit—the cortex, brainstem, cerebellum, and spinal cord—that underlies the processing of inputs and outputs; a motor plan (usually the limb), or the effector of the output of the neural circuit; and the environment, in which movement takes place, shaping the interplay between the neural circuit and the motor plan. We shall see in the next paragraphs the interplay among these elements in the generation of movement.

Movement generation can be described as a sensorimotor loop[38] (ie, a series of transformations between sensory signals and motor commands, or a chaining of one sensorimotor event to another). It has been said that learning has occurred when patients gain consistency and efficiency over the control of the elements needed to generate the movement. As Albert Einstein once said, nothing happens until something moves. To make something happen is the driving force of all the complex movements we humans have learned to do—and do well. Time and again, humans have been able to master highly complex movements. And it is primarily because people are endowed with an amazing neural circuitry that underlies the processing of sensory inputs and motor outputs.

Many of the simple functional movements that humans carry out on a daily basis require complex control and networking among areas of the CNS, the neural circuit. The control of movement, to some extent, can be likened to the coordinated action of each of the instrument players in a symphony orchestra. There are different instrument players, and one's performance affects others' performances. It is not enough to know how to play well; one must also know how to take signals from the conductor and be aware of the others' performances. The same thing occurs when the CNS generates body movements. Many CNS structures are involved, and each one effectively communicates with other CNS structures to deliver a smooth and well-coordinated movement.[2,39-43]

Figure 4-1 illustrates the processes involved in movement generation.[44] Everyone's movements are goal-oriented. Given a task goal (eg, reaching for a coffee mug off to the left side of one's body), the control system chooses a control policy. This is a mapping of the task goal to motor commands of turning the head toward the cup, lifting the arm, and grasping the coffee mug. This choice is made based on some criteria such as the expected cost (eg, the level of difficulty to get to the coffee mug) and reward (eg, drinking coffee). Then, the control system generates the motor command, which is a particular way of activating groups of muscles to move the hand in a certain trajectory from its starting location to where the coffee mug is. For this, the system has taken in some knowledge of the motor

Box 4-1

A Clinician's Perspective

In the late 1960s, one author started working with individuals diagnosed with severe head injury with resultant vegetative states for more than 8 months. The first client, CH, taught the physical therapist that there was more flexibility in the CNS than known at the time.

The author worked with CH for a month, then the patient came out of his vegetative state and regained and maintained consciousness, but had severe movement problems with limitations in range of motion and motor control. The physical therapist worked on attaining bed mobility, coming to sit, sitting, and early standing. CH regained normal range of motion but, if triggered, had various reflexive responses, such as severe positive supporting reaction in his lower extremities (LE) if pulled to standing with weight on his forefoot. However, the patient could come to assisted standing with normal LE tone and a foot-flat position.

A famous surgeon hired by CH's insurance company evaluated CH and determined—after pulling him to standing and triggering severe plantar flexion and inversion of the feet, knee extension, and hip internal rotation and adduction—that the best way to treat this patient was major surgery. That surgery would cut his heel cords, release his knee extensors, and release his hip internal rotators, adductors, and hip extensor. The result would allow him to function sitting in the wheelchair.

The physician responsible for CH in the rehabilitation and long-term care facility asked the physical therapist her opinion. The physical therapist stated that the physician had triggered a strong reflex, but CH had full range of motion. The physical therapist did not feel surgery was needed. The physician denied CH's surgery.

The surgeon returned 5 months later when CH was walking independently in the parallel bars and almost ready to walk without assistance. The doctor's first statement was that the patient could not do that. Then he tested the patient for proprioceptive awareness in space while in the prone position. CH was able to place his contralateral limb and mirror the position that the doctor has used with the other leg. The doctor again stated that the patient could not do that. He then told the physical therapist that he would show her that the damage was there. They both went up to the ward with the patient. The surgeon injected the patient with valium, and the original tonal patterns of arching extension in supine with arms and legs stuck in abnormal patterns presented themselves. He then offered the physical therapist a job and told her that he could convince her that early surgery was the only way to treat these patients. The physical therapist thanked him but denied the job offer.

Three months later, CH walked out of the hospital without observable motor deficits. He did have some perceptual problems, but he was working on learning to regain that function. He went back to a fairly normal quality of life.

That patient taught the physical therapist, who in time became a neuroscientist and a movement specialist, that, if given the correct environment, there was potential in the CNS to learn. This required that both the physical therapist and patient were working on movement within the patient's CNS ability, both were motivated to improve, and both were enjoying the activities. It demonstrated that with repetition of practice, motor control and learning were attainable, and motor learning was maintained as long as the patient kept practicing and learning during daily living, and was motivated to retain and gain movement control. She believed that there was some ability of the CNS to relearn in spite of existing pathology or disease. As a clinician, she never thought that health care practitioners heal the pathology, only that the CNS has the ability to learn. In 1968, that patient showed the physical therapist all the current concepts taught today, but it took 40 years for the research to explain how CH, using normal movement patterns, walked out of the hospital. The patient demonstrated motor control, motor learning, and neuroplasticity, although at the time those terms were not yet used, because the science was years from being discovered.

plan. This is the current body configuration (eg, trunk and arm posture) relative to the position of the coffee mug. The way one reaches for the cup will be different if the cup is nearby or at some distance to the left. For these reaches, different joint movements and muscle activation patterns are required, and, consequently, different biomechanical forces are generated.

Lastly, the system has to take into consideration the environment in which reaching takes place (eg, on a cluttered desk or cleared table or in a dark room). The control of reaching is different when it takes place in a dark room, because one cannot rely on visual feedback to guide one's movement, and must instead rely on another sensory modality, such as proprioception. While sensory feedback is not necessary to perform some movements, the control system relies on sensory information of past movements to guide upcoming movement and online sensory feedback for ongoing movement. Thus, whether the coffee cup is on a cluttered or cleared table creates different perceptual challenges to the CNS, which has the potential to change the motor response. The motor command is also mapped to a set of predicted sensory outcomes, referred to as the

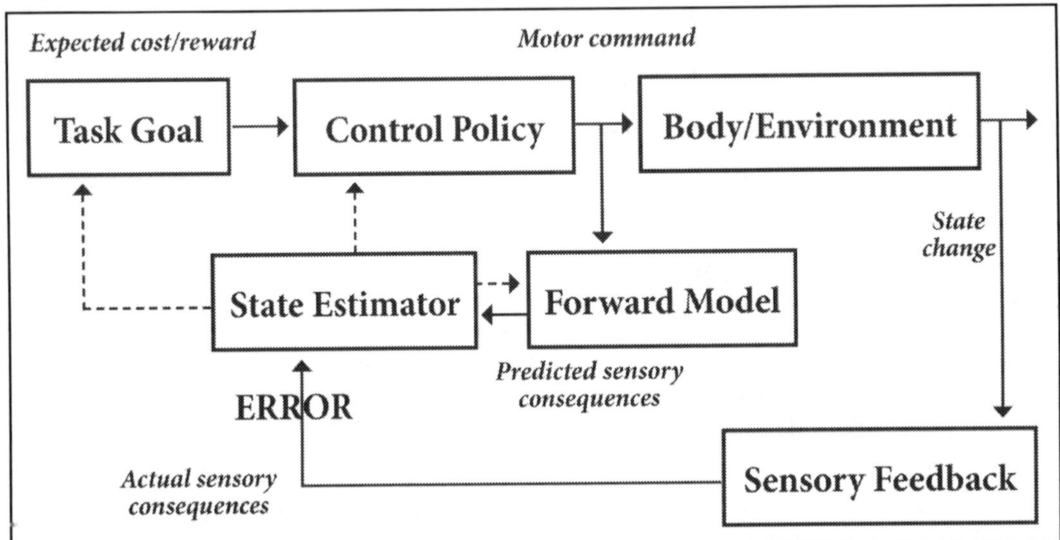

Figure 4-1. General schema for the control of movement. (Adapted from Shadmehr R, Krakauer JW. A computational neuroanatomy for motor control. *Exp Brain Res*. 2008;185[3]:359-381. doi:10.1007/s00221-008-1280-5.)

sensory forward model. This refers to what a person expects to feel on accomplishing the task. Now, imagine a scenario when, on lifting up the coffee mug, the person overshoots the grip force by lifting an empty mug instead of a full one. The system had planned for a grip force appropriate for a mug filled with coffee and relied on a forward model that predicted sensory outcomes of lifting a full mug. Fortunately, most individuals' systems are able to take in the new information, calculate an error, and modify the movement plan so that the next time the cup is picked up, the right grip force should be generated. When the motor command leads to success in achieving the goal, it produces the expected change in the performer and/or the environment. When the motor command fails to do so, there is an error associated with the predicted sensory outcomes: "I expected my hand to reach the cup if I moved this way, but instead my hand ended in a completely different place." This task of comparing the predicted with the measured sensory consequences has been attributed to a state estimator. In the presence of error, modifications may take place in the control policy (ie, changing the way one activates muscles), the forward model (ie, changing the predicted sensory outcomes based on new sensory input), or the task goal (ie, making new coffee or changing the weight of the fluid).

Perturbation studies give therapists a window into the nature of the controlled movement parameters and adaptive strategies.[45] Numerous motor control studies have used perturbed arm reaching (eg, loads or visuomotor rotations), walking, and posture. An example of widely used perturbation in motor control studies is the application of force fields during reaching movements.[46,47] Subjects are asked to move a cursor to a target displayed on a screen by moving a robotic manipulandum. Hand trajectories during unperturbed reaching typically follow a straight path from the start hand position to the end target position. After performing some trials of unperturbed reaching, subjects are exposed to a force field. It is a velocity-dependent force whose direction is always perpendicular to the direction of hand movement. Figure 4-2 illustrates how hand trajectories change in the presence of unexpected perturbations. Early in adaptation, the subject's hand is pushed to the side and misses reaching the target. The hand trajectory shows a huge deviation from the intended straight trajectory (*trajectory errors*) to the target location (*endpoint errors*). With practice, the subject learns to compensate for the force field, as can be observed in the reduction in the trajectory and endpoint errors. Thus, motor errors like the initial trajectory errors and endpoint errors drive adaptation and the return to straight-hand trajectories. At this stage, the subject has learned to control movements predictively rather than through successive late-feedback corrections.

These studies and others have shown that straightness of the hand trajectory and minimum endpoint variability are invariant features of arm-reaching movements. What happens if the subject has no access to error information (eg, because of a loss of sensation or brain injury leading to an inability to predict sensory states associated with a motor command)? How does the system control movements in such contexts? One way to simulate this in an experimental setup is to withdraw the sensory feedback on the cursor position so subjects are no longer able to see their trajectory and endpoint errors.[46] Subjects in both feedback conditions were able to correct their trajectory and endpoint errors. However, trajectories became straight with visual feedback, but remained curved without it. The different trajectories suggest differences in the information conveyed by vision and proprioception. As illustrated in Figure 4-1, our sensorimotor system relies on sensory information before, during, and after the generation of movement. Effective

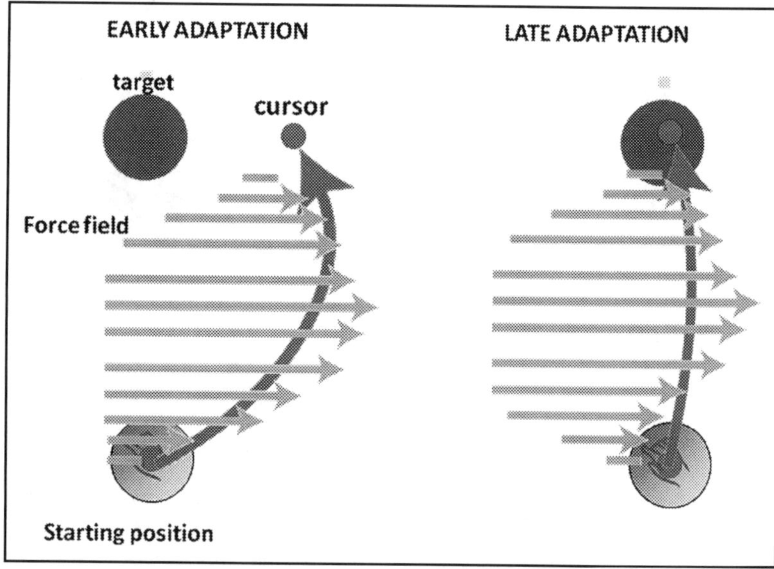

Figure 4-2. Changes in hand trajectories from early to late exposures to a force field perturbation. (Reprinted with permission from Dr. Fritzie Arce-McShane.)

communication between sensory and motor areas of the cerebral cortex is critical. Indeed, our recent neurophysiological studies provide evidence of synchronized activity of neurons in the sensorimotor cortex that point to reciprocal interactions between sensory and motor areas of the cortex (Figure 4-3). That is, the primary motor cortex (MI) modulates sensory processing in the primary somatosensory cortex (SI), and that the primary SI transmits to the primary MI the sensory information critical for successful task performance.[1,2]

It is not the physical therapist assistant's responsibility to know what movement dysfunctions correlate with what types of lesions, the locations of lesions, or the status of a lesion, but it is the responsibility of the physical therapist assistant to recognize a change in the control of a pattern or functional skill, and inform the physical therapist. This can be a critical health issue when the change seems to be toward dysfunction vs function. One of the challenges in understanding motor control is realizing that the physical therapist's or the physical therapist assistant's motor control over his or her body affects feedback to the patient. The patient's ability to perform a task depends on inherent mechanisms, which may vary from the therapist's regardless of a CNS lesion.[48] One of the most obvious differences is probably anthropometric. The clinician's height, weight, flexibility, strength, endurance, and other traits affect the motions that can be reinforced through feedback to the patient. In addition, these same body parameters affect how a patient can perform movement. The easiest example to articulate is observing how a short vs a tall person comes out of a chair. Observe your fellow classmates or clinicians, and you will be surprised at the difference.

When analyzing motor control of a specific movement, such as walking, the therapist will look at many motor programs that are running simultaneously. These programs include automatic walking, postural control of the head, axial muscles and trunk in open and closed chain environments, balance programs from heel strike to heel strike of both legs, arm swing and how it perturbs the patient, and the environment within which the patient is walking (eg, wood floor, shag rugs, cement walkway, or grass on level ground vs up and down inclines). Each one of these programs is a movement sequence being controlled by the CNS. The CNS must control and modify all of these programs simultaneously for a clinician to observe normal walking within the environment specified. Some patients may lose one of the multitudes of programs, and therefore a physical therapist assistant could be expected to help train the patient to run a complex program such as walking. The activity may be performed under a variety of controlled environments, such as with a body weight–bearing overhead suspension system, an exoskeleton, or another assistive device such as a cane or walker. The decision as to which mechanism to use with the patient may depend more on available tools and the environment within which the training is done. A body weight–support system and a treadmill reduce the individual's need to run adequate postural programs and reduce the variable power production used throughout the gait cycle. The frequency of stepping can be controlled externally, while a physical therapist assistant can help with foot placement. As the patient gains control of posture, walking, balance power, stepping frequency, and symmetrical stride length, the amount of suspension can be reduced, which demands more motor control by the patient (see Chapters 5 and 19). Similarly, an exoskeleton can reduce the demands on the patient, but is still a very expensive rehabilitation tool not found in every facility. For the patient to gain motor control, the environ-

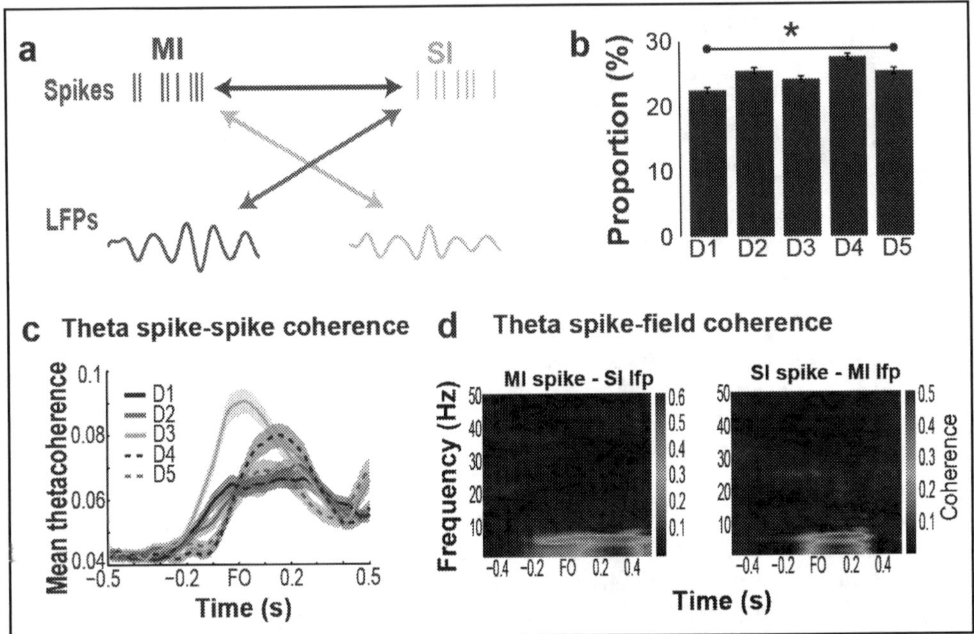

Figure 4-3. Cortico-cortical coherence in sensorimotor cortex. (A) Schema of paired cortical neuronal spikes and local field potentials (LFPs) between the primary MI and the primary SI used in coherence analyses: paired spikes from MI and SI, paired MI spikes and SI LFPs, and paired SI spikes and MI LFPs. (B) Proportion of neuronal pairs with significant modulation of theta spike-spike coherence showed day-to-day (D1-D5) changes and significant increase from D1 to D5. (C) Day-to-day changes in the modulation of theta spike-spike coherence during ±0.5 s relative to the onset of force (FO). Shown as mean (±1 SEM) coherence across pairs of neurons. Coherence exhibited peak magnitude on D3. (D) Each coherogram shows the magnitude of spike-field coherence (color scale) of a single pair of signals as a function of frequency and time relative to FO. (Adapted from Arce-McShane FI, Ross CF, Takahashi K, Sessle BJ, Hatsopoulos NG. Primary motor and sensory cortical areas communicate via spatiotemporally coordinated networks at multiple frequencies. *Proc Natl Acad Sci USA*. 2016;113[18]:5083-5088. doi:10.1073/pnas.1600788113.)

ment must allow the patient to achieve the desired movement outcomes. Thus, control on a hard surface is easier than control on a compliant surface such as grass or deep carpeting. Often, removal of unneeded sensory stimuli (such as noise, excessive colors, and people moving within the environment) can allow the CNS to focus and control movement such as walking. To say that control is independent, the therapist needs to reintroduce that sensory information while the patient is running the programs.

Many aspects of CNS function lead to motor control. Sensory processing is critical for motor learning and becomes vital if the program being run needs changing. Thus, not only systems considered motor (eg, the basal ganglia, cerebellum, and frontal lobes) are necessary when a patient is performing functional activities. Perception of the environment plays a key role in determining what control is necessary to succeed in a task. If a patient has sensory or perceptual dysfunctions, the result may be motor control problems, although the deficit may not be within the motor system. The physical therapist assistant is not responsible for analyzing all these perceptual motor problems, but should be able to evaluate whether a patient is failing at the task or becoming frustrated because of errors. The control of movement and posture is a complex interaction of many systems. In the case of a child who has never learned those motor programs, motor control will start with initial motor learning, which will lead to control. Following CNS injury, the control over those systems can become compromised. It is up to the physical therapist and the physical therapist assistant to create the optimal environments for the patient to gain or regain the control necessary for functional activities.

Motor Learning

Motor control and motor learning are basically 2 sides of the same coin. Learning how the brain learns is especially important when there is injury in the neural circuitry. The system may have to initially learn or, in the case of injury, relearn motor skills. This is the scenario clinicians face in the rehabilitation setting. Physical therapists and physical therapist assistants train patients to gain or regain functional skills, initially assisting them and then taking them to optimal levels of performance. Therapists want functional skills gained or achieved in one session to be carried over to other practice environments and with longer periods in between practice.[48] By assuming there will be carryover into future sessions, clinicians are often frustrated at the next session. Motivation on the part of the patient plays another very important role in whether they regain and are willing to learn. Thus, the activity must be something the individual wants to learn or relearn to regain function. In addition, the concept of priming the nervous system to learn has recently become a topic of discussion.[16,49] Byl in 2017 stressed the importance of variables that affect the environment and learning. These variables include "use it or loss it," "make learning fun," "progress task specificity," and other variables that the therapist can introduce during treatment. With an understanding of these motor learning principles, carryover will mean that the patient regains more quickly what he demonstrated in the previous session.

Motor learning is the study of how individuals acquire, modify, and retain motor memories so they can be used, reused, and modified during functional activities. Examples of functional motor memory patterns include rolling, postural control of the head and trunk in all planes of movement, coming to stand, toilet training, feeding, walking, running, skiing, mountain climbing, spelunking, playing group sports, or engaging in any other combination of simple to complex motor behaviors synthesized to allow for success at the motor task that the patient has identified as something valued and important to quality of life. In that way, the limbic emotional system helps drive that learning through motivation and the chemistry it activates.

Principles of motor learning can be summarized in 4 major points:

1. Learning is a process of acquiring the capability for skilled action.
2. Learning results from experience or practice.
3. Learning cannot be measured directly—instead, it is inferred based on behavior.
4. Learning produces relatively permanent changes in behavior; thus, short-term alterations are not thought of as motor learning.[29]

Motor learning is a complex process reflecting the nervous system's response to a task-specific activity that emerges from an interaction between the need to perform the task and the environment within which the task is being performed.[48,50-53] The difference between a short-term change in behavior and motor learning can be demonstrated when a physical therapist assistant is working with a patient on rolling from supine to side-lying. At the beginning of the treatment session, the patient may need both verbal and physical assistance to complete the task, yet, by the end of the session, is able to roll independently. The next day, the patient may not roll independently from supine to side-lying even with verbal cueing, but is more quickly able to roll without assistance. This is an example of a short-term alteration in which permanent motor learning has not occurred. When the patient is consistently capable of rolling independently over time (a relatively permanent change in behavior), motor learning has occurred.

A variety of components affect motor learning, or how movement is expressed is a result of the interaction of all the components. These components include the context within which a motor program is practiced, the schedule of practice, the stage of motor learning of the behavior (whether learning a new program or relearning an old one), how feedback is applied, and the type of feedback applied. Each is discussed separately.

Practice Context

Practice context refers to the way a therapist chooses to teach the motor activity. There are 4 practice context categories: whole learning, pure-part learning, progressive/sequential-part learning, and whole-part-whole learning.

Whole Learning

Whole learning refers to practicing a behavior or task in its entirety. Simple and discrete motor tasks (ie, activities that have a definite beginning and end), such as rolling over in bed, moving from sit-to-stand, or scratching one's head, generally require whole learning. Asking an individual to stand up from a chair is a whole program. The physical therapist assistant may break the activity into 4 steps by asking that individual to scoot forward, place both feet 6 inches apart, shift weight over the feet, and then stand up. When breaking down the task, the patient may have more difficulty following the instructions than if he or she were asked to just stand up. Asking an individual to stand up requires one program that incorporates all the steps but is best practiced as a whole activity. When a specific impairment such as strength, range, or balance is identified, a physical therapist may ask a physical therapist assistant to treat the impairment or impairment train first (eg, strengthening, increasing range of motion, or balance training under specific environments), but then the activity must be practiced as a whole program for motor learning to occur. It is incorrect to assume that strengthening a muscle will automatically lead to an individual being able to perform a functional skill such as standing up from a chair.

Pure-Part Learning

Pure-part learning is used for complex activities where the component parts are discrete motor programs in and of themselves. When learning a tennis serve, an individual needs to learn how to throw the ball into the air vertically with a specific height expected and using the nondominant arm, and how to traject the dominant arm while holding the racket for the face of the racket to hit the ball overhead with a specific angle and force. It does not matter whether the individual is taught first how to throw and second how to traject the racket. Ultimately, both need to be learned and then practiced together as a whole activity for motor learning to occur. As a clinical example, a physical therapist asks a physical therapist assistant to teach an individual to stand up from and sit down onto a chair.

The first part of the activity, to attain and stop at the vertical upright standing pattern, requires the strength, range, postural control, and balance to shift one's weight over one's feet; concentric contractions from sit-to-stand using posture, balance, and movement patterns; initiation programming to begin the activity; and knowledge of where vertical is in space. The second discrete part of this motor program requires going from stand-to-sit. Eccentric control over the same patterns is required; thus, the 2 movements are unique in their programming. At times, a physical therapist assistant may assist the patient to standing and then practice one-quarter of both parts of the pattern (eg, sit down a little onto a bar stool, and then rise to stand with control). Once the patient can easily do these movements, the physical therapist assistant can increase the range within which the patient practices. This represents 2 unique programs. What determines the amount of range is the ease and fluidity of the patient's movements. Once the patient can lower to the height of a normal seat and return to standing, the physical therapist assistant needs to have the patient sit down, relax, and then stand up. The goal is to have the patient practice the whole program once both parts are learned. This is an example of pure-part learning, even though only one-quarter of both patterns is initially practiced. The decision to start in standing could be made because the patient was not able to generate enough force to come to stand or the force generated was excessive. There are many reasons why a patient might be asked to begin in standing. The physical therapist assistant could collaborate with the physical therapist to decide whether training the patient to independently come to standing is an appropriate approach for a specific patient. Starting in sitting or in standing will lead to the patient's independence in the sit-to-stand-to-sit program as a whole, but one way may be easier for the patient to learn initially, and this may reduce the time needed to learn the skill.

Progressive/Sequential-Part Learning

Progressive/sequential-part learning is employed when teaching intermediate skills and serial tasks (which are composed of several discrete tasks) that require many steps that must be performed in a specific sequence to be considered successful. When practiced, the learning always begins with the same initial step and follows in sequence with additional steps. Line dancing is an example of a sequential part task. If the components of the dance are taught to individuals as unique parts, different groups of people will put those parts together in different sequences, thus creating chaos on the dance floor. In a therapeutic environment, a physical therapist assistant may want to teach a patient how to stand up from a wheelchair. This task consists of 3 activities: lock the brake on the wheelchair, pick up the foot pedal, and then come to stand. Although these 3 activities are separate parts of the whole, teaching the patient to perform them in a specific sequence or order will help the patient to learn not only the activity but also the sequential series within which it should be performed. This is especially true when patients have specific types of perceptual impairment. Again, collaboration with the physical therapist will assist in determining whether this approach may be beneficial for a specific patient. Every physical therapist and physical therapist assistant has or will have a patient who stands up and then tries to either lock the brake or pick up the foot pedals. Often, the result is the practitioner writing up an incident report because the patient falls.

Whole-Part-Whole Learning

Whole-part-whole learning is the most frequently used in the clinical environment. An individual is first asked to perform the whole task; the clinician then breaks down the task into separate components and reconstitutes the entire program. The purpose is to have the patient execute the whole task so that a complete task analysis can be made. In a task analysis, the clinician needs to recognize what parts of the task are missing, what components of the movement are functioning, and what parts function intermittently and in limited ranges or positions in space. From this analysis, the results should help the physical therapist assistant determine what components need to be practiced when or in what sequence. Also, when some improvement is achieved by the patient, the physical therapist assistant could determine if it is appropriate to practice the whole task. This type of practice generally incorporates impairment training, which needs to then be incorporated into the program as a whole.

If there is some uncertainty as to whether the task should be taught through whole, pure-part, progressive/sequential-part, or whole-part-whole learning, consulting and collaborating with the supervising physical therapist is appropriate before beginning the intervention. If the physical therapist has not learned to articulate this type of analysis into the clinical decision-making, then the physical therapist assistant can help the physical therapist by asking the clinician to verbally explain this analysis and resulting approach to intervention. If neither feels totally comfortable, then using a book similar to this one can help both clinicians analyze the situation and determine what is best for the patient. Whether physical therapists or physical therapist assistants, many clinicians make decisions based on experience or gut feeling. Encouraging these individuals to clearly articulate their clinical decisions using accepted terminology helps reduce miscommunication and facilitate achievement of desired outcomes in an efficient manner (Box 4-2).

Practice Schedule

This motor learning component refers to the nature and frequency at which the patient practices the task. As practice is a critical element to motor learning, identifying which practice schedule best matches the task is important. There are 3 categories of practice schedule: mass, variable, and random practice.

Mass Practice

Mass practice is characterized by the individual practicing a particular skill in its entirety. This type of practice schedule is used to learn or relearn a skill that is essential for ADL. Regardless of how simple or complex the functional task, initially the individual needs to perform mass practice of the whole task. Thus, if parts of the task need to be learned as discrete components, they can be taught using pure-part, progressive/sequential-part, or whole-part-whole learning. However, to achieve permanent motor learning, the entire pattern/motor task must be practiced frequently enough for the CNS to learn the pattern as a whole. A physical therapist assistant may need to guide or instruct the patient to practice any or all components of the whole task or the whole activity itself, but for the learner to initially retain the learning, mass practice is essential. In an inpatient rehabilitation level of care, a patient comes to the physical therapist clinic once, twice, or 3 times a day to practice the functional skills within a mass-practice clinical environment. A physical therapist may need to determine the skill level at which the patient is performing to decide whether it is appropriate to delegate the intervention to a physical therapist assistant. If the only way a patient can perform a task is with constant correction of error and constant manual contact, then the physical therapist assistant needs to develop the skills necessary to initially guide the patient in the motor tasks, or the task should remain within the scope of the physical therapist. If, on the other hand, the patient needs to either practice with guidance to stay within the motor task or needs to work on specific components or impairments, these activities are well within the scope of practice of the physical therapist assistant.

Mass practice, from a practical perspective, is the opportunity for the patient to repetitively practice a motor pattern or functional movement with few interruptions; this helps limit distractions that can hinder the CNS from remembering the motor task being taught. Normal motor development, as discussed in Chapter 3, is an excellent illustration of the role of mass practice in a child's development of functional movement. For example, a child may try to succeed at a movement task such as rolling over. Once the child experiences success, the child will practice this activity repeatedly. The parents may become frustrated because the child may roll off a bed or will try to roll when being bathed or having a diaper changed. The child's CNS knows that, to learn that motor task, this type of practice is critical. Once the motor memory is consolidated, the individual will no longer need to mass practice unless the external environment changes. For example, if an individual learns through mass practice to walk on a hard, flat surface, that person should be able to automatically use that motor memory within that environment. If the person now wishes to walk on grass or up or down a hill, the environment for walking has changed, and mass practice will again be necessary to learn the variations of walking as an automatic adaptation. As an individual begins to automatically retrieve motor memories during ADL, the amount of practice needed is reduced. Similarly, the number of tasks the CNS might be asked to do, whether motor or cognitive, should increase between practicing the specific functional movements. Motor learning requires mass practice, but the

Box 4-2
Summary of Practice Context

- Whole learning: Motor program is practice as a whole. Whole learning should be taught for simple programs, such as rolling over, coming to sit, coming to stand, and walking. If the program is not available to the patient, then the physical therapist assistant must break it into usually sequential parts. For example, when coming to stand from a chair, the patient is asked to come to stand in one fluid program. If the patient does not have enough power, then strengthening is appropriate. Once there is enough muscle power, again instruct the patient to come to stand incorporating the gained power.
- Pure-part learning: Pure-part learning means that 2 or more parts make up a program. Both parts are essential, but it is not important to teach one before the other. Cutting vegetables for a soup might be an example. It does not matter which vegetable is cut first, but all must be cut before cooking.
- Progressive/sequential-part learning: Progressive/sequential-part learning is based on the requirement that the motor programs needed to carry out the skill have a sequential nature. If that sequence is mixed up, the skill will either fail or the end result could cause a fall. Once a patient comes into the clinic in a wheelchair and needs to transfer onto the mat, there is a sequential process for that activity. Once at the mat, the patient must first lock the brakes and pick up the footrests before standing, pivoting, and sitting down. Without using that sequence, the patient may stand, pivot, and fall because either the wheelchair moved or the foot pedals caused a trip.
- Whole-part-whole learning: Most physical therapists/physical therapist assistants use this type of learning when teaching a motor skill. First the patient is asked to perform an activity as a whole (eg, coming to stand from the chair), then the therapist will identify what parts or impairments need to be practiced or regained, and that will become part of the plan of care. As the patient regains control over the impairments, the activity is reintroduced and practiced as a whole activity. At times, the clinician will also use sequential parts along with the activity to make sure the patient has corrected both the parts and the sequence needed to succeed in the task.

Box 4-3

Stages of Motor Learning

- Stage 1: Cognitive stage/acquisition of a motor skill
- Stage 2: Associative stage/refinement
- Stage 3: Autonomous stage/retention

physical therapist must realize that if the individual stops practicing a task, then future performance of the skill may deteriorate.

Distributed Practice

Distributed practice is used when the patient has acquired a motor memory of the task, but impairment errors occur and practice is still needed to ensure long-term motor memory. With distributed practice, there are intervals between practice that are equal to or greater than the time spent practicing. This type of practice is generally used in situations or environments when patients do not require a high level of care or assistance in performing the activity. The specific frequency of intervention and practice should correlate with the needs of the patient and proceed from more frequent to less frequent as the patient progresses with independence. When practicing a large number of activities, with limited time to truly embed the learning of any motor task, the patient may not gain long-term independence in anything. Thus, selecting functional activities that gain the greatest independence for the patient is very important. Those programs or activities need to be valued by the patient to create the motivation to practice. The decision about what to practice may fall into the responsibility of the physical therapist; the practice itself certainly is within the scope of practice of the physical therapist assistant. There may be certain functional activities that the patient is mass practicing, while others are on a distributed practice schedule. An example of distributed practice might be ambulating with a walker. Initially, the patient would need to spend a lot of time just practicing using the walker. Once on a distributed schedule, the patient may still need standby assistance but is not expected to practice every hour; instead, the patient practices sometime in the morning and afternoon, but in between works on other functional activities.

Random Practice

Random practice refers to practice performed independently without a scheduled frequency or order. Random practice is, ultimately, the responsibility of the patient and/or caregiver. Once the patient can practice independently or with standby assistance, the activity must become part of that individual's daily-living life skill. Generally, neither the physical therapist nor the physical therapist assistant must be present during random practice; however, follow-up visits may be indicated to ensure that practice has been incorporated into the patient's lifestyle. The arrangement of a daily-living random practice schedule should be part of a home program, and the physical therapist assistant may be given the responsibility of monitoring these ADL. For example, a patient may be independently coming out of the chair and walking to the bathroom or kitchen, but be losing that ability over time because of lack of practice, according to his spouse. Simultaneously, because of a medical condition, the man may need to drink a glass of water hourly. That water can be made accessible to the individual on a table by his chair or at the water source such as a sink. If the patient is told that he needs to get up and go to the kitchen or bathroom for a glass of water every hour, he will automatically practice sit-to-stand, walking a certain distance, and then returning to his chair and sitting back down. The patient is empowered to the responsibility of drinking the water, but the whole activity incorporates functional movements that are practiced automatically as part of the daily routine. If he misses getting up once or twice a day, it will not affect his motor learning because he is randomly practicing the activity independently.

Stages of Motor Learning

Many authors have described the critical junctures in the process where an individual learns a specific task, and they generally follow a 3-stage sequence. Learning a motor skill usually starts with an individual cognitively thinking and practicing the tasks frequently, with a considerable amount of errors in performance, improving to a point at which the activity is performed automatically and with very few, if any, errors (Box 4-3).

Stage 1: Cognitive Stage/Acquisition of a Motor Skill

At Stage 1, the patient is learning a new skill or relearning an old one as a whole activity. At this stage, an individual needs to practice often and needs a lot of external feedback from the clinician to be successful. The more the patient recognizes the importance of the activity as improving independence or quality of life, the greater the compliance. However, allowing the patient to practice and recognize errors in task performance and then self-correct during the subsequent practice are important during this initial stage. For example, if a patient is coming to stand and shifts weight to the lateral aspect of the foot, then there is a greater likelihood of falling; however, if he or she is allowed to recognize the error in weight-bearing and then self-corrects the activity, then the boundaries of the activity are being practiced and learned. The patient would then be using both postural and balance programs to maintain control over the weight-bearing leg. Giving the patient time to self-correct before providing the external feedback is important. For example, allowing the patient to continue performing the task without self-correcting the movement results in the reinforcement of the wrong motor program.

Consider a situation in which a physical therapist asks a patient to stand. The patient executes the task, starts to fall, is unable to self-correct, then performs the task again with the same result. In this case, the patient is no longer in the coming to stand pattern. The patient is then practicing falling! In this example, the appropriate thing to do is to provide feedback to the patient as to the performance, determine a way for the patient to recognize the errors internally if appropriate and possible, and then allow the patient to perform the activity of coming to stand again with the appropriate amount of assistance. The physical therapist assistant would need to prevent the individual from falling and help the patient stay within the coming to stand pattern.

There are many ways to encourage an individual to stay within the pattern. Teaching the patient to respond to inherent/intrinsic feedback from within the body is a critical component of this stage of learning. When in the acquisition stage of motor learning, the environment used for practice should be consistent, and the type of practice is generally mass practice. In this stage, the motor skill is typically under conscious control; automaticity of the movement performance is not yet achieved. Once a patient begins to automatically respond to the demands of the external environment by the use of an appropriate control policy (eg, automatically stepping when the weight of the body is forward enough on the foot to trigger a stepping reaction), the patient executes movements in a feedforward pattern. This feedforward pattern means that the individual no longer needs feedback or sensory input for the CNS to know that walking is the appropriate response. As an example, the feedforward mechanism is similar to that of a DVD player. Once the equipment is told to run the movie, the player will continue running the movie until it is told to stop. Likewise, when the motor system, because of either the external environment or internal environment of the individual (eg, motivation or cognitive decision), is told to walk, the person will walk until a change is required. That motor system will continue to walk the musculoskeletal system until some aspect of the CNS changes that decision. Feedback to the CNS is often the critical component of the CNS's decision to change a control policy. Thus, as a physical therapist assistant begins to understand the stages of motor learning, consideration of feedback variables will need to be incorporated into these appropriate stages.

Stage 2: Associative Stage/Refinement

In Stage 2, a patient can execute movements within specific environmental constraints, decrease the number of errors during the activity, and apply less effort during performance. Generally, the environment used during performance is consistent, although variance in the specific components is present. For example, if a patient is able to sit on a hard surface as long as the patient does not reach and perturb him- or herself more than 20 degrees, then the task is learned, but it is limited in range, power, and/or balance when perturbed beyond range. The patient is in the refinement phase. A physical therapist assistant may want to add an activity of reaching for objects in space slightly beyond the 20-degree mark. The physical therapist assistant may want to retain the same environment (eg, a hard surface) while allowing the patient to refine the movement and self-correct. Then the patient may be asked to sit on a compliant surface but only move within the original 20 degrees. As the patient gains control reaching beyond 20 degrees while on a compliant surface, the therapist can enlarge or refine the activity. At this stage, a patient is enlarging control within a specific environment.

Stage 3: Autonomous Stage/Retention

At Stage 3, the patient moves to a variety of different environments and retains control of the whole task. Continuing the previous example, once the patient has learned to sit on a hard surface, the physical therapist assistant may move to a compliant surface, such as a gymnastic ball, and ask the patient to throw and catch an obstacle. The true hallmark of learning is the ability to retain the skill and transfer the skill into different settings and under different conditions and environmental and cognitive challenges.[52]

Feedback

There are 2 types of feedback: intrinsic and extrinsic. Feedback depends on sensory input. When patients have sensory loss, feedback mechanisms are often lost or inconsistent, and compensation through alternative sensory systems is indicated.[54-58]

Intrinsic Feedback

Intrinsic feedback is based on sensory responses inherent to the patient's body as part of the desired movement itself. For example, the muscles and joints tell the CNS where the trunk and limbs are in space and which limbs are in an open or closed chain. The vestibular system in the inner ear tells the CNS where the head is in space. Both sensory mechanisms are inherent and are the primary input for refinement and retention of posture and movement. This input is ongoing, and the motor system may use a feedforward mechanism. The physical therapist should determine whether there is conflict or loss in inherent feedback. If deficits exist, the physical therapist may delegate the specific activities that allow the patient to regain accurate sensory awareness during the activity or substitute another sensory system. For example, if, in sitting, the patient is unable to equally bear weight on both ischial tuberosities because of a decreased sense of pressure or proprioception, the physical therapist assistant may place a mirror to allow the patient to self-correct using vision (assuming that the patient's visual perception is intact). If the lack of appropriate intrinsic feedback or an alternative compensatory input system is unavailable, then error in the movement cannot be corrected and may lead to failure in obtaining functional independence.

Extrinsic Feedback

Extrinsic feedback is based on an outside source providing feedback. Biofeedback, auditory feedback from a therapist's voice, use of a mirror, and touch, pressure, and proprioceptive input feedback that the therapist uses during handling techniques are a few of the many extrinsic feedback mechanisms physical therapists and physical therapist assistants use. This type of feedback can lead to better performance during a motor activity, but until the patient self-corrects using inherent feedback, independence is not obtained. There are 2 types of extrinsic feedback.[59-63]

Knowledge-of-performance feedback uses a sensory system (such as the therapist's voice) to inform the patient as to whether the quality or efficiency of the movement pattern is achieved. This type of feedback is given as the person is performing the task and generally at critical times to ensure the individual accomplishes the task. A physical therapist assistant may say, "You are doing fine, Mr. B, but you need to keep your balance over your feet," "You need to push down on your walker," or "Put your foot farther forward."

Knowledge-of-results feedback informs the patient as to whether the task is accomplished or how close the movement comes to accomplishing the task. The type of feedback is given at the end of the task and truly gives feedback as to the entire activity or task performed. The physical therapist assistant may say, "Mrs. J, you came to standing without my help," or "You should not sit down without looking because you just sat on Mr. M." Both types of feedback give the learner information regarding error. Constant feedback leads to immediate behavioral performance, but the patient will learn to rely on external feedback and will not develop a need to process inherent information necessary to learn the task independently.

As an example, a physical therapist assistant verbally corrects many aspects of walking, and the patient does very well by the end of the morning session. In the afternoon, when the patient is asked to walk again, the patient's performance is the same as at the beginning of the morning and does not show the changes made by the end of the morning session. Obviously, the patient is depending on external feedback from the physical therapist assistant and not learning to perform the task independently. There is a fine line between whether the patient is depending on the external feedback to functionally move or is using that feedback to develop an internal awareness.[64] The physical therapist assistant can determine this difference by withdrawing the feedback and observing whether the patient can retain the motor skill both during treatment and at the following session.

External feedback can be provided in several ways. *Summary feedback* is when the feedback is given after a set number of trials of the task (eg, after every other or every third trial). *Faded feedback* initially provides feedback after every trial, then decreases to every other trial, every third, every fourth, and so on. During *delayed feedback*, the clinician withholds the feedback for a short time (eg, a 5-second delay) after the task has been performed.[65] When facilitating motor learning, faded feedback appears to be most effective, as the feedback becomes increasingly intermittent throughout patient trials (practice), and therefore the patient has to rely more on internal feedback and self-correction to perform the task safely and efficiently. Delayed feedback also allows for improved motor learning by providing the patient time to self-assess performance.

However, the specific feedback schedule depends on the patient and the task to be learned and practiced. This is another area in which the physical therapist/physical therapist assistant collaboration and communication are important in setting up optimal feedback and practice parameters. But, whether under the direct supervision of a physical therapist or within an environment where the physical therapist assistant has some autonomy, there is clear evidence to show that physical therapist interventions following CNS damage does lead to motor learning and consequent improvement in an individual's ability to perform functional activities.[66] Those data clearly identify the need for physical therapy interventions in individuals following CNS damage (Table 4-2). Indeed, human subjects who had their arm moved passively along reach trajectories and received visual feedback on movement success showed performance gains that were at par with participants in a matched active condition.[67]

Physical Therapist/Physical Therapist Assistant Collaboration in Relation to Motor Learning Activities

Approaches to facilitate learning or relearning of a motor skill are a critical component when providing interventions aimed at optimizing function. Remember that a complex motor activity may consist of a variety of motor programs. Following injury to the brain, the memory of each program may need to be evaluated by the physical therapist. It is the physical therapist's decision to run certain aspects of an entire program. Delegation of any of those activities can be given to the physical therapist assistant.

For example, an individual who has suffered a traumatic brain injury may need to relearn specific components of a task. The physical therapist may ask the physical therapist assistant to bring the patient to standing using the right lower extremity. If both legs are used, then the left leg may go into a strong extensor pattern, such as hip extension and adduction, knee extension and ankle inversion, and plantar flexion. Thus, the right leg would be ready to stand, but the left would not. The physical therapist assistant may be instructed to bring the patient to stand on the right foot, but bend the left lower extremity at the knee and place the left knee on a stool. In this way, the right leg could practice

Table 4-2
Summary of Motor Learning Concepts

Type of Learning	*Practice Parameters*	*Feedback Schedule*
Initial learning	Mass practice of motor program or functional skill. Reintroduction of corrections of impairments into the functional skill. Will begin with block design.	Needs knowledge of both performance and results. Initial reinforcement is immediate, thus showing high performance but lower retention.
Learning shows programming, but with large number of errors	Practice will go from mass to distributed as the patient begins to self-correct errors. Widening of the window of range within the program can increase. Design will move from block to random as program becomes more automatic. Mental practice can be used to encourage internal repetition.	May still use knowledge of performance during times when patient's error exceeds the range of the program, but knowledge of results will in time become the most important feedback. As the physical therapist assistant moves to variability of practice, the program will become more generalizable. Reinforcement becomes more intermittent with a higher degree of retention.
Learning shows motor program has been established	Practice schedule should go from distributed to random with the patient being motivated to run the correct procedure. Patient is self-motivated to perform the programs as part of daily living and social responsibilities.	Patient internally corrects using inherent mechanisms and no longer needs the physical therapist assistant to reinforce motor learning, except for social reasons. We all like to hear we are doing well.

all components of standing and the left leg could still practice postural control of the hip without going into a strong extensor pattern. This delegation to the physical therapist assistant is appropriate, and many physical therapist assistants may also be given the responsibility to transition the patient to bilateral standing as long as the left leg has developed the necessary postural control to inhibit a total extensor synergy.

Neuroplasticity

Neuroplasticity is defined as cellular adaptations in the CNS that allow an individual to learn novel skills or relearn functions previously lost because of cellular death by trauma or disease at any age.[68-71] The changes occur in response to external and internal demands placed on the individual's CNS, and the feedback the brain receives from those demands. Within an optimal treatment environment, the resultant behavior leads to functional recovery and allows the individual to regain or attain a higher quality of life. In reality, neuroplasticity occurs throughout life. Internal adaptations of the CNS to height, weight, endurance, acute and chronic disease, and cellular death over a lifetime allow all of us to maintain function as our bodies change. Similarly, over a lifetime, there will be variations in external environments such as climate, exercise level, dietary demands, and habitat. The CNS has to adapt to these changes as well. When trauma or disease causes dramatic, observable changes in behavior, then everyone around becomes aware of those variances. Theory from the early- to mid-20th century led therapists to believe that once cellular death had occurred, nothing could be done except to compensate for lost function. It was believed that plasticity within the CNS was not possible. Therapists working with patients with CNS disease or trauma could not reconcile the discrepancy between theory and patient recovery following disease or trauma. Therapists have always dealt with function, and physicians with pathology. Often, the pathology, according to the physician or basic scientist, would indicate that function was impossible, yet therapists dealing with behavior found that patients often got better and regained lost motor function.

In the past 3 decades, with the advent of better measurement tools and research on human and animal models, scientists and researchers have discovered that the brain is much more plastic than previously thought. It has been found that, given an appropriate environment to learn in, the brain can learn or relearn despite cellular damage.[72-83] Indeed, network connectivity among motor cortical neurons in the hemisphere contralateral to the amputated arm was modified following learning.[3] Neuroplasticity provides an explanation at the basic science level for behavior that therapists have observed since the beginning of the profession. Previously, clinicians, especially master clinicians, had difficulty explaining or could not explain how patients regained function; however, they could observe and measure those behaviors. As a clinician and therapist, Umphred always believed that if a motor behavior looked right to her or other people, was easy and enjoyable for the patient, then somehow the intervention was creating change in the direction of normality and functional recovery, no matter the theory.

Neuroplasticity helps explain why patients were regaining function even though the medical system of the time said they could not. This theory has helped guide therapists with intervention delineation. The CNS will always try to succeed at a task presented, as long as the individual is motivated to succeed.[48] If the environment used to teach a task is too difficult, then a patient will find other ways to try to succeed. For example, if a patient cannot flex the hip at push-off, he or she will circumduct the hip or use some alternative movement pattern to succeed at bringing the limb forward. These alternatives are easily identified and, if practiced, will become a new movement pattern for the patient; they will, however, require more energy because they are less efficient. They will affect synergy patterns, postural control, balance, and needed power throughout the range.

Therefore, it would be better to try to trigger the patient's normal walking patterns before choosing some compensatory solution. The complex theory and its relationship to function often fall into the responsibility of the physical therapist and not the physical therapist assistant, but that does not mean that the physical therapist assistant will not discover the movement patterns that lead to normal function. The physical therapist assistant has sensory input to the eyes and ears and kinesthetic feelings from touch and pressure that can help lead to solutions to a patient's functional recovery. Thus, it is the physical therapist assistant's job to become a keen observer of functional movement and report changes in those behaviors to the physical therapist. A patient's movement or postural problems are usually answered by the patient's own motor responses and truly reflect the plasticity of the CNS.

Kleim and Jones[84] synthesized the pertinent research on neuroplasticity in a way that provides specific suggestions in the application of neuroplasticity in rehabilitation practice. For more information, the reader is encouraged to review this research article. The following principles have direct implications in physical therapist assistant practice:

1. "Use it or lose it."[84] The physical therapist assistant must encourage the patient to acquire and practice normal movements that improve functional performance. Movements and functional patterns that are not performed or practiced are lost, including the motor circuitry responsible for that movement in the CNS. For example, following a stroke, a patient may have a reduced ability to use an arm or leg. Without rehabilitation, over time, the patient will learn not to use the affected extremity, leading to the concept of learned non-use. Because of this, the neuronal circuitry responsible for the movement occurring on the affected extremities also disappears. It is difficult to overcome learned non-use, but more recent research states that it is possible.
2. "Use it and improve it."[84] It is not sufficient to just encourage use of the affected extremity. Specific training to improve function on that limb consequently drives the changes in the brain that reinforce this improvement.
3. "Specificity."[84] The training to improve function has to be specific. This means that the physical therapist assistant must choose activities that will directly improve the quality and efficiency of the desired movement. For example, if the goal is to strengthen the lower extremities to improve the performance of sit-to-stands, then the physical therapist assistant must practice the particular activity with the patient. Performing open-chain strengthening exercises for the lower extremities may improve strength, but will not necessarily translate to the patient's improved ability to stand up from the sitting position. In addition to specificity, the activity must be meaningful for the patient (see #5, "Saliency matters").
4. "Repetition and intensity matter."[84] The practice of a particular activity must include the appropriate amount of intensity to drive the needed neuroplastic changes to regain the movement or function. Most recent research on this topic clearly shows that the intensity of therapy that we currently provide the majority of our patients/clients is ***not*** sufficient to drive these changes. It is therefore important to maximize practice by optimizing the patient's adherence to his or her home program. Additional approaches to optimizing repetition in practice include the use of a patient contract, an activity log to document performance of a home program, and activities to encourage or force the use of the more affected extremities.
5. "Saliency matters."[84] The chosen activity being practiced must be meaningful for the patient. This means that the patient perceives the importance of the movement or task and sees how practicing this task leads to the attainment of goals and functions that he or she desires.

Conclusion

If a patient has never learned normal motor patterns (eg, in the case of trauma in utero or at birth), the movement pattern must be mass-practiced in an environment where success is possible, reinforcement accurate, and potential actualized. To get internal motivation, the brain needs to recognize that the movement being introduced is easier than the one previously learned, and that easier movement leads to greater functional progression. If the individual has already learned a movement strategy, such as walking, and suffers a traumatic incident, such as traumatic head injury or stroke, the potential exists to regain a previously learned pattern or to learn a new one in the intervention environment of the therapist. An individual must first learn a pattern or task-specific program, and then practice enough for the control over that program to become automatic, as in the feedforward motor program.

A learned program is similar to a disc placed in a DVD player. The CNS determines the pattern and will run the program (or disc) until the CNS is told to change it. As an example, the therapist places the client in an environment where the patient's CNS determines that walking is the appropriate program to play. The type of walking observed tells the therapist what programs are interacting and being controlled by the patient. That person runs the motor control of walking until either the CNS tells it to do something else or the motor control of that individual cannot self-correct the error, and the environment forces a new pattern. A person falling because of a surface change for which the person cannot compensate is an example of external environmental change that forces a loss of motor control over walking. Understanding motor learning and what patterns the CNS can use to control the motor system's response to a required movement can give tremendous insight into the prognosis of a patient with movement dysfunction following insult to the CNS. How the map fits together will be influenced by the physical therapist, the physical therapist assistant, the patient, and the environments within which the patient can learn. The following case examples should help the physical therapist assistant understand the theoretical principles presented in this chapter.

Case Studies

The following case studies are patient examples similar to those discussed in later chapters. The physical therapist assistant is not expected to be able to answer clinical questions after reading this chapter. Instead, the physical therapist assistant can use these cases to help integrate the information presented in all the chapters that discuss specific clinical problems. It is recommended that the learner read this chapter, the case examples, and the questions to identify appropriate questions regarding motor control, motor learning, and neuroplasticity as they relate to patient care. After reading and analyzing any chapter dealing with a clinical problem, the physical therapist assistant can return to this chapter, find an appropriate case, and then progress through the questions and answers to better integrate this material into decisions on clinical management.

Case #1

The patient is a 6-month-old child diagnosed with spastic diplegia. She was born 8 weeks premature and was extremely flaccid (low tone) at that time. The child's gestational age would be placed at 4 months, giving the child the 8 weeks she should have remained in utero. However, the child's tonal characteristics are extensor-dominant in the trunk and lower extremities. The child has more control over the arms than the legs, but loses function of the arms when placed in positions that require a lot of trunk stability, such as sitting or putting pressure on the feet in standing. The child does not have adequate head control and is unable to roll over, come to sitting, or sit independently.

The physical therapist has asked the physical therapist assistant to use a handling technique with rotation of the trunk initially in side-lying. The physical therapist assistant should rotate the child's lower trunk on the upper trunk to facilitate rolling and have one of the patient's lower extremities lead with hip and knee flexion (without holding the ball of the foot). As the child begins to respond to rolling, the physical therapist assistant encourages the child to assist with the movement itself.

Second, the child should be placed on the physical therapist assistant's bent knees with the head in vertical and, with small-degree changes of the trunk, the physical therapist assistant should facilitate small movements of the head and thus assist the child in gaining head control. As the child responds with head movement that brings the head to face vertical, the physical therapist assistant enlarges the degrees of motion. The physical therapist assistant works from vertical toward horizontal (both toward prone and supine) and back to vertical. The physical therapist assistant only goes as far as the child's postural responses to head control are observed. Thus, the physical therapist assistant is given the responsibility of working on both rolling activities and development of head control.

Questions

1. Why has the physical therapist asked the physical therapist assistant to perform these activities? Why were those activities important in improving the child's movement abilities?
2. Is the request within the domain of the physical therapist assistant?
3. At what stage of motor learning is the child?
4. What type of practice context would you choose? The response needs to relate to whole, pure-part, progressive/sequential-part, and whole-part-whole learning.
5. What type of practice schedule would you expect the physical therapist assistant to use? When considering the practice schedule, what type of feedback would be used initially, and how would that feedback be changed as the patient improves?
6. Why would you expect change, and what might it look like? When or why would you ask the physical therapist to change the interventions delegated?

Case #2

The patient is a 5-year-old boy who suffered an anoxic event due to drowning. Before the injury, he was an active, healthy child in kindergarten, and doing very well. The child was in a coma for 1 week and in a vegetative state for 3 weeks. He is now medically stable and has been sent to neurorehabilitation for physical therapy. The patient can roll and come to sitting, although his trunk tone is low. He can be placed in sitting and remain there independently as long as he is not perturbed or asked to move. He cannot stand up from sitting and does not control going from sit toward horizontal.

The physical therapist has asked the physical therapist assistant to work on sitting balance and strengthening of the postural extensors of the trunk and hips. The physical therapist assistant has placed herself in kneeling behind the child, using her own leg to support the boy's trunk from behind. This brings the boy into a vertical postural pattern while sitting. The physical therapist assistant then asks the child to reach for toys and hand them to his mother. Once the child begins to hold and respond with balance reactions, the physical therapist assistant moves the child to sitting on a gymnastic ball and continues to work on sitting and balance control. Next, using the same gymnastic ball, the physical therapist assistant rolls the child toward prone and then into a vertical kneeling posture, using the ball to help support the trunk extensors. Then, using toys and manipulating the ball, the physical therapist assistant increases the demand on the child's motor system to maintain and/or regain upright posture during play.

Questions

1. Why has the physical therapist asked the physical therapist assistant to perform these activities? Why were those activities important in improving the child's movement abilities?
2. Is the request within the domain of the physical therapist assistant?
3. At what stage of learning is the child?
4. What type of environmental context would you choose?
5. What type of feedback/reinforcement schedule would you expect the physical therapist assistant to use?
6. Why would you expect change, and what might it look like? How would you as a physical therapist assistant examine this child's motor control and determine that a change in intervention would be appropriate?

Case #3

The patient is a 27-year-old man who suffered a traumatic brain injury following a head-on collision while driving his car without a seat belt. He has been in the intensive care unit for 4 days and has been transferred to the rehabilitation unit today. The physical therapist has performed the initial evaluation of the patient. He is conscious but has extremely low tone. He is unable to come to sitting or standing independently, and he does not have enough tone to sit independently.

The physical therapist has asked the physical therapist assistant to sit the patient on the side of the bed with the feet supported, by first raising the head of the bed, then guiding the patient into sitting. Either the physical therapist assistant can kneel behind the patient on the bed with a ball in the patient's lap and the patient's arms over the ball, or the physical therapist assistant can sit in front of the patient and make sure his weight is forward over his pelvis with his arms on the physical therapist assistant's shoulder. The goal is to increase the length of time the patient is able to sit semi-independently. As the patient gains control and strength, the physical therapist assistant has him begin to reach for real targets, such as a cup or ball, while maintaining trunk and pelvic control. The goal is to gain independent sitting. This is accomplished through the patient being challenged by perturbation of his weight over his hips during reaching or regaining balance if shoved. The physical therapist assistant is also asked to work on transfers between the bed and the wheelchair and back to reduce the total dependency he now has when performing transfers.

Questions

1. Why has the physical therapist asked the physical therapist assistant to perform these activities? Why were those activities important in improving the person's movement abilities?
2. Is the request within the domain of the physical therapist assistant?
3. At what stage of learning is the patient concerning sitting?
4. Is the physical therapist assistant working on new learning or relearning an old program?
5. What type of environmental context would you choose (eg, quiet or noisy, and hard or soft surface)?
6. What type of feedback/reinforcement schedule would you expect the physical therapist assistant to use?
7. Why would you expect change, and what might it look like? When or why would you ask the physical therapist to change the interventions delegated?

Case #4

The patient is a 59-year-old man with the medical diagnosis of Parkinson's disease. He is able to perform all functional activities at a certain rate, but he has great difficulty regaining his balance if he trips, and difficulty initiating changes such as sit-to-stand and stand-to-walk. He especially complains of problems turning (eg, turning into the bathroom, or turning and walking back to the dining room with his food).

First, the physical therapist asks the physical therapist assistant to teach the patient to use a partial rotation pattern when coming to sit, vs the adult sitting pattern he is using. The physical therapist also asks the physical therapist assistant to have the patient practice going from sit-to-stand-to-sit on a variety of surfaces, with the chair or stool at a variety of levels. The physical therapist delegates placing this patient on the treadmill, first at his normal gait pattern and then changing the settings to encourage fluctuation in walking speed and height of incline. The fourth task for the physical therapist assistant is to create a maze for the patient to walk through that requires him to turn at each corner. Initially, he should be instructed to just walk, and then he should progress to walking through the maze facing a specific direction. Once he can do this independently, the activities will become his home exercise program, which he must practice to maintain function for as long as possible. Additionally, the physical therapist may delegate other activities to the patient's significant other or other caregiver because the patient still needs to continue practicing but does not need a physical therapist or a physical therapist assistant to help with these functions at this time.

Questions

1. Why has the physical therapist asked the physical therapist assistant to do these activities? Why were those activities important in improving the person's movement abilities?
2. Is the request within the domain of the physical therapist assistant?
3. At what stage of learning is the adult in relation to walking?
4. Is the physical therapist assistant working on new learning or relearning an old program?
5. Why did the physical therapist select the specific environmental context, and why should it work?
6. What type of reinforcement schedule would you expect the physical therapist assistant to use?
7. Why would you expect change, and what might it look like? When or why would you ask the physical therapist to change the interventions delegated?

Case #5

The patient is a 71-year-old man with the medical diagnosis of a mild right cerebrovascular accident with resulting left hemiplegia. He can sit independently but does not have equal weight-bearing on the left hip. With assistance, he can come to standing with the majority of weight on his right leg.

The physical therapist has delegated to the physical therapist assistant the activity of weight-shifting in sitting. Specifically, the physical therapist assistant is to have the patient reach with his right arm over to the left side as far as possible and increase that range as the patient improves. If he can use the left arm to do the same, then the physical therapist assistant is to also include that extremity. Second, the physical therapist assistant is to assist the physical therapist in placing the patient in a harness to do supported weight-bearing on the treadmill. Once the patient is in the position and the physical therapist determines the pace and degree of body weight–support, the physical therapist assistant will be assisting the patient with his left leg to practice walking.

Questions

1. Why has the physical therapist asked the physical therapist assistant to do these activities? Why were those activities important in improving the person's movement abilities?
2. Is the request within the domain of the physical therapist assistant?
3. At what stage of learning is the adult concerning walking?
4. Is the physical therapist assistant working on new learning or relearning an old program?
5. Why did the physical therapist select the specific environmental context?
6. What type of reinforcement schedule would you expect the physical therapist assistant to use?
7. Why would you expect change, and what might it look like? When or why would you ask the physical therapist to change the interventions delegated?

References

1. Arce-McShane FI, Hatsopoulos NG, Lee J-C, Ross CF, Sessle BJ. Modulation dynamics in the orofacial sensorimotor cortex during motor skill acquisition. *J Neurosci.* 2014;34(17):5985-5997. doi:10.1523/JNEUROSCI.4367-13.2014
2. Arce-McShane FI, Ross CF, Takahashi K, Sessle BJ, Hatsopoulos NG. Primary motor and sensory cortical areas communicate via spatiotemporally coordinated networks at multiple frequencies. *Proc Natl Acad Sci USA.* 2016;113(18):5083-5088. doi:10.1073/pnas.1600788113
3. Balasubramanian K, Vaidya M, Southerland J, et al. Changes in cortical network connectivity with long-term brain-machine interface exposure after chronic amputation. *Nat Commun.* 2017;8(1):1796. doi:10.1038/s41467-017-01909-2
4. Ethier C, Oby ER, Bauman MJ, Miller LE. Restoration of grasp following paralysis through brain-controlled stimulation of muscles. *Nature.* 2012;485(7398):368-371. doi:10.1038/nature10987
5. Mohanty R, Sinha AM, Remsik AB, et al. Machine learning classification to identify the stage of brain-computer interface therapy for stroke rehabilitation using functional connectivity. *Front Neurosci.* 2018;12:353. doi:10.3389/fnins.2018.00353
6. Ostry DJ, Gribble PL. Sensory plasticity in human motor learning. *Trends Neurosci.* 2016;39(2):114-123. doi:10.1016/j.tins.2015.12.006
7. Roemmich RT, Long AW, Bastian AJ. Seeing the errors you feel enhances locomotor performance but not learning. *Curr Biol.* 2016;26(20):2707-2716. doi:10.1016/j.cub.2016.08.012
8. Scott SH. A functional taxonomy of bottom-up sensory feedback processing for motor actions. *Trends Neurosci.* 2016;39(8):512-526. doi:10.1016/j.tins.2016.06.001
9. Galea MP. Physical modalities in the treatment of neurological dysfunction. *Clin Neurol Neurosurg.* 2012;114(5):483-488. doi:10.1016/j.clineuro.2012.01.009

10. dos Santos Mendes FA, Pompeu JE, Modenesi Lobo A, et al. Motor learning, retention and transfer after virtual-reality-based training in Parkinson's disease—effect of motor and cognitive demands of games: a longitudinal, controlled clinical study. *Physiotherapy*. 2012;98(3):217-223. doi:10.1016/j.physio.2012.06.001
11. Schenkman M, Hall DA, Barón AE, Schwartz RS, Mettler P, Kohrt WM. Exercise for people in early- or mid-stage Parkinson disease: a 16-month randomized controlled trial. *Phys Ther*. 2012;92(11):1395-1410. doi:10.2522/ptj.20110472
12. Heba S, Lenz M, Kalisch T, et al. Regionally specific regulation of sensorimotor network connectivity following tactile improvement. *Neural Plast*. 2017;2017:5270532. doi:10.1155/2017/5270532
13. Ismail FY, Fatemi A, Johnston MV. Cerebral plasticity: windows of opportunity in the developing brain. *Eur J Paediatr Neurol*. 2017;21(1):23-48. doi:10.1016/j.ejpn.2016.07.007
14. McLaughlin KA, Sheridan MA, Nelson CA. Neglect as a violation of species-expectant experience: neurodevelopmental consequences. *Biol Psychiatry*. 2017;82(7):462-471. doi:10.1016/j.biopsych.2017.02.1096
15. Bao T, Carender WJ, Kinnaird C, et al. Effects of long-term balance training with vibrotactile sensory augmentation among community-dwelling healthy older adults: a randomized preliminary study. *J Neuroeng Rehabil*. 2018;15(1):5. doi:10.1186/s12984-017-0339-6
16. Byl N. A review and perspective on maximizing brain plasticity: priming the nervous system to learn. *Int Phys Med Rehab J*. 2017;1(5):124-126. doi:10.15406/ipmrj.2017.01.00027
17. Liang N, Funase K, Narita T, Takahashi M, Matsukawa K, Kasai T. Effects of unilateral voluntary movement on motor imagery of the contralateral limb. *Clin Neurophysiol*. 2011;122(3):550-557. doi:10.1016/j.clinph.2010.07.024
18. Schmidt L, Lebreton M, Cléry-Melin ML, Daunizeau J, Pessiglione M. Neural mechanisms underlying motivation of mental versus physical effort. *PLoS Biol*. 2012;10(2):e1001266. doi:10.1371/journal.pbio.1001266
19. Mastos M, Miller K, Eliasson AC, Imms C. Goal-directed training: linking theories of treatment to clinical practice for improved functional activities in daily life. *Clin Rehabil*. 2007;21(1):47-55. doi:10.1177/0269215506073494
20. Merrett DL, Kirkland SW, Metz GA. Synergistic effects of age and stress in a rodent model of stroke. *Behav Brain Res*. 2010;214(1):55-59. doi:10.1016/j.bbr.2010.04.035
21. Liddell EG. Cajal and Sherrington. *Lect Sci Basis Med*. 1956-1958;6:100-115.
22. Knott M, Voss DE. *Proprioceptive Neuromuscular Facilitation*. New York, NY: Harper & Row; 1968.
23. Bobath B. *Abnormal Postural Reflex Activity Caused by Brain Lesions*. 3rd ed. Frederick, MD: Aspen Publications; 1985.
24. Rood M. The use of sensory receptors to activate, facilitate, and inhibit motor response, autonomic and somatic, in developmental sequence. In: Scattely C, ed. Approaches to Treatment of Patients With Neuromuscular Dysfunction. Third International Congress, World Federation of Occupational Therapists. Dubuque, IA: William Brown Group; 1962.
25. Ayres AJ. *The Development of Sensory Integration Theory and Practice*. Dubuque, IA: Kendall/Hunt Publishing; 1974.
26. Johnstone M. *Restoration of Normal Movement After Stroke*. New York, NY: Churchill Livingstone; 1995.
27. Brunnstrom S. *Movement Therapy in Hemiplegia*. 2nd ed. Philadelphia, PA: JB Lippincott; 1992.
28. Carr JH, Sheperd RB. *Movement Science: Foundations for Physical Therapy in Rehabilitation*. Frederick, MD: Aspen Publishers; 1987.
29. Umphred DA. *Neurological Rehabilitation*. St. Louis, MO: CV Mosby; 1985.
30. Sherrington CS. *The Integrative Action of the Nervous System*. New York, NY: Cambridge University Press; 1947.
31. Bernstein N. *Coordination and Regulation of Movement*. New York, NY: Pergamon Press; 1967.
32. Tuller B, Turvey MT, Fitch HI. The Bernstein perspective II: the concept of muscle linkage or coordinative structure. In: Kelso JAS, ed. *Human Motor Behavior. An Introduction*. Hillsdale, NJ: Erlbaum; 1982.
33. Brooks VB. *The Neural Basis of Motor Control*. New York, NY: Oxford University Press; 1986.
34. Horak F. Assumptions underlying motor control for neurological rehabilitation. In: Contemporary Management of Motor Control Problems: Proceedings of the II STEP Conference. Alexandria, VA: Foundation for Physical Therapy; 1991.
35. Gordon J. A top-down model for neurologic rehabilitation. Presented at: III Step Conference: Linking Movement Science and Intervention; 2005, Salt Lake City, UT.
36. Cramer SC, Sur M, Dobkin BH, et al. Harnessing neuroplasticity for clinical applications. *Brain*. 2011;134(Pt 6):1591-1609. doi:10.1093/brain/awr039
37. Connell LA, McMahon NE, Tyson SF, Watkins CL, Eng JJ. Mechanisms of action of an implementation intervention in stroke rehabilitation: a qualitative interview study. *BMC Health Serv Res*. 2016;16(1):534. doi:10.1186/s12913-016-1793-8
38. Ghahramani Z, Wolpert D, Jordan M. Computational models of sensorimotor integration. In: Morasso P, Sanguineti V, eds. *Self-Organization, Computational Maps, and Motor Control*. Amsterdam, The Netherlands: Elsevier; 1997:117-147. doi:10.1016/S0166-4115(97)80006-4
39. Bastos AM, Vezoli J, Fries P. Communication through coherence with inter-areal delays. *Curr Opin Neurobiol*. 2015;31:173-180. doi:10.1016/j.conb.2014.11.001
40. Fries P. A mechanism for cognitive dynamics: neuronal communication through neuronal coherence. *Trends Cogn Sci*. 2005;9(10):474-480. doi:10.1016/j.tics.2005.08.011
41. Koralek AC, Costa RM, Carmena JM. Temporally precise cell-specific coherence develops in corticostriatal networks during learning. *Neuron*. 2013;79(5):865-872. doi:10.1016/j.neuron.2013.06.047
42. Soteropoulos DS, Baker SN. Cortico-cerebellar coherence during a precision grip task in the monkey. *J Neurophysiol*. 2006;95(2):1194-1206. doi:10.1152/jn.00935.2005
43. Witham CL, Wang M, Baker SN. Corticomuscular coherence between motor cortex, somatosensory areas and forearm muscles in the monkey. *Front Syst Neurosci*. 2010;4:38. doi:10.3389/fnsys.2010.00038
44. Shadmehr R, Krakauer JW. A computational neuroanatomy for motor control. *Exp Brain Res*. 2008;185(3):359-381. doi:10.1007/s00221-008-1280-5

45. Mansfield A, Schinkel-Ivy A, Danells CJ, et al. Does perturbation training prevent falls after discharge from stroke rehabilitation? A prospective cohort study with historical control. *J Stroke Cerebrovasc Dis.* 2017;26(10):2174-2180. doi:10.1016/j.jstrokecerebrovasdis.2017.04.041
46. Arce F, Novick I, Shahar M, Link Y, Ghez C, Vaadia E. Differences in context and feedback result in different trajectories and adaptation strategies in reaching. *PLoS One.* 2009;4(1):e4214. doi:10.1371/journal.pone.0004214
47. Shadmehr R, Mussa-Ivaldi FA. Adaptive representation of dynamics during learning of a motor task. *J Neurosci.* 1994; 14(5 Pt 2):3208-3224. doi:10.1523/JNEUROSCI.14-05-03208.1994
48. Roller P, Lazaro R, Byl N, Umphred D. Motor control, motor learning and neuroplasticity. In: Umphred D, Lazaro R, Roller P, Burton G, eds. *Umphred's Neurological Rehabilitation.* 6th ed. St. Louis, MO: Elsevier; 2012:69-97.
49. Mezzarobba S, Grassi M, Pellegrini L, et al. Action observation plus sonification. a novel therapeutic protocol for Parkinson's patient with freezing of gait. *Front Neurol.* 2018;8:723. doi:10.3389/fneur.2017.00723
50. Shumway-Cook A, Wollacott M. *Motor Control: Translating Research Into Clinical Practice.* 4th ed. Philadelphia, PA: Lippincott Williams & Wilkins; 2011.
51. Candia V, Wienbruch C, Elbert T, Rockstroh B, Ray W. Effective behavioral treatment of focal hand dystonia in musicians alters somatosensory cortical organization. *Proc Natl Acad Sci USA.* 2003;100(13):7942-7946. doi:10.1073/pnas.1231193100
52. Goh HT, Sullivan KJ, Gordon J, Wulf G, Winstein CJ. Dual-task practice enhances motor learning: a preliminary investigation. *Exp Brain Res.* 2012;222(3):201-210. doi:10.1007/s00221-012-3206-5
53. Spampinato DA, Block HJ, Celnik PA. Cerebellar-M1 connectivity changes associated with motor learning are somatotopic specific. *J Neurosci.* 2017;37(9):2377-2386. doi:10.1523/JNEUROSCI.2511-16.2017
54. Kuo AD. The relative roles of feedforward and feedback in the control of rhythmic movements. *Mot Contr.* 2002;6(2):129-145. doi:10.1123/mcj.6.2.129
55. Sullivan KJ, Knowlton BJ, Dobkin BH. Step training with body weight support: effect of treadmill speed and practice paradigms on poststroke locomotor recovery. *Arch Phys Med Rehabil.* 2002;83(5):683-691. doi:10.1053/apmr.2002.32488
56. Winstein CJ. Knowledge of results and motor learning—implications for physical therapy. *Phys Ther.* 1991;71(2):140-149. doi:10.1093/ptj/71.2.140
57. Vahdat S, Darainy M, Milner TE, Ostry DJ. Functionally specific changes in resting-state sensorimotor networks after motor learning. *J Neurosci.* 2011;31(47):16907-16915. doi:10.1523/JNEUROSCI.2737-11.2011
58. Wong JD, Kistemaker DA, Chin A, Gribble PL. Can proprioceptive training improve motor learning? *J Neurophysiol.* 2012;108(12):3313-3321. doi:10.1152/jn.00122.2012
59. Schmidt RA, Lee TD. *Motor Control and Motor Learning: A Behavioral Emphasis.* 3rd ed. Champaign, IL: Human Kinetics; 1999.
60. Lehrer N, Attygalle S, Wolf SL, Rikakis T. Exploring the bases for a mixed reality stroke rehabilitation system, part I: a unified approach for representing action, quantitative evaluation, and interactive feedback. *J Neuroeng Rehabil.* 2011;8(1):51. doi:10.1186/1743-0003-8-51
61. Lehrer N, Chen Y, Duff M, L Wolf S, Rikakis T. Exploring the bases for a mixed reality stroke rehabilitation system, Part II: design of interactive feedback for upper limb rehabilitation. *J Neuroeng Rehabil.* 2011;8(1):54. doi:10.1186/1743-0003-8-54
62. Rikakis T. Utilizing media arts principles for developing effective interactive neurorehabilitation systems. *Conf Proc IEEE Eng Med Biol Soc.* 2011;2011:1391-1394. doi:10.1109/IEMBS.2011.6090327
63. Carr JH, Sheperd RB. *Neurological Rehabilitation: Optimizing Motor Performance.* Philadelphia, PA: Elsevier Limited; 1998.
64. Fairbrother JT, Laughlin DD, Nguyen TV. Self-controlled feedback facilitates motor learning in both high and low activity individuals. *Front Psychol.* 2012;3:323. doi:10.3389/fpsyg.2012.00323
65. O'Sullivan SB, Schmitz TJ. *Physical Rehabilitation: Assessment and Treatment.* 5th ed. Philadelphia, PA: FA Davis; 2007.
66. Hollands KL, Pelton TA, Tyson SF, Hollands MA, van Vliet PM. Interventions for coordination of walking following stroke: systematic review. *Gait Posture.* 2012;35(3):349-359. doi:10.1016/j.gaitpost.2011.10.355
67. Bernardi NF, Darainy M, Ostry DJ. Somatosensory Contribution to the Initial Stages of Human Motor Learning. *J Neurosci.* 2015;35:14316 LP-14326.
68. Komiyama T, Sato TR, O'Connor DH, et al. Learning-related fine-scale specificity imaged in motor cortex circuits of behaving mice. *Nature.* 2010;464(7292):1182-1186. doi:10.1038/nature08897
69. Petreanu L, Gutnisky DA, Huber D, et al. Activity in motor-sensory projections reveals distributed coding in somatosensation. *Nature.* 2012;489(7415):299-303. doi:10.1038/nature11321
70. Xu T, Yu X, Perlik AJ, et al. Rapid formation and selective stabilization of synapses for enduring motor memories. *Nature.* 2009;462(7275):915-919. doi:10.1038/nature08389
71. Yang G, Pan F, Gan WB. Stably maintained dendritic spines are associated with lifelong memories. *Nature.* 2009;462(7275):920-924. doi:10.1038/nature08577
72. Asboth L, Friedli L, Beauparlant J, et al. Cortico-reticulo-spinal circuit reorganization enables functional recovery after severe spinal cord contusion. *Nat Neurosci.* 2018;21(4):576-588. doi:10.1038/s41593-018-0093-5
73. Jain N, Qi HX, Collins CE, Kaas JH. Large-scale reorganization in the somatosensory cortex and thalamus after sensory loss in macaque monkeys. *J Neurosci.* 2008;28(43):11042-11060. doi:10.1523/JNEUROSCI.2334-08.2008
74. Jarosiewicz B, Chase SM, Fraser GW, Velliste M, Kass RE, Schwartz AB. Functional network reorganization during learning in a brain-computer interface paradigm. *Proc Natl Acad Sci USA.* 2008;105(49):19486-19491. doi:10.1073/pnas.0808113105
75. Johansson BB. Brain plasticity and stroke rehabilitation. The Willis lecture. *Stroke.* 2000;31(1):223-230. doi:10.1161/01.STR.31.1.223

76. Kambi N, Halder P, Rajan R, et al. Large-scale reorganization of the somatosensory cortex following spinal cord injuries is due to brainstem plasticity. *Nat Commun.* 2014;5(1):3602. doi:10.1038/ncomms4602
77. Nudo RJ. Functional and structural plasticity in motor cortex: implications for stroke recovery. *Phys Med Rehabil Clin N Am.* 2003;14(1)(suppl):S57-S76. doi:10.1016/S1047-9651(02)00054-2
78. Ward NS, Brown MM, Thompson AJ, Frackowiak RS. Neural correlates of motor recovery after stroke: a longitudinal fMRI study. *Brain.* 2003;126(Pt 11):2476-2496. doi:10.1093/brain/awg245
79. Das A, Franca JG, Gattass R, et al. The brain decade in debate: VI. Sensory and motor maps: dynamics and plasticity. *Braz J Med Biol Res.* 2001;34(12):1497-1508. doi:10.1590/S0100-879X2001001200001
80. Hoshino O. Neuronal bases of perceptual learning revealed by a synaptic balance scheme. *Neural Comput.* 2004;16(3):563-594. doi:10.1162/089976604772744910
81. Jackson PL, Lafleur MF, Malouin F, Richards C, Doyon J. Potential role of mental practice using motor imagery in neurologic rehabilitation. *Arch Phys Med Rehabil.* 2001;82(8):1133-1141. doi:10.1053/apmr.2001.24286
82. Kandel ER, Schwartz JH, Jessel TM, Siegelbaum SA, Hudspeth AJ. *Principles of Neural Science.* 5th ed. New York, NY: McGraw-Hill; 2012.
83. Arya KN, Verma R, Garg RK, Sharma VP, Agarwal M, Aggarwal GG. Meaningful task-specific training (MTST) for stroke rehabilitation: a randomized controlled trial. *Top Stroke Rehabil.* 2012;19(3):193-211. doi:10.1310/tsr1903-193
84. Kleim JA, Jones TA. Principles of experience-dependent neural plasticity: implications for rehabilitation after brain damage. *J Speech Lang Hear Res.* 2008;51(1):S225-S239. doi:10.1044/1092-4388(2008/018)

Please visit www.routledge.com/9781630915650 to access additional material.

Chapter 5
Intervention Procedures

Darcy A. Umphred, PT, PhD, FAPTA and Jan Black, PT, MSPT

KEY WORDS Augmented interventions | Evidence-based intervention | Functional training | Impairment training | Motor programs | Patient participation in quality of life activities | Priming the nervous system | Sensory retraining

Chapter Objectives

- Distinguish among intervention categories, including functional training, impairment training, hands-on guidance, robotics, virtual reality, and sensory or somatosensory retraining.
- Recognize when an intervention is not resulting in progression toward stated goals.
- Recognize successful and independent performance of functional activity.
- Understand the role of self-motivated participation training in optimizing patient quality of life.
- Identify and use different learning environments to optimize patient participation.

Intervention, as defined in the *Guide to Physical Therapist Practice*, is "purposeful and skilled interaction of the (physical therapist) with the patient/client to produce change."[1] Although the definition of intervention continues to define the role of the physical therapist, intervention is intertwined in the role of the physical therapist assistant. To the physical therapist, intervention incorporates the following: coordination, communication, and documentation of services; patient- or client-related instruction; and direct patient intervention. Within these 3 categories, coordination of services is the only area that should never be delegated to the physical therapist assistant. Therefore, the physical therapist assistant needs to develop skills in communication with the physical therapist, other health care practitioners, the patient, and caregivers.

Documentation skills, when appropriately delegated, are a critical form of communication with other individuals on the patient's team and with outside organizations such as accreditation organizations and third-party payers.[2] All documentation done by the physical therapist assistant needs to be co-signed by the physical therapist, which clearly shows that communications are open. Although portions of the reexamination could be part of the physical therapist assistant's delegated responsibilities, it is not within the role of the physical therapist assistant to interpret the examination results unless the physical therapist has clearly identified a plan of care that incorporates change in relation to patient test results. The physical therapist assistant begins practice with intervention, and then may be asked to follow up with reexamination using the original tools or other methods of examination. It is within the physical therapist assistant's scope of practice to teach patients and families functional skills; use of adaptive equipment such as walkers, canes, braces, robotics, and other augmented devices; home programs; and discharge programs only if the physical therapist has taken the responsibility of clearly identifying what those skills or programs are.

Within the framework of physical therapist assistant practice, intervention precedes reexamination. This book reflects that same model, and thus this chapter precedes the chapter on examination. Specific examinations procedures for movement dysfunctions can be found within

Lazaro RT, Umphred DA, eds.
Umphred's Neurorehabilitation for the Physical Therapist Assistant, Third Edition (pp 83-125).

specific chapters regarding medical diagnoses that cause those movement problems. The physical therapist assistant should not be asked to perform an initial examination on the patient and interpret the result, to establish the initial treatment protocol, or to determine that the patient no longer needs service. The physical therapist assistant may be asked to perform follow-up examinations and to write a discharge summary and follow-up recommendations, as long as the physical therapist co-signs that information. Clearly differentiating actions that are the physical therapist's responsibility and those that can be delegated to a physical therapist assistant are legally binding according to state laws. If the physical therapist assistant is asked to perform activities that are outside the physical therapist assistant's scope of practice, then it could place the patient (consumer of a product) at risk, and both the physical therapist and the physical therapist assistant can be held liable. Given the previous scenario, a physical therapist assistant would be misused, and the patient would be given an incorrect perception of the services being provided. This particular issue, with the problems it creates, is becoming a basis for claims denial, malpractice, and consumer fraud.

It is the physical therapist assistant's responsibility to identify the proper scope of practice, and to recognize when the patient is at risk, even when components of intervention have been delegated. The primary role of the physical therapist assistant within the therapeutic community is direct intervention with the patient under the direction of the physical therapist. It is appropriate to delegate treatment interventions to the physical therapist assistant when the services of the physical therapist assistant will positively affect patient progress and when the role of either physical therapist or physical therapist assistant would, similarly, enhance that progress. It is not unusual that part of the intervention would be delegated while other parameters stay within the scope of the physical therapist.

Physical therapy interventions encompass a vast area of techniques that incorporate interactions with the cardiopulmonary, integumentary, musculoskeletal, and neuromuscular systems.[1] Although the specific pathology or disease identified by the physician may fall within one of these body systems, physical therapists and physical therapist assistants do not treat disease or pathology; rather, they treat the impairments, activity limitations, and participation restrictions caused by those diseases or pathologies. For that reason, similar physical therapy techniques may be used for multiple medical diagnoses, or multiple physical therapy interventions may be incorporated into a patient's treatment plan although that individual has one specific disease. For the physical therapist assistant to identify risk factors or contraindications and abnormal signs exhibited by the patient during a physical therapy session, knowledge of human anatomy, physiology, and disease processes is always an important part of the physical therapist assistant's education.

It is the primary responsibility of the physical therapist, when delegating portions of the plan of care to the physical therapist assistant, to have adequate knowledge of the patient's status and abilities, as well as the abilities of the physical therapist assistant to whom patient care is being delegated. To assist physical therapists as well as physical therapist assistants in understanding the complex decision-making required to determine that direct patient intervention can be delegated to a physical therapist assistant, the American Physical Therapy Association has created a physical therapist assistant Direction Algorithm (Figure 5-1). Physical therapist assistants can use this algorithm to identify areas of change or uncertainty regarding the patient's status, ranging from the scope of physical therapist assistant work, patient condition, specific outcomes to be addressed by direct physical therapist assistant intervention, abilities/knowledge/skills of the physical therapist assistant, liabilities and risk, and payers. Often, especially in people with neurological dysfunction, changes in the patient's presentation or medical status may be first noted by the physical therapist assistant during an intervention. It is the physical therapist assistant's responsibility to report to the physical therapist any questionable behaviors of the patient at the beginning of, during, or at the conclusion of an intervention. If the physical therapist assistant has any question or concern regarding the health of the patient and/or appropriateness of the intervention itself, that physical therapist assistant is bound by law and ethics to communicate that concern to the physical therapist as quickly as possible. For that reason, the physical therapist assistant is often asked to check heart rate, blood pressure, skin color, pain levels, depth and rate of breathing, levels of consciousness, and cognitive response patterns of patients. These assessments become a part of ongoing intervention and are discussed in Chapter 6 on examination. Before the patient interventions are delegated, the physical therapist has the legal responsibility to check all contraindications and risk factors to guarantee that the patient can safely receive treatment. Even though this check should make the physical therapist assistant feel safe that a patient will not be harmed by intervention, monitoring patient signs is a critical component to maintaining that safety parameter.

This text discusses patients and clients who have had some form of central nervous system (CNS) disease, pathology, or trauma with resultant motor dysfunction. The chapter on motor learning and motor control provides important background information on how individuals learn a motor skill and how therapeutic interventions can be optimized to facilitate return of function. Specific intervention recommendations for specific medical diagnoses can be found in Chapters 8 through 19 of this text. In addition, a chapter on cardiopulmonary impact on motor dysfunction will also lead the physical therapist assistant to avenues of intervention interactions, strategies, and ways to enhance patient performance (see Chapter 16). The concept of intervention through direct patient contact will be

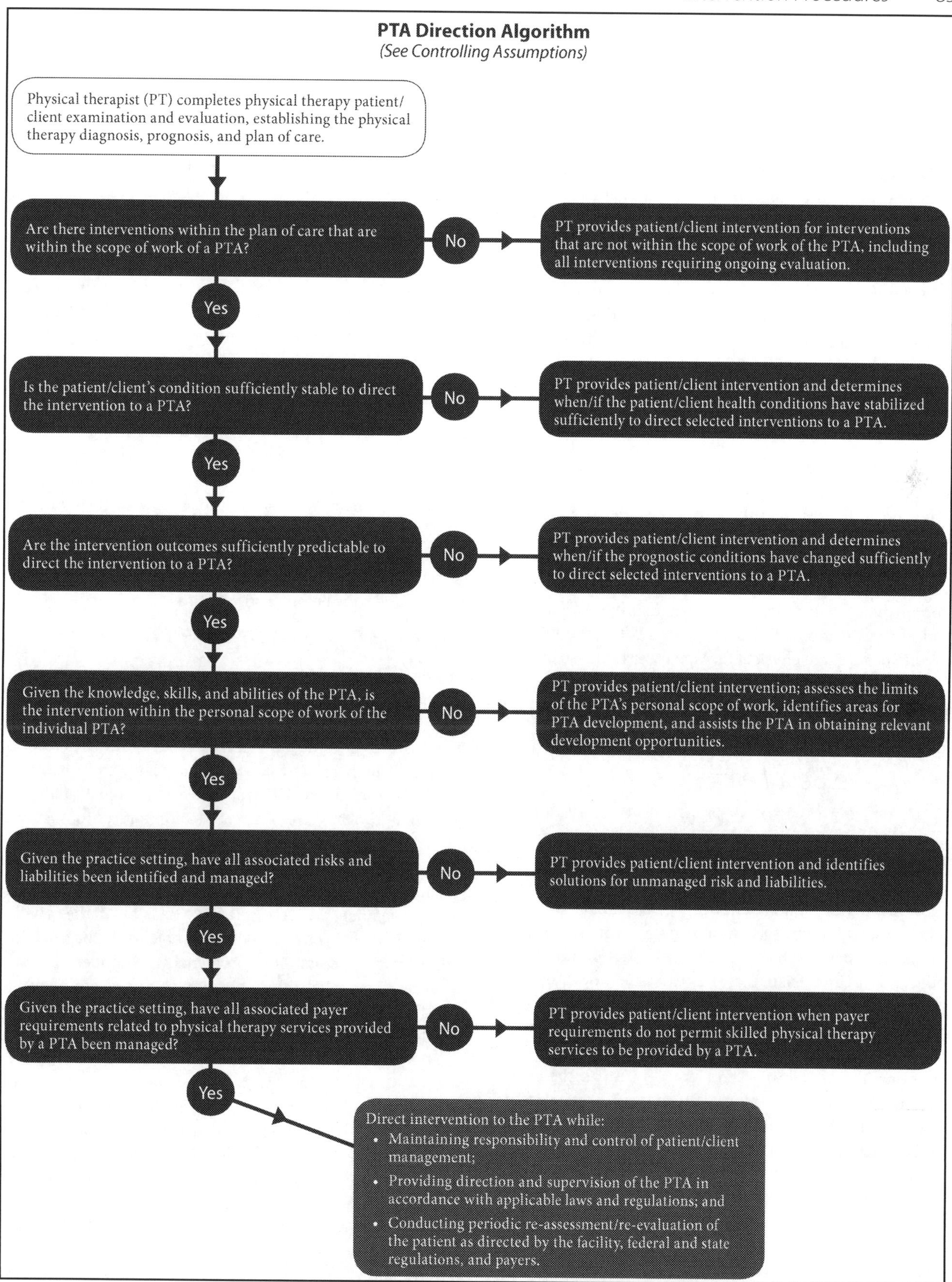

Figure 5-1. Algorithm used to determine whether an intervention should be delegated to the physical therapist assistant. (Reprinted from www.apta.org/PTinMotion/2010/9/PTAsToday, with permission of the American Physical Therapy Association. Copyright © 2010 American Physical Therapy Association.)

the focus of this chapter. In Chapter 18 of this book, additional discussions of alternative intervention strategies and approaches considered as complementary therapies are also presented to widen the physical therapist assistant's understanding of possible intervention strategies. To gain skills in any of these complementary therapies, additional education is needed before application is appropriate. Within this third edition of this text, new relevant chapters will also help the physical therapist practitioner in neurorehabilitation. The physical therapist assistant may not be asked to work in acute care, with technology, or with chronic illnesses today, but the possibility of moving into those areas is realistic. Thus, all therapeutic tools should be considered as part of the physical therapist assistant's toolbox.

Designing Successful Interventions: Things to Consider

The ultimate goal of any physical therapy intervention is to optimize activity and participation and help the patient achieve the highest quality of life possible. Interventions must be thoughtfully designed, carefully monitored, and assessed for effectiveness. When designing these interventions, the physical therapist needs to consider the patient's cognitive understanding of the task, and the patient's attitude or motivation toward the activity. To maintain this quality of care, the physical therapist assistant also needs to be able to understand the cognitive and the emotional level at which the patient interacts.

Cognitive Understanding of the Task: How One Best Learns

There are areas of CNS processing that are not considered motor but directly affect motor performance. Perception, levels of consciousness, and distractibility all affect motor control. The perceptual problems and residual movement dysfunction following CNS damage are huge. The physical therapist assistant is not expected to evaluate or analyze these problems and their impact on movement, but rather to appreciate that they exist and how they affect the presented movement problems. For example, if a patient post-head injury overshoots a target and then self-corrects to the target, it is a perceptual problem (praxis) and falls into the area of cognitive problems. If instead the patient tries to self-correct the movement throughout a trajectory toward the target, it is a motor control problem (ataxia) and a sign of cerebellar involvement. The physical therapist assistant needs to recognize the difference between these 2 movement problems, but the physical therapist needs to determine the interpretation of its consequences. The physical therapist assistant needs to recognize when the patient changes behaviors or motor responses, and whether those responses seem better or worse than when first observed, then communicate those changes to the physical therapist. The causation of the changes could be perceptual learning and improvement, motor control itself, or some other problem, but that determination is not the physical therapist assistant's responsibility.

One additional cognitive area the physical therapist assistant should consider when working with a patient is how both the therapist and the patient learn, or their *preferred learning style*. You as a clinician enjoy learning, and often in specific ways. Some of you love to read, while others of you would rather be out playing a physical activity, while still others would prefer visualizing how to interpret art or some beautiful scene in the wild. These styles often reflect whether you prefer to use language and think linearly, use kinesthesis and learn about the world through those feelings, or use spatial thought and visualize many things at the same time. Your patients are no different, except that they have CNS problems and many may not be as adaptable at using alternative learning styles. So, talk to your patients, ask them what they like to do for enjoyment, such as reading, gold panning, or bird watching; and what they do for work, such as being a teacher, a bank teller, a writer, an artist, or an engineer. Each one of those answers gives you, the physical therapist assistant, a window into how that person thinks and what modalities (eg, language, movement itself, or demonstration) might make the learning easier for the patient, and thus be more successful.

Attitude Toward the Activity

The patient's emotional system plays a key role in regulation of muscle tone, in adherence to performance of the activity, in the belief of the importance of the activity and its relationship to life, and in his or her confidence toward the physical therapist assistant as a health care provider. Similarly, the physical therapist assistant must acknowledge that those 4 areas affect the motor responses and attitudes of the practitioner. Throughout a stressful day, many individuals, including patients and practitioners, radiate tension into their shoulders and necks, which a family member can recognize at the end of the day. A patient who has motor control problems to begin with will often exaggerate those problems when under pressure or upset. These behaviors are not triggered consciously; it is the emotional system's response to the interactions, whether it is increased tension after a day of work or exaggerated movements following an interactive day. Similarly, when individuals are depressed, their motor system is also depressed, and movement is more difficult and tiring. The physical therapist assistant needs to be aware of the emotional responses of individuals during therapy. Many times, following CNS insults, patients have less control of their emotional reactions; thus, they may get angry more easily, cry more often, and laugh inappropriately. Many of these patients recognize the behaviors as inappropriate but cannot control the emotional or limbic system. It is very important that the physical therapist assistant create environments within which the patient can develop motor control of the neuromuscular and the emotional environment.

If lack of success in a task creates anger, then it may be important for the physical therapist assistant to articulate and highlight what the patient did right and was successful in performing, rather than the mistakes that the patient made. Understanding the emotional reactions of a patient and the stimulus that triggered that response, and determining whether it helps or hurts the learning, is a skill that all clinicians need to develop. If, during a transfer, a therapist demands that a patient stand up, the patient may stand due to feeling angry, feeling disempowered or humiliated and being treated like a child, or just wanting the activity to finish so the therapist will go away. The patient's emotional reaction will create extensor tone, and that tone will help generate the force needed to stand, but teaching someone to stand on top of anger or another strong emotional response means that every time the individual wants to stand, that emotional reaction will need to be triggered.

By controlling the noise, distractions, and rate of success or failure, the physical therapist assistant can allow the patient to practice the movement activities successfully, without the influence of the emotional system. Once the motor programs are established, reintroducing emotional and perceptual challenges can be integrated into the functional activity as impairment training. The physical therapist assistant is responsible for carrying out the established program designed by the physical therapist. When the patient is ready or the CNS seems capable of handling additional stress, the physical therapist assistant should recognize that information and give it to the physical therapist. The decision to change the environment and make it more complex is the physical therapist's responsibility, unless the physical therapist assistant has been given clear parameters to identify and document specific changes in behavior and the activity or components to be changed. Patients will go through phases of adjustment to their respective CNS disease or trauma. Similarly, families will be going through adjustments. There is no guarantee that the patient, the family, or the health care providers will be adjusting in a similar manner or time sequence. Thus, the physical therapist assistant needs to have some understanding of how adjustments or emotional liability affects motor performance (see Chapter 7). Interacting with the patient in a friendly, respectful way helps the patient feel respected and seen as a person, and not a system problem with movement dysfunction.[3]

Priming the Nervous System

New evidence, being presented at conference as well as in literature, suggests that the nervous system benefits from being primed before interventions are initiated.[4-7] Byl stressed that the brain has plasticity throughout our lifetime, but one critical factor to plasticity is maintaining our physical, emotional, and cognitive balance throughout that time frame.[4] Although the causations of disease may be genetic, environmental, or habit, regaining that balance can at least begin to reestablish the potential for positive change. Thus, exercising the physical body, eating a balanced diet, challenging cognitive thought processes through fun activities, and approaching life with a positive attitude no matter what can lead to priming the nervous system to growth and change.

As a physical therapist assistant, you have an opportunity to encourage your patients to participate in life. You can show them the positive attitude toward engaging in physical activities, which promotes cardiovascular and pulmonary health along with engaging the nervous system in repair. Thus, your attitude toward each day will affect the emotional health of your patients and can facilitate both your and their neuroplasticity in the present and the future. To keep the brain priming for motor, emotional, or cognitive learning, all individuals in the environment need to be having fun, enjoying the learning, and actively interacting and participating.[4]

Dosing in Treatment of Patients With Movement Dysfunction

At present, there is no substantial research to guide physical therapists or physical therapist assistants when treating neurological movement problems across the age spectrum. Some discussion of dosage can be found in the literature and is often delineated by the age of the individual and the movement dysfunction.

Specific dosage indication for the pediatric population cannot be identified due to the complexity of the specific patient population. Pediatric physical therapy promotes independence, increases participation, facilitates motor development and function, improves strength and endurance, enhances learning opportunities, and eases challenges with daily caregiving. However, the specific treatments will focus upon the type of physical therapy practice setting and the specific needs of the child. Whether the treatment is for an acute condition, a long-term medical problem, or a progressive neurological condition will also play a factor in dosage recommended and the treatment protocol selected, such as constraint-induced therapy, bracing and orthotics, use of high-tech equipment, or therapeutic horseback riding (see Chapters 9 and 10). The pediatric section has developed some guidelines for colleagues treating children in the school systems,[8] but consideration then must be made whether the child is being treated for medical or health-related movement problems, or for educational reasons, which then fall under the individual education plan and within the law according to the Individual Disability Education Act. The physical therapist assistant will need to depend upon the physical therapist to determine specific dosage for each child.

For the young adult, middle-aged, and geriatric populations, specific dosage for specific movement dysfunctions after identification of a movement problem from a neurological condition have yet to be clearly identified, reported, or established for reliability and validity, although national health organizations are looking into these questions. The

Box 5-1

Additional National Resources Regarding Interventions and Potential Guidelines

- Physical Therapy. https://multiplesclerosis.net/treatment/physical%20-therapy/
- Post-Stroke Rehabilitation. https://stroke.nih.gov/materials/rehabilitation.htm
- Guidebook on Parkinson's Disease. https://www.medifocus.com/parkinsonsMedifocus
- Practice and Patient Care. https://www.apta.org/Practice/
- Research & Training. https://www.nih.gov/research-training

physical therapist assistant will depend upon the physical therapist for guidance in this area until clear protocols have been established, tested, researched, and reported in the literature. Today, state laws, insurance mandates, location of the services, and needs of the patient will continue to guide any dosage recommendations vs available research. The physical therapist can always seek out national organizations to read and understand where this concept is going and whether new guidelines have been developed (Box 5-1).

Categories of Intervention

Delegated intervention to a physical therapist assistant will fall within 1 of 5 categories, each having a slightly different focus:

1. Functional activity training
2. Impairment training
3. Hands-on guidance by the therapist or the use of augmented equipment
4. Somatosensory retraining
5. Participation training

The first 3 categories primarily reflect function within the motor system and movement dysfunction of the patient. The fourth category encompasses individuals with sensory or processing problems that result in motor dysfunction. The fifth area addresses life and those activities the individual values and wants to participate in during the transition from rehabilitation back to life's demands and activities. If the goal of physical therapy treatment is purposeful and meaningful functional movement activities, then the ultimate goal of every treatment program should be empowering the patient to achieve independent functional control over movement within the respective environment whenever possible. It is just as much the physical therapist assistant's responsibility to identify competencies in intervention procedures as it is for the physical therapist to acknowledge those competencies when delegating intervention within the plan of care. If the physical therapist assistant is unfamiliar or lacks the necessary skills to provide the identified interventions, then it is important to discuss that with the physical therapist and ask for assistance or guidance within any specific area.

Functional Training

Functional training interventions focus on 3 areas: activities of daily living (ADL), such as bed mobility or ambulation; instrumental activities of daily living (IADL), which include activities that an individual does after waking up, dressing, and eating, such as shopping, using a computer or phone, cooking, and managing money or medications; and participation and leisure activities that are self-selected and considered to give a person quality of life, such as group activities (eg, attending worship services, and going shopping), group sports (eg, basketball, baseball, shuffle board, and pickle ball), individual sports (eg, golfing, swimming, running, and fly fishing), and group or individual physical enhancement activities (eg, martial arts training, water aerobics, treadmill, and elliptical training). All 3 areas fall within the category of functional training. When intervention focuses on specific activities, the patient needs repetitive practice of that activity to regain or maintain skill in the functional motor strategies needed to perform the activity (see Chapter 4). If the goals of the intervention include performance of any one of these skills, then the functional motor plan is already available to the patient, and only practice and variance within the environment is needed for perfection. In this case, a physical therapist should definitely delegate this activity to the physical therapist assistant. As the patient improves skill in these activities, delegation may be given to family members or caregivers, when those people are available and willing.

Functional training in ADL includes achieving bed mobility, coming to sit and stand from surfaces, transferring onto and from chairs (eg, a wheelchair [w/c] or a toilet), transferring into and out of a shower or tub, ambulation on all types of surfaces with visual environments (eg, normal lighting, darkened environment, or a crowded street), dressing and undressing, and using ambulatory aids (eg, crutches, a cane, or a walker with or without a brace or exoskeleton). In a home health environment, the physical therapist assistant may be asked to perform additional functional training, such as teaching and practicing bathing, eating, and cooking. However, more often, the occupational therapist and/or a certified occupational therapy assistant will be responsible for the patient's practice with these activities. The goal of functional activity training is not to guide the patient with the hands-on skill of the therapist, but rather to guarantee that the patient is performing these activities safely and with repetitive practice. Repetitive and random practice schedules will solidify responses to these activities as automatic, with the patient no longer needing to think through the steps of the movement and, instead, performing the activity without effort in a feedforward program (see Chapter 4).

Many times, patients will desire a high level of motor performance as their goal and become frustrated that the treatment program focuses on activities that individuals assume they can do or should be able to do. For example, if an individual wants to return to fly fishing at his cabin on a lake, determining how he will get from his cabin to the beach and whether he will sit or stand while fishing will help the therapist communicate to the patient why he is practicing sit-to-stand and ambulation activities. Once the patient understands that practice will lead to the ultimate goal of fly fishing, the individual usually becomes motivated and adherent. Having patients determine what activities they view as part of normal life will generally generate individuals who no longer think of these activities as therapy but rather as life choices. Functional training should be the ultimate goal of any sequential treatment plan. Understanding the components critical for any functional movement leads to the second category of intervention strategies.

When a physical therapist assistant is practicing functional training, the entire movement may be broken down into smaller components, with the easiest aspects practiced first to have the patient realize that the activity is possible, and success is within reach. For example, if independent sit-to-stand-and-back-to-sit is identified as a goal in the plan of care, the physical therapist assistant has the option of how the patient will initially practice that activity. The activity could begin once the patient was assisted to stand by having him first begin to lower his body onto a bar stool or a chair or a high/low table or mat that has been raised up. This type of activity decreases the need for full power, postural integrity, and changing from relaxed sitting in flexion to standing with postural stability.

Once the patient can lower onto the edge of the higher stool or mat and reverse the motion and come to stand, 3 additional aspects of the activity can be changed. First, the object used as a chair/mat can be lowered so additional range and power are required to accomplish the activity. Second, the patient can be asked to lower to sit, relax on the edge, and then come back to stand. Third, the patient can be asked to lower to the seat, move back into sitting, and then come back to stand. Each of these activities creates additional demands on the motor system and enlarges the patient's ability to gain control over that specific movement pattern of coming to standing and reversing the activity with control.

All functional activities need core body stability or postural stabilization to hold the body in space as the individual moves from one functional position to another, as well as maintaining the body against gravity when just sitting or standing. Thus, teaching the individual to move the trunk and lower limb or trunk and upper limb combines an extremity with the trunk, which provides the postural or core stabilization. Rolling requires head, upper body, and trunk as a pattern for rolling or when leading from the lower extremity (LE) using with one leg that goes into hip flexion and internal rotation along with knee flexion as the trunk and head follow the movement. These patterns teach bed mobility. Often the patient needs to begin normal functional movement while in sitting vs supine before being independent in the category of bed mobility because of the tone problems in the supine position that arise after CNS deficits. For that reason, functional training may need to begin in vertical sitting. This position provides the greatest base of support (BOS) outside of horizontal and the least amount of power needed to maintain the trunk in an erect posture. Having the patient work on small postural adjustments off vertical while using an upper extremity (UE) to reach toward a target, or rotating across the chest to touch something on the other side, will strengthen the muscles being activated. These movements also incorporate balance activities when sitting and require the integration of an upper limb with the trunk movement. Similar activities can be performed with the LE by asking the patient to shift weight and begin to stand up or reach one leg across the other toward a target. As a functional activity, the physical therapist assistant should be observing movement that looks normal and integrated. The range of motion (ROM) can be enlarged as the patient initiates and controls postural adjustment off midline until the patient can go from sit to supine or sit-to-stand. If these activities trigger abnormal tone, then potential impairment training may be needed before the patient would be expected to control normal movement from one spatial position to another.

Progressing the Functional Training Activities: Rate of Movement and the Ability to Alter Rate

As individuals grow and learn to control their functional movements, they simultaneously learn to control the rate or speed of those movements. For example, as children learn to walk, they also learn to walk slower and faster. As the rate increases, the walking will turn into running. A physical therapist assistant may be instructed to teach a patient walking using a walker. Initially, the patient will walk very slowly and should progress to better control and a faster progression. With CNS damage and relearning, often the patient is taught to walk while cognitively thinking about each aspect of the program: pick up the walker, step with the right foot, pick up the walker, and then step with the left foot. As the patient has never walked with a walker, this is a new motor program. The physical therapist assistant needs to remember that the patient once had a rate of walking that was normal for that individual. It might have been as slow as the movement when using the walker, but more often, it would have been faster. If the physical therapist assistant needs to impairment-train in this area, then the patient needs to practice the movement at various speeds. This impairment training can be accomplished by using a metronome or a forced stepping environment such as a treadmill, or by the physical therapist assistant holding onto the walker and pulling the patient forward, triggering a stepping reaction to increase the rate of the walking.

Impairment Training

This category is associated with interventions that are system-specific and that focus on a component of a movement that has resulted in dysfunction within the functional activity. This area of treatment has many subcategories. Impairments may be the direct result of musculoskeletal problems such as ROM limitations, muscle weakness due to disuse, biomechanical misalignment due to joint problems, or leg-length discrepancy. A plan of care that eliminates or minimizes these impairments certainly would be appropriate to delegate to a physical therapist assistant.

Similarly, cardiopulmonary or peripheral vascular disease can create many types of pain, poor endurance to exercise, and even lightheadedness and confusion when the oxygen levels drop. For that reason, the physical therapist assistant will often be asked to monitor breathing, heart rate, blood pressure, and oxygen saturation level using a fingertip oximeter and pain scales, regardless of the patient's medical diagnosis. If physical therapist assistants ever have concerns about the cardiopulmonary/peripheral vascular system, they should communicate those concerns to the physical therapist of record. If that physical therapist is unavailable, concerns should be shared with another physical therapist, nurse, or physician.

Areas of integumentary problems encompass medical complications from ulcers, burns, or reddened areas, or any unusual reactions of the skin before, during, or following a therapeutic intervention. These impairments are especially important to understand if the patient is being asked to practice specific activities that entail movement across a surface (eg, rolling, coming to sit, or sitting for an extended period of time). Similarly, if a scar limits ROM and thus movement function itself, then interventions that mobilize the tissue using therapeutic modalities to increase tissue elasticity may be delegated to the physical therapist assistant. The physical therapist assistant must then be aware that those modalities can also burn the patient, especially if the skin or vascular system cannot accommodate the modality. Patients with long-term contractures following CNS injury often have skin integrity problems. The skin becomes very fragile and thin, and thus splits easily if ROM over the joint creates too much stretch at too high a rate. If the skin splits at the joint, it will cause not only pain but also an open wound. The physical therapist assistant will need to work slowly and pay constant attention to the skin reaction when treating most patients with contractures and limited skin mobility after neurological insults.

Interventions to Improve Joint Mobility (Range of Motion)

In many physical therapy clinics, exercises that improve joint ROM are delegated to a physical therapist assistant. When the only limitation is musculoskeletal, the complexity and skill of performing ROM on a patient need not be difficult. However, when treating a patient with ROM limitation possibly secondary to a neurological dysfunction, a variety of parameters must be considered before delegation:

- During the ROM, does the joint stay in a correct biomechanical position throughout the range?
- Is the limitation of range due to hypertonicity around the joint? If so, what muscles are hypertonic and how are they interacting in patterns of movement? With introduction of a rotatory pattern, can the limb be moved into and out of the areas of limitation?
- What rotatory patterns are limited? If rotation is incorporated into the ROM exercise, does the hypertonicity decrease? If so, does the patient have a stable joint, or are muscles around the joint hypotonic?

The physical therapist should consider these questions before delegating this activity. Once the responsibility has been delegated, the physical therapist assistant should continue to ask these questions. When the range increases and/or the tone around the joint changes, the physical therapist assistant should report that change to the physical therapist, and potential intervention strategies for impairment training may need to be modified.

The physical therapist assistant must always remember to stabilize the joint throughout the motion. The physical therapist assistant must make sure the pattern of motion used by the patient to perform the activity is normal without substitutions of muscles not normally engaged during the specific motion. The physical therapist assistant may be asked to instruct the patient to perform the activity within a certain degree of motion and to slowly increase that range as the patient demonstrates normal motor control. If the patient complains of pain, often the cause of pain is misalignment of the joint, and this can be corrected by moving the joint into a better biomechanical position. As long as the patient is able to correct the joint alignment, then the physical therapist assistant is impairment training. Once the physical therapist assistant does the correction for the patient, it is no longer impairment training but hands-on intervention. Fear of pain during ROM often causes muscle splinting, which leads to incorrect alignment of the joint(s). That fear is often associated with the memory of some other health care practitioner having moved the limb when the patient did not have any control. That movement might then create an initial pain response as well as the memory of the experience. The physical therapist assistant needs to teach the patient that pain is not acceptable and that the patient needs to tell the practitioner when it hurts. The physical therapist assistant must recognize a pain grimace response in addition to requesting verbal communication of pain. If the patient is being assisted through part of the range that may have pain, the patient must trust that the physical therapist assistant will stop once pain is present. If not, the patient will continue splinting or guarding the joint. Gaining the patient's trust often results in eliminating splinting because of fear of pain and simultaneously causes a gain in ROM.

Interventions to Improve Neuromuscular System Impairments

Impairments within the neuromuscular system include activity states of the spinal motor generators (eg, hyper- or hypotonicity and rigidity), stereotypic or reflexive patterns within functional movement (eg, flexion and extension synergies, reflexive response such as asymmetrical and symmetrical tonic neck reflexes, and positive supporting reactions), resting fluctuation in motor tonicity (eg, non-intentional tremor), fluctuation in motor tonicity on purposeful activity (eg, athetosis or ataxia), balance problems (eg, sensory input and balance synergy problems), reaction time to perturbations, rate of movement (ie, how fast or slow the CNS will run a program), cognitive understanding of the task (eg, perception, levels of consciousness, and distractibility), and attitude toward the activity (eg, motivation, levels of emotional stability, and ethnic bias). A brief description and some intervention suggestions will be included within each subsection of this practice pattern.

States of the Spinal Motor Generators (Hyper- or Hypotonicity and Rigidity)

A common impairment seen in patients with CNS damage is an altered state of the spinal motor generators. This altered state can create movement dysfunctions. When the motor generators are firing at too high a rate, the result will create muscle reactions that are hypertonic and/or reactive to stretch. Usually, when these generators are firing and causing hypertonicity, the response is not seen in an individual muscle, but rather is seen in patterns of muscle interactions referred to as synergies. An agonist, or isolated muscle, is naturally linked to other muscles (*agonistic synergy*) that work closely with a particular muscle to perform specific functional movements.

Similarly, if the generators are not firing adequately in one muscle group, then the behavioral response will often be hypotonicity within a pattern of movement. Except in specific peripheral nervous system injury or disease, behavior responses are more likely to be seen in patterns. At times, a limb may have a hypertonic agonistic synergy, while the antagonistic synergy is hypotonic or seems low-toned or weak. If both the agonistic synergy and the antagonistic synergy are hypertonic, then movement in both directions is limited, and the person may exhibit rigidity. Hypertonicity is an abnormal state of the motor generators and usually follows hypotonicity within muscle groups and instability of the joint. Because of hypotonicity, the body will naturally try to maintain joint integrity and create additional tone in other muscles around the joint structure. Instructing the patient to perform slow, relaxing rotation away from the tight pattern, along with deep breathing, often lowers the state of the motor pool and decreases the hypertonicity. An example may be seen in a patient with Parkinson's disease who demonstrates trunk rigidity. An appropriate intervention that the physical therapist assistant can perform is having the patient in hook-lying position, then performing slow and gentle lower trunk rotations to decrease tone, in preparation for functional activities such as rolling, coming to sit, transfers, and ambulation.

The physical therapist assistant must remember that decreasing hypertonicity does not guarantee stability of the joint(s) or volitional control over movement. Many times, decreasing hypertonicity forces the therapist into a hands-on approach to intervention vs impairment training because of the decreased state of the motor pool resulting in hypotonicity or weakness and joint instability.

Stereotypic or Reflexive Patterns Within Functional Movement

Patients' movement responses following CNS injury often include stereotypic or reflexive patterns of movement (eg, flexion and extension synergies, reflexive response such as asymmetrical and symmetrical tonic neck reflexes, and supporting reactions such as coming up on the toes and ball of the foot instead of standing with pressure through the heel). These programs are often the only patterns available to the patient's CNS when an external or peripheral stimulus demands or requires a motor response. Similarly, when neuronal loops within the CNS trigger involuntary motor response patterns, the motor system drives those available programs. Thus, individuals in lowered states of consciousness may exhibit hypertonic synergistic patterns of motor responses (eg, extension synergies incorporating hip and knee extension, internal rotation, adduction of the hip, plantarflexion, and pronation of the foot). Most synergies and reflexive patterns are inherent or preprogrammed within the CNS and have been incorporated and integrated within the CNS in early motor development. These patterns reflect combinations of movement patterns in response to demands placed on the CNS from peripheral input systems and internal feedback loops. Specific reflex responses are identified in Chapter 6. Specific impairment training techniques that discourage repetitive practice of these stereotypic patterns can be found in Chapters 8 through 17. An easy concept to remember is that the opposite movement pattern from the involuntary pattern is often the solution to gaining or regaining motor control. Adding rotation away from either synergy pattern can lead to more functional movement. By activating the antagonistic synergy, the hypertonic synergy or reflex pattern will often automatically be dampened through the interaction of motor programs within the CNS.

The physical therapist assistant must be cautioned that by triggering the antagonistic synergy, what may happen is just a shift from one synergy to another. If the patient is able to independently run these antagonistic programs or components of these programs, then the therapeutic environment is considered impairment training. The patient's CNS must be able to control both agonistic and antagonistic synergy patterns and combinations of muscle patterns within those synergies to move to functional training. If the patient's motor programming is stuck in synergy or stereotypic patterns, the patient will be limited in responses to the demands of life. These stereotypic patterns often force the biomechanical position of joints to be misaligned, leading to future secondary musculoskeletal impairments.

A physical therapy goal will generally encompass reduction of hypertonicity and obligatory responses of stereotypic programs. The physical therapist assistant needs to remember that the causation of hypertonicity synergies is often instability within joint structures. Similarly, the use of reflexive or stereotypic patterns is the CNS's response to environmental demands, which require gravitational postural responses. To empower the patient's CNS to gain or regain the fluid control over multiple patterns of movement, the environment must be modified so that the response can be appropriate to the demand within the environment. This may require environmental adaptation and/or hands-on guidance to guarantee the CNS is in control of the programs, regardless of how limiting that might be early in the therapeutic intervention process. Again, if by adapting or limiting the environment the patient is capable of initiating and maintaining a normal movement sequence, then the physical therapist assistant is impairment training. Once the physical therapist assistant adds hands-on control of the movement itself, the activity is no longer impairment training, and then falls under the next section for categories of intervention.

Resting Fluctuation in Motor Tonicity (Nonintentional Tremor)

Patients with diseases within the basal ganglia or associated pathways often have what is referred to as *resting tremors* in the hands, tongue, and even the feet. Within the hands, this nonintentional movement is often referred to as a pin-rolling pattern (see Chapter 14). Whether the patterns are in the hands, feet, or tongue, these movements are involuntary and in a specific flowing movement pattern and illustrate a lack of control or inhibition by the CNS to some automatic motor programming. The tremors are often exaggerated when the patient has strong emotional reactions to the environment, but sometimes can be controlled upon intentional movement. Often, the tremors can be decreased with slow, deep breathing; visualization by the patient of a relaxing environment (eg, picturing a waterfall or watching the wave action of the ocean); and weight-bearing of the extremities. Nonintentional tremors usually do not limit function. The patient must determine whether the movement is socially limiting. Refer to Chapter 14 for specific recommendations for intervention ideas for individuals with basal ganglia movement type problems.

Fluctuation in Motor Tonicity Upon Purposeful Activity

Patients who have cerebellar problems or motor control problems associated with cerebellar disease may exhibit fluctuation in muscle tone when moving. If a patient lacks the postural programming to stabilize the joints during movement but has the power and range to generate the movement program, the patient will have problems controlling the rate or speed of the movement and the ability to slow down or reverse the movement during functional activities. Thus, the physical therapist assistant will observe a lack of axial and trunk stabilization when the patient is moving, especially when the distal segment is non–weight-bearing, such as the swing phase of gait. Movements often seem too powerful for the activity, and the patient often overshoots the target.

The movements themselves are less exaggerated during weight-bearing activities because of the increase in proprioceptive input through approximation and the normal postural patterns required. For that reason, patients can practice movements with weighted vests or exercise tubing to add resistance and compression during activities such as reaching or during the swing phase of gait. If the patients can put on or don the weighted vest or belt themselves and the physical therapist assistant is to observe and guard during the activity, this intervention would be impairment training. If the physical therapist assistant needs to apply the resistance and/or compression during a movement, then it is hands-on intervention and not considered impairment training. Hands-on intervention can lead to impairment training, which in turn can lead to functional independence as long as the functional activity is practiced and incorporated into life activities.

Interventions That Improve Balance and Postural Control

Balance is an important component of critical functional activities. Balance is required for the patient to control all programs needed to either maintain the body's BOS over its center of gravity (COG) or to replace the body's COG back under its BOS (Figures 5-2A and B). Balance can also be considered a component of a larger movement, such as the postural stability needed to reach an object, come to standing, walk, sit and eat, or dress. Providing interventions that improve balance impairments could be delegated to physical therapist assistants.

Balance training can focus on maintaining or regaining balance once an anticipated or unexpected perturbation occurs. A perturbation occurs when a directional force causes the body to react to maintain or regain COG over a specific BOS. That BOS may be one foot, both feet, a foot and a knee (one-half kneel), both hips in the sitting position, or the entire body (the trunk, head, and hips) when a person is lying down and rolling from side-to-side. The ability to react to the perturbation is based on sensory

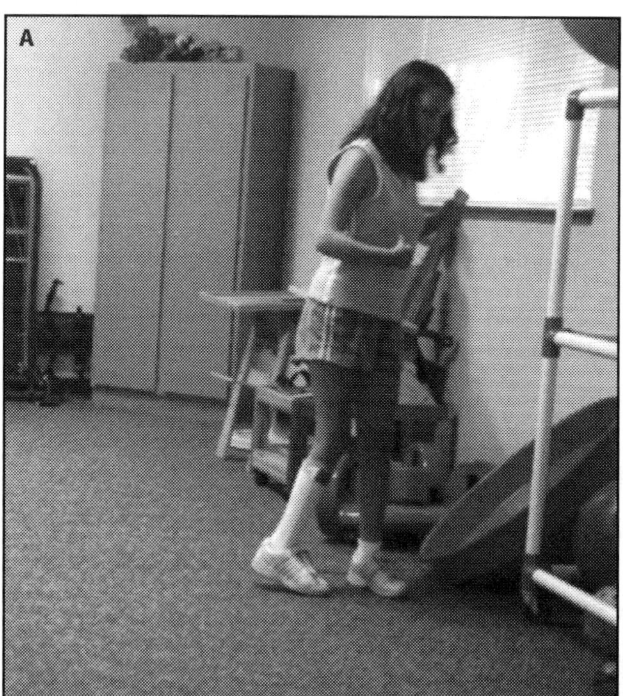

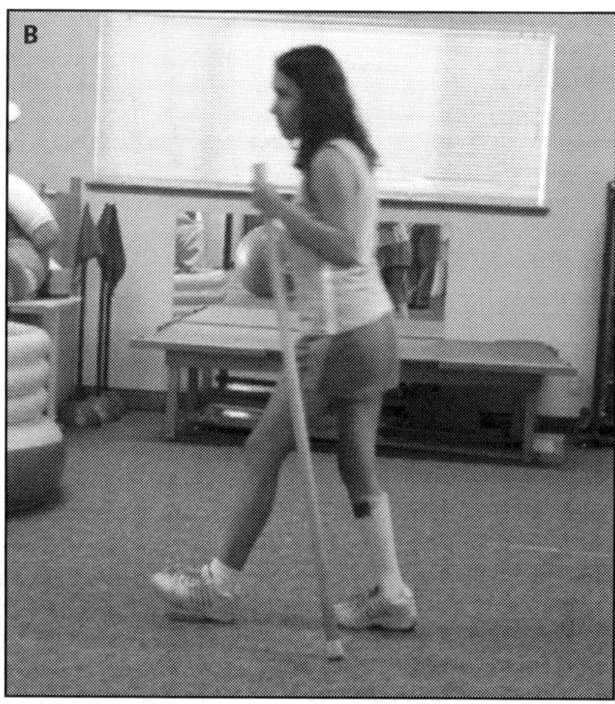

Figure 5-2. Balance: Maintaining COG within the existing BOS. (B) Balance: Replacing the BOS back under the COG, stepping.

input from the proprioceptive, vestibular, and visual systems and inherent balance synergy programs involving the ankle, hip, and stepping. In addition, when the patient is instructed in the use of a support system (eg, a cane, walker, or transfer bar), a therapist needs to consider the balance within the points of support used by the individual for ambulation or movement from one base to another. Generally, there is a balance aspect to all movement and, thus, a patient will incorporate balance programming as part of the functional activity while moving. Balance training includes creating environments in which the patients will perturb themselves (eg, by weight-shifting during reaching or walking), perturb and replace their COG (eg, by stepping or protecting themselves with their arms when falling), and regain balance when an external force, either anticipated (recognized that the perturbation will occur, such as a child running without looking toward you) or unanticipated (it just happens), perturbs them during a movement activity (eg, being bumped or shoved by someone else while walking). The physical therapist assistant is often asked to encourage patients to automatically react to weight-shifting during reaching, transferring, and ambulating. The only way those automatic reactions can be observed is when the physical therapist assistant either distracts the patient's attention during a movement or perturbs the COG without notice.

There are many ways to enhance balance reactions.[9] Incorporating the 3 sensory modalities of proprioceptive, vestibular, and vision will often help the patient respond adequately to perturbations.[10,11] Obviously, balance reactions can be facilitated in sitting by asking the patient to reach toward objects in various directions. Similarly, the physical therapist assistant can give gentle perturbations to the patient while sitting and see whether normal balance responses are present. If so, more forceful pushes can be given to facilitate both balance and strengthening. By adding weight at the shoulders or hips, proprioception is enhanced and will add important sensory input to the CNS. The physical therapist assistant must simultaneously be aware that adding weight means the patient will need additional power or strength to move. Similarly, increasing resistance to forward movement when walking by using an exercise band around the waist again increases the proprioceptive input. The therapist can increase and decrease that resistance, which changes the perturbation of the forward movement. Similarly, if the physical therapist assistant shifts diagonally behind the patient, the specific perturbation changes.[12]

If the physical therapist assistant asks the patient to close his or her eyes and then perturbations are given, only proprioception and vestibular systems are available to the patient with regard to balance. The physical therapist assistant can observe and see whether the patient's balance responses remain intact or diminish once vision is taken away. This determination is important. If the patient does not have adequate balance with vision occluded, then walking or moving at night may become dangerous and place the patient at a high risk of falling. Recommendations that direct the family to place nightlights in hallways and any room that might be used by the patient are very important to help avoid falling at night. These sensory changes not

Box 5-2

Case Example: Incorporating Normal Activities Into Balance and Strength Training

A vice president of the university where physical therapist Umphred taught asked her to come to her home and help with her husband's continued rehabilitation. The vice president explained that her husband had a stroke but did very well. He had proceeded with inpatient rehabilitation for 3 weeks, then outpatient physical therapy for another 4 weeks, beginning with 3 times a week and tapering to once a week the last week. He then had home health care for 4 weeks, with the physical therapist coming twice a week. He used a cane but had now gone back to the walker. He had been able to function independently at the time the therapy was stopped. It had been a month, and he was now having balance problems, was not safe walking independently around the house, and had stopped walking outside. He needed assistance getting out of his chair and spent the day reading. His wife came home at lunch to make sure he had food and to walk him to the bathroom. She was concerned about his decline in function and wondered whether he needed to be placed in a care facility or whether she should retire to take care of him.

The physical therapist went to the home and observed the individual move. He was able to stand up independently but was unsteady, weak, and concerned he would fall. He was able to walk with the cane or walker, but again was fearful of falling and complained that his leg muscles felt tired. The therapist noticed a water pitcher and glass by the chair and asked why they were there. The individual explained that he had been a diabetic for more than 20 years and needed to drink a glass of water every hour to maintain control over his diabetes. The therapist asked him if he could walk the 35 feet to the kitchen sink, and if so, to demonstrate. He did so without any signs of falling. The therapist then recommended that his wife no longer leave a pitcher of water with him when she went to work, and that he should get up every hour and go to the sink to get his water. She also said she would be back in a couple of days to see how he was doing. Within the first week, he was no longer having difficulty getting out of the chair, no longer had a fear of falling, and had given up the walker and was using a cane for balance assistance. By the end of the second week, he was going outside and walking around on the sidewalk. He began by walking 10 to15 feet and turning around, and then increased that distance as he felt stronger. By the end of the month, he was again going to the store with his wife and walking around, interacting with her and with life.

All the therapist did was change one thing in the environment that forced balance and strength training as part of daily living, and used a motivator (ie, getting a glass of water hourly) that he had already incorporated into his living style. He did his own therapy without anyone identifying that he needed to keep practicing strength and balance activities as part of his daily living. Once they were incorporated into his life, he once again regained all of the function he had worked so hard to regain during rehabilitation.

only occur following CNS damage they also change as individuals age.[13]

Asking the patient to sit or stand on compliant surfaces such as foam (see Figure 12-7) or rocker boards challenges the proprioceptive system and forces the patient to use vestibular and vision as the sensory input for balance. Practicing walking on these types of surfaces will determine whether the individual can safely walk on grass or outdoor surfaces that are uneven. If going to the park with grandchildren or playing with friends at the beach is important to the individual, then practicing on uneven and compliant surfaces needs to be incorporated into the plan of care. Also, going outside and practicing on the specific type of surface that the individual will be walking on, such as grass or sand, will further enhance the training and link the function to the environment in which the patient will perform once out of the therapy situation (Box 5-2).

There are certain situations in which subsystem problems cause balance impairments, and, therefore, working on that specific impairment may improve balance. For example, standing balance may be impaired by lack of ankle dorsiflexion mobility, either by dorsiflexor weakness or tight gastrocsoleus muscle. In this case, strengthening the ankle dorsiflexors or stretching the gastrocsoleus (or both) could improve balance. Another subsystem problem might be the respiratory system (Box 5-3). Lack of adequate oxygen exchange can also cause weakness especially in postural stabilization and control over movement. Thus, the physical therapist assistant may be asked to use aerobic activities as part of or prior to training to improve both endurance and balance and other movement problems.[14,15] The importance of the physical therapist assistant recognizing early fatigue in patients cannot be overemphasized.

A specialized aspect of balance training addresses interventions that improve the function of the vestibular system. The vestibular system's primary responsibility is to maintain clear vision during head movement. It also assists in orienting the head and trunk to vertical in relationship to gravity. The vestibular system is one of the sensory receptors responsible for balance and is located within the inner ear. Although the vestibular system is not the most important sensory modality for balance, when dysfunctional, it can cause severe balance problems. The vestibular system is a highly sensitive end organ that reports head movement in all directions using the labyrinths of both inner ears along with the utricle and saccule, which identify the head

Box 5-3

Example of a Patient With Pulmonary Issues That Limit Function

In 1968, at Umphred's first job, she was evaluating and treating a patient who had a stroke 5 weeks earlier. Another therapist had treated him at a rehabilitation facility for more than 3 weeks, but his endurance to walking was very poor. He was unable to walk 10 feet without being exhausted. His LE strength was good, but it fatigued quickly. She realized by listening to his breathing in a quiet environment that he was wheezing and had no diaphragmatic breathing on his right side. She worked with him on triggering his diaphragm on the right by using a pneumatic belt that forced his diaphragm up into his chest and then released it quickly to stretch the diaphragm muscles. Within 2 weeks of working with him on this quick stretch technique for enhancing motor function of the diaphragm, this patient was able to walk approximately a mile without resting. He taught her not only that patients will become her teachers, but also that every patient, no matter the movement problem, needs adequate ventilation to functionally move or interact in daily living with any quality of life. When a patient seems to have poor endurance in spite of physical therapy intervention, then both the physical therapist and the physical therapist assistant should always make sure ventilation is adequate. A quick way to check breathing is to use a spirometer. Ask the patient to breathe in and blow or exhale into the spirometer. As a physical therapist or physical therapist assistant, you may be shocked at what you find.

position in space whether the person is lying down supine or prone, side-lying, sitting, or standing. Individuals with vestibular problems often have signs of vertigo, dizziness, nausea, poor posture control, rapid movement (*nystagmus*) of the eyes, and complaints of falling.

Vestibular problems can be central or peripheral in origin. The most common peripheral vestibular problem is *benign paroxysmal positional vertigo*. In this condition, a calcium carbonate crystal (*otoconia*) collects and lodges within the semicircular canals. When this happens, the sensory receptors in these canals send false signals to the brain, causing the symptoms mentioned here. A common physical therapist intervention for this problem is called *canalith repositioning* to move the otoconia out of the way. This repositioning can reset the vestibular system and clear the semicircular canals of any obstructions, but that procedure is not delegated to the physical therapist assistant because of the constant reassessment that needs to occur initially and throughout the procedure.

The vestibular and auditory systems both share the eighth cranial nerve to communicate with the CNS. The eighth cranial nerve enters the nervous system in the lower brainstem. Individuals with a medical disease referred to as *Ménière's disease*[16] will complain of ringing of the ears along with presenting vestibular signs, especially vertigo and nausea. Given ringing sounds (auditory) and vertigo (vestibular), the connection between the auditory and vestibular sensory systems through the eighth cranial nerve can be clearly shown. This disease would be considered an external vestibular problem because the disease is located external to the CNS. Acute/chronic labyrinthitis and unilateral peripheral vestibular hypofunction[17] are other external vestibular problems that cause the patient to demonstrate similar clinical symptoms. To a physical therapist assistant, the symptoms can be the same, and the greatest concern is the patient's falling.[9]

The vestibular problem could also be central in origin. Individuals who have damage to the brainstem from meningitis, tumors, cerebellar issues, brainstem strokes, or spinal/head trauma will often demonstrate vestibular dysfunction. This may involve the vestibular nuclei, cerebellum, midbrain, and higher cortical centers. In central vestibular problems, interventions often include exercises that gradually habituate the vestibular system to the movements or situations that trigger the dizziness or disequilibrium response. The patient's CNS must learn to readapt to vestibular stimulation. Several interventions could be delegated to the physical therapist assistant in this situation; examples include VOR X1 and X2 exercises. In the VOR X1 exercise, the patient is positioned in the sitting position (then progressed to standing as able) and holds an index card with a printed "X" (the target) in the middle. The patient holds this card at eye level and is asked to move the head from side-to-side and told to keep the "X" in clear focus. If the patient is able to maintain a clear focus, then the patient is asked to increase the speed of the side-to-side movement. Next, the same exercise is performed, but this time the head is moved up and down. This exercise is performed in 1-minute bouts. As the patient improves, he or she can progress to the VOR X2 exercise. It is basically the same as the X1 exercise, but this time, the patient moves the head side-to-side while simultaneously moving the index card from side-to-side in the opposite direction as the movement of the head. Again, the patient is asked to keep a clear focus of the target. If the target becomes blurry or jumps around, the speed is decreased (Figures 5-3A and B).

Another goal of vestibular rehabilitation is to challenge the vestibular system during standing and gait. When the body seems to be in motion, one primary goal of the vestibular information is to determine whether the motion is caused by the body swaying on a hard surface (movement over one's BOS) or whether the surface itself is causing the perturbations (standing on a compliant surface such

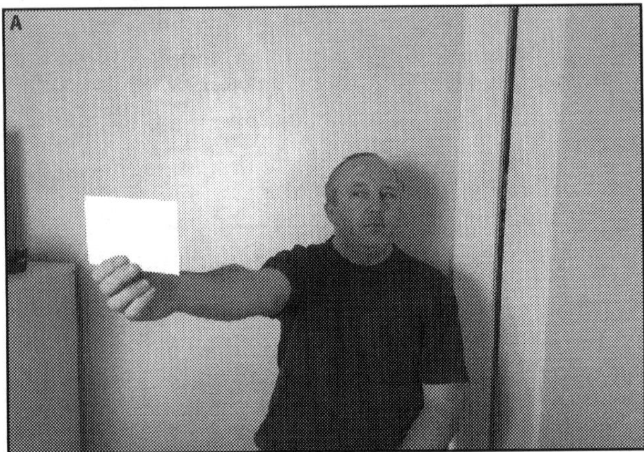

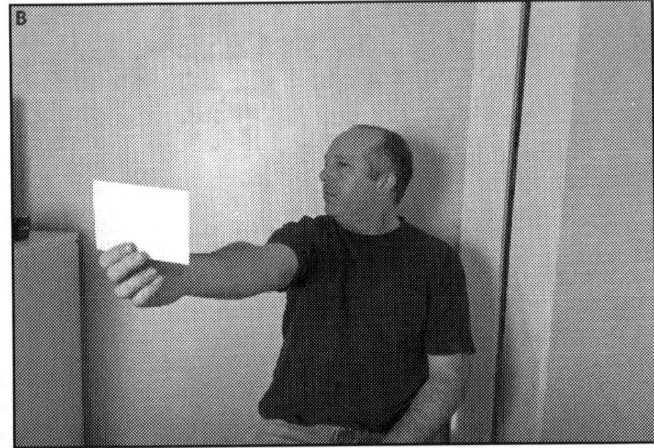

Figure 5-3. (A) VOR exercises. Both exercises may be progressed by increasing the speed of movement while the focus is maintained on the target. VOR X1: The card remains stationary and the person moves his head from side-to-side, keeping his eyes on the target on the card. (B) VOR X2: The head and the card are moved in opposite directions at the same time, while the person keeps his eyes on the target on the card.

as a pillow or being shoved by something such as a dog). Thus, with vestibular rehabilitation, one primary goal is adaptation of the vestibular input so the patient can once again tolerate this information. Once that is achieved, then creating activities that help the CNS process vestibular input along with somatosensory and vision can become an objective. Introducing activities that encourage the person to walk through obstacle courses that have compliant and noncompliant surfaces, then adding throwing and catching balls or striking at objects such as balloons, can further enhance the use of all 3 sensory modalities to optimize balance. Any activity that encourages normal balance reactions can be used sequentially as part of vestibular rehabilitation and balance training. Vestibular exercises can be found online and incorporated into a therapy session or set up for practice at home once the patient is capable of performing home exercises.[18,19] Interventions may be delegated to the physical therapist assistant. An example of a patient with vestibular dysfunction can be found online under the examination section of Chapter 6.

Balance problems caused by the vestibular system can often be modified by using both vision and proprioception input to facilitate balance reactions. The patient can use electronic tools such as the Wii (Nintendo) balance system or other electronic devices to increase the proprioceptive feedback as well as the visual recognition of successfully completing the task presented. These tools can be used to enhance proprioception and vision and modify the sensitivity of the CNS to vestibular problems. Computerized environments such as virtual reality or immersive environments can also be successfully used as part of vestibular rehabilitation.[20,21] The use of these types of environments for training will become more common and may be delegated by the physical therapist to the physical therapist assistant in the future. (Refer to the section on technology later in this chapter as well as Chapter 19.)

Another important aspect of balance training is *dual tasking*, or performing 2 tasks simultaneously. This type of training forces the motor system to respond with adequate balance reaction while the patient is concentrating on a specific task. There are an infinite number of activities a physical therapist can perform that are considered dual tasking. For example, if the patient is asked to walk and count backward by 3 starting at 100, the activity is considered dual tasking. Dual tasking just means that the patient's attention needs to be on some cognitive activity while the motor system is running a movement such as walking, eating, or brushing one's hair. Often therapists think a patient has adequate balance, but once the individual's attention is placed on something other than reacting to a perturbation, the patient will fall. If a patient is practicing a transfer while the television is on and something on the television draws the patient's attention, the question would be: "Does the patient stop the transfer and sit back down, fall during the transfer, or automatically continue with the motor activity while attending to what was on the television?" This dual tasking is the only way a therapist can have confidence that the patient will respond adequately when perturbed during everyday life.[21-28] In many neuromuscular conditions, the ability of the patient to successfully dual-task may be impaired. This is a very important skill to teach the patient to provide the opportunity to again participate in normal life activities, which require an individual to take on multiple tasks. For example, increasing cognitive load by asking the patient to walk and talk at the same time or by having the patient perform 2 motor tasks like walking while carrying a cup full of water are common interventions that may improve dual task performance.

In addition to dual tasking, the therapist can increase the difficulty of the activity itself. Asking the patient to walk down a hallway with no obstacles still requires balance. Asking the patient to walk through an obstacle course that has turns and a lot of visual distortions such as mirrors or toys to step over creates additional difficulties. Asking the patient to walk sideways through the same maze while singing "Happy Birthday" or listing the names of his or

Box 5-4

Examples of Activities That Could Be Used in a Group Balance Class

- Station 1: Have 2 individuals perform stand-to-sit while throwing a light ball back and forth. Increase the activity by either increasing the weight of the ball to cause greater perturbations or increasing the distance between the 2 chairs.
- Station 2: Have 2 individuals walk down a rug that has objects such as tubes, foam, egg cartons, or balls underneath. Increase the difficulty by having the patients either talk to each other while walking, walk while blindfolded, or walk carrying a tray initially with a glass only and then with a glass with water. If a patient has vestibular problems, do not use a blindfold for this activity because the individual will likely fall.
- Station 3: Have each participant practice hitting a hanging ball with a plastic bat or a long cardboard tube. Increase the difficulty by having the hanging ball move.
- Station 4: Have each patient walk up and over 2 steps or up and down a few steps. Increase the activity by having them talk to each other.
- Station 5: Have each patient sit on a chair that has a compliant surface, such as a seat on a rocker or soft form, so the patient's weight will not allow feeling the horizontal surface. Have the patients throw and catch plastic balls. To increase the difficulty, make the balls smaller and heavier.
- Station 6: Have 2 people hit a balloon back and forth with their hands while standing. Increase the difficulty by having the pair increase the distance between them.

The physical therapist may recommend that the physical therapist assistant record what is happening at each station. This can be performed by having the pair of individuals write down or check off how many times they completed the task, as well as the difficulty level achieved. The participants can see their improvement when they are asked to record. The physical therapist assistant can observe whether any patients are decreasing their accomplishments, which might mean a developing problem such as progressive deterioration, a new health issue, a depressed patient, or some other body system problem.

her closest friends increases the difficulty of the motor requirements and also is dual tasking. When the physical therapist assistant has a group of individuals who need or would benefit from balance training and who have similar balance impairments, a group class can be created. Using stations and pairing the individuals as partners can create a fun and social experience (Box 5-4).

Reaction Time to Perturbations

Reaction time to a perturbation is based on 3 important aspects of the CNS. First, the brain must receive accurate and nonconflicting sensory information from proprioceptive, vestibular, and visual peripheral receptors. Second, the brain must process this information at various levels. Third, the CNS must select and control the correct motor programs to respond appropriately. Thus, the physical therapist assistant may be instructed in the direction and force of perturbations within specific positions to impairment train this function. If the physical therapist assistant is providing perturbations as a means of training the patient to improve balance reactions, then the physical therapist assistant must start with light perturbations, then progress to greater forces as the patient is able to successfully maintain balance following these activities. The physical therapist assistant can then alter the direction of force (eg, forward-backward, side-to-side, or diagonal) and then also the rate of perturbations. This will improve not just anticipatory reactions, but also reactive control.

Hands-On Therapeutic Intervention or Augmented Treatment Intervention

In the therapeutic environment, situations often require the therapist to provide additional assistance whether using hands or other devices to allow the patient to succeed in the task being practiced. Although hands-on therapeutic intervention or augmented treatment intervention is not necessarily exclusive of functional or impairment training, it is presented as a separate category so the physical therapist assistant will understand more clearly the options available with regard to providing additional assistance that may allow for more successful outcomes.

The goals of using the therapist's hands during therapeutic interventions are as follows:

1. To guide or assist patients during functional movements
2. To control specific patterns of movement while preventing stereotypic patterns
3. To give patients the sensory input as feedback for correct movement control
4. To allow patients to experience the functional movements that will encourage them to move from one spatial position to another
5. To create a limited environment where patients can succeed at the desired task

6. To motivate patients by letting them experience some aspect of success and potential accomplishment toward a desired function

The physical therapist may instruct the physical therapist assistant to teach the patient by verbally describing, visually demonstrating, or kinesthetically handling through a movement. The physical therapist gives those instructions because the best way for the patient to learn has been identified. This is referred to as a *learning style*. If this has not been identified, the physical therapist assistant can try instructing the patient using each style or a combination of the 3. It is very important that the physical therapist assistant know his or her own learning style, because all of us tend to teach through the style with which we are most comfortable. The preferential style of the physical therapist assistant may not be the best for the patient. All health care practitioners must create the optimal environment for learning, which means, initially, to teach through the style of the patient and then progress to less optimal styles to allow the patient to adapt to the external world.

Relaxation Techniques

The physical therapist assistant can use many techniques to teach or encourage a patient to relax. The one approach that will not work, but is often used, is asking the patient to relax. This is especially true with patients who have increased tone or hypertonicity. The presence of hypertonicity points out the fact that the person is unable to decrease the tone voluntarily, or the patient would.[29,30]

Slow, deep breathing encourages the patient to use the diaphragm, which will relax the autonomic system and generally relax tension and tone.[31,32] If the patient can follow commands, then having the patient practice this type of breathing will help relax the system and reduce tone. This can be practiced in supine, side-lying, sitting, or even standing positions. Asking the patient to participate in this type of breathing can empower the patient to a technique that will help reduce tension and tone when life or the internal or external environment triggers the motor response.[12]

The environment within which the patient is living, whether in a rehabilitation center, a skilled nursing facility, or at home, can often be used to decrease the tension or tone. Many types of music will relax individuals, and the physical therapist assistant can determine the best music to use by asking the patient or the patient's family. Having calm, soft music in the background can help bring the emotional system into balance, and that system often creates tension or tone in muscles.[30] Similarly, lighting in the room can affect the tone of patients. Bright lighting or darkness can be very alerting and often will increase tone. Soft, natural lighting from the sun is the best, if available. Similarly, the physical therapist assistant's voice can be a critical factor in teaching relaxation. If the physical therapist assistant has a high-pitched voice, the voice itself can often increase tone, while a soft, monotone voice can lead to relaxation.[12]

When touching the patient, the physical therapist assistant should use firm or constant pressure vs a light touch to use deep proprioception vs cutaneous receptors in the skin. Light touch is very alerting and often creates a protective response that, when a patient cannot control tone, will only increase that tone. Thus, when moving from one point on the body to another, do not let go of the first hold until the second spot on the skin/body has been touched with deep pressure. Once the initial touch is accepted and the patient relaxes, the physical therapist assistant should not let go and retouch because the patient will again need to relax to the new touch. If the initial deep pressure touch is held as the new touch is applied, the patient often does not interpret the new touch as threatening and thus has no need to elicit a protective reaction. It is often recommended that the physical therapist assistant also inform the patient before changing holds, allowing the patient's CNS time to adjust to the fact that new sensory information will be applied from the second touch. The physical therapist assistant needs to use observational skill to identify the responses of the patient and how the patient responds to the touch.

Another way to help decrease tone or elicit relaxation can be used when the patient is supine. Take hold of the heel of a foot with one hand while placing the second hand under the back of the knee, placing the knee in slight flexion. If one of the patient's legs is more involved or has higher tone than another, start with the least involved leg. Then gently use a pushing motion up through the leg, causing slight compression and oscillations that travel up the leg into the spine and neck regions. The speed of the oscillations is patient-dependent. Always begin with slow, gentle oscillations, then, increase the speed and force slightly and see whether the patient's body shows more relaxation. The patient's response to the oscillations will tell the physical therapist assistant the best amount of force and speed to use. This approach should never be very forceful or performed at a high speed. If the patient can follow commands, have him or her take slow, deep breaths as the physical therapist assistant oscillates from the leg. This will combine the diaphragmatic breathing and the gentle oscillation, causing even more relaxation. This approach should never cause pain. The physical therapist assistant may observe oscillations through the leg and lower spine and then, as the movement approaches the higher spinal segments, those segments may move as one unit. This may be an indication of tightness within the spine and should be reported to the physical therapist to determine whether additional spinal treatments need to be applied. These restrictions may also be the site of pain in a patient because those segments move as one unit, are tight, and may be compressed. Again, discussion with the physical therapist is appropriate.

When confronted with a patient who has very high extensor tone when supine, this technique is often very effective prior to having the patient roll. Once the tone begins to decrease, the physical therapist assistant can easily flex the knee and hip with rotation, triggering a body-on-body righting reaction and thus beginning the motion of rolling. The patient can more easily take control of the movement once the hypertonicity has been reduced. Thus, the physical therapist assistant is assisting with the movement but always allowing the patient to take as much normal effortless control as possible as the movement is occurring.

The same type of oscillations can be performed from the head, but the physical therapist assistant is cautioned first to ask the physical therapist whether it is appropriate, and then, if told to incorporate it into the plan of care, to begin very gently, holding the head with both hands. Make sure hands do not cover the ears because that will take away auditory sound and often causes the patient to become alert and anxious, which increases tone. The physical therapist assistant needs to use observational skills as well as tactile and proprioceptive feedback to determine the speed and intensity of the oscillations. The patient's response to the gentle movements will determine the rate and amount of gentle compression. Again, the patient can be asked to breathe deeply while the oscillations are performed. Often, the physical therapist assistant can observe specific areas of tightness once the patient begins to relax. The oscillations should cause gentle movement within the entire body of the patient. There may be joints, especially in the spine, that are restricted, and those joints will move as one unit. If the physical therapist assistant does not understand something, reporting and discussing those findings with the physical therapist is appropriate. The physical therapist can be asked for guidance to determine the best way to handle the restrictions. When oscillating from the head, the physical therapist assistant should never try to trigger a neck-on-body right reaction, because the weight of the body is too great. The physical therapist may use this technique to begin head-on-body righting with a small child, but it takes tremendous skill and should not be performed by the physical therapist assistant until those skills have been learned and the physical therapist has given that aspect of intervention to the physical therapist assistant. Relaxation can be part of using handling techniques but, again, high tone is often generated because of a lack of stability within the joints themselves, so the physical therapist assistant must exercise caution when handling after relaxation is triggered. The goal is normalizing muscle tone using relaxation techniques, not taking away hypertonicity and replacing it with hypotonicity.

To encourage postural extension of the trunk, gentle oscillations from slight compression to distraction can be applied through the knee when the patient is in the sitting position to encourage postural extension of the trunk. Another way to facilitate the same postural extension is by having the patient sit on the side of the mat while the physical therapist assistant is sitting on a therapy ball behind the patient. The ball can be placed against the trunk to provide stability and facilitate postural extension while the physical therapist assistant slips 2 legs along the lateral aspects of both sides of the patient's trunk and under the arms. The physical therapist assistant can slowly bring the patient's arms into abduction and slight external rotation of the shoulder by slowly rocking on the ball from side-to-side. This abduction and external rotation will also facilitate postural extension of the trunk. The physical therapist assistant can slowly shift weight on the ball from side-to-side, which will cause the patient to laterally move from one hip to another. If capable, the patient can be asked to reach with one hand toward a target as the physical therapist assistant shifts weight onto the hip that would naturally bear weight as the patient reaches toward the target. This technique will cause reduction or relaxation of high tone and facilitate balance reactions and postural extension of the trunk. These techniques can be combined as the patient begins to take control over the movement itself.[4] Examples of these relaxation techniques can be found on the video site that accompanies this text. The physical therapist assistant should practice these skills with another physical therapist assistant. In that way, the physical therapist assistant, acting as the patient, can provide feedback to the individual performing the techniques. Individuals with normal tone will still relax when these approaches are applied. The physical therapist assistant can observe how different people react differently given the same relaxation techniques.

Handling Techniques

Techniques that are used to guide a movement from one position to another are considered *handling techniques*. There are many ways to guide or facilitate movement.[33-39] Techniques such as proprioceptive neuromuscular facilitation (PNF)[33] were designed to focus on motor impairments within specific patterns of movement or diagonal patterns. The focus of this approach is often strengthening muscle groups; increasing range within specific functional patterns; facilitating agonistic and antagonistic patterns to gain coactivation or stability around joints during both weight-bearing and non–weight-bearing activities (ie, closed- and open-chain activities); and guiding the patient within patterns to move in rolling, coming to sit, standing, and ambulating. A physical therapist assistant may be introduced to these patterns during school, but developing a high level of skill requires additional training and many hours of practice. A section of this chapter specifically discusses PNF and its application to patients with CNS dysfunction.

The approach that originally used the term *handling techniques* was the Bobath approach,[34,35] which, within the United States today, has evolved into a methodology known as Neuro-Developmental Treatment (NDT).[20] Although specific aspects of the approach have changed and the theoretical constructs behind the methodology have incorporated more current theories of motor control, motor learning, and neuroplasticity, many of the techniques remain the

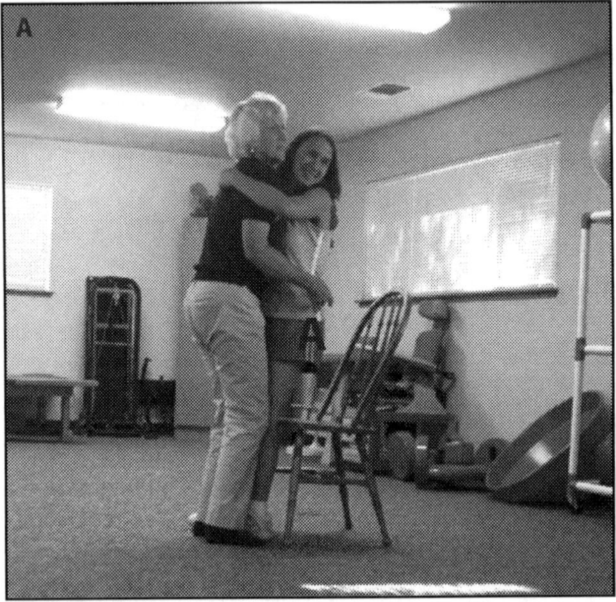

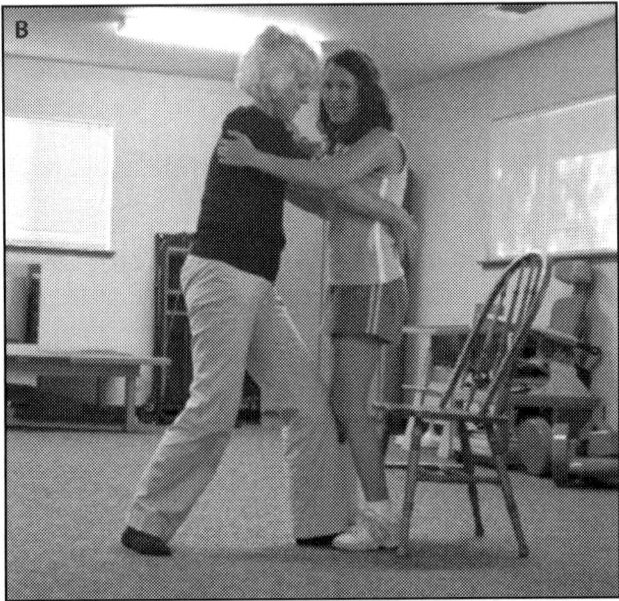

Figure 5-4. Handling a dependent patient when coming to stand for a transfer. (A) Incorrect: The therapist is vertical, and the patient is off vertical and falling backward. (B) Correct: The therapist is slightly off vertical, and the patient has the opportunity to feel vertical or upright posture.

same. For specific information on NDT, please refer to the NDT section later in this chapter.

In general, a physical therapist assistant will need to learn how to "handle" or guide a patient in performing the following activities:

1. Rolling over or from side-to-side in bed
2. Coming to sit from the horizontal position whether on the floor or in bed
3. Moving over one's BOS in sitting to independently sit for activities such as reaching, feeding, and donning clothes
4. Coming to stand from both a horizontal position when on the floor or bed (half-kneel to stand or squat to stand) or while rising from a chair (partial squat to stand) to reach or prior to initiating walking
5. Overcoming inability to perform an activity because of abnormal muscle function (eg, weakness, hypertonicity, or fluctuations in the state of the motor pool)
6. Dealing with perceptual/cognitive problems that create movement distortions or level of consciousness prevents interactions
7. Helping the patient participate in a successful movement response to realize potential within the motor control system

Although entire textbooks[36,40,41] discuss specific handling techniques and patterns of movement to be used to assist patients following a CNS insult, the physical therapist assistant is encouraged to watch individuals move, to shut one's eyes, and to feel the movement as the body rolls over, comes to sit, moves in sitting, rises to standing, and walks. If a therapist is guiding a patient through a movement, the therapist needs to differentiate feedback that relates where the therapist is in space from where the patient's body is in space. For example, if a physical therapist assistant is guiding a patient to standing from a w/c or chair and is guarding the patient by limiting flexion of the patient's knees, then the feet of the therapist and the patient will occupy space close to each other. If the therapist is feeling totally stable and vertical, the patient's body cannot be in the same vertical position, and generally, the patient will be leaning backward and have a sense of falling. If, on the other hand, the therapist feels slightly off-balance posterior, then the patient has an opportunity to stand erect. Once the patient is erect, there will be little need to grab the therapist, the patient's biomechanical system will be stacked optimally, the feedback to the patient will be accurate with regard to verticality, and the entire environment will often become more relaxed for both individuals (Figures 5-4A and B).

Handling techniques are often used to help a patient roll over. That patient may be at a low state of consciousness, may have flaccid or hypertonic extremities, may not be able to follow a command, or may not want to move. Generally, it is easiest to assist a patient to roll by handling an LE. If the patient is in supine (on the back) and needs to roll to the side (to relieve body pressure, to change sheets, to prepare to come to sit, or some other functional activity), the physical therapist assistant will often handle the patient from one LE. The extremity of choice will be the leg that needs to move to attain a side-lying position. That is, if the patient needs to roll to the right, the left leg will need to flex, slightly abduct, and externally rotate initially, followed by flexion and internal rotation to guide the pelvis onto the right side. The opposite would be true if rolling to the left. The specific amount of flexion, abduction, and external rotation needed initially depends on the patient's muscle tone and

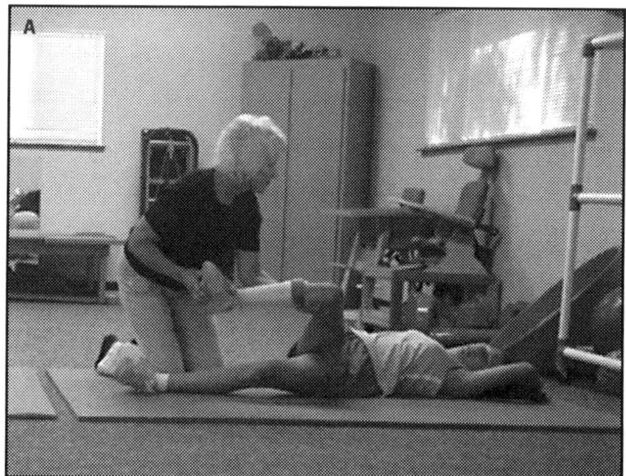

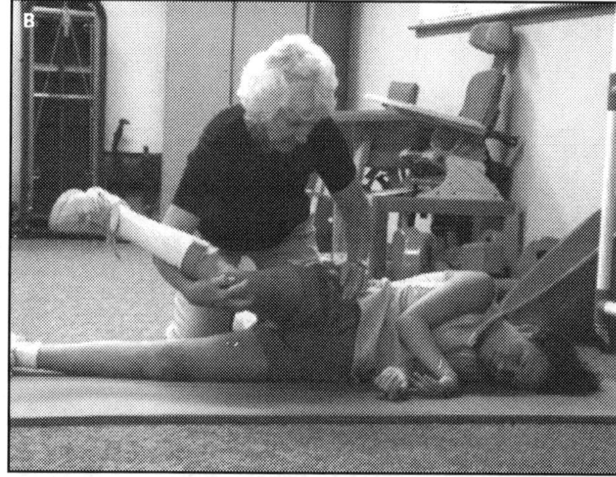

Figure 5-5. (A) Rolling the patient to the side using the leg or foot as the point of control. Initially handle leg into flexion, slight abduction, and external rotation. (B) Handle the rotation at the pelvis by maintaining flexion of the hip with slight abduction while guiding into internal rotation.

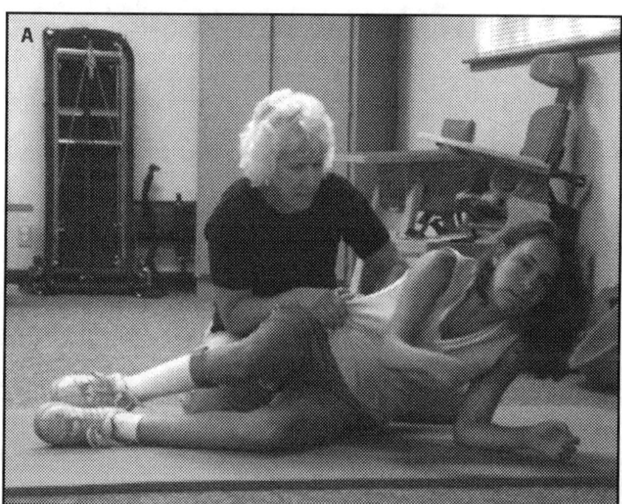

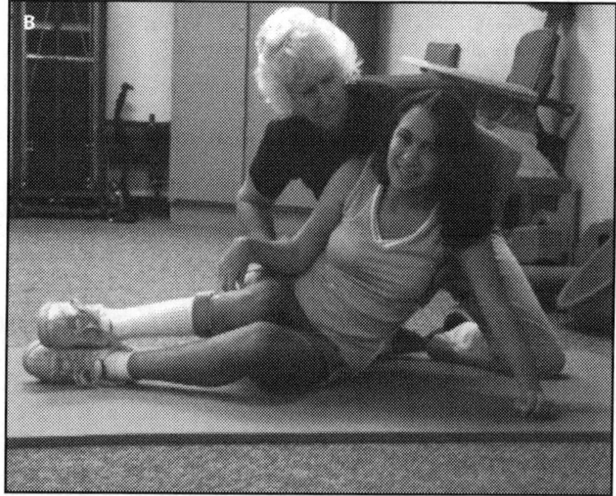

Figure 5-6. (A) Handling from side-lying to sitting. Pressure is placed in a downward and posterior direction on the topside anterior iliac crest to guide the topside hip into sitting. (B) The patient's upper body and head are guided to vertical by supporting the patient's trunk under the brachial plexus and head from the back on the bottom side.

ROM. The physical therapist assistant should guide or control the pelvis at the hip, using the entire leg while moving the leg toward the desired side (Figures 5-5A and B). The trunk will follow the pelvis either through a body-on-head or a body-on-body-on-head righting reaction.

Handling an individual from side-lying to sit is easily performed by applying pressure to the patient's topside anterior iliac crest in a downward and posterior direction (Figure 5-6A). The physical therapist assistant may need to assist the patient's upper body and head. This can be performed by supporting the patient from the back, under the bottom side arm (brachial plexus) and head (Figure 5-6B).

Once the patient is in a sitting position, a large variety of movement activities can be guided and practiced. The physical therapist assistant can support the patient from the back while sitting on a ball (Figure 5-7A). In this position, the physical therapist assistant can control both UEs as well as the trunk to assist in activities such as weight-shifting and reaching. The physical therapist assistant can work on similar activities while in the half-kneel position (Figure 5-7B). The leg that the therapist is using to kneel on can also be used to support the patient's trunk, while the half-kneeling leg can be used to direct the patient's UE during reaching and hand-to-mouth activities. When the therapist is approaching the patient from the front, many patterns can be facilitated through handling. In Figure 5-7C, the therapist is supporting the patient's arm with a half-kneeling leg. Using the therapist's leg gives the patient a feeling of safety because the arm is resting on a solid body part vs being suspended in space either by the patient's muscle power and ligaments or being held by the therapist. With the therapist's leg supporting the patient's arm, both of the therapist's hands are free to work on activities such as inhibition of tone in the scapula, shoul-

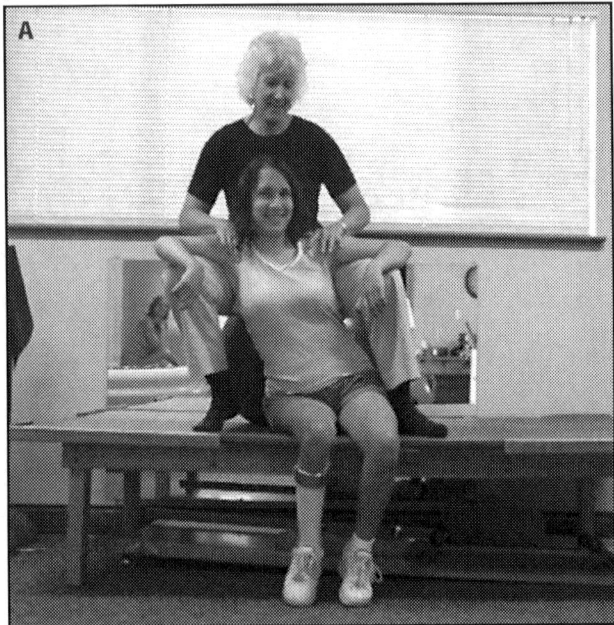

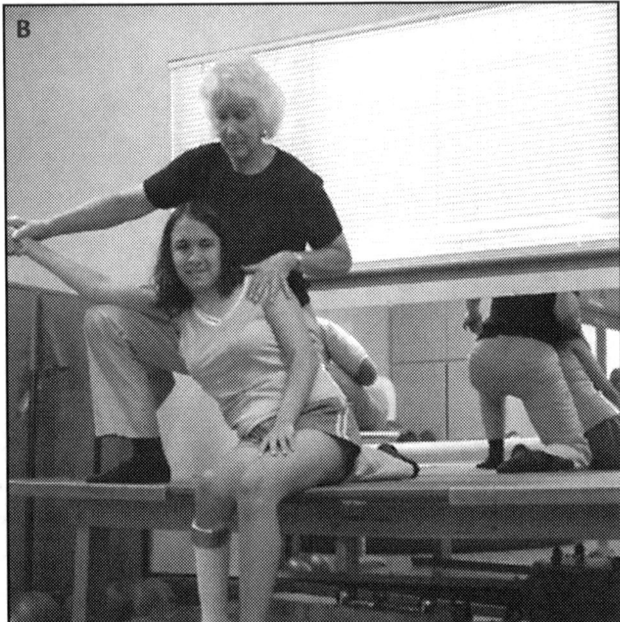

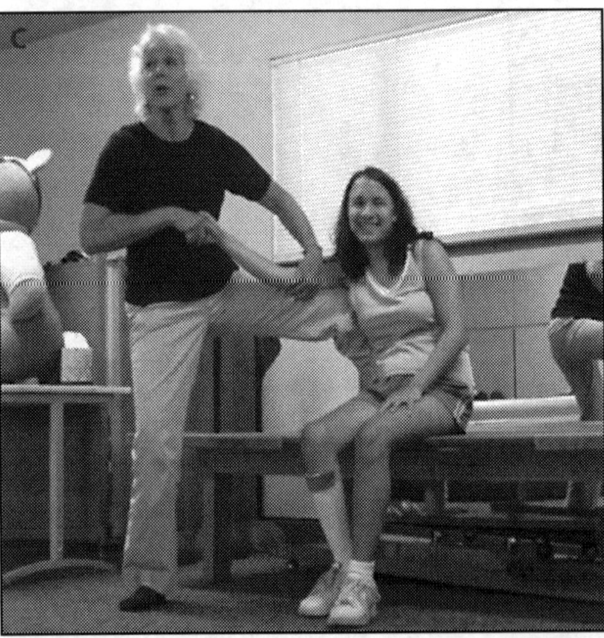

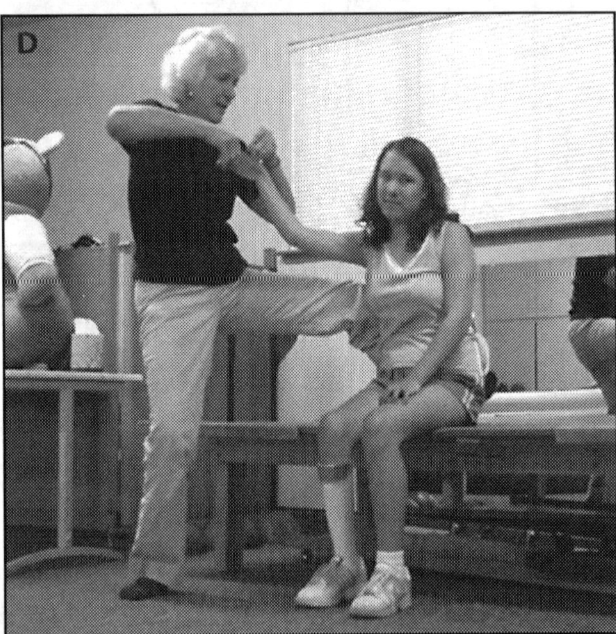

Figure 5-7. (A) Handling while in sitting. The therapist sits on a ball while supporting the trunk while placing the arms/shoulder girdle in flexion, abduction, external rotation, and scapular protraction. (B) The therapist supports the patient's trunk with the leg that is kneeling while using the half-kneeling leg to support a shoulder allowing the patient's arm to elevate; externally rotate with shoulder protraction. (C) While the patient is in sitting, the therapist supports the patient's involved UE and slowly assists in shoulder elevation, external rotation, and shoulder protraction and retraction. (D) Handling from the front. The therapist handles the patient from the hand and posterior hip. These handling positions should be changed frequently enough to keep the patient from becoming dependent upon the therapist's hands.

der elevation, external rotation, and elbow extension with wrist and finger extension. This UE pattern is usually the antagonistic pattern to that seen in involved UEs of patients following head injuries and strokes.

Once high-tone agonistic patterns are relaxed, the physical therapist assistant can encourage the patient to assist in control over the antagonistic patterns. The goal is ease of movement, not force production. It would be better to assist the ROM activity while having the patient control or assist as much as possible vs having the patient try so hard that abnormal synergistic patterns of movement are responding in relation to the demand. Remember, movement is effortless. Feel yourself move, and you will recognize how easy it is. The patient should practice that same effortless movement. Handling encourages practice in a movement controlled by the patient. The entire goal of therapy is always to empower the patient to gain control over all functional activities. Teaching patients to try as hard as they can will generally create a large amount of hypertonicity, and thus limit functional control. The physical therapist assistant can handle the patient's pelvis and pelvic movement by handling the anterior hip through downward and posterior pressure on one side while applying downward and anterior pressure on the opposite posterior pelvic rim. This pressure will facilitate postural extension of the trunk and encourage the patient to sit up and weight-shift (Figure 5-7D).

Patients can be brought to standing in many ways. The patient can be guided to standing from sitting with the therapist guiding from one UE. Usually, the physical therapist assistant should guide from the more involved UE (Figures 5-8A and B). If the patient needs maximal assistance to come to stand, then a ball and a high/low mat or table can be used effectively. First, bring the patient forward in the chair. Next, place his or her UEs over a medium-sized ball, which can then be placed on the edge of the high/low mat. Next, bring the patient forward over the ball as the ball rolls onto the mat. The patient's COG should now be over the feet, with the hips flexed and the trunk supported by the ball. Next, the physical therapist assistant can press on the high/low mat control device and begin to raise the mat/table. The table will bring the patient to stand in a relaxed manner with maximal support. The arms should remain relaxed in shoulder elevation and scapular protraction. Once the trunk is stacked into a biomechanical position, the physical therapist assistant may need a counterforce in front of the ball to avoid the ball slipping away from the patient and therapist. Initially, the handling techniques will need to be from the side of the patient. As soon as the patient is relaxed with the trunk resting over the ball with the feet flat, the therapist can reposition his or her body to the rear of the patient. At that time, the therapist can reach under the patient's upper trunk and guide the upper body toward a vertical posture. Generally, the head will right after the shoulders, and the patient will be standing in a normal upright position. The patient will feel stabilized between the therapist and the ball. Weight-shifting can be practiced to encourage body support over the feet. If the patient slowly rolls the ball from side-to-side, forward, and backward, this facilitates perturbations for balance and postural reactions. The physical therapist assistant can also practice partial stand-to-squat by having the patient or therapist control the table mat's position as it goes up and down. Once the patient can go from stand-to-sit and back up again, the patient will usually have the sit-to-stand pattern within the CNS motor control. Therapists often use this same approach on children, using a ball that is large enough to bring the child into standing off the ball (Figures 5-8C and D).

The physical therapist may ask the physical therapist assistant to begin ambulation training before the patient comes to standing independently. The physical therapist assistant must remember that ambulation uses different combinations of motor programs than the sit-to-stand or stand-to-sit. The physical therapist assistant may be asked to stabilize the ankle/knee interactions using an orthotic device. Similarly, the physical therapist may want the physical therapist assistant to instruct the patient in the use of either a walker or a cane to assist in balance and stability during gait. The physical therapist assistant must emphasize an erect posture of the patient's trunk and head. If the patient is encouraged to stand and walk on bent hips, the patient will need more power to remain upright, will fatigue more quickly, and will limit the types of balance reactions available to the CNS. Additional recommendations for handling children, adolescents, and adults can be found in Chapters 9 through 14. A recording of handling techniques that illustrate rolling, coming to sit, sit-to-kneel, kneel-to-half-kneel, and half-kneel-to-stand can be found online to complement this text.

Use of Assistive Devices While Handling

A physical therapist assistant may use pulleys, exercise tubing, bolsters, wedges, balls, foam, and taping to limit or encourage specific movement patterns while preventing others. For the patient to be considered functionally independent, the physical therapist assistant and/or physical therapist must remove the patient's need for handling techniques and/or the need for therapeutic/adaptive equipment. The continued use of adaptive equipment may allow the patient to be functional without another person assisting, but that equipment often limits the environment within which the patient can function. Body weight–supported treadmill training (BWSTT) is considered an augmented approach.

The degree of augmentation may assist when the physical therapist or physical therapist assistant needs to better control a motor response of a leg, such as placement of the foot after the swing phase of gait. This augmentation is performed to drive an appropriate motor response and, thus, keep the LE kinematics within an acceptable parameter of performance during gait.[42-45] Additional information regarding BWSTT can be found later in this chapter.

Using the Sensory System to Enhance/Reinforce or to Retrain Function

Following CNS insults, many patients have decreased sensory awareness and/or sensory processing problems.[46-50] It is the physical therapist's responsibility to evaluate for these deficits, but delegation of training may be given to the physical therapist assistant. Thus, the physical therapist assistant needs to be aware of each sensory system and how intervention may increase or decrease input to any one of these systems. Similarly, some patients develop sensory processing problems because of overuse, as seen in dystonia. Understanding the sensory systems and their function is critical:

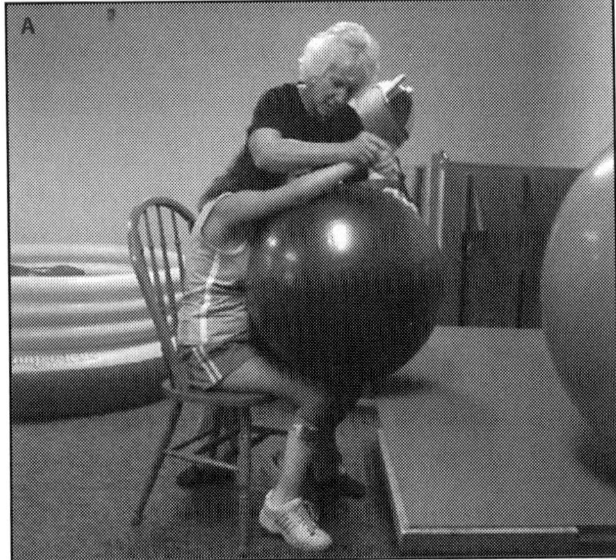

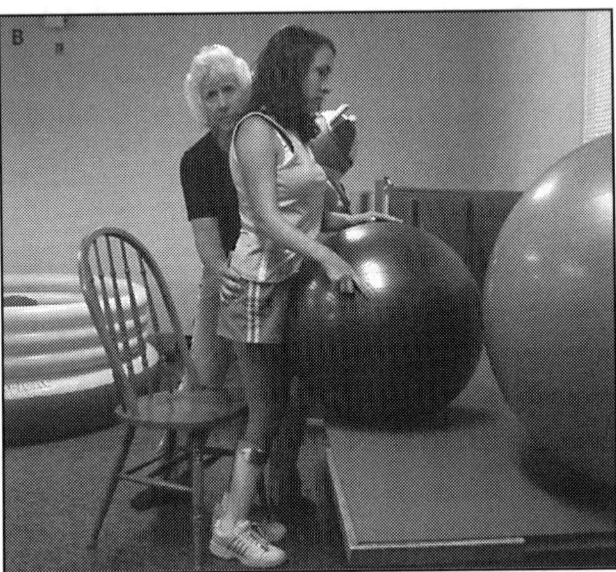

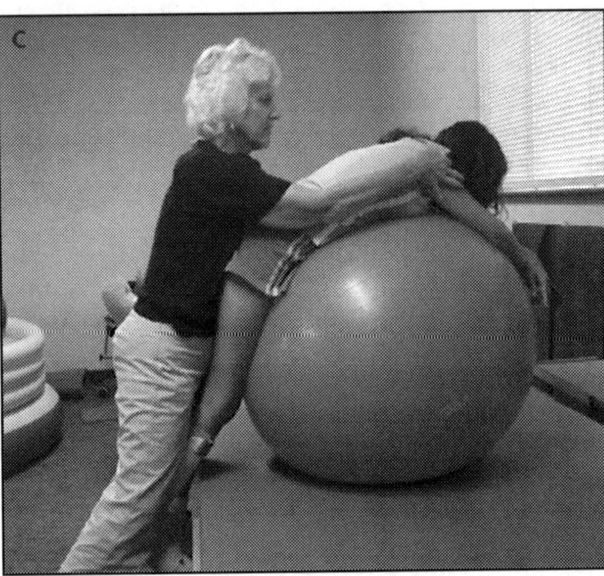

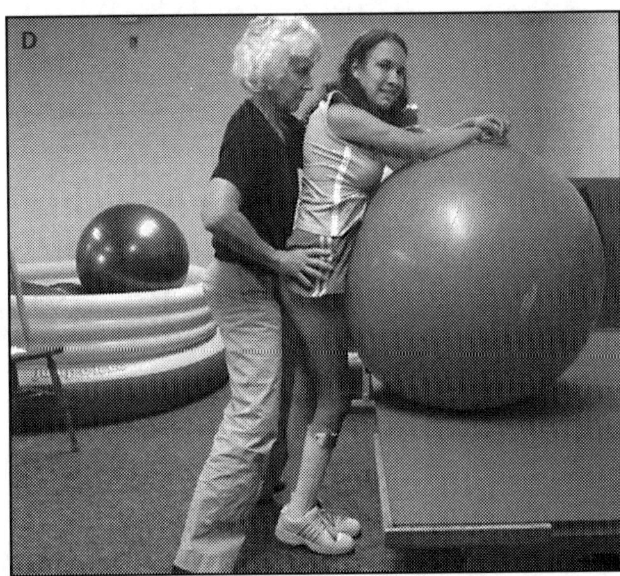

Figure 5-8. (A) Guiding to stand from the more involved side. The ball is positioned in front of the patient within the patient's lap. (B) The patient and the ball are guided to roll the patient's COG over her feet before bringing her to upright. (C) The patient is guided onto a large ball. Slow rocking can be done in this position to increase relaxation. (D) Roll the patient onto her feet while relaxed to maintain normal postural extension without causing extensor hypertonicity.

- To use them appropriately as part of treatment in the clinical environment
- To identify when the patient is negatively reacting to that input
- To understand how sensory retraining can lead to functional ability as seen in patients with dystonia or any sensory deficit that affects movement

The auditory system was already discussed in relation to the use of voice as a therapeutic tool. Similarly, when the physical therapist assistant demonstrates to the patient, the patient's visual system is engaged to receive and interpret the visual array. At times, the environmental input of either or both auditory and visual sensory information may be overwhelming to the CNS and actually decrease function. Thus, the physical therapist assistant may be asked to intervene initially in a quiet environment in a room where the walls are painted a solid color without pictures or windows. Once the patient begins to improve in motor function, the auditory and visual environments can become more complex and more demanding of the CNS to continue to run appropriate motor programs while the world bombards the brain with sensory information. The physical therapist assistant also needs to remember that when working with the elderly, these systems may have changed over the lifetime, and an increase in the amount of specific input may be necessary to facilitate learning.[51,52]

Similarly, proprioception and vestibular information can be increased or decreased depending on the intervention environments the therapist creates. Often, having the patient supine in a quiet environment can lead to a high awareness of proprioceptive information at joints and muscles using assistive motions and joint compression and traction. Once the patient begins to feel those sensations, the physical therapist assistant can move the patient to more physically demanding environments, such as sitting, and have the patient again become aware of the sensory input. These types of treatment environments would be considered *sensory training* or *sensory processing training*. They can often be performed during the patient's rest periods, because they require relaxation and, when accompanied by deep breathing, will often decrease the state of the motor generators, thus dampening inappropriate proprioceptive information from the muscles and joints. Many philosophies and/or intervention suggestions[37,53-56] learned through readings and course attendance emphasize this type of sensory training.

Having patients differentiate sensory objects with their vision shielded is a way to help them develop or relearn sensory discriminations. Initially, the patient may need to kinesthetically feel and see the object. Then, the object is shielded from sight, and the patient is asked to recognize what is being felt. That recognition can be through verbal responses or pointing to pictures of similar objects. Patients can be taught to process sensory information in many ways. Some of those possibilities will be taught in school, some taught by other therapists in the clinic, some taught in courses, and some discovered by the physical therapist assistant. This process of learning will continue as long as the physical therapist assistant remains open to learning new skills.

Obviously, the sensory systems are part of learning and are critical to relearning functional movement. When a sensory system itself is damaged, the function may be lost or diminished or even cause additional problems to the motor system. This damage can be due to a stroke, head injury, degeneration, or demanding repetitive activity over a long period of time. Dystonia is considered a problem in kinesthetic sensory processing. It is often considered a problem of overuse of a system that has led to dysfunction or inappropriate processing of that specific sensation.[57-65]

Dystonia is often seen in individuals who repetitively and often use a specific motor pattern at a high speed. Musicians, typists, and computer users all repetitively use specific motor patterns as part of daily living. The result can lead to the somatosensory system no longer being able to differentiate slight differences in input, and the end result is a mass motor response to activity. When the individual wants to type specific letters on a computer, all fingers type simultaneously, thus causing tremendous error in the motor response. A musician who uses rapidly changing motor responses within a small ROM demands fine gradation and can overuse the system, with the result that the somatosensory system can no longer differentiate those fine changes in input.[57,61,62]

Dystonia can also be due to a genetic predisposition that develops as the person ages. No matter the causation, sensory retraining begins by having the individual practice some of the same patterns of movement but in different spatial positions, which triggers different sensory neurons both peripherally and on the primary and secondary sensory cortices.[55,57,64] There is a lot of research on dystonia, and the physical therapist assistant needs to be aware that this problem can exist and that treatment protocols can help the individual retrain the sensory cortices.[42,43,48,49,66-71] The physical therapist assistant will know that the treatment objectives are being met by the patient's success at doing the IADL or participation activity that has been set as the goal.

Participation Training

The World Health Organization's International Classification of Functioning, Disability and Health model, as discussed in Chapter 1, stresses that problems with functional activities often decrease an individual's ability to participate in life. Thus, prior to beginning intervention, it is very important to determine those activities that the individual values and hopes to resume once rehabilitation has been completed. An individual may want to go fly fishing, bird watching, golfing, gold panning, or ballroom dancing[72]; go to religious services; or participate in some other type of activity. Those activities fall under the category of participation and lead to improved quality of life. Any activity that might be considered a high level of motor function will most likely incorporate postural function, reciprocal limb movements, ambulation, and many other motor programs that blend together to create the activity the individual values. For that reason, the physical therapist assistant should ask what the individual hopes to someday be able to accomplish. After the individual describes what is needed to perform that activity, the therapist needs to create an environment that will lead to accomplishment of that activity. For example, assume an individual wants to fly fish, but has had a stroke in the left hemisphere and thus shows signs of right hemiplegia. His sitting balance is poor, he has moderate use of his right UE, and his right LE has developed an extensor synergy typically seen post-stroke.

The therapist should never tell the patient that his fly fishing days are over, because no one knows that. Instead, ask the patient what he has to do when he is fly fishing. Assume initially that he is going to perform this activity while sitting. Ask him or a family member to bring in his fishing rod. The base of the rod can be placed in a weighted can, which will hold the rod vertical. Then, have the patient sit on the side of a mat with a gym ball supporting his right shoulder. Use a Velcro (Velcro) glove to secure his right hand to the rod. Ask the patient to slowly move the rod back and forth similarly to part of the ROM he might use to cast the rod. The range can be enlarged as the shoulder function returns. This activity will automatically perturb his sitting balance, and neuroplasticity should help with regaining that function. The physical therapist assistant can sit behind the patient on another gym ball or in the kneeling position and maintain the patient's trunk in postural extension while moving his right arm back and forth as if he were casting. The activity is not yet fly fishing, but as a physical therapist assistant, you are providing the environment that will lead to participation in that activity.

The patient determines the specific activity (in this case, fly fishing). The creativity of the physical therapist assistant encourages the patient to regain the motor function needed to maintain hope that the patient will again participate in those activities that were loved prior to the stroke. The physical therapist assistant can use a variety of measures (see Chapter 6) to reassess the patient's gains in muscle strength, postural control, balance, and UE mobility, all of which are important attributes of fly fishing. The same activity analysis needs to be performed with each activity the patient chooses. Do not select an activity that you as a physical therapist assistant *think* would be good for this patient. Instead, *empower* patients to those activities they want to do. The internal motivation will lead to practice. Repetitive practice leads to motor learning and then to motor control (see Chapter 4). Getting the emotional commitment from the patient is a key to succeeding and obtaining positive outcomes following physical therapy. If the physical therapist assistant feels uncomfortable or does not understand the goal or activity the patient is requesting, it is appropriate to discuss the activity with the physical therapist. The physical therapist may also be unfamiliar with the desired activity of the patient, but 2 professionals will be able to come up with many more components within the activity and thus break the task down into a sequential process of learning that can be used to guide the patient toward the desired motor skills. Doing exercises or impairment training that will be integrated into the function activity identified by the patient will lead to participation.[73,74]

Telehealth: A Future for Physical Therapy Practice

The use of telehealth is and will continue to be more a part of physical therapy services as the profession broadens in its scope of providing the best care for patients, especially those individuals who cannot access typical service institutions, and those living environments that providers cannot easily access. The US Veterans Administration is expanding the use of telehealth services across state lines to all eligible beneficiaries. These services could be provided in nonfederal sites including physical therapy practices and homes of patients. This may be the beginning of a new service provider system and may reach into all areas of physical therapy practice from pediatrics through geriatrics.[75-77]

The physical therapist assistant may be asked to participate in online programs in which the patient participates from home and is not in the clinic with the therapist.[78-82] The specifics are determined by the needs of the patient and the available resources. But the concepts and analysis of motor learning, motor control, and neuroplasticity will remain the same. Only the mechanism for how the service is delivered will be modified.

Similarly, patients who reenter society may ask the physical therapist assistant what they should do to maintain their gained function. There are many places where the patient can exercise to maintain physical skills. But if the patient only practices specific exercises such as strength training, there may not be carryover into maintaining functional skills.[74] Activities that are functionally based and work on all components of movement simultaneously should have a better chance of maintaining and improving function.[83-86] Refer to Chapter 18 for additional information on these alternative approaches to maintaining motor function.

Limiting Environmental Parameters and Using Adaptive Equipment to Enhance Training

The physical therapist may ask the physical therapist assistant to conduct a home visit to evaluate environmental factors that will limit functional independence. For example, a patient may be able to walk on a hard surface while in the rehabilitation center, but the patient's home may have thick pile carpeting with soft foam support. These 2 environments are not compatible. Either the patient needs to learn to walk on compliant surfaces while under the care of physical therapy, or the physical therapist needs to recommend that the family pull up the carpet and replace the floor with a noncompliant surface. If the patient needs to stand and take a step or 2 prior to transferring onto the toilet in the bathroom, then that pattern of movement of stepping, turning, and sitting needs to be emphasized as part of the intervention program, vs transferring on and off a toilet to a chair.

Similarly, if a patient has difficulty rising from a 90-degree angle in sitting, such as from a toilet or lounge chair, a raised toilet seat or a chair that raises the patient to vertical can assist in making the individual more independent within the home environment. The use of adaptive equipment for feeding, long shoehorns for donning shoes, and Velcro for ties can give an individual more freedom in ADL. The reality is that even if a patient has the potential and neuroplasticity to regain total independence, the physical therapist must set priorities and discuss them with the physical therapist assistant. Patients often have limited funding and a defined number of visits available. Thus, if a patient is no longer eligible for physical therapy services, the physical therapist and the physical therapist assistant need to empower that individual to continue learning and regaining function. This does not mean unrealistic expectations. On the contrary, it means setting goals and identifying the steps that the patient can safely follow to regain functional tasks that are important to them. This should include a long-term home program that turns into everyday life activities.

The physical therapist assistant needs to remember that every time the therapist's voice reinforces a patient, feedback is being given. The use of voice has many effects on the patient's CNS. A loud voice, unless the patient is hard-of-hearing, can be perceived as yelling at or speaking down to the patient. High pitches can become irritating, whereas very low pitches can be relaxing. Physical therapist assistants need to learn how to modulate their voice to optimize the motor responses of the patient. As the patient regains motor control during intervention, the physical therapist assistant needs to change volume and pitch to allow the patient's CNS to practice control under a variety of environmental circumstances.

One very important environmental adaptation for the patient is positioning between therapy sessions. Correct positioning of the limbs and trunk should be a team decision so that consistency is practiced throughout the day. It is very important that the limbs do not hang passively against gravity. This is one of the primary reasons a flaccid shoulder will begin to sublux. The response of the CNS to subluxation is to create stability, and thus, hypertonicity generally develops. That hypertonicity is in patterns or synergistic programs, and those programs can continue to sublux the shoulder because of asymmetry across the shoulder girdle. Some subluxations of the shoulder can be prevented by placing pillows under the arm so that the pull of gravity is not vertical. The limb can be placed on a lapboard to support the shoulder. Tape can be used to maintain shoulder alignment. There are many ways to position limbs while sitting and lying down. Pillows, splints, or cones for the hand are often used between therapy sessions. If the physical therapist assistant is not sure of correct positioning, it is appropriate to ask the physical therapist for suggestions. The physical therapist assistant needs to remember that no clinician has all the best answers to the best intervention for each patient. As a physical therapist assistant, you may find something that works better for the patient. It is your job to show the physical therapist. It is the physical therapist's job to try to figure out why it works.

Equipment such as canes, w/cs, walkers, transfer boards, shower chairs, and raised toilet seats are often needed when teaching individuals ADL and IADL, and are often used during interventions as part of a physical therapist assistant's skills. Measuring the appropriate length of a quad cane or a regular cane is within the scope of the physical therapist assistant's practice, and whether the patient is safe to move from a quad cane to a regular cane may also be expected to be within the parameters of the function of a physical therapist assistant. Even if the physical therapist assistant does not feel comfortable making those decisions early in the clinical career and asks for guidance from the physical therapist, with clinical experience, many of these decisions will be delegated to the physical therapist assistant.

In some skilled nursing facilities, the physical therapist assistant orders equipment for the patient to take home when discharged from the facility. Again, the physical therapist assistant can determine the appropriate measurements of an adjustable shower chair, raised toilet seat, or walker. Which w/c to order can be much more complex, but today, the physical therapist often uses the w/c vendor to help make those decisions. The vendor often has a variety of w/cs and will measure the patient's body dimensions prior to a therapist making any of those decisions. In time, this responsibility may fall to the physical therapist assistant's scope of practice, but again, the vendor and physical therapist should always be available for recommendations.

Special Focus Areas: Emerging Evidence-Based Treatment Approaches

Constraint-Induced Movement Therapy

Constraint-induced movement therapy (CIMT) has been developed as an intervention to improve individuals' functional ability. Most research and applications of CIMT are directed to the UEs, although the principles and techniques are being applied to the LEs as well. CIMT was developed based on several principles: learned non-use, task-specific training, intense practice that drives neuroplasticity, and behavioral interventions that optimize compliance to a specific exercise regimen.[87-89] In its basic format, CIMT consists of restraining the less-involved extremity (eg, for the UE, through the use of a mitt, sling, or glove) for 90% of the day, thereby forcing the individual to use the affected arm in specific tasks.

"Shaping" or *adapted-task practice* is task-oriented training that involves timed trials that ask the patient to perform a particular movement in successive repetitions. The intent of shaping is to drive specific neuroplastic changes in the cortex and to overcome learned non-use. These timed trials could involve 10 trials of 30 seconds each, with the therapist providing encouragement and feedback during this portion of the training.

The next component is called *task practice*, during which the patient performs functional, meaningful, and salient activities for 15 to 20 minutes at a time. The goal of this training is to perform functional activities that are challenging and important for the patient. The last component includes the behavioral strategies, which are aimed at optimizing practice of the home program. This includes the development of a behavioral contract, a daily exercise journal in which the patient documents the activities performed at home, and periodic assignments of skills to be performed at home. The training is usually performed in a rehabilitation environment where assistance is available and the restraint monitored, and practice is performed up to 6 times/day for at least 2 weeks.

Because this type of therapy requires one functional upper limb and one upper limb that show deficits within the motor system, this type of therapy is generally used with individuals post-stroke.[90] A minimum criterion of motor function (eg, 10 degrees of finger and 20 degrees of wrist extension) has been shown to be necessary to gain functional control over the hand.[90] The literature is mixed when this type of treatment is initiated in patients soon after their stroke; for this reason, it is not recommended that the physical therapist delegate this intervention if CIMT is used with a patient who is earlier than 3 months post-stroke.[91-95] In contrast, the literature supports CIMT for individuals who had their stroke 3 to 6 months prior to beginning this therapy.[90,96-100] Although most patients who receive this intervention are found within a rehabilitation environment, some literature supports this treatment approach with children within the home environment.[101,102]

Whether in inpatient acute rehabilitation or in rehabilitation training within skilled nursing facilities, physical therapist assistants may be asked to perform components of this intervention. The physical therapist should initiate the plan of care and then delegate appropriate tasks to the physical therapist assistant. The shaping and task-practice components of the intervention could be supervised by the physical therapist assistant. Initially the physical therapist assistant may need to assist the extremity in the task-specific movement(s), but the patient is also expected to force the use of the involved extremity. The physical therapist assistant may need to use handling to facilitate normal movement, but should move to have the patient initiating and controlling the movement. The patient is expected to participate actively during each session, and each session should focus on intensive, repetitive, task-specific training. Whether the intensive training is at home or in the clinic, it can lead to long-term functional recovery.[103-105] The physical therapist of record should identify this specific training in the plan of care.[88-90]

Neuromuscular Electrical Stimulation: An Old Treatment Concept With New Applications and Research

The use of neuromuscular electrical stimulation (NMES) has always been a part of physical therapy practice, and today it is certainly within the scope of the physical therapist assistant as long as it is under the guidelines and guidance of the supervising physical therapist. The National Institute of Health has conducted clinical research trials related to the use of NMES for strokes,[69,106] while de Freitas and colleagues conducted a systemic review on the use of NMES following spinal cord injuries.[107] Although the evidence does not show that with total paralysis NMES will automatically help in relearning of muscle function, there certainly is literature to suggest that with incomplete injuries or partial paralysis of movement, it does help to regain strength.[107] Pain management is another area in which NMES has been used extensively and shown to be a viable treatment alternative, especially when home units are used, application taught, and the control of the unit empowered by the patient.[108]

The specific application of NMES units will depend upon the patient diagnosis, the units available to the patient and the physical therapist assistant, and the receptiveness of the patient to the treatment.[109] As the physical therapist will establish frequency, type of modulation, dosage, and the specific application site(s) of the electrodes, adequate guidance to the physical therapist assistant should always be available. NMES should never cause additional pain, and the physical therapist assistant should always stop treatment and report to the physical therapist if the patient complains of additional pain, whether in the specific site location or somewhere else in the body. Unless, the physical therapist instructs the physical therapist assistant to change any of the protocol when reduction of pain is reported, those decisions should remain the responsibility of the physical therapist. Today's patients easily access the internet looking for ideas for pain reduction. A patient or respective family members may come to the physical therapist assistant and ask if you recommend the use of a NMES or transcutaneous electrical nerve stimulation unit to reduce pain. The physical therapist assistant must always remember that state law regulates practice, and you will always be held to that law, regardless of whether your opinion regarding any NMES unit might prompt you to encourage its use. To protect yourself and your practice, always ask the physical therapist.

Integrating Technology Into Clinical Practice: Body Weight–Supported Treadmill Training, Exoskeletons, Robotics, and Virtual Reality Environments

Technology takes many forms today and will be used more often in the future. This topic covers the use of body weight–support systems, exoskeletons on either UEs or LEs, virtual reality, visual adaptive environments, balance equipment, computer technology for cognitive and motor training, and training using interactive gaming programs. This technology has many uses during intervention activities, and a physical therapist assistant might be expected to use it in therapy.

The use of BWSTT is one way to decrease the demand for trunk and axial postural control while practicing ambulation (see Figures 9-12A and B, Figure 12-10, Figure 13-7, and Figure 19-1). The amount of power the patient needs for trunk or core postural function can be controlled through suspension, while the treadmill simultaneously triggers normal walking patterns. There are various ways to unweight an individual. Some systems use a harness suspended over a treadmill, some are support systems that allow overground training ambulation, and others suspend a patient using air and an inflatable suit that the patient dons.[110] Suspension systems can be placed on tracks within a home or physical therapy clinic to allow the individual to practice walking. As the core trunk or postural muscles gain power and endurance, the amount of body weight–support can be reduced. Simultaneously, the therapist can demand the patient respond to different speeds and inclines of the treadmill itself. The goal certainly is walking without the need for suspension at all if this is a possibility. Some patients never gain that motor control, but exercising using BWSTT will keep other muscles strong and provide cardiopulmonary and circulatory function. Functional electrical stimulation could also be used to augment motor output and facilitate movement. Many of these systems can also allow therapists to work on both sitting and standing balance without requiring the patient to control full body weight. This encourages the patient to activate motor control to tolerance and triggers postural coactivation without eliciting abnormal tone.[110,111] (Chapters 9, 12, 13, and 18 offer illustrations on BWSTT.) BWSTT has been shown to be effective in patient populations, including individuals who have been diagnosed with stroke,[112-116] cerebral palsy,[117,118] Parkinson's disease,[119] multiple sclerosis,[120] incomplete spinal cord injury,[121,122] and traumatic brain injury.[123,124]

The physical therapist assistant must always remember that for a patient to become functionally independent, the individual will still need to gain internal postural stability, strength, range, and motor programs without the use of a support system such as an overhead harness. If the physical therapist assesses how much unweighting, or which equipment is needed, or which program to run (eg, walking, running, or obstacles overground), a physical therapist assistant can be responsible for the training. Whether the equipment is accessible in a clinic often limits its use. But these may become very commonly used due to reduction of cost of technology, the consistency of the training, and the variability of practice with controls that they provide. When equipment is available, physical therapist assistants certainly could be expected to train individuals using BWSTT. Physical therapists also use these systems to obtain reliable measures for establishment of specific plans of care. Physical therapist assistant may be asked to use these same tools to measure ongoing gains following treatment, as well as measures of outcomes following interventions.[125-131]

The following is a specific example of the role of the physical therapist assistant in this intervention approach. At times, the physical therapist will delegate to the physical therapist assistant a functional activity that incorporates impairment training and control over specific aspects of a motor program. An example would be using a body weight–support harness while having a client walk on a treadmill (see Figures 9-12A and B, Figure 12-10, and Figure 13-7). The functional activity practiced is walking, varying the rate and incline of the treadmill-walking track to accommodate impairment problems. The motion itself should trigger a stepping program; the physical therapist assistant should not need to assist in the walking. The body weight–support system eliminates the need for full power and programming for posture and movement during the functional activity. By having the body weight partially supported, the patient is expected to control the entire feed-forward walking program and all its component programs within the patient's capability limits. The physical therapist assistant can change the rate of walking, the power needed to generate force during walking, the incline or decline of the movement, and other components of walking (eg, hard and soft surfaces of the shoe). All these aspects are considered impairment training because the patient is forced to self-correct the programming within the limits of the impairments.

As soon as the physical therapist assistant needs to guide the movement itself (eg, picking up the foot and placing it in its correct biomechanical position), the body-support intervention is not impairment training, but would instead be considered within the third category of intervention. In this third area, considered *hands-on guidance* by therapists, the physical therapist or physical therapist assistant may need to use hands-on control to guide motor responses to keep the patient within an acceptable parameter of performance. At the beginning of training, the patient may need help using the involved LE in push-off, swing phase, and heel striking. With repetitive practice, the patient should regain control over that specific pattern of movement. Given the intervention example of body weight–supported walking, the physical therapist assistant might be delegated both impairment and functional training within the patient's control parameters.[15,21]

Another type of technology that a physical therapist assistant may see in the clinic is an exoskeleton. Exoskeletons provide joint stability and are used to assist individuals who have limb-specific stabilization problems, such as someone who has suffered a stroke. Many of these exoskeletons are expensive and are being used for research only. The exoskeleton's computer program is sensitive to the force, range, and task-specific movement needed by the patient during the activity. The UE exoskeletons are primarily used in patients post-stroke, whereas the LE technology has been used with individuals who have had a stroke, a spinal cord injury, multiple sclerosis, or Parkinson's disease.[110,132-135] Exoskeletons are often seen in physical therapy clinics, and their use is becoming more frequent as the demand increases and the cost becomes more affordable. As the frequency increases, the physical therapist assistant may be expected to train individuals using an exoskeleton. Many of these devices can be found on the internet, as well as information regarding the manufacturer's recommendation of the exoskeleton's primary use.

Virtual reality and interactive gaming are quickly becoming intervention approaches used in stroke rehabilitation and other types of CNS involvement. Virtual reality creates a visual world that represents the environment within which the specific task is used. It has been used effectively with individuals post-stroke,[136-140] individuals with multiple sclerosis[141,142] or traumatic brain injury,[143] children who have cerebral palsy,[144,145] and children who have developmental delays.[146] As an example of the use of a virtual reality environment for an adult, consider the physical therapist assistant as working on teaching the IADL of grocery shopping using a cart while the patient is on a treadmill. The patient would hold onto a rail at the front of the treadmill. As the patient applies pressure on the support structure, which visually looks like the handle of a grocery cart, and starts walking within the virtual reality environment visually shown in front, the patient perceives the scene of walking down an aisle in a grocery store. When the patient stops to determine whether to get X vs Y items in the grocery aisle, the treadmill will also stop. The treadmill is driven by the movement of the patient's walking. Using these types of environments, the patient can be monitored for balance, motor coordination, and any other motor impairment that might be a critical factor related to independence and fall risk.[142] For a child, the virtual reality may be a playground or a fantasy world.[145] The complexity of virtual reality programming has rapidly expanded in play, and new research will constantly be available with the enjoyment people are finding in use of technology.

Gaming programs that require physical interactions have become a part of clinical practice and are considered technology available within a physical therapy environment. The Wii and the PlayStation (Sony) gaming programs that can facilitate balance, strength, and ROM, along with other motor strategies, have quickly become part of the physical therapist's toolbox related to intervention ideas.[147-149] A patient can be supported using a harness to prevent any chance of falling while actively participating in the activity shown on a television using one of the gaming programs. The patients can be bowling, skiing, sailing, playing golf, or practicing any other motor skill they value as quality of life participation activities that they plan to resume in the future. For patients of any age, these activities can be fun, competitive with other individuals, and social, and they provide immediate feedback as to success. The programs can store memory of the participant's successes from day to day and objectively show rates of improvement. For individuals whose recovery seems very slow, it can be hard to see these improvements, and this is one way to give concrete, positive feedback regarding their recovery.[27,142,145,150,151] One very important aspect of gaming is the interaction of the patient with the game. Once the patient is interacting with the game, self-motivation can easily become the motivator to participate with these games especially as they are available for home use.

Obviously, the use of technologies can be combined. The BWSTT can be used in a virtual environment. The gaming programs can be used as part of telecommunication from a distance.[152] Where technology will take therapy is open to the imagination. The one thing that seems predictable is that physical therapist assistants will be using these technologies as part of their scope of practice.

Aquatic Therapy Integrated Into Physical Therapy

Aquatic therapy is yet another specialized evidence-based intervention that the physical therapist assistant, under the direction of the physical therapist, can provide. Aquatic therapy can be used with a variety of both medical and movement-based diagnoses seen across the lifespan.[153,154] Aquatic therapy intervention can be used to treat patients who could benefit from the physical properties of water, such as buoyancy, hydrostatic pressure, and/or resistance. Physical therapy interventions often add manual resistance, weights, or TheraBand products to improve strength and progress challenges to movement. The viscosity or resistance of the water producing similar challenges can become additive and increases the flexibility and variety during practice. Alternatively, the water can provide a gravity-eliminated medium for weaker individuals to help initiate early movement similar to using a powder board or other antigravity tools.

Research has shown using body weight–support devices to be a benefit to assisting patients in movement activities. Body weight–support devices are used to encourage or challenge functional mobility skills such as standing, dynamic balance, and ambulation on and off the treadmill. The use of a pool and its buoyancy can provide similar assistance. A patient might present with a traumatic brain injury and a fear of falling due to impaired protective responses. Putting that individual in a pool can provide a safe environment to challenge the patient's balance reactions to activities with the added input of the water, its resistance, and resultant support to the intervention. If the patient enjoys being in the water, this environment can produce an opportunity for greater independence of movement without assistance, which can certainly motivate the individual to participate not only initially, but also in future interventions. If a patient is fearful of water, then the clinician needs to respect that fear and make sure the patient feels safe throughout the entire treatment.

Patients who participate in aquatic therapy interventions can expect the water to have an effect on the major biological systems. When treating an aquatic patient, a clinician can expect physiological effects to the cardiovascular, pulmonary, musculoskeletal system, and renal systems.[155] The physical therapist should give the physical therapist assistant strict treatment guidelines based on each individual patient, the medical presentation, and what impact the water could have. For instance, an individual with a spinal cord injury could have a compromised circulatory system, which impacts body temperature regulation or heart rate responses to the aquatic intervention. Providing the right exercise intensity, monitoring heart rate, and modifying the water temperature could make a big difference in the safety and effectiveness of a treatment session.[156]

The pool can provide a fun, beneficial treatment intervention with benefits such as promoting muscle relaxation, increased ease of movement, reduced gravitational forces, stability, and improved confidence. However, the physical therapist assistant should also be aware of the contraindications and communicate any observations or concerns directly to the physical therapist. These could include a patient with an infectious disease, new or ongoing integumentary issues, incontinence, cardiac failure, low vital lung capacity, or abnormal blood pressure. These contraindications are not absolute and may depend on facility policy as well as individual presentation. A patient may develop problems that would make water therapy contraindicated even after the physical therapist has delegated the intervention to the physical therapist assistant.

Interventions in the pool, similar to those on land, can include therapeutic exercise, functional mobility training, manual and respiratory therapies all with the goal of improving patient function. Whether the water is indicated as a sound intervention is based on patient evaluative findings by the physical therapist, goals, and tolerance to the water.[156] The physical therapist assistant will be given the intensity, duration, and frequency of land-to-aquatic treatment ratios, as well as appropriate outcome measures to demonstrate progress and advance the patient through the plan of care. Research has certainly identified that aquatic therapy can be beneficial for patients with movement problems arising from neurological insults. Whether the focus is on strengthening, increasing movement function, decreasing fatigue while participating in movement, decreasing fear and anxiety, changing environment within which the person moves, or generally increasing physical fitness, the evidence substantiates integrating this type of intervention into physical therapy management whenever possible or realistic.[157-167]

Historical documentation of the use of water as a healing medium can be traced as far back as 2400 BC. It wasn't until the late 1890s that aquatic therapy moved from a simple passive immersion to a treatment technique.[168] Unfortunately, the use of water for rehabilitation is vastly underused despite an increase in popularity and advances in aquatic technology. The advancement of aquatic technology such as specialized floatation devices, resistive jets, underwater cameras for visual feedback, and treadmills continues to advance the use of water as an effective intervention and provide the clinician endless treatment options (Figure 5-9). Aquatic facilities continue to become more widely available and have improved the means by which today's aquatic therapy is provided. Patients can transition from skilled aquatic therapy under the direction of a clinician to a community-based program to continue to enjoy the water and its benefits as a life activity that can produce fun, social interaction, and improved movement and quality of life.

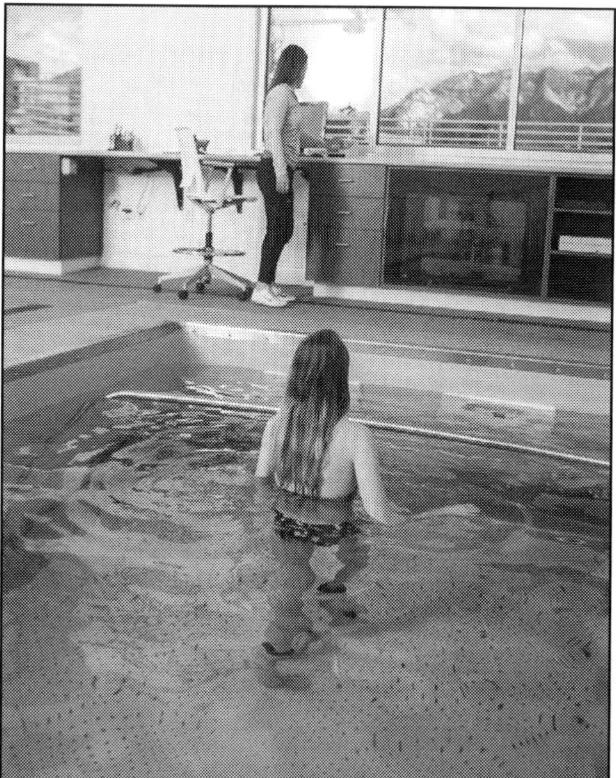

Figure 5-9. Use of an underwater treadmill, variable depth adjustable floor, and computer technology to enhance patient participation and motivation.

Specific Intervention Techniques: Proprioceptive Neuromuscular Facilitation and Neuro-Developmental Treatment

This section will discuss 2 specific intervention approaches that have been used in populations with movement dysfunctions due to neurological problems. These 2 techniques involve all categories of intervention: functional training, impairment training, augmented (hands-on) intervention, and even somatosensory retraining. The pervasive use of these approaches in neurological rehabilitation necessitates the discussion of these approaches in detail.

Many critics of these approaches cite the lack of solid scientific evidence behind their use. While that may be currently true, many factors—such as the variability in the use and application of these techniques, the complexity of research methodologies that involve neurological intervention studies, and the lack of valid, reliable, sensitive, and specific tools to assess progress—are major considerations.

It is important to incorporate the principles of neuroplasticity when performing these interventions. This includes selecting activities that are salient, meaningful, and functional for the patient, considering the number of repetitions and the context by which these interventions are used.

Proprioceptive Neuromuscular Facilitation

PNF uses movement patterns incorporating multiplanar, diagonal, and functional movement with rotation and inhibition/facilitation principles to affect muscle coordination, strength, and/or length.[33,169] PNF has applications to orthopedic and neuromuscular populations because of its versatility as an intervention.[170-172] PNF combines patterns, either for the limbs, the trunk, or the whole body, with techniques that can address passive, active-assisted, isometric, concentric, and/or eccentric muscle activity.[169] By combining the movement pattern with the appropriate technique, PNF can be used with multiple types of patient impairments ranging from difficulty initiating movement, movement timing, coordination, co-contraction, static holding, stretching, and strengthening.

PNF was developed based on the neurophysiological principles of muscles discovered by Sherrington in the 1900s and Sister Kenney's manual therapy techniques.[173] Herman Kabat, a neurophysiologist and physician, with Margaret Knott and Dorothy Voss, both physical therapists, worked in the 1950s to further develop PNF techniques and nomenclature at Kasier Vallejo in California. Knott and Voss published the first book describing PNF in the 1960s.[33] The initial population of patients who drove the development of this technique suffered from the motor impairments caused by polio. This disease attacked the alpha motor neuron, and this approach is especially effective when considering alpha motor neuron involvement. Polio did not affect upper motor neurons, so these individuals maintained their original motor learning and could draw on those programs to assist in regaining motor function. This approach is especially effective with individuals with orthopedic complications or spinal cord injury, because those individuals exhibit impairments of sensory and motor neurons coming to and from the spinal column as well as the peripheral system itself. Today, Kasier Foundation Hospital in Vallejo, California, has an internationally recognized residency program for physical therapists wishing to study PNF intensively.

The most common PNF patterns are those addressing the limbs, pelvis, or scapulae (Table 5-1).[169] While the patient is moving through these patterns, the therapist implements sensory inputs to facilitate movement. Verbal directions are given in a loud, encouraging voice with short commands such as "Push, now, harder." The therapist's manual contacts are very precise, with the hands over muscles to be activated during the pattern using a supportive grip. These manual contacts can be used to provide resistance or support, as needed, depending on the goal of the PNF intervention and the patient's level of motor impairment. Additionally, the therapist can apply joint distraction to facilitate flexion or joint approximation to facilitate extension. To facilitate initiation of the movement, the therapist may deliver a quick stretch to the muscles performing the movement.

The therapist then combines the facilitation techniques and the movement pattern with PNF techniques addressing how the muscles are contracting and the timing of movements. Common PNF techniques are shown here[170]:

- **Rhythmic initiation:** Begins with the therapist moving the patient through the desired movement using passive ROM, followed by active-assistive ROM, active ROM, and finally providing resistance through the ROM.
- **Contract relax and hold relax:** Techniques used either for stretching or for short-duration change to abnormal muscle tone. By using either the Golgi tendon organs or reciprocal inhibition, the patient contracts selected muscles followed by a sustained passive stretch provided by the therapist (*contract relax*), or passive stretch provided by the therapist is followed by an isometric holding contraction by the patient (*hold relax*).
- **Rhythmic stabilization:** The patient holds a position while the therapist applies manual resistance. No motion should occur from the patient. The patient should simply resist the therapist's movements. The therapist holds this resistance, and then switches to the alternate pattern, again with the patient holding. Usually rhythmic stabilization is performed in the direction of rotation.
- **Alternating isometrics:** Similar to rhythmic stabilization, but the resistance is applied to both sides of the joint, usually not in the direction of rotation.

For example, the patient may have weakness of the right dorsiflexors due to a stroke. Because of this weakness, the patient demonstrates gait deviations such as shortened right step length, toe contact on the right during initial contact in stance phase, and a foot drop. PNF intervention may be used to strengthen the dorsiflexors while also working on timing and coordination of dorsiflexion in relation to the knee and hip joint. Intervention may start with a limb pattern ending in the right LE in hip flexion, knee flexion, and dorsiflexion. To start, rhythmic initiation may be used to acquaint the patient with the PNF pattern and to allow for passive and active-assisted dorsiflexion, depending on the extent of the patient's weakness. The therapist can increase the resistance to the dorsiflexors as the patient's strength increases to add more challenge. Initially the patient may be positioned in left side-lying and transition to supine, sitting, and standing as the ability to handle the extra

Table 5-1

Proprioceptive Neuromuscular Facilitation Patterns for Extremities and Trunk

	Start Position	***End Position***
Upper Extremity		
D1 flexion	• Shoulder: Extension-adduction-internal rotation • Elbow: Extension • Forearm: Pronation • Wrist: Extension • Fingers: Extension	• Shoulder: Flexion-adduction-external rotation • Elbow: Flexion • Forearm: Supination • Wrist: Flexion • Fingers: Flexion
D1 extension	• Shoulder: Flexion-adduction-external rotation • Elbow: Flexion • Forearm: Supination • Wrist: Flexion • Fingers: Flexion	• Shoulder: Extension-adduction-internal rotation • Elbow: Extension • Forearm: Pronation • Wrist: Extension • Fingers: Extension
D2 flexion	• Shoulder: Extension-adduction-internal rotation • Elbow: Extension • Wrist: Extension • Finger: Extension	• Shoulder: Flexion-abduction-external rotation • Elbow: Flexion • Wrist: Flexion • Finger: Flexion
D2 extension	• Shoulder: Flexion-adduction-external rotation • Elbow: Flexion • Wrist: Flexion • Finger: Flexion	• Shoulder: Extension-abduction-internal rotation • Elbow: Extension • Wrist: Extension • Finger: Extension
Lower Extremity		
D1 flexion	• Hip: Extension-adduction-internal rotation • Knee: Extension • Ankle: Plantar flexion	• Hip: Flexion-adduction-external rotation • Knee: Flexion • Ankle: Dorsiflexion
D1 extension	• Hip: Flexion-adduction-external rotation • Knee: Flexion • Ankle: Dorsiflexion	• Hip: Extension-adduction-internal rotation • Knee: Extension • Ankle: Plantar flexion
D2 flexion	• Hip: Extension-adduction-internal rotation • Knee: Extension • Ankle: Plantar flexion	• Hip: Flexion-abduction-external rotation • Knee: Flexion • Ankle: Dorsiflexion
D2 extension	• Hip: Flexion-abduction-external rotation • Knee: Flexion • Ankle: Dorsiflexion	• Hip: Extension-adduction-internal rotation • Knee: Extension • Ankle: Plantarflexion

(continued)

Table 5-1 (continued)

Proprioceptive Neuromuscular Facilitation Patterns for Extremities and Trunk

	Start Position	*End Position*
Pelvis		
Anterior elevation	Pelvis: Depression-posterior rotation	Pelvis: Elevation-anterior rotation
Posterior depression	Pelvis: Elevation-anterior rotation	Pelvis: Depression-posterior rotation
Anterior depression	Pelvis: Elevation-posterior rotation	Pelvis: Depression-anterior rotation
Posterior elevation	Pelvis: Depression-anterior rotation	Pelvis: Elevation-posterior rotation
Scapula		
Anterior elevation	Scapula: Depression-downward rotation	Scapula: Elevation-upward rotation
Posterior depression	Scapula: Elevation-upward rotation	Scapula: Depression-downward rotation
Anterior depression	Scapula: Elevation-downward rotation	Scapula: Depression-upward rotation
Posterior elevation	Scapula: Depression-upward rotation	Scapula: Elevation-downward rotation

resistance of gravity and the challenge of trunk control/balance increases. As the patient masters the PNF pattern motorically and strength improves, then other techniques such as rhythmic stabilization or alternating isometrics can be added or substituted. At an advanced level, the therapist can resist the pattern while the patient ambulates (in the parallel bars if extra stability and UE support are needed).

PNF interventions can also assist in retraining activities such as transfers and gait. Patients with poor trunk control, particularly poor ability to stabilize the trunk via co-contraction during other dynamic movements such as sit-to-stand transfers, may benefit from PNF interventions. In sitting, the therapist can use rhythmic stabilization with manual contacts at the scapulae and anterior shoulder to work on maintaining an engaged co-contraction (coactivation) of the trunk and increase strength and endurance for maintaining an upright and midline trunk position. This can then be put into a functional task such as sit-to-stand by applying resistance to the upper trunk through the anterior lean needed at the beginning of the transfer and changing the resistance to more approximation through the shoulder girdle during the lift-off portion of the transfer. The approximation during lift-off will facilitate the patient's trunk and LE extensors, the muscle groups needed to successfully perform lift-off and achieve standing.

Pelvic PNF intervention is commonly employed in gait training. The pelvic PNF patterns can be used selectively to assist the patient with specific phases of gait. For example, should the patient demonstrate a posteriorly rotated pelvis during the swing phase, the pelvic anterior elevation pattern may be used as an intervention. Starting in the side-lying position, the pelvic anterior elevation pattern may be practiced with rhythmic initiation first to familiarize the patient with the pattern and allow the therapist to see what pelvic ROM the patient has, and then the therapist can apply resistance that the patient's strength can tolerate. The therapist can also adapt the resistance to have the patient work on either concentric or eccentric pelvic motor control. This can then be transitioned to gait, as the therapist applies the same resistance to the pelvis during the transition from stance to swing phase of gait.

Full body patterns, such as mass flexion, incorporate multiple PNF patterns and techniques into functional movements such as rolling, allowing for more complex movements and requiring more motor control from patients. Mass flexion is a PNF full-body pattern that combines the pelvic anterior elevation pattern with the scapular anterior depression pattern, requiring the whole length of the trunk on one side to be active. Mass flexion pattern can be used as an intervention to help a patient with rolling from supine to side-lying.

For example, your patient has had a stroke causing left-sided hemiparesis. PNF intervention may begin with the patient in the right side-lying position practicing the pelvic and scapular patterns individually.[33,174] Once the patient can perform each of these 2 patterns with sufficient control, the patterns can be combined and performed simultaneously to produce the mass flexion pattern. To progress this intervention, the patient can be positioned in a quarter roll position and perform mass flexion with a rolling motion. As the patient gains competence, the patient can be positioned in supine and perform mass flexion with the complete rolling motion.

PNF is immensely flexible in application with patients.[92] Therapists can adapt the PNF patterns to work on only one joint to target isolated areas of deficits. Because the patterns and techniques can be interchanged to address specific patient goals and can be advanced within and across treatment sessions, PNF is a valuable intervention to work on a variety of motor system and motor control impairments.[170-172] The physical therapist assistant needs to be familiar with basic PNF patterns and techniques, as these may be part of the plan of care determined by the physical therapist.

Neuro-Developmental Treatment: Based on Sequential Movement Analysis and Its Progression as the Central Nervous System Learns—Not Just Child Development

NDT is an intervention approach, commonly used with people of all ages who have neurological dysfunction, that uses facilitation and inhibition techniques provided in a direct, hands-on approach.[34,40] NDT is based on sequential movement analysis and its progression as the CNS learns. Its sequences are not based on specific sequences of child development, but rather on why a child or adult may use specific patterns of movement or movement progression against gravity or with gravity eliminated to help the CNS gain function. These interventions are individualized based on the patient's impairments and activity limitations and are guided during sessions by the patient's response to treatment.[34] NDT is used in both physical therapy and occupational therapy treatment.

The NDT approach was developed by Berta (physiotherapist) and Karel Bobath (psychiatrist/neurophysiologist) in Germany in the mid-20th century, and is sometimes still referred to as the *Bobath concept*.[34,175,176] Developed for adults with hemiplegia after stroke and children with cerebral palsy, today NDT is used for many neurological diagnoses. The early theoretical basis of NDT surrounded the restoration of normal postural reflexes progressing rigidly through the developmental sequence to normalize movement. The theoretical basis for NDT has progressed as our understanding of the CNS, motor learning and motor control, and neuroplasticity have evolved. Today, NDT aims to achieve the goal of developing optimal movement patterns through the use of orthotics and appropriate compensations, instead of aiming for completely "normal" movement patterns. The NDT approach is promoted through the Neuro-Developmental Treatment Association,[177] which also provides continuing education specific to NDT, including extensive courses of study for treatment of babies, children, and adults.

Concepts key to the NDT approach include patient handling techniques to facilitate and/or inhibit movement interfering with normal movement patterns using key points of control.[34,40] Handling, in the NDT approach, is therapeutic in nature and uses the therapist's hands and body to provide manual contact and directional cues to the patient's body. The touch used, as light as possible to encourage the best patient response and most movement possible from the patient, is specific to the impairments demonstrated by the patient. Although the touch is light in pressure, it is proprioceptive and does not elicit a light touch withdrawal. Patients with touch sensitivity need deeper touch to facilitate postural patterns and functional movement. The specific touch depends on the reaction of the patient and should be enough to cause appropriate facilitation or inhibition to the patient's muscles, while also providing cues as to the direction of movement.[40,175,176]

Therapists analyze postures and movements, looking for movement dysfunctions present when the individual is asked to move. The NDT approach requires active participation from the patient and the therapist, as the therapist must perform ongoing assessments of the success of the handling in normalizing the patient's movement while the patient must be actively performing the posture or movement.[40] Depending on the patient, rehabilitation goals may work to improve postural control, coordination of movement sequences, movement initiation, body alignment or posture, abnormal muscle tone, and/or muscle weakness.

Handling should be provided using key points of control.[34,40] Any part of the patient's body may be a key point of control; this distinction is related to what joint or body segment is required for performance of the selected activity. For example, using the NDT approach to achieve midline trunk orientation in sitting may use key points of control at the patient's sides (above the hip bones), with the therapist keeping an open hand with the fingers spread wide apart. This key point of control allows the therapist manual contact with the abdominal muscles as well as the lower ribs and extensor muscles. As key points of control move farther away from the body segment initiating the movement, the response of the patient may be delayed. For example, the therapist may select the shoulder girdle region of the patient as a key point of control for midline trunk orientation, by placing a hand over the top of the shoulder, with the open hand contacting the clavicles and the scapular spines. This allows the therapist to facilitate left-right orientation, as well as anterior-posterior orientation. Because this point of control is farther away from the abdominal and back extensor muscles, the response seen in the patient may be delayed. The specific response will also require more motor control on the part of the patient, because the handling is more removed from the specific region of the lower trunk and abdominals.

The NDT approach uses many contact points and not just the hands/fingers to provide manual facilitation. One example commonly encountered in the neurological population involves placing the therapist's tibia in contact with the patient's tibia to provide manual and directional cues for knee control during standing, transfers, and gait. This key point of control allows the therapist to simultaneously use both hands to provide input in other areas, while also providing important handling to the patient's LE.[175] Likewise, the therapist may use the forearm against other body segments of the patient while the hands are also providing handling. This adaptation is common to control the position of the UE in support during sitting. The therapist faces the patient and uses the forearm on the posterior region of the patient's elbow to provide input to keep the elbow extended and pushing into the surface, while the therapist's hand is on the patient's trunk to provide input about trunk control.

The NDT approach also stresses the importance of the trunk in the patient's ability to sustain postural control in a vertical position (such as sitting or standing) and for normal movement (such as walking).[176] Many NDT sessions will include portions that focus on the patient's ability to maintain upright postural trunk control in quiet vertical activities and during dynamic movement. Additionally, to address abnormal muscle tone, the NDT approach uses weight-bearing postures to facilitate coactivation around joints, which pulls in postural function. For patients with hypotonic limbs, weight-bearing can also facilitate normal joint alignment, such as in the glenohumeral joint, while also facilitating the limb extensor muscles by way of joint approximation. Weight-bearing can also facilitate more normal muscle tone in patients with hypertonicity and/or spasticity by using reciprocal inhibition.[34] Although many colleagues think that NDT was based on incorrect understanding of the brain, in fact it was based on movement and what has become movement science. The founders of these techniques were not neuroscientists, but were physical therapists and analyzed movement at a finite level. They saw not only a large visual picture of sequential movement, but also the connections between what we might call positions in space. They used that movement understanding and sequences to develop their approaches. Then, they tried to explain what they saw using science of that time, which was incorrect. Throwing all those tools away because colleagues thought the approaches were based on neuroscience vs movement science would be tragic and a disservice to our profession. There is new research emerging on how NDT approaches are based on today's neuroscience, which makes the tools and sequences much more realistic and easier to understand.[178,179]

Conclusion

Intervention possibilities are numerous,[180] and many are yet to be discovered.[181] The ultimate goal of physical therapy intervention is the patient regaining all movement function as an effortless and enjoyable motor experience. This goal may often be unrealistic given the extent of the lesion, the potential of the patient, and the time available to the physical therapist or physical therapist assistant for treatment. As a result, decisions need to be made and goals established based on the specific needs of the patient and family given the environmental restraints of the home, the support systems, the number of visits, the motivation of the patient, and the total health of the individual.

The physical therapist assistant may be delegated many aspects of the intervention program, and the physical therapist may retain certain components. It is the physical therapist's responsibility to delegate appropriately. If the physical therapist assistant is unsure of the delegated intervention strategies, then the physical therapist assistant must ask for help. In that way, the physical therapist will develop better communication strategies, and the physical therapist assistant will develop better intervention skills.

This chapter presented 5 categories of intervention: functional training, impairment training, hands-on therapeutic or adaptive intervention, somatosensory retraining, and participation training. The ultimate physical therapy goal is functional motor recovery in all aspects of life activities. Although the intervention may need to begin with sensory training and hands-on intervention, the goal is to work toward independent functional motor control by the patient. During physical therapy treatment, often specific impairment training needs to be incorporated, such as increasing ROM, decreasing hypertonicity while increasing muscle strength, or increasing respiratory input and exhalation for better oxygenation of the muscle tissues and better endurance.

Once a patient can independently run motor programs in a feedforward fashion, the practice needs to become a life activity to retain the skill. At this time, practice needs to be delegated to family, friends, caregivers, and the patient. Transferring throughout the day, brushing teeth, washing hair, and getting from bed to living room to kitchen to outside are a child's and an adult's everyday expectations. Generally, if the patient is empowered to learn or relearn those functional skills no matter the age, the patient will continue to move and practice these skills as part of daily life. If, on the other hand, those activities are thought of as therapy and something that has to be done to get out of the hospital or health care services, then the empowerment of those patients to their own motor potential has not been accomplished, and often, carryover into life activities is not actualized. As soon as the patient stops practicing, skill can be lost and function decreased. A clinician may find the same patient returning to therapy due to lost function, but in reality, the patient has lost or never obtained the motivation to continue what was learned during the initial physical therapy intervention period.

There are many additional reasons why a patient may lose function over time. He may become ill and thus lose muscle endurance, and it becomes too hard to do those daily activities. She may have another insult to her CNS or have a progressive problem. None of those medical conditions are within the power of the physical therapist or physical therapist assistant to control, but helping empower the patient to realistic possibilities is critical for motivation. It is not acceptable for the daily therapeutic program to be satisfying to the therapist without those feelings of accomplishment extending to the patient. Patients need the feeling of success to continue on a road of learning. Empowering the patient to his or her potential is a critical aspect of intervention and certainly part of the physical therapist assistant's role during intervention. Life changes from day to day, but all of us want to feel that, no matter where we are on this path of learning, we have more potential to learn and grow each day. A patient is no different.

Case Studies

Case #1

Mrs. Jones is a 78-year-old woman who has a history of falling. She has a history of diabetes and knows she is to drink water once an hour. After magnetic resonance imaging scans, blood studies, and other medical examinations, the physician could not make a definitive diagnosis regarding her falling. The patient was sent to physical therapy to determine whether interventions might help. At the initial visit, Mrs. Jones had a black eye and informed the physical therapist that she had fallen into her closet when she tried to get a shoe. After a thorough balance assessment, the physical therapist determined that Mrs. Jones had all balance strategies, adequate ROM, and knew when she was falling. She used to swim daily with her friends at her senior living facility's inside pool but had stopped after an episode of pneumonia. During that episode, she stayed at her daughter's apartment next to hers. She remained in bed the majority of the day for slightly more than 4 weeks. She has become very inactive, lives in a small apartment, and goes out only when her daughter takes her to the doctor. She no longer drives, and her daughter does all her grocery shopping. She usually heats a microwave dinner in the evening and has cereal and fruit or cheese for her breakfast and lunch. Her daughter often brings a meal and eats with her. Mrs. Jones is weak, especially in her ankles, knees, and hips bilaterally. That weakness is especially true in her postural muscles in both legs and her back. She spends the majority of the day sitting in her rocking chair, watching television or reading. She has a large pitcher of water by her chair, which allows her to have her hourly glass of water. She also speaks in short sentences. She fatigues quickly during physical activity and has a slowed reaction time to perturbations. The physical therapist has delegated 5 interventions to the physical therapist assistant before a reassessment. The physical therapist gave the physical therapist assistant the following instructions:

1. Have Mrs. Jones practice getting up and down from her chair at least once an hour by telling her to go to the kitchen and get a glass of water instead of using a pitcher by her chair. Give the responsibility to Mrs. Jones, because she is independent in this activity and has walls to stop her falling if she loses her balance.
2. Have Mrs. Jones practice reaching for her shoes and donning them:
    a. First, sitting from her chair: Session 1.
    b. Second, standing with a support arm holding onto a table, a chair, or some other stable piece of furniture: Sessions 2 and 3.
    c. Third, standing with a shoe directly within her BOS: Sessions 3 and 4.
    d. Fourth, standing, moving her shoe sequentially farther and farther away from her limits of stability. Progress to reaching into the closet by Session 5. Progress through this sequence as she increases her tolerance to moving over her COG without falling. She may progress faster or slower depending on her endurance and fear of falling.
3. Teach Mrs. Jones diaphragmatic breathing:
    a. First, while lying on her bed: Session 1.
    b. Second, when standing or walking. Count the number of syllables she uses in a sentence at the beginning of therapy and at the end. Document and report those numbers to the physical therapist following each session: Session 2.
4. After you, the physical therapist assistant, can walk with Mrs. Jones 25 yards (the distance to the mailbox and back), instruct the daughter to walk with her mother daily to the mailbox. The daughter should be told that the goal is to increase that distance on a weekly basis. She might walk with her mother to the pool, rest, and walk back. Once she can do that easily, have her mother begin swimming on a daily basis.

Questions

1. What clinical symptoms would the physical therapist assistant want to immediately discuss with the physical therapist?
2. Under which area of intervention does this program fall?
3. Are all activities appropriate to be delegated to the physical therapist assistant?

Case #2

Charley is an 8-year-old who was diagnosed with cerebral palsy at 3 months of age. His family has been told he has spastic diplegia. He was in therapy as an outpatient in a developmental program until age 5 and now receives physical therapy 2 times/week while in school. Charley recently underwent heel-cord lengthening. The child was initially placed in casts to maintain ROM and allow healing. The casts have now been bivalved and will be used as night splints. The child has been referred to the outpatient clinic to regain functional use of his LEs for gait. The physical therapist has delegated strengthening exercises of the gastrocsoleus muscles to the physical therapist assistant. The physical therapist assistant is instructed to do passive stretching to the ankles with a focus of gaining approximately 5 degrees beyond 90 degrees at each session with the goal of gaining and maintaining 110 degrees of ankle ROM for ambulatory activities. The physical therapist also wants the physical therapist assistant to do strengthening exercises in patterns that encourage the child to break up the extensor synergy (+ supporting reaction) while incorporating ankle function both in weight-bearing and non–weight-bearing positions. These activities can be encouraged in sit-to-stand, side-stepping, half-knee-to-stand, and kicking a ball with one foot while maintaining balance and support.

Questions

1. Are these interventions within the scope of practice of the physical therapist assistant?
2. Under which area of intervention does this program fall?
3. How would the physical therapist assistant document change in range and power of the LEs, and how is that affecting functional behavior?

Case #3

The patient is a 28-year-old man who suffered a head trauma following an auto accident 10 days previously. No orthopedic or integumentary problems exist. The patient has a tracheotomy and is intubated for feeding. He lost consciousness immediately, and the paramedics had to resuscitate him following a cardiac arrest. He was without oxygen for only 2 minutes, and the doctors do not anticipate any severe anoxic injury. The patient was in the intensive care unit for 2 days and has been transferred to a subacute rehabilitation unit. The patient is in a vegetative state, considered Level III on a Rancho scale. The physical therapist is working with the patient on a ball in the vertical position sitting and kneeling to try to facilitate automatic postural trunk and head control. The physical therapist has delegated ROM exercises, as well as horizontal rolling and bed mobility, to the physical therapist assistant. The physical therapist wants the physical therapist assistant to encourage rolling by handling from the LEs. Initial handling should begin with the patient in the side-lying position and should facilitate rolling toward prone and back toward supine. As the patient begins to automatically respond, the physical therapist assistant is to increase the ROM of the rolling activity with the hopes that the patient will begin to roll. The physical therapist has instructed the physical therapist assistant to work in the patient's bed in the morning and on the mat in the physical therapy clinic in the afternoon. Following the physical therapist assistant's intervention, the physical therapist will work on sitting and kneeling, with the physical therapist assistant helping by guarding the patient (controlling the roll of the ball) and encouraging interactions with the patient while in the patient's visual gaze.

Questions

1. Are these interventions within the scope of practice of the physical therapist assistant?
2. What clinical signs would the physical therapist assistant want to report immediately to the physical therapist?
3. How would the physical therapist assistant document change?
4. Under which area of intervention does this program fall?

Case #4

The patient is a 58-year-old woman who suffered a left cerebrovascular accident 2 weeks ago. She is a chief executive officer of a large corporation and suffered her stroke following a 22-hour air flight returning from a business trip to East Asia. She has minimal speech involvement and has functional motor use of her right UE and LE; however, she has significant loss in sensation. She has normal sensation in her face, trunk, shoulders, and hips, but has poor proprioception in her right knee and ankle and no proprioception or tactile sensation in her right elbow, wrist, or hand. She is right-hand dominant. Because of the poor sensation, she is unable to use proprioception to anticipate a perturbation, which could cause a fall in standing or during ambulation. She uses her visual and vestibular system to compensate for poor proprioception, but when distracted in standing or during ambulation, she is slow to react and tends to fall. She has automatic protective extension in a feedforward UE movement, but without vision, has little idea where her arm is in space or whether her hand is functionally doing anything. The physical therapist has delegated to the physical therapist assistant UE sensory awareness exercises with the patient, with and without vision. The physical therapist has instructed the physical therapist assistant to:

1. Have the patient hold various objects first in the left hand and then in the right. The patient is first asked to look at the object while it is in the left hand, manipulate it, and then visualize what it looks like.
2. Have the patient first find an object (eg, spoon, marble, comb, sandpaper, or cotton) in sand and rice with visual assistance, then perform the same activity without vision. If she cannot perform this activity initially, the physical therapist assistant will tell her what the object is, then have her look at it, shut her eyes, and visualize the form while manipulating it.

The physical therapist performs sensory awareness retraining first in the supine position, moving to sitting, and ending in standing to facilitate bilateral integration and better somatosensory cortical awareness. Once the patient has some awareness of the right LE, the physical therapist delegates to the physical therapist assistant bilateral LE weight-bearing activities in a body weight–supported harness over the treadmill. The physical therapist assistant is instructed to:

1. Have the patient practice rocking on her feet, visualizing the symmetrical movement at both ankles.
2. Have the patient practice weight-shifting onto and off the right LE, then shift to the same activity on the left.
3. Have the patient begin ambulation while in the harness on a treadmill while visualizing the movement in her right LE. Once she acknowledges that she feels her right LE and is able to ambulate on the treadmill with only 10% of her body weight supported, the physical

therapist should be told to begin gait training in various sensory environments without body support. The physical therapist will use the virtual reality program to assist the patient in IADL. Once the patient is able to successfully complete the tasks using virtual reality, the physical therapist will use the Wii balance program to have the patient practice those motor activities she enjoyed doing prior to the stroke. The physical therapist assistant will be responsible for guarding the patient once she begins using the Wii to guarantee that she does not fall.

Questions

1. Are these interventions appropriate to delegate to the physical therapist assistant?
2. What clinical symptoms would the physical therapist assistant want to immediately discuss with the physical therapist?
3. How would the physical therapist assistant document change in the areas of intervention?
4. Under which area of intervention does this program fall?

References

1. American Physical Therapy Association. Guide to Physical Therapist Practice 3.0. http://guidetoptpractice.apta.org/. Accessed August 1, 2018.
2. Erickson ML, McKnight R. *Documentation Basics for the Physical Therapist Assistant.* 3rd ed. Thorofare, NJ: SLACK Incorporated; 2018.
3. Koloroutis M, Trout M. *See Me As Person: Creating Therapeutic Relationships with Patients and Their Families.* Minneapolis, MN: Creative Health Care Management, Inc; 2012.
4. Byl N: A review and perspective on maximizing brain plasticity: priming the nervous system to learn. *Int Phys Med Reh J.* 2017;1(5).
5. Doidge N. *The Brain That Changes Itself.* New York, NY: Penguin Group; 2015.
6. Hassanzahraee M, Zoghi M, Jaberzadeh S. How different priming stimulations affect the corticospinal excitability induced by noninvasive brain stimulation techniques: a systematic review and meta-analysis. *Rev Neurosci.* 2018;29(8):883-899. doi:10.1515/revneuro-2017-0111
7. Merzenich M. *Soft Wired.* San Francisco, CA: Parnassus Publishing LLC; 2013.
8. Antoszyk S, Devenport G, Grabinski T, James D, Moore J, Phillis LN. Dosage Considerations: Recommending School-Based Physical Therapy Intervention Under IDEA Resource Manual Dosage Considerations: Recommending School-Based Physical Therapy Intervention Under IDEA. Dosing of School Based Special Interest Group; Section on Pediatric. https://pediatricapta.org/includes/fact-sheets/pdfs/15DosageConsideration ResourceManual.pdf. Accessed August 19, 2018.
9. Allison L, Fuller K. Balance and vestibular dysfunction. In: Umphred D, Lazaro R, Roller M, Burton G, eds. *Umphred's Neurological Rehabilitation.* 6th ed. St. Louis, MO: Elsevier; 2013. doi:10.1016/B978-0-323-07586-2.00031-5
10. Connors KA, Galea MP, Said CM, Remedios LJ. Feldenkrais Method balance classes are based on principles of motor learning and postural control retraining: a qualitative research study. *Physiotherapy.* 2010;96(4):324-336. doi:10.1016/j.physio.2010.01.004
11. Kesten A. Gait paradigm. Accessed March 21, 2020.
12. Umphred D, Lazaro R, Roller P, Byl N. Intervention techniques for clients with movement disorders. In: Umphred D, Lazaro R, Roller M, Burton G, eds. *Umphred's Neurological Rehabilitation.* 6th ed. St. Louis, MO: Elsevier; 2013. doi:10.1016/B978-0-323-07586-2.00018-2
13. Kalisch T, Kattenstroth JC, Noth S, Tegenthoff M, Dinse HR. Rapid assessment of age-related differences in standing balance. *J Aging Res.* 2011;2011:160490. doi:10.4061/2011/160490
14. Menezes KK, Nascimento LR, Ada L, Polese JC, Avelino PR, Teixeira-Salmela LF. Respiratory muscle training increases respiratory muscle strength and reduces respiratory complications after stroke: a systematic review. *J Physiother.* 2016;62(3):138-144. doi:10.1016/j.jphys.2016.05.014
15. Valkenborghs SR, Visser MM, Nilsson M, Callister R, van Vliet P. Aerobic exercise prior to task-specific training to improve poststroke motor function: A case series. *Physiother Res Int.* 2018;23(2):e1707. doi:10.1002/pri.1707
16. Arroll M, Dancey CP, Attree EA, Smith S, James T. People with symptoms of Ménière's disease: the relationship between illness intrusiveness, illness uncertainty, dizziness handicap, and depression. *Otol Neurotol.* 2012;33(5):816-823. doi:10.1097/MAO.0b013e3182536ac6
17. Brodovsky JR, Vnenchak MJ. Vestibular rehabilitation for unilateral peripheral vestibular dysfunction. *Phys Ther.* 2013;93(3):293-298. doi:10.2522/ptj.20120057
18. Hain TC. Vestibular Rehabilitation Therapy (VRT). Chicago Dizziness and Hearing. www.dizziness-and-balance.com/treatment/rehab.html. Accessed February 6, 2013.
19. 4 Awesome Exercises for Balance and Leg Strength #64. RenegageHealth.com. www.youtube.com/watch?v=e6pnogAnKFU. Accessed February 6, 2013.
20. Gottshall KR, Sessoms PH, Bartlett JL. Vestibular physical therapy intervention: utilizing a computer assisted rehabilitation environment in lieu of traditional physical therapy. *Conf Proc IEEE Eng Med Biol Soc.* 2012;2012:6141-6144. doi:10.1109/EMBC.2012.6347395
21. An HJ, Kim JI, Kim YR, et al. The effect of various dual task training methods with gait on the balance and gait of patients with chronic stroke. *J Phys Ther Sci.* 2014;26(8):1287-1291. doi:10.1589/jpts.26.1287
22. Crowner B, Kelly VE, Lee YA. Dual-task and context-dependent learning to modify functional motor performance, balance, and fall risk. Part 1: theoretical background and interpretive considerations. In: Combined Sections Meeting of the American Physical Therapy Association; January 21-24, 2013; San Diego, CA.
23. Doyle MS, Hershberg JA, Howard R, Osborn MB, Wagner JM. Dual-task and context-dependent learning to modify functional motor performance, balance, and fall risk. Part 2: clinical implications and applied interventions. In: Combined Sections Meeting of the American Physical Therapy Association; January 21-24, 2013; San Diego, CA.

24. Fritz NE, Basso DM. Dual-task training for balance and mobility in a person with severe traumatic brain injury: a case study. *J Neurol Phys Ther.* 2013;37(1):37-43. doi:10.1097/NPT.0b013e318282a20d
25. Yogev-Seligmann G, Giladi N, Gruendlinger L, Hausdorff JM. The contribution of postural control and bilateral coordination to the impact of dual tasking on gait. *Exp Brain Res.* 2013;226(1):81-93. doi:10.1007/s00221-013-3412-9
26. Fernandes Â, Rocha N, Santos R, Tavares JM. Effects of dual-task training on balance and executive functions in Parkinson's disease: A pilot study. *Somatosens Mot Res.* 2015;32(2):122-127. doi:10.3109/08990220.2014.1002605
27. Lee MM, Lee KJ, Song CH. Game-based virtual reality canoe paddling training to improve postural balance and upper extremity function: a preliminary randomized controlled study of 30 patients with subacute stroke. *Med Sci Monit.* 2018;24:2590-2598. doi:10.12659/MSM.906451
28. Fritz NE, Cheek FM, Nichols-Larsen DS. Motor-cognitive dual-task training in persons with neurologic disorders: a systematic review. *J Neurol Phys Ther.* 2015;39(3):142-153. doi:10.1097/NPT.0000000000000090
29. Park ER, Traeger L, Vranceanu AM, et al. The development of a patient-centered program based on the relaxation response: the Relaxation Response Resiliency Program (3RP). *Psychosomatics.* 2013;54(2):165-174. doi:10.1016/j.psym.2012.09.001
30. Umphred D, Thompson MH, West TM. Limbic systems influence over motor control and learning. In: Umphred DA, Lazaro R, Roller M, Burton G, eds. *Umphred's Neurological Rehabilitation.* 6th ed. St. Louis, MO: Elsevier; 2013. doi:10.1016/B978-0-323-07586-2.00014-5
31. Busch V, Magerl W, Kern U, Haas J, Hajak G, Eichhammer P. The effect of deep and slow breathing on pain perception, autonomic activity, and mood processing—an experimental study. *Pain Med.* 2012;13(2):215-228. doi:10.1111/j.1526-4637.2011.01243.x
32. Iglesias SL, Azzara S, Argibay JC, et al. Psychological and physiological response of students to different types of stress management programs. *Am J Health Promot.* 2012;26(6):e149-e158. doi:10.4278/ajhp.110516-QUAL-199
33. Knott M, Voss DE. *Proprioceptive Neuromuscular Facilitation.* New York, NY: Harper & Row; 1968.
34. Bobath B. *Adult Hemiplegia: Evaluation and Treatment.* 2nd ed. London, England: William Heinemann Medical Books; 1978.
35. Bly L. A historical and current view of the basis of NDT. *Pediatr Phys Ther.* 1991;3(3):131-135. doi:10.1097/00001577-199100330-00005
36. Brunnstrom S. *Movement Therapy in Hemiplegia.* 2nd ed. Philadelphia, PA: JB Lippincott; 1992.
37. Feldenkrais M. *Awareness Through Movement.* New York, NY: Harper & Row; 1977.
38. Goff B. The application of recent advances in neurophysiology to Miss M. Rood's concept of neuromuscular facilitation. *Physiotherapy.* 1972;58(12):409-415.
39. Johnstone M. *Restoration of Normal Movement After Stroke.* New York, NY: Churchill Livingstone; 1995.
40. Bobath B. *Abnormal Postural Reflex Activity Caused by Brain Lesions.* 3rd ed. Frederick, MD: Aspen Publications; 1985.
41. Bly L. *Baby Treatment Based on NDT Principles.* San Antonio, TX: Therapy Skill Builders; 1999.
42. Barbeau H, Visintin M. Optimal outcomes obtained with body-weight support combined with treadmill training in stroke subjects. *Arch Phys Med Rehabil.* 2003;84(10):1458-1465. doi:10.1016/S0003-9993(03)00361-7
43. Hesse S, Werner C. Partial body weight supported treadmill training for gait recovery following stroke. *Adv Neurol.* 2003;92:423-428.
44. Hicks AL, Adams MM, Martin Ginis K, et al. Long-term body-weight-supported treadmill training and subsequent follow-up in persons with chronic SCI: effects on functional walking ability and measures of subjective well-being. *Spinal Cord.* 2005;43(5):291-298. doi:10.1038/sj.sc.3101710
45. Stein J. Motor recovery strategies after stroke. *Top Stroke Rehabil.* 2004;11(2):12-22. doi:10.1310/RK4A-6ETG-K8RL-3XA7
46. Carey LM, Matyas TA. Frequency of discriminative sensory loss in the hand after stroke in a rehabilitation setting. *J Rehabil Med.* 2011;43(3):257-263. doi:10.2340/16501977-0662
47. Chabok SY, Kapourchali SR, Saberi A, Mohtasham-Amiri Z. Operative and nonoperative linguistic outcomes in brain injury patients. *J Neurol Sci.* 2012;317(1-2):130-136. doi:10.1016/j.jns.2012.02.009
48. Schabrun SM, Hillier S. Evidence for the retraining of sensation after stroke: a systematic review. *Clin Rehabil.* 2009;23(1):27-39. doi:10.1177/0269215508098897
49. Tyson SF, Hanley M, Chillala J, Selley AB, Tallis RC. Sensory loss in hospital-admitted people with stroke: characteristics, associated factors, and relationship with function. *Neurorehabil Neural Repair.* 2008;22(2):166-172. doi:10.1177/1545968307305523
50. Sinanović O, Mrkonjić Z, Zukić S, Vidović M, Imamović K. Post-stroke language disorders. *Acta Clin Croat.* 2011;50(1):79-94.
51. Goble DJ, Coxon JP, Wenderoth N, Van Impe A, Swinnen SP. Proprioceptive sensibility in the elderly: degeneration, functional consequences and plastic-adaptive processes. *Neurosci Biobehav Rev.* 2009;33(3):271-278. doi:10.1016/j.neubiorev.2008.08.012
52. Shaffer SW, Harrison AL. Aging of the somatosensory system: a translational perspective. *Phys Ther.* 2007;87(2):193-207. doi:10.2522/ptj.20060083
53. Ayres A. Sensory Integration and Praxis Test (SIPT) Manual. Los Angeles, CA: Western Psychological Association; 1989.
54. Byl NN. Focal hand dystonia may result from aberrant neuroplasticity. *Adv Neurol.* 2004;94:19-28.
55. Byl N, Roderick J, Mohamed O, et al. Effectiveness of sensory and motor rehabilitation of the upper limb following the principles of neuroplasticity: patients stable poststroke. *Neurorehabil Neural Repair.* 2003;17(3):176-191. doi:10.1177/0888439003257137
56. Byl NN, Nagarajan SS, Merzenich MM, Roberts T, McKenzie A. Correlation of clinical neuromusculoskeletal and central somatosensory performance: variability in controls and patients with severe and mild focal hand dystonia. *Neural Plast.* 2002;9(3):177-203. doi:10.1155/NP.2002.177
57. Altenmüller E, Jabusch HC. Focal dystonia in musicians: phenomenology, pathophysiology, triggering factors, and treatment. *Med Probl Perform Art.* 2010;25(1):3-9.
58. Byl NN. Diagnosis and management of focal hand dystonia in a rheumatology practice. *Curr Opin Rheumatol.* 2012;24(2):222-231. doi:10.1097/BOR.0b013e32835007ce

59. Coq JO, Barr AE, Strata F, et al. Peripheral and central changes combine to induce motor behavioral deficits in a moderate repetition task. *Exp Neurol.* 2009;220(2):234-245. doi:10.1016/j.expneurol.2009.08.008
60. Dolberg R, Hinkley LB, Honma S, et al. Amplitude and timing of somatosensory cortex activity in task-specific focal hand dystonia. *Clin Neurophysiol.* 2011;122(12):2441-2451. doi:10.1016/j.clinph.2011.05.020
61. Hinkley LB, Dolberg R, Honma S, Findlay A, Byl NN, Nagarajan SS. Aberrant oscillatory activity during simple movement in task-specific focal hand dystonia. *Front Neurol.* 2012;3:165. doi:10.3389/fneur.2012.00165
62. McKenzie AL, Goldman S, Barrango C, Shrime M, Wong T, Byl N. Differences in physical characteristics and response to rehabilitation for patients with hand dystonia: musicians' cramp compared to writers' cramp. *J Hand Ther.* 2009;22(2):172-181. doi:10.1016/j.jht.2008.12.006
63. Rosenkranz K, Butler K, Williamon A, Cordivari C, Lees AJ, Rothwell JC. Sensorimotor reorganization by proprioceptive training in musician's dystonia and writer's cramp. *Neurology.* 2008;70(4):304-315. doi:10.1212/01.wnl.0000296829.66406.14
64. Rosenkranz K, Butler K, Williamon A, Rothwell JC. Regaining motor control in musician's dystonia by restoring sensorimotor organization. *J Neurosci.* 2009;29(46):14627-14636. doi:10.1523/JNEUROSCI.2094-09.2009
65. Steeves TD, Day L, Dykeman J, Jette N, Pringsheim T. The prevalence of primary dystonia: a systematic review and meta-analysis. *Mov Disord.* 2012;27(14):1789-1796. doi:10.1002/mds.25244
66. Hinkley LB, Dolberg R, Honma S, Findlay A, Byl NN, Nagarajan SS. Aberrant oscillatory activity during simple movement in task-specific focal hand dystonia. *Front Neurol.* 2012;3:165. doi:10.3389/fneur.2012.00165
67. Kattenstroth JC, Kalisch T, Kowalewski R, Tegenthoff M, Dinse HR. Quantitative assessment of joint position sense recovery in subacute stroke patients: a pilot study. *J Rehabil Med.* 2013;45(10):1004-1009. doi:10.2340/16501977-1225
68. Kattenstroth JC, Kalisch T, Peters S, Tegenthoff M, Dinse HR. Long-term sensory stimulation therapy improves hand function and restores cortical responsiveness in patients with chronic cerebral lesions. Three single case studies. *Front Hum Neurosci.* 2012;6:244. doi:10.3389/fnhum.2012.00244
69. Kattenstroth JC, Kalisch T, Sczesny-Kaiser M, Greulich W, Tegenthoff M, Dinse HR. Daily repetitive sensory stimulation of the paretic hand for the treatment of sensorimotor deficits in patients with subacute stroke: RESET, a randomized, sham-controlled trial. *BMC Neurol.* 2018;18(1):2. doi:10.1186/s12883-017-1006-z
70. Katz M, Byl NN, San Luciano M, Ostrem JL. Focal task-specific lower extremity dystonia associated with intense repetitive exercise: a case series. *Parkinsonism Relat Disord.* 2013;19(11):1033-1038. doi:10.1016/j.parkreldis.2013.07.013
71. Voos MC, Oliveira TP, Piemonte ME, Barbosa ER. Case report: physical therapy management of axial dystonia. *Physiother Theory Pract.* 2014;30(1):56-61. doi:10.3109/0959 3985.2013.799252
72. Kattenstroth JC, Kalisch T, Kolankowska I, Dinse HR. Balance, sensorimotor, and cognitive performance in long-year expert senior ballroom dancers. *J Aging Res.* 2011;2011:176709. doi:10.4061/2011/176709
73. Cohen JW, Ivanova TD, Brouwer B, Miller KJ, Bryant D, Garland SJ. Do performance measures of strength, balance, and mobility predict quality of life and community reintegration after stroke? *Arch Phys Med Rehabil.* 2018;99(4):713-719. doi:10.1016/j.apmr.2017.12.007
74. Dorsch S, Ada L, Alloggia D. Progressive resistance training increases strength after stroke but this may not carry over to activity: a systematic review. *J Physiother.* 2018;64(2):84-90. doi:10.1016/j.jphys.2018.02.012
75. American Physical Therapy Association. *PT in Motion News.* May 11, 2018. http://www.apta.org/PTinMotion/. Accessed August 9, 2019.
76. Simkins J. Innovations in telehealth: As telehealth moves from theory to practice, here's an update. PT in Motion. 2017. http://www.apta.org/PTinMotion/. Assessed August 19, 2018.
77. WebPT. How Can Physical Therapists Use Telehealth? https://www.webpt.com/blog/post/how-can-pts-use-telehealth. 2017. Accessed August 19, 2018.
78. Agostini M, Moja L, Banzi R, et al. Telerehabilitation and recovery of motor function: a systematic review and meta-analysis. *J Telemed Telecare.* 2015;21(4):202-213. doi:10.1177/1357633X15572201
79. Chen J, Jin W, Zhang XX, Xu W, Liu XN, Ren CC. Telerehabilitation approaches for stroke patients: systematic review and meta-analysis of randomized controlled trials. *J Stroke Cerebrovasc Dis.* 2015;24(12):2660-2668. doi:10.1016/j.jstrokecerebrovasdis.2015.09.014
80. Dobkin BH. A rehabilitation-internet-of-things in the home to augment motor skills and exercise training. *Neurorehabil Neural Repair.* 2017;31(3):217-227. doi:10.1177/1545968316680490
81. Putrino D. Telerehabilitation and emerging virtual reality approaches to stroke rehabilitation. *Curr Opin Neurol.* 2014;27(6):631-636. doi:10.1097/WCO.0000000000000152
82. Hsieh YW, Chang KC, Hung JW, Wu CY, Fu MH, Chen CC. Effects of home-based versus clinic-based rehabilitation combining mirror therapy and task-specific training for patients with stroke: a randomized crossover trial. *Arch Phys Med Rehabil.* 2018;99(12):2399-2407. doi:10.1016/j.apmr.2018.03.017
83. Cramer H. Yoga Therapy in the German Healthcare System. *Int J Yoga Therap.* 2018;28(1):133-135. doi:10.17761/2018-00006
84. Keay L, Praveen D, Salam A, et al. A mixed methods evaluation of yoga as a fall prevention strategy for older people in India. *Pilot Feasibility Stud.* 2018;4(1):74. doi:10.1186/s40814-018-0264-x
85. Rhee TG, Marottoli RA, Van Ness PH, Tinetti ME. Patterns and perceived benefits of utilizing seven major complementary health approaches in U.S. older adults. J *Gerontol A Biol Sci Med Sci.* 2018;73(8):1119-1124. doi:10.1093/gerona/gly099
86. Zou L, Sasaki JE, Zeng N, Wang C, Sun L. A systematic review with meta-analysis of mindful exercises on rehabilitative outcomes among post-stroke patients. *Arch Phys Med Rehabil.* 2018;99(11):2355-2364. doi:10.1016/j.apmr.2018.04.010
87. Oujamaa L, Relave I, Froger J, Mottet D, Pelissier JY. Rehabilitation of arm function after stroke. Literature review. [in English and French]. *Ann Phys Rehabil Med.* 2009;52(3):269-293. doi:10.1016/j.rehab.2008.10.003

88. Sunderland A, Tuke A. Neuroplasticity, learning and recovery after stroke: a critical evaluation of constraint-induced therapy. *Neuropsychol Rehabil.* 2005;15(2):81-96. doi:10.1080/09602010443000047
89. van der Lee JH. Constraint-induced movement therapy: some thoughts about theories and evidence. *J Rehabil Med.* 2003;35(41)(suppl):41-45. doi:10.1080/16501960310010133
90. Wolf SL, Winstein CJ, Miller JP, et al; EXCITE Investigators. Effect of constraint-induced movement therapy on upper extremity function 3 to 9 months after stroke: the EXCITE randomized clinical trial. *JAMA.* 2006;296(17):2095-2104. doi:10.1001/jama.296.17.2095
91. Boake C, Noser EA, Ro T, et al. Constraint-induced movement therapy during early stroke rehabilitation. *Neurorehabil Neural Repair.* 2007;21(1):14-24. doi:10.1177/1545968306291858
92. Dromerick AW, Edwards DF, Hahn M. Does the application of constraint-induced movement therapy during acute rehabilitation reduce arm impairment after ischemic stroke? *Stroke.* 2000;31(12):2984-2988. doi:10.1161/01.STR.31.12.2984
93. Dromerick AW, Lang CE, Birkenmeier RL, et al. Very early constraint-induced movement during stroke rehabilitation (VECTORS): a single-center RCT. *Neurology.* 2009;73(3):195-201. doi:10.1212/WNL.0b013e3181ab2b27
94. Humm JL, Kozlowski DA, James DC, Gotts JE, Schallert T. Use-dependent exacerbation of brain damage occurs during an early post-lesion vulnerable period. *Brain Res.* 1998;783(2):286-292. doi:10.1016/S0006-8993(97)01356-5
95. Kozlowski DA, James DC, Schallert T. Use-dependent exaggeration of neuronal injury after unilateral sensorimotor cortex lesions. *J Neurosci.* 1996;16(15):4776-4786. doi:10.1523/JNEUROSCI.16-15-04776.1996
96. Lin KC, Wu CY, Wei TH, Lee CY, Liu JS. Effects of modified constraint-induced movement therapy on reach-to-grasp movements and functional performance after chronic stroke: a randomized controlled study. *Clin Rehabil.* 2007;21(12):1075-1086. doi:10.1177/0269215507079843
97. McIntyre A, Viana R, Janzen S, Mehta S, Pereira S, Teasell R. Systematic review and meta-analysis of constraint-induced movement therapy in the hemiparetic upper extremity more than six months post stroke. *Top Stroke Rehabil.* 2012;19(6):499-513. doi:10.1310/tsr1906-499
98. Peurala SH, Kantanen MP, Sjögren T, Paltamaa J, Karhula M, Heinonen A. Effectiveness of constraint-induced movement therapy on activity and participation after stroke: a systematic review and meta-analysis of randomized controlled trials. *Clin Rehabil.* 2012;26(3):209-223. doi:10.1177/0269215511420306
99. Treger I, Aidinof L, Lehrer H, Kalichman L. Modified constraint-induced movement therapy improved upper limb function in subacute poststroke patients: a small-scale clinical trial. *Top Stroke Rehabil.* 2012;19(4):287-293. doi:10.1310/tsr1904-287
100. Myint JM, Yuen GF, Yu TK, et al; Chun Por Wong. A study of constraint-induced movement therapy in subacute stroke patients in Hong Kong. *Clin Rehabil.* 2008;22(2):112-124. doi:10.1177/0269215507080141
101. Chen CL, Kang LJ, Hong WH, Chen FC, Chen HC, Wu CY. Effect of therapist-based constraint-induced therapy at home on motor control, motor performance and daily function in children with cerebral palsy: a randomized controlled study. *Clin Rehabil.* 2013;27(3):236-245. doi:10.1177/0269215512455652
102. Lin KC, Wang TN, Wu CY, et al. Effects of home-based constraint-induced therapy versus dose-matched control intervention on functional outcomes and caregiver well-being in children with cerebral palsy. *Res Dev Disabil.* 2011;32(5):1483-1491. doi:10.1016/j.ridd.2011.01.023
103. Bang DH, Shin WS, Choi SJ. The effects of modified constraint-induced movement therapy combined with trunk restraint in subacute stroke: a double-blinded randomized controlled trial. *Clin Rehabil.* 2015;29(6):561-569. doi:10.1177/0269215514552034
104. Chen HC, Chen CL, Kang LJ, Wu CY, Chen FC, Hong WH. Improvement of upper extremity motor control and function after home-based constraint induced therapy in children with unilateral cerebral palsy: immediate and long-term effects. *Arch Phys Med Rehabil.* 2014;95(8):1423-1432. doi:10.1016/j.apmr.2014.03.025
105. Park H, Kim S, Winstein CJ, Gordon J, Schweighofer N. Short-duration and intensive training improves long-term reaching performance in individuals with chronic stroke. *Neurorehabil Neural Repair.* 2016;30(6):551-561. doi:10.1177/1545968315606990
106. Knutson, JS, Fu MJ, Sheffler LR, Chae J. Neuromuscular Electrical Stimulation for Motor Restoration in Hemiplegia. *Phys Med Rehabil Clin N Am.* 2015;26(4):729-745.
107. de Freitas GR, Szpoganicz C, Ilha J. Does neuromuscular electrical stimulation therapy increase voluntary muscle strength after spinal cord injury? A systematic review. *Top Spinal Cord Inj Rehabil.* 201;24(1):6-17.
108. Deer TR, Mekhail N, Provenzano D, et al; Neuromodulation Appropriateness Consensus Committee. The appropriate use of neurostimulation of the spinal cord and peripheral nervous system for the treatment of chronic pain and ischemic diseases: the Neuromodulation Appropriateness Consensus Committee. *Neuromodulation.* 2014;17(6):515-550. doi:10.1111/ner.12208
109. Maffiuletti NA, Gondin J, Place N, Stevens-Lapsley J, Vivodtzev I, Minetto MA. The clinical use of neuromuscular electrical stimulation for neuromuscular rehabilitation: what are we overlooking? *Arch Phys Med Rehabil.* 2018;99(4):806-812.
110. Byl K, Byl N, Byl M, et al. Integrating technology into clinical practice in neurological rehabilitation. In: Umphred D, Lazaro R, Roller M, Burton G, eds. *Umphred's Neurological Rehabilitation.* 6th ed. St. Louis, MO: Elsevier; 2013. doi:10.1016/B978-0-323-07586-2.00047-9
111. United States Department of Veterans Affairs. Journal of Rehabilitation Research and Development. www.rehab.research.va.gov/jour/11/484/hidler484.html. Accessed July 31, 2013.
112. Combs SA, Dugan EL, Ozimek EN, Curtis AB. Effects of body-weight supported treadmill training on kinetic symmetry in persons with chronic stroke. *Clin Biomech (Bristol, Avon).* 2012;27(9):887-892. doi:10.1016/j.clinbiomech.2012.06.011

113. Duncan PW, Sullivan KJ, Behrman AL, et al; LEAPS Investigative Team. Body-weight-supported treadmill rehabilitation after stroke. *N Engl J Med.* 2011;364(21):2026-2036. doi:10.1056/NEJMoa1010790
114. Fluet GG, Merians AS, Qiu Q, et al. Robots integrated with virtual reality simulations for customized motor training in a person with upper extremity hemiparesis: a case study. *J Neurol Phys Ther.* 2012;36(2):79-86. doi:10.1097/NPT.0b013e3182566f3f
115. Høyer E, Jahnsen R, Stanghelle JK, Strand LI. Body weight supported treadmill training versus traditional training in patients dependent on walking assistance after stroke: a randomized controlled trial. *Disabil Rehabil.* 2012;34(3):210-219. doi:10.3109/09638288.2011.593681
116. Kelley CP, Childress J, Boake C, Noser EA. Over-ground and robotic-assisted locomotor training in adults with chronic stroke: a blinded randomized clinical trial. *Disabil Rehabil Assist Technol.* 2013;8(2):161-168. doi:10.3109/17483107.2012.714052
117. DiBiasio PA, Lewis CL. Exercise training utilizing body weight-supported treadmill walking with a young adult with cerebral palsy who was non-ambulatory. *Physiother Theory Pract.* 2012;28(8):641-652. doi:10.3109/09593985.2012.665983
118. Kurz MJ, Wilson TW, Corr B, Volkman KG. Neuromagnetic activity of the somatosensory cortices associated with body weight-supported treadmill training in children with cerebral palsy. *J Neurol Phys Ther.* 2012;36(4):166-172. doi:10.1097/NPT.0b013e318251776a
119. Rose MH, Løkkegaard A, Sonne-Holm S, Jensen BR. Improved clinical status, quality of life, and walking capacity in Parkinson's disease after body weight-supported high-intensity locomotor training. *Arch Phys Med Rehabil.* 2013;94(4):687-692. doi:10.1016/j.apmr.2012.11.025
120. Swinnen E, Beckwée D, Pinte D, Meeusen R, Baeyens JP, Kerckhofs E. Treadmill training in multiple sclerosis: can body weight support or robot assistance provide added value? A systematic review. *Mult Scler Int.* 2012;2012:240274. doi:10.1155/2012/240274
121. Behrman AL, Harkema SJ. Locomotor training after human spinal cord injury: a series of case studies. *Phys Ther.* 2000;80(7):688-700. doi:10.1093/ptj/80.7.688
122. Harkema SJ, Schmidt-Read M, Lorenz DJ, Edgerton VR, Behrman AL. Balance and ambulation improvements in individuals with chronic incomplete spinal cord injury using locomotor training-based rehabilitation. *Arch Phys Med Rehabil.* 2012;93(9):1508-1517. doi:10.1016/j.apmr.2011.01.024
123. Esquenazi A, Lee S, Packel AT, Braitman L. A randomized comparative study of manually assisted versus robotic-assisted body weight supported treadmill training in persons with a traumatic brain injury. *PM R.* 2013;5(4):280-290. doi:10.1016/j.pmrj.2012.10.009
124. Moriello G, Frear M, Seaburg K. The recovery of running ability in an adolescent male after traumatic brain injury: a case study. *J Neurol Phys Ther.* 2009;33(2):111-120. doi:10.1097/NPT.0b013e3181a6ab6b
125. Betschart M, McFadyen BJ, Nadeau S. Repeated split-belt treadmill walking improved gait ability in individuals with chronic stroke: A pilot study. *Physiother Theory Pract.* 2018;34(2):81-90. doi:10.1080/09593985.2017.1375055
126. Combs-Miller SA, Kalpathi Parameswaran A, Colburn D, et al. Body weight-supported treadmill training vs. overground walking training for persons with chronic stroke: a pilot randomized controlled trial. *Clin Rehabil.* 2014;28(9):873-884. doi:10.1177/0269215514520773
127. Day KA, Leech KA, Roemmich RT, Bastian AJ. Accelerating locomotor savings in learning: compressing four training days to one. *J Neurophysiol.* 2018;119(6):2100-2113. doi:10.1152/jn.00903.2017
128. Kang TW, Oh DW, Lee JH, Cynn HS. Rhythmic arm swing integrated into treadmill training in patients with chronic stroke: A single-subject experimental study. *Physiother Theory Pract.* 2018;34(8):613-621. doi:10.1080/09593985.2017.1423430
129. Kim KH, Lee KB, Bae YH, Fong SSM, Lee SM. Effects of progressive backward body weight suppoted treadmill training on gait ability in chronic stroke patients: A randomized controlled trial. *Technol Health Care.* 2017;25(5):867-876. doi:10.3233/THC-160720
130. Srivastava A, Taly AB, Gupta A, Kumar S, Murali T. Bodyweight-supported treadmill training for retraining gait among chronic stroke survivors: A randomized controlled study. *Ann Phys Rehabil Med.* 2016;59(4):235-241. doi:10.1016/j.rehab.2016.01.014
131. Yokoyama H, Sato K, Ogawa T, Yamamoto SI, Nakazawa K, Kawashima N. Characteristics of the gait adaptation process due to split-belt treadmill walking under a wide range of right-left speed ratios in humans. *PLoS One.* 2018;13(4):e0194875. doi:10.1371/journal.pone.0194875
132. Calabrò RS, Naro A, Russo M, et al. Shaping neuroplasticity by using powered exoskeletons in patients with stroke: a randomized clinical trial. *J Neuroeng Rehabil.* 2018;15(1):35. doi:10.1186/s12984-018-0377-8
133. Cramer SC. Brain repair after stroke. *N Engl J Med.* 2010;362(19):1827-1829. doi:10.1056/NEJMe1003399
134. Lo AC, Guarino PD, Richards LG, et al. Robot-assisted therapy for long-term upper-limb impairment after stroke. *N Engl J Med.* 2010;362(19):1772-1783. doi:10.1056/NEJMoa0911341
135. Veerbeek JM, Langbroek-Amersfoort AC, van Wegen EE, Meskers CG, Kwakkel G. Effects of robot-assisted therapy for the upper limb after stroke. *Neurorehabil Neural Repair.* 2017;31(2):107-121. doi:10.1177/1545968316666957
136. Bergmann J, Krewer C, Müller F, Koenig A, Riener R. Virtual Reality to control active participation in a subacute stroke patient during robot-assisted gait training. *IEEE Int Conf Rehabil Robot.* 2011;2011:5975407. doi:10.1109/ICORR.2011.5975407
137. Laver KE, George S, Thomas S, Deutsch JE, Crotty M. Virtual reality for stroke rehabilitation. *Cochrane Database Syst Rev.* 2011;(9):CD008349.
138. Lucca LF. Virtual reality and motor rehabilitation of the upper limb after stroke: a generation of progress? *J Rehabil Med.* 2009;41(12):1003-1100. doi:10.2340/16501977-0405
139. Piron L, Turolla A, Agostini M, et al. Exercises for paretic upper limb after stroke: a combined virtual-reality and telemedicine approach. *J Rehabil Med.* 2009;41(12):1016-1102. doi:10.2340/16501977-0459
140. Cano Porras D, Siemonsma P, Inzelberg R, Zeilig G, Plotnik M. Advantages of virtual reality in the rehabilitation of balance and gait: systematic review. *Neurology.* 2018;90(22):1017-1025. doi:10.1212/WNL.0000000000005603

141. Fulk GD. Locomotor training and virtual reality-based balance training for an individual with multiple sclerosis: a case report. *J Neurol Phys Ther.* 2005;29(1):34-42. doi:10.1097/01.NPT.0000282260.59078.e4

142. Jonsdottir J, Bertoni R, Lawo M, Montesano A, Bowman T, Gabrielli S. Serious games for arm rehabilitation of persons with multiple sclerosis. A randomized controlled pilot study. *Mult Scler Relat Disord.* 2018;19:25-29. doi:10.1016/j.msard.2017.10.010

143. Mumford N, Duckworth J, Thomas PR, Shum D, Williams G, Wilson PH. Upper-limb virtual rehabilitation for traumatic brain injury: a preliminary within-group evaluation of the elements system. *Brain Inj.* 2012;26(2):166-176. doi:10.3109/02699052.2011.648706

144. Green D, Wilson PH. Use of virtual reality in rehabilitation of movement in children with hemiplegia—a multiple case study evaluation. *Disabil Rehabil.* 2012;34(7):593-604. doi:10.3109/09638288.2011.613520

145. Gagliardi C, Turconi AC, Biffi E, et al. Immersive virtual reality to improve walking abilities in cerebral palsy: a pilot study. *Ann Biomed Eng.* 2018;46(9):1376-1384. doi:10.1007/s10439-018-2039-1

146. Salem Y, Gropack SJ, Coffin D, Godwin EM. Effectiveness of a low-cost virtual reality system for children with developmental delay: a preliminary randomised single-blind controlled trial. *Physiotherapy.* 2012;98(3):189-195. doi:10.1016/j.physio.2012.06.003

147. Deutsch JE, Borbely M, Filler J, Huhn K, Guarrera-Bowlby P. Use of a low-cost, commercially available gaming console (Wii) for rehabilitation of an adolescent with cerebral palsy. *Phys Ther.* 2008;88(10):1196-1207. doi:10.2522/ptj.20080062

148. Saposnik G, Teasell R, Mamdani M, et al; Stroke Outcome Research Canada (SORCan) Working Group. Effectiveness of virtual reality using Wii gaming technology in stroke rehabilitation: a pilot randomized clinical trial and proof of principle. *Stroke.* 2010;41(7):1477-1484. doi:10.1161/STROKEAHA.110.584979

149. Flynn S, Palma P, Bender A. Feasibility of using the Sony PlayStation 2 gaming platform for an individual post-stroke: a case report. *J Neurol Phys Ther.* 2007;31(4):180-189. doi:10.1097/NPT.0b013e31815d00d5

150. Nuic D, Vinti M, Karachi C, Foulon P, Van Hamme A, Welter ML. The feasibility and positive effects of a customised videogame rehabilitation programme for freezing of gait and falls in Parkinson's disease patients: a pilot study. *J Neuroeng Rehabil.* 2018;15(1):31. doi:10.1186/s12984-018-0375-x

151. Rand D, Givon N, Bar A. Michal A video-game group intervention: experiences and perceptions of adults with chronic stroke and their therapists. *Can J Occup Ther.* 2018;85(2):158-168. doi:10.1177/0008417417733274

152. Lewis JA, Deutsch JE, Burdea G. Usability of the remote console for virtual reality telerehabilitation: formative evaluation. *Cyberpsychol Behav.* 2006;9(2):142-147. doi:10.1089/cpb.2006.9.142

153. Bandy WD, Sanders B. *Therapeutic Exercise: Techniques for Intervention.* Philadelphia, PA: Lippincott Williams & Wilkins; 2001.

154. Becker BE. Aquatic therapy: scientific foundations and clinical rehabilitation applications. *PM R.* 2009;1(9):859-872. doi:10.1016/j.pmrj.2009.05.017

155. Becker BE. Biophysiologic aspects of hydrotherapy. In: Becker BE, Cole AJ, eds. *Comprehensive Aquatic Therapy.* Boston, MA: Butterworth-Heinemann; 1997:17-48.

156. Black J, Hansen M. Neurologic Physical Therapy: Aquatic Therapy and Lab. In: *Neuromuscular Management Course.* University of Utah; November 2018.

157. Aidar FJ, Gama de Matos D, de Souza RF, et al. Influence of aquatic exercises in physical condition in patients with multiple sclerosis. *J Sports Med Phys Fitness.* 2018;58(5):684-689.

158. Depiazzi JE, Forbes RA, Gibson N, et al. The effect of aquatic high-intensity interval training on aerobic performance, strength and body composition in a non-athletic population: systematic review and meta-analysis. *Clin Rehabil.* 2019;33(2):157-170. doi:10.1177/0269215518792039

159. Ellapen TJ, Hammill HV, Swanepoel M, Strydom GL. The benefits of hydrotherapy to patients with spinal cord injuries. *Afr J Disabil.* 2018;7(0):450. doi:10.4102/ajod.v7i0.450

160. Güeita-Rodríguez J, García-Muro F, Rodríguez-Fernández ÁL, Lambeck J, Fernández-de-Las-Peñas C, Palacios-Ceña D. What areas of functioning are influenced by aquatic physiotherapy? Experiences of parents of children with cerebral palsy. *Dev Neurorehabil.* 2018;21(8):506-514. doi:10.1080/17518423.2017.1368728

161. Kargarfard M, Shariat A, Ingle L, Cleland JA, Kargarfard M. Randomized controlled trial to examine the impact of aquatic exercise training on functional capacity, balance, and perceptions of fatigue in female patients with multiple sclerosis. *Arch Phys Med Rehabil.* 2018;99(2):234-241. doi:10.1016/j.apmr.2017.06.015

162. Pérez de la Cruz S. A bicentric controlled study on the effects of aquatic Ai Chi in Parkinson disease. *Complement Ther Med.* 2018;36:147-153. doi:10.1016/j.ctim.2017.12.001

163. Pérez de la Cruz S. Effectiveness of aquatic therapy for the control of pain and increased functionality in people with Parkinson's disease: a randomized clinical trial. *Eur J Phys Rehabil Med.* 2017;53(6):825-832.

164. Severin AC, Burkett BJ, McKean MR, Wiegand AN, Sayers MGL. Effects of water immersion on squat and split-squat kinematics in older aged adults. *J Aging Phys Act.* 2019;27(3):398-405. doi:10.1123/japa.2018-0166

165. Wheeler S, Acord-Vira A, Davis D. Effectiveness of interventions to improve occupational performance for people with psychosocial, behavioral, and emotional impairments after brain injury: a systematic review. *Am J Occup Ther.* 2016;70(3):7003180060p1-9.

166. Xu GZ, Li YF, Wang MD, Cao DY. Complementary and alternative interventions for fatigue management after traumatic brain injury: a systematic review. *Ther Adv Neurol Disorder.* 2017;10(5):229-239. doi:10.1177/1756285616682675

167. Zhu Z, Yin M, Cui L, et al. Aquatic obstacle training improves freezing of gait in Parkinson's disease patients: a randomized controlled trial. *Clin Rehabil.* 2018;32(1):29-36. doi:10.1177/0269215517715763

168. Irion JM. Historical overview of aquatic rehabilitation. In: Ruoti R, Morris P, Cole A, eds. *Aquatic Rehabilitation.* Philadelphia, PA: Lippincott Williams & Wilkins; 1997.

169. Voss DE, Ionta MK, Myers BJ. *Proprioceptive Neuromuscular Facilitation: Patterns and Techniques.* 3rd ed. Philadelphia, PA: Lippincott Williams & Wilkins; 1985.

170. Adler SS, Beckers D, Buck M. *PNF in Practice: An Illustrated Guide*. 4th ed. Berlin, Germany: Springer-Medizen; 2014. doi:10.1007/978-3-642-34988-1
171. Hindle KB, Whitcomb TJ, Briggs WO, Hong J. Whitcomb TJ, Briggs WO, Hong J. Proprioceptive neuromuscular facilitation (PNF): its mechanisms and effects on range of motion and muscular function. *J Hum Kinet*. 2012;31(1):105-113. doi:10.2478/v10078-012-0011-y
172. Guiu-Tula FX, Cabanas-Valdés R, Sitjà-Rabert M, Urrútia G, Gómara-Toldrà N. The Efficacy of the proprioceptive neuromuscular facilitation (PNF) approach in stroke rehabilitation to improve basic activities of daily living and quality of life: a systematic review and meta-analysis protocol. *BMJ Open*. 2017;7(12):e016739. doi:10.1136/bmjopen-2017-016739
173. IPNFA. Historical perspective of PNF. http://www.ipnfa.org/index.php?id=113. Updated January 10, 2013. Accessed January 15, 2013.
174. Baum N. Proprioceptive neuromuscular facilitation shoulder progression for patients with spinal cord injury resulting in quadriplegia. *Phys Ther Case Reports*. 1998;1(6):296-300.
175. Smedal T, Lygren H, Myhr KM, et al. Balance and gait improved in patients with MS after physiotherapy based on the Bobath concept. *Physiother Res Int*. 2006;11(2):104-116. doi:10.1002/pri.327
176. Lennon S. Gait re-education based on the Bobath concept in two patients with hemiplegia following stroke. *Phys Ther*. 2001;81(3):924-935. doi:10.1093/ptj/81.3.924
177. Neuro-Developmental Treatment Association. SLP & NDT. http://www.ndta.org/. Accessed July 31, 2013.
178. Corrado B, Sommella N, Ciardi G, et al. Can early physical therapy positively affect the onset of independent walking in infants with Down syndrome? A retrospective cohort study. *Minerva Pediatr*. 2018.
179. Tekin F, Kavlak E, Cavlak U, Altug F. Effectiveness of neuro-developmental treatment (Bobath concept) on postural control and balance in cerebral palsied children. *J Back Musculoskeletal Rehabil*. 2018;31(2):397-403. doi:10.3233/BMR-170813
180. Umphred DA, Lazaro R, Roller M, Burton G, eds. *Neurological Rehabilitation*. 6th ed. St. Louis, MO: Elsevier; 2013.
181. III STEP: symposium on translating evidence into practice. University of Utah, July 15-22, 2005. Special Editions: *Phys Ther*. 2006;86(4,5,6).

Please visit www.routledge.com/9781630915650 to access additional material.

Chapter 6

Examination Procedures

Irwin S. Thompson, PT, MPT, EdD; Patricia Harris, PT, MS; and Lisa Ferrin, PTA, AS

KEY WORDS Balance testing | Examination | Examination of the neuromuscular system | Functional testing/testing for activity limitations | Impairment testing | Pain assessment | Participation | Sensory testing

Chapter Objectives

- Discuss the purposes of a neuromuscular examination.
- Identify the responses expected from specific neuromuscular examinations.
- Identify and discuss the role of the physical therapist assistant in assessing patients with central nervous system (CNS) movement problems by using follow-up tests and measures.
- Identify and discuss what assessment tools a physical therapist assistant should be competent to administer in relation to the established plan of care and physical therapy prognosis.
- Clarify and discuss when and why it is appropriate for the physical therapist assistant to perform the neuromuscular follow-up examination and when the test procedures should be performed by the physical therapist.

The *Guide to Physical Therapist Practice* (the *Guide*) defines *examination* as "a comprehensive screening and specific testing process leading to diagnostic classification or, as appropriate, to a referral to another practitioner."[1] *Evaluation* is defined as "a dynamic process in which the physical therapist makes clinical judgments based on data gathered during the examination.... The initial examination is required prior to the initial intervention and is performed for all patients/clients.... *Reexamination* is the process of performing selected tests and measures after the initial examination to evaluate progress and to modify or redirect interventions."[1] The physical therapist assistant may identify when a reexamination is indicated based on "new clinical findings or failure to respond to physical therapy interventions."[1] This chapter follows the chapter on intervention to be consistent with the process used by a physical therapist assistant. Within the physical therapist's frame of reference, examination and evaluation precede development of a plan of care and the intervention process. Within the paradigm of the physical therapist assistant, reexamination follows initiation of intervention strategies identified within the plan of care. Thus, the order of the first section of this book is aligned closely with the professional role of the physical therapist assistant. There are typically 3 types of formal examinations and evaluations a physical therapist uses when a patient receives physical therapy: an initial examination/evaluation, a reexamination/reevaluation, and a discharge examination/evaluation. Not all components of an initial examination are repeated for subsequent examinations. Typically, data is collected to inform further clinical decision-making.

Based on the findings of an initial examination, the physical therapist establishes a physical therapy diagnosis, which "indicates the primary dysfunctions toward which the physical therapist directs interventions."[1] The physical therapy diagnosis informs the development of a prognosis

Lazaro RT, Umphred DA, eds. *Umphred's Neurorehabilitation for the Physical Therapist Assistant, Third Edition* (pp 127-154).

Box 6-1

Categories to Be Included in the Patient History

- General demographics: age, sex, race/ethnicity, primary language, and education
- Social history: cultural beliefs and behaviors, family and caregiver resources, social interactions, social activities, and support systems
- Employment: work, job, school, play
- Developmental history
- Living environment: devices and equipment, living environment and community characteristics, and projected discharge destination
- General health status
- Social/health habits (past and current)
- Family history
- Medical/surgical history
- Current conditions/chief complaints that led the patient/client to seek physical therapy
- Functional status and activity level
- Patient's treatment goals
- Medications: over-the-counter and prescriptions
- Results of other clinical tests: laboratory and diagnostic tests

that is "the determination of the predicted optimal level of improvement in function and the amount of time needed to reach that level."[1] The physical therapist then establishes the plan of care, which is the "culmination of the examination, diagnostic, and prognostic processes."[1] The plan of care includes anticipated goals and expected outcomes (long- and short-term goals); physical therapy interventions, including duration and frequency; prognosis; and discharge plans.[1] The plan of care must also include communication and coordination activities with other professionals as appropriate, and the development of a home program.

A complete examination allows the identification of movement problems that can be appropriately managed through physical therapy intervention (see Figure 1-3). In addition, the evaluation enhances the patient's achievement of optimal health and well-being by identifying the interactions of body systems as they relate to the patient's signs, symptoms, and progress with rehabilitation. The process also protects the patient by identifying potential life-threatening or emergency conditions and/or the need to refer to other individuals who will be able to better manage aspects of the patient's care. The physical therapist assistant uses the information obtained by the physical therapist to guide delivery of patient intervention. Each time the patient is seen, the physical therapist assistant must review body systems and identify any change in those systems. This is a critical aspect of patient care, and a life-threatening situation can emerge if a problem develops that is not identified during any treatment session.

This chapter will focus on the initial examination process performed by the physical therapist and will include a discussion of the role of the physical therapist assistant in the reexamination and discharge examinations. Following the *Guide*,[1] the neuromuscular examination should consist of the patient/client history, a review of systems and system review, and tests and measures appropriate for the medical diagnosis and movement dysfunctions identified by the physical therapist.

It is important for the physical therapist assistant to be familiar with the components of the neuromuscular examination. An understanding of its components guides delivery of the interventions included in the physical therapist's treatment plan. The physical therapy examination begins with the patient history.

Patient History

The patient's history is the starting point for the physical therapist's initial examination. The patient's history is obtained through the patient's medical record, intake forms, questionnaires, and an interview (which may include the patient's interpretation of why the services of a physical therapist are required, and the patient's goals for therapy). According to the *Guide*,[1] the patient history should include many, if not all, of the components in Box 6-1.

The patient interview is performed in a private area to protect the patient's privacy and allow the patient to feel comfortable and open when answering questions. The physical therapist gathers the initial patient history. Additional information pertinent to the medical history may become evident during subsequent visits with the physical therapist assistant, who would then report and document new findings to the supervising physical therapist.

Systems Review

The next portion of the patient examination is the review of systems. The *systems review* examines the influence of body systems (Box 6-2) on the patient's complaint.[1]

The purpose of the systems review is to determine whether a referral to other medical professionals is needed. It is also used to assess the influence of the status of the systems on the patient's prognosis and plan of care. If the physical therapist assistant is providing intervention, then a brief systems review prior to beginning any treatment may be the first time early identification of a system problem becomes evident. Thus, the physical therapist assistant needs to understand not only why the physical therapist performed the systems review initially, but also how to review these systems before beginning any intervention to identify when a patient needs to be seen by a medical provider or other health professional.

Box 6-2

List of Body Systems Screened by the Physical Therapist and Physical Therapist Assistant

- Musculoskeletal
- Neuromuscular
- Cardiovascular
- Pulmonary
- Integumentary
- Gastrointestinal
- Endocrine
- Visual
- Ear/nose/throat
- Urogenital
- Hematologic/lymphatic
- Psychological

Tests and Measures

Tests of Body Functions and Structures

There are tests and measures specific to each of the areas of the physical therapy examination. These tests and measures assist the physical therapist in interpreting the patient's status. According to the *Guide*,[1] tests and measures are used to identify signs and symptoms, to determine the physical therapy diagnosis and prognosis, to establish the plan of care, to determine changes in the patient's status, and to identify the progression toward or the achievement of goals. Certain portions of the tests that were performed by the physical therapist during the initial examination may be assigned to the physical therapist assistant for reexamination during the course of treatment. If the physical therapist assistant identifies additional clinical signs and symptoms, these findings must be communicated to the physical therapist to determine whether additional tests are needed.

Observation

Observation of each patient occurs continually throughout the examination and treatment by the physical therapist and the physical therapist assistant. Observation involves using the senses of vision, hearing, and smell to identify potential abnormalities. Some of the areas the physical therapist assistant should observe are the patient's appearance, general movement patterns, posture, areas of swelling/edema, facial expression, breathing pattern, body odors, and ability to communicate. Observation of any of these areas, especially if they have changed, can guide the physical therapist assistant and the physical therapist in the need for further examination.[2]

Vital Signs

Monitoring vital signs is essential for safe patient treatment. There are 5 vital signs[3]: heart rate, respiration rate, blood pressure, temperature, and pain. Vital signs screen for potential medical complications and establish the ability of the patient to tolerate physical therapy intervention. Vital signs need to be assessed before each treatment and, depending on the patient's medical status, during the treatment session to determine the patient's ability to tolerate therapy. In addition, oxygen saturation rates may be taken via pulse oximetry to determine the patient's blood oxygenation level, as indicated.[4]

Heart Rate/Pulse

Heart rate refers to the number of heart beats per minute (bpm), and is an indirect measure of left ventricular contraction.[4] It can be measured during rest and with activity, and is useful for assessing a patient's readiness for or response to therapeutic intervention.[5] Heart rate can also be used as part of a comprehensive evaluation of a patient's cardiovascular fitness level, and can help determine effective training zones for aerobic exercise.[6] For patients with cardiovascular compromise, monitoring heart rate becomes part of the regular assessment protocol during each patient treatment. This is done to ensure the safety of the patient, and to recognize any changes in patient status.

Normal resting heart rate is between 60 and 100 bpm.[5] A resting heart rate below 60 bpm is documented as *bradycardia*, or slow heart rate. A resting heart rate above 100 bpm is *tachycardia*, or fast heart rate.[5] Qualitative aspects of a patient's pulse may also be assessed. The rate, rhythm, and volume of pulse may be described with the following terms[4]:

- Strong and regular: a strong force to each beat with a regular rhythm
- Weak and regular: a weak force to each beat with a regular rhythm
- Irregular: a strong force to each beat with an irregular rhythm
- Thready: a weak force to each beat with an irregular rhythm

Bradycardic or tachycardic heart rates, or abnormal pulses, may indicate underlying cardiac pathology.[7] In such instances, the physical therapist assistant should consult with the supervising physical therapist or a qualified medical professional before initiating treatment. Some individuals may exhibit heart rates that fall outside of these norms without pathology being present. For instance, well-conditioned athletes or very relaxed individuals may demonstrate resting heart rates below 60 bpm.[6] Certain medications—such as calcium channel blockers, bronchodilators, or antidepressants—may also contribute to depressed or accelerated heart rates.[8,9,10] A review of the patient's medical history coupled with a patient's heart rate measurement should assist in determining whether it is safe to initiate treatment.

To measure a patient's heart rate, a stopwatch or clock with a second hand is required.[6] The most common area to

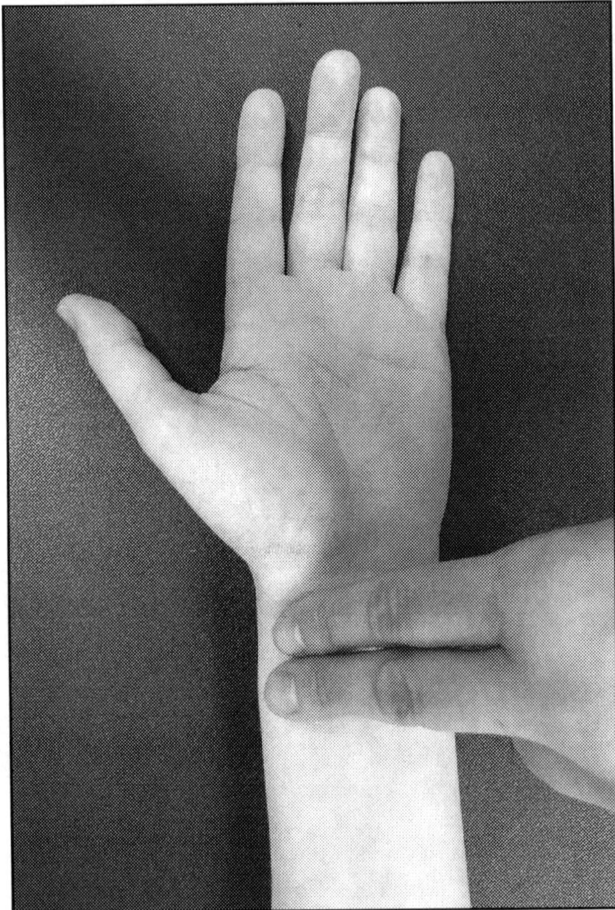
Figure 6-1. Assessing the radial pulse.

measure a patient's heart rate is on the radial pulse, though the carotid, brachial, femoral, or dorsalis pedis pulses may also be used.[5] The physical therapist assistant palpates the radial pulse on the lateral and volar aspect of the forearm, just proximal to the wrist (Figure 6-1). The number of heart beats in a 15-second period is counted and multiplied by 4 to determine the patient's heart rate. An error of +/- 4 bpm is possible with this type of measurement.[6]

Respiration Rate

Respiration rate measures the number of breaths per minute.[11] It is helpful in determining a patient's respiratory function, and is often assessed in patients with respiratory conditions.[11] A normal resting respiration rate is between 12 and 20 breaths per minute.[11] A respiration rate that falls outside of these values may indicate respiratory complications.[12] The physical therapist assistant should consult with the supervising physical therapist or a qualified medical professional before initiating treatment if a patient exhibits signs or abnormal respiration. To assess respiration, the physical therapist assistant observes the chest or abdomen and counts the number of rises and falls for 60 seconds.

Box 6-3

Blood Pressure Guidelines From the American Heart Association

- Normal: less than 120/80 mm Hg
- Elevated: systolic between 120 and 129, and diastolic less than 80
- Stage 1: systolic between 130 and 139, or diastolic between 80 and 89
- Stage 2: systolic at least 140, or diastolic at least 90
- Hypertensive crisis: systolic over 180 and/or diastolic over 120, with patients needing prompt changes in medication if there are no other indications of problems, or immediate hospitalization if there are signs of organ damage

Source: American Heart Association, 2017.

Blood Pressure

Blood pressure is the measurement of the force of blood against the arteries.[11] It is regularly relied upon as an indicator of cardiovascular health.[11] It should be monitored in patients with suspected cardiovascular deficits before and during physical therapy interventions to determine appropriateness of and response to treatment.[13] Blood pressure is typically recorded using a *sphygmomanometer* (blood pressure cuff) and a stethoscope, though automatic blood pressure monitors are witnessing more widespread use in clinical settings.[5] A patient's blood pressure is recorded as 2 numbers: systole and diastole.[5] Systole refers to the pressure that occurs when the heart's left ventricle contracts.[11] Diastole is the peripheral pressure during heart relaxation.[11] The American Heart Association published new blood pressure guidelines in 2017 (Box 6-3).[14]

The physical therapist assistant must regularly monitor blood pressure, as indicated, and report changes in a patient's status to the supervising physical therapist. Abnormal blood pressure responses to activity, such a diastolic blood pressure that is elevated greater than 10 mm Hg, or a depressed systolic blood pressure, warrant cessation of the intervention and communication with the supervising physical therapist or a qualified medical professional.[13]

Temperature

Body temperature represents the balance between heat production and loss.[15] It is affected by both intrinsic and extrinsic factors. Homeostasis maintains core body temperatures within a normal range, accepted as between 36°C and 37.50°C (96.80°F to 99.50°F).[16] Changes in body temperature may indicate abnormal neurologic or metabolic activity.[17] Most commonly, elevated temperatures, particularly those above 38.80°C (100.0°F), may be evidence

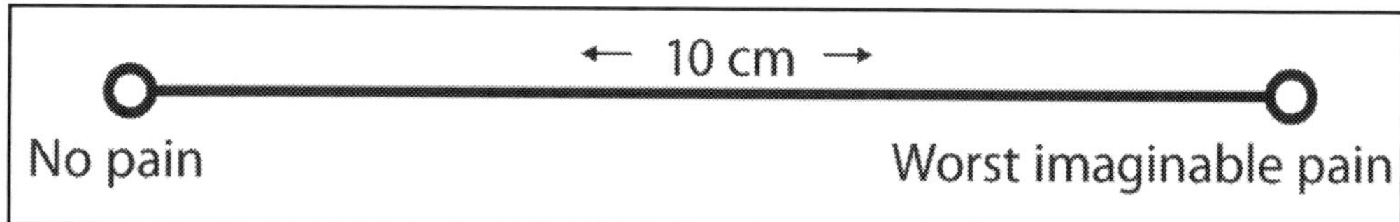

Figure 6-2. Visual analog pain scale.

of fever.[15] Consequently, knowledge of patient body temperature is useful in informing clinical decision-making in physical therapy care.

Body temperature is typically measured sublingually or rectally, as these are the most accurate areas for assessment. Tympanic or axillary temperatures readings, though convenient, lack validity and are not recommended.[15] Irrespective of location, the physical therapist assistant must document the site of measurement for consistency across subsequent measurements.[15]

Oxygen Saturation

Though not one of the 5 vital signs, oxygen saturation, measured via pulse oximetry, is regularly assessed in patients with cardiorespiratory conditions.[12] Oxygen saturation measures the percentage of oxygen in the blood compared to the amount it can carry.[12] It is easily assessed via a portable pulse oximeter attached to the index finger.[12] Normal oxygen saturation is greater than 89%.[12] At lower oxygen saturation levels, the patient should be restricted from physical activity.

Pain Assessment

Assessment of pain can be particularly problematic in a patient with a neurological condition, namely due to issues of comprehension and expression. According to the Commission on Accreditation in Physical Therapy Education, the physical therapist assistant should be able to "administer standardized questionnaires, graphs, behavioral scales, or visual analog scales for pain" as well as recognize "activities, positioning, and postures that aggravate or relieve pain or altered sensations."[18]

The following are commonly used pain scales:

- The Numerical Rating Scale[19]: The patient is asked to rate the pain from 0 (no pain) to 10 (worst pain possible).
- Visual analog pain scale[19]: This is a 10-cm line with the left-hand side representing no pain and the right-hand side indicating the worst imaginable pain. The patient marks a point along the line to indicate the level of pain (Figure 6-2). This scale has been found to be unreliable for individuals with impaired abstract reasoning skills.[20]
- McGill Pain Questionnaire: This is a self-reported assessment instrument containing 3 categories of word descriptors: sensory, affective, and evaluative. It contains a pain intensity scale to help determine the properties of the pain experience. The questionnaire provides quantitative pain information that can be treated statistically.[21]
- Wong-Baker FACES Pain Rating Scale[22]: This scale (www.WongBakerFaces.org) is a series of 6 faces ranging from a smiley face for 0, or no hurt, to a distraught face for 10, or worst hurt. It requires little instruction and does not require verbal instruction.
- Checklist of Nonverbal Pain Indicators (CNPI)[23]: This is a list of 6 pain indicators (ie, verbal complaints, facial grimaces and winces, bracing, restlessness, rubbing, and vocal complaints) that are scored as 0 if the behavior is not observed and 1 if the behavior is observed even briefly. The CNPI is reliable and valid for older adults with acute or chronic pain, patients in critical care units, and patients with dementia.
- Pain Assessment in Advanced Dementia[24]: This assesses 4 pain indicators (ie, breathing, negative vocalization, facial expression, and consolability). Each item is scored from 0 to 2, with 0 indicating no pain and 2 indicating considerable discomfort.
- Pediatric pain scales[25]:
    - Crying Requires Increased Vital Signs Expression Sleeplessness: Appropriate for use with neonatal infants in the first month of life. This assesses 5 variables: crying, oxygen requirements, facial expression, vital signs, and sleeping pattern. The variables are scored from 0 to 2, with a maximum possible score of 10. Higher pain expression is indicated by a higher score.
    - Neonatal Infant Pain Scale: Appropriate for use with infants, this assesses 6 variables (facial expression, crying, breathing pattern, arms, legs, and state of arousal) that are scored in 1-minute intervals before, during, and after a painful intervention. The variables are scored from 0 (no pain) to 2 (pain).
    - Face, Legs, Activity, Crying, Consolability Scale: This is used to measure post-procedural pain intensity in young children. It ranks 5 indicators (face, legs, activity, crying, and consolability) on a 3-point severity scale (0 to 2), with a maximum total score of 10.

Facial expression scales, such as the Wong-Baker FACES Pain Rating Scale, are commonly used with children age 5 or older when they are able to rate pain intensity.[22]

Table 6-1

States of Altered Consciousness

Coma	A state of unresponsiveness from which the patient cannot be aroused even with strong stimuli. The patient's eyes are closed.[26]
Stupor	Arousable only by continuous, vigorous stimuli.[26]
Obtunded	Slower psychological response to stimulation with an increased need for sleep. Difficult to arouse from sleeping. Confusion and drowsiness is noted when awake.[26]
Vegetative State	Cycling of arousal states with periods of eye opening in an unresponsive patient.[26] Regular sleep-wake cycles and normal respiratory patterns are also present.[27] If the vegetative state lasts longer than 30 days, the term *persistent vegetative state* is used.[12]
Minimally Conscious State	Severely impaired consciousness in which there is behavioral evidence of minimal but definite presence of self- or environmental awareness.[26] Evidence may include the ability to follow simple commands, the presence of gestural or verbal yes/no responses, intelligible speech, and nonreflexive movements or affective behaviors.[27]
Syncope	Fainting; a temporary loss of consciousness frequently as a result of a drop in blood pressure.[27]
Delirium	Not oriented to time, place, and people in the environment, but still oriented to self. Delusions or hallucinations may be present.[26]

Adapted from Lundy-Ekman L. *Neuroscience: Fundamentals of Rehabilitation.* St. Louis, MO: Elsevier: 2013 and Posner JB, Saper CB, Schiff N, Plum F. *Plum and Posner's Diagnosis of Stupor and Coma.* New York, NY: Oxford University Press; 2007.

Mental Status

Mental status includes consciousness and arousal, orientation, attention, and higher cognitive functions. Understanding the patient's mental status is important in determining the patient's ability to function in the physical therapy setting. According to the Commission on Accreditation in Physical Therapy Education,[18] the physical therapist assistant should be able to recognize "changes in the direction and magnitude of patient's state of arousal, mentation, and cognition." Understanding the patient's mental status allows the physical therapist assistant to appropriately deliver physical therapy interventions and to accurately document the patient's response to treatment.

Consciousness and Arousal

Arousal is the patient's responsiveness to stimulation and indicates readiness for activity.[1] Arousal is an important component in identifying the state of consciousness (Table 6-1). A change in arousal, attention, and/or cognition must be communicated to the physical therapist or appropriate medical professionals.

Orientation

Orientation is the ability of an individual to cognitively adapt within an unfamiliar environment, allowing for accurate awareness of person, place, time, and situation. The individual is assessed according to either 3 domains (ie, orientation to person, place, and time), abbreviated as "oriented × 3/3" or 4 domains (ie, orientation to person, place, time, and situation), abbreviated as "oriented × 4/4." When a patient is not oriented to one or more domains, it is documented with the domains that were correctly identified listed within parentheses (eg, "oriented × 2/4 [person, place]").[26]

Attention

Attention is the patient's ability to stay focused on a task. There are several categories of attention: selective attention, sustained attention, alternating attention, and divided attention (Box 6-3).[26]

A common test used to examine aspects of arousal, attention, and cognition is the Mini-Mental State Exam.[27] It is a proprietary test[28] composed of 8 sections:

1. Orientation
2. Immediate recall
3. Attention
4. Delayed verbal recall
5. Naming
6. Three-stage command
7. Reading
8. Writing

Results of the Mini-Mental State Exam are important when planning interventions. Patients who demonstrate deficits in immediate recall may have difficulty following directions. The patient who has difficulty with 3-stage commands may have difficulty learning the proper technique for wheelchair (w/c) transfers. Instructing the patient to "position the w/c next to the bed, apply the locks, scoot forward, lean forward, and transfer" would contain too many commands for the patient with sequencing problems to follow. If the patient has delayed verbal recall, listing total hip precautions may be difficult.

The Cognitive Abilities Screening Instrument[29] is a nonproprietary test that examines 6 key cognitive abilities: digit span or other mental tracking; verbal fluency; reasoning/judgment; expressive language; visual construction;

and immediate free verbal recall, delayed free verbal recall, or cued verbal recall.

Sensation

A patient's sensory status provides valuable information to the physical therapist and physical therapist assistant. First, specific patterns of sensory impairment indicate possible damage from any number of areas in the CNS or peripheral nervous system.[30] For example, patients with radial nerve impairment will experience sensory loss along the radial side of the dorsal aspect of the hand while patients with median nerve impairment will experience sensory loss along the radial side of the palmar surface of the hand. Second, impaired sensation may result in specific movement impairments, such as a wide base of support (BOS) when walking secondary to impaired sensation in the feet in individuals with peripheral neuropathies. Finally, impaired sensation may predispose patients to injuries such as sprained ankles or decubitus ulcers.[31]

Sensation can be divided into 3 major categories.[32] *Exteroceptive sensation* (superficial sensation) refers to receptors located in the skin and the mucous membranes. Exteroceptive sensation includes tactile or touch sensation, pain sensation, and temperature sensation. *Proprioceptive sensation* (deep sensation) refers to receptors located in muscles, tendons, ligaments, and joints. Proprioceptive sensation includes proprioception (joint position sense), vibratory sense, and kinesthesia (movement sense). *Combined cortical sensory function*, which requires interpretation in the brain, includes stereognosis, graphesthesia, 2-point discrimination, touch localization, and double simultaneous stimulation.

Sensation can also be divided into 5 categories[33]:

1. Discriminative touch (primary sensation), which includes location of touch and tactile thresholds
2. Discriminative touch (cortical sensation), which includes 2-point discrimination, bilateral simultaneous touch, and graphesthesia
3. Conscious proprioception, which includes joint movement, joint position, and vibration, discriminative touch, and stereognosis
4. Fast pain (lateral pain system), which is sharp, prickling pain
5. Discriminative temperature, which is heat or cold

Sensory Testing

Several principles apply to sensory testing[32]:

- It should be determined whether the patient is able to understand the testing procedure.
- The patient needs to be positioned comfortably, and the areas to be tested should be accessible.
- The testing procedure should be explained prior to testing.
- The patient's vision should be obscured during the examination.

Box 6-3

Definitions of Types of Attention

- Selective attention: The patient's ability to concentrate on a task while screening out unnecessary information. One method of testing selective attention is the Digit Span Test, in which the therapist gives the patient a short list of numbers to recall either forward or backward.
- Sustained attention (vigilance): The patient's ability to maintain time on task. Sustained attention is tested by observing the patient's ability to remain on task, and documenting the type of task and the amount of time the patient was able to sustain attention to the task.
- Alternating attention (attention flexibility): The patient's ability to shift attention between tasks. Alternating attention is tested by examining the patient's ability to shift between tasks.
- Divided attention: The patient's ability to perform 2 tasks simultaneously (eg, to walk and talk at the same time [Walkie-Talkie Test]).

- The examination begins with the areas where sensation is unimpaired, to be used as reference points and to make sure that the patient understands the test. The examiner then completes the rest of the examination in areas of suspected impairment.
- Sensation is documented as normal (100% accuracy), impaired (more than 50% but less than 100% accuracy), absent (less than 50% accuracy), or unable to test.[34] A diagram of the dermatomes or sensory distribution of the peripheral nerves may be used to illustrate the pattern of sensory impairment.[29] Figures 6-3A and B illustrate the dermatome level of innervation on the left and identification of the specific peripheral nerves on the right.

Discriminative Touch (Primary Sensation)

- **Light touch[35]:** A wisp of cotton is used for testing light touch (Figure 6-4). A wisp is obtained by pulling a cotton ball apart or by pulling off the end of a cotton swab. The wisp is touched to the skin without swiping, and the patient is asked to identify when the stimulus is felt. Swiping the cotton wisps across the skin may give an inaccurate response, as swiping may stimulate the hair follicles or be interpreted as tickling.
- **Location of touch[33]:** The examiner lightly touches the patient with the fingertips or a wisp of cotton. The patient is asked to point to the area or tell the examiner where the stimuli is felt.
- **Tactile thresholds[33]:** Semmes Weinstein monofilaments may be used to test tactile thresholds and pro-

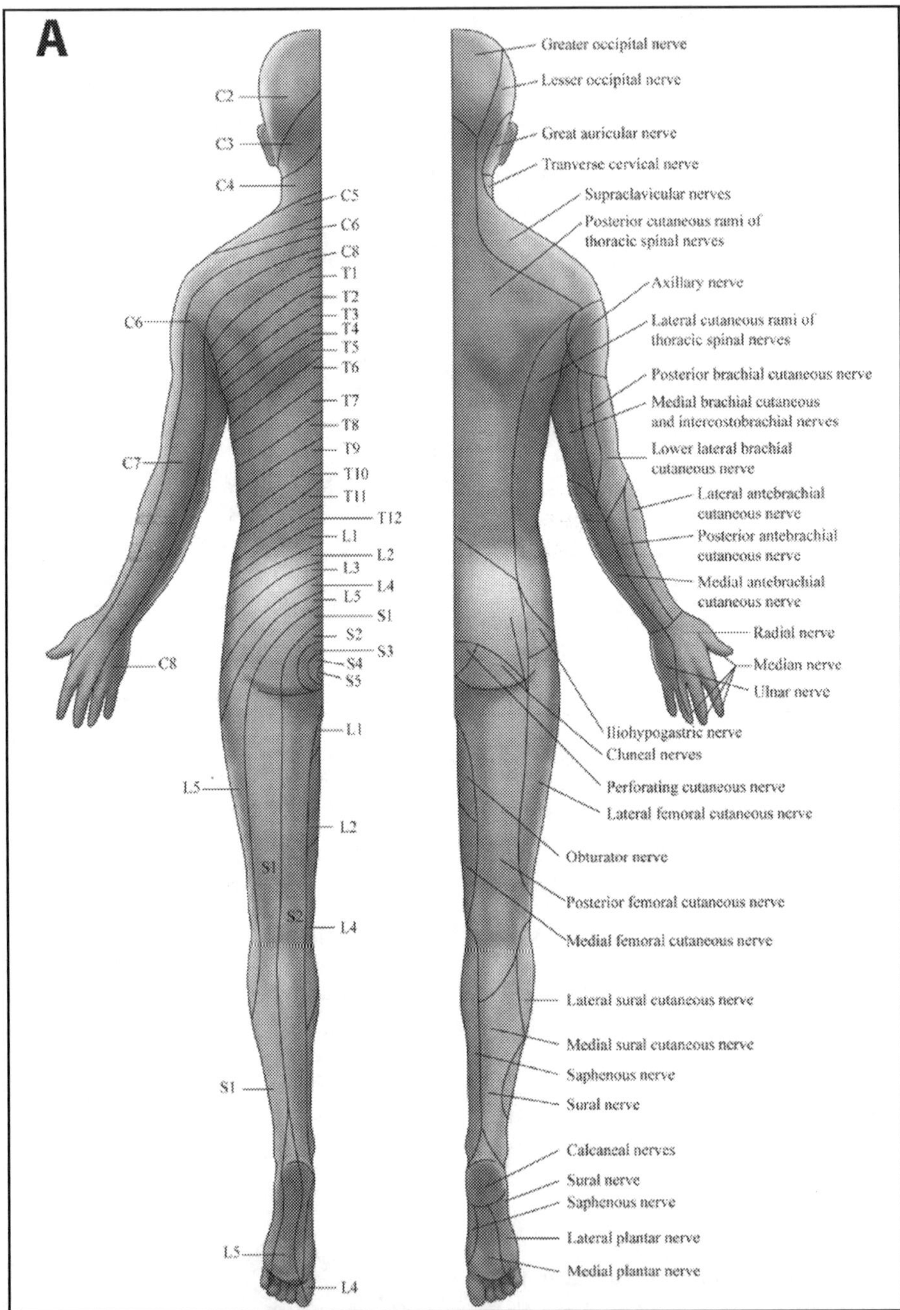

Figure 6-3A. Example of pattern of sensory distribution (dermatome) or level of innervation on the left with the peripheral nerve name on the right. Posterior view.

vide specific information about the degree of sensory loss (Figure 6-5). The monofilament is applied perpendicularly to the skin. Adequate pressure is applied to cause the filament to bend. The patient indicates whether the touch is felt. A patient with normal sensation of the foot can feel the 6-g filament everywhere on the foot. The inability to respond to a 10-g or greater filament may indicate a loss of protective sensation. This is particularly important for patients with peripheral neuropathies, often associated with diabetes, who may have decreased protective sensation. Loss of protective sensation places the patient at greater risk for formation of a pressure ulcer.

Discriminative Touch (Cortical Sensation)[33]

- **Two-point discrimination:** A 2-point discriminator is used (Figure 6-6) and set at distances appropriate for the area being tested, with the 2 points being moved closer and closer together until the subject is unable to distinguish the 2 points as separate.

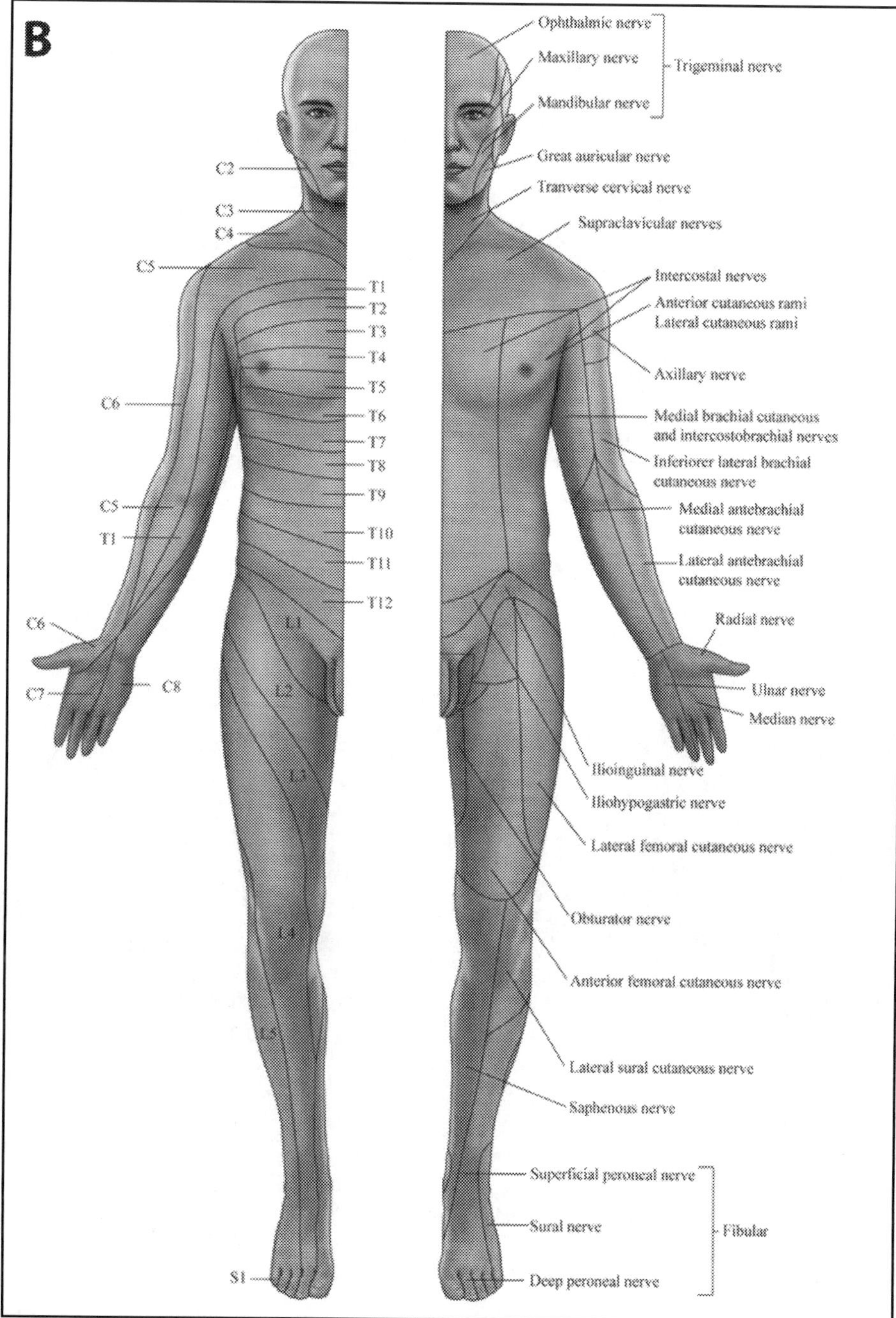

Figure 6-3B. Anterior view.

- **Bilateral simultaneous touch:** Usually the forearms and shins are tested. The tester asks the subject to identify whether the tester is lightly touching one limb, the opposite limb, or both sides of the body at the same time. This test determines whether a person can attend to information coming from 2 areas at the same time.
- **Graphesthesia:** The subject is positioned with his or her palm facing the examiner and fingers pointed upward. The examiner uses the eraser end of a pencil or similar object to trace a letter on the palm of the subject's hand. The subject is then asked to identify the letter.

Conscious Proprioception[33]

- **Joint movement (kinesthesia):** The examiner, using a fingertip grip, grasps the lateral surfaces of the subject's limb. The joint is passively moved in small increments. The subject is instructed to tell the examiner whether the joint is being "bent" or "straightened." Errors would indicate that the subject does not reliably

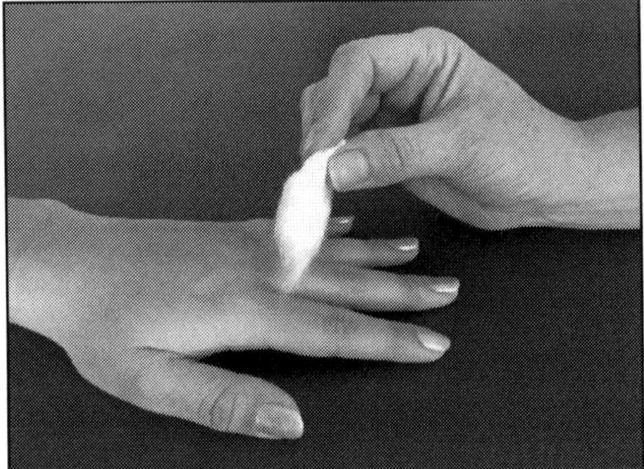

Figure 6-4. Using a cotton wisp to test light touch.

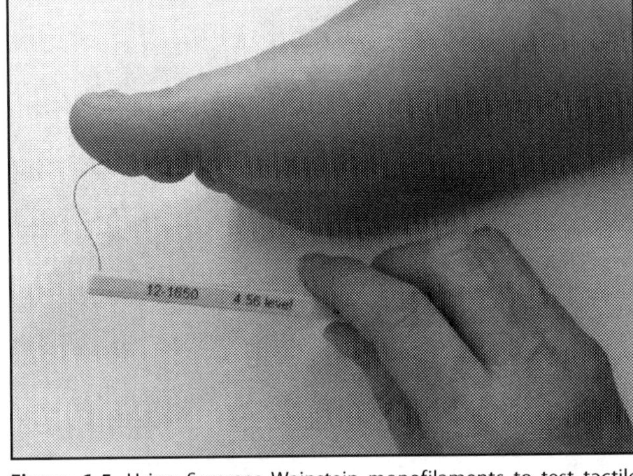

Figure 6-5. Using Semmes Weinstein monofilaments to test tactile thresholds.

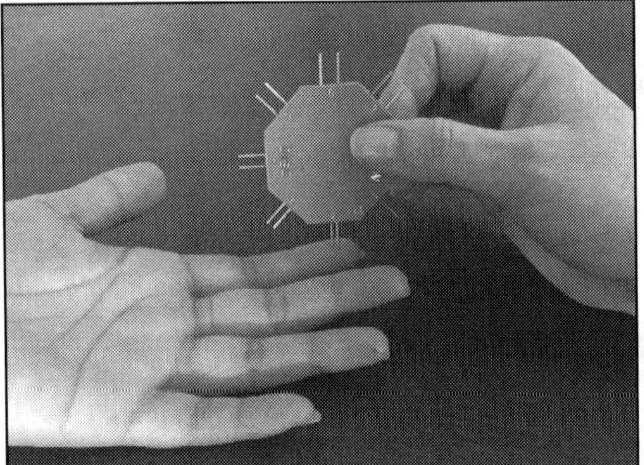

Figure 6-6. Using a 2-point discriminator to test for 2-point discrimination.

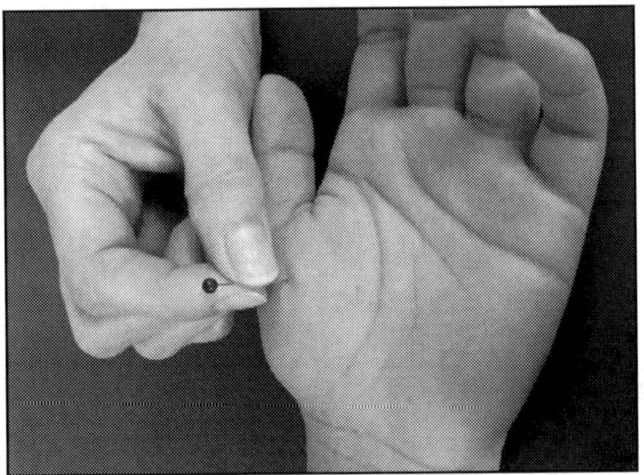

Figure 6-7. Using a pin to test pain sensation.

know when a joint is moving, which is significant during movement activities.

- **Joint position (proprioception):** The examiner, using a fingertip grip, grasps the lateral surfaces of the subject's limb. The examiner moves the joint and holds it in a static position. The subject is asked to either replicate the position with the opposite limb or describe the position of the joint. Errors would indicate that the subject does not know where the limb is in space, which can have significance during functional activities.
- **Vibration:** The examiner uses as tuning fork that vibrates at 128 Hz. The tuning fork is struck to create a vibration. The end of the vibrating tuning fork is then placed on a bony prominence. The subject is asked to report whether the vibration is felt or to indicate when the vibration stops.
- **Stereognosis:** The examiner places a common object, such as a paper clip or key, in the subject's hand. The subject is allowed to manipulate the object and then is asked to identify it. Errors would indicate that the subject with diminished vision would have difficulty selecting objects.

Fast (Superficial) Pain (Lateral Pain System)

A clean, unused safety pin is used to test pain sensation and to differentiate between sharp and dull. To test sharp, the sharp end of the safety pin is placed against the patient's skin, and enough pressure is applied to indent but not puncture the skin (Figure 6-7). Sliding the examiner's fingers down the pin ensures the correct amount of pressure. The rounded end of the safety pin is used to provide dull stimuli, which is alternated randomly with the sharp stimulus. The examiner then asks the patient to identify whether the sensation feels sharp or dull.[36] To map an area of impaired sensation, a pinwheel may be used. The handle of the pinwheel is held lightly between the examiner's thumb and index finger, and the pinwheel is rolled lightly across the subject's skin, circling the circumference of the limb. Specific patterns of sensory loss may indicate lesions in specific peripheral nerves.[33]

Discriminative Temperature (Heat or Cold)[36]

Two test tubes are used, 1 filled with hot water (the temperature should not exceed 45°C to avoid the possibility of a burn) and the other filled with crushed ice and water. The examiner touches the subject's skin with the test tubes in a random fashion and asks the subject to identify whether the test tube is hot or cold. Note that pain sensation and temperature sensation are carried in the same pathway in the spinal cord, so testing of both sensations may not be necessary, although loss of temperature sensation may precede the loss of pain sensation.

Motor Examination

The motor examination involves several components as identified in Box 6-4.

Box 6-4

Motor Examination Components

- Examination of ROM
- Examination of muscular tone
- Examination of strength
- Examination of phasic stretch reflexes
- Examination of synergy

Range of Motion

Range of motion (ROM) refers to the available movement of the joints. Generally, goniometric measurements are used to indicate the available ROM of a joint. Note that accurate ROM measurement may be difficult to obtain if the patient has cognitive impairments or abnormal muscle tone. Limited ROM will adversely affect the patient's postural alignment and ability to move in a biomechanically correct manner. For example, lack of adequate ankle dorsiflexion may cause the patient's knee to hyperextend during the stance phase of gait. A patient who lacks adequate hip flexion will have difficulty maintaining a sitting position. A patient with limited shoulder flexion may have difficulty dressing.

Muscular Tone

Many terms are used for motor examination (Table 6-2). Several tests are used to examine muscle tone. The Tardieu Rating Scale[37] and Modified Ashworth Scale[38] test the patient's degree of spasticity. When using the Tardieu Rating Scale, the patient is placed in the supine position, and the limb that is being tested is moved at different velocities. The amount of resistance is scored on a scale of 0 to 5, with 0 indicating that there was no resistance to passive movement and 5 indicating that the joint was immovable.

When using the Modified Ashworth Scale (Table 6-3), the limb is moved passively, and the amount of resistance is scored on a scale of 0 to 4, with 0 indicating no increase in muscle tone and 4 indicating the limb was rigid. The type of muscle tone varies with the area of injury to the nervous system. For example, injury to a peripheral nerve results in low or no tone in the muscle (*hypotonia*), while injury to the spinal cord usually results in hypertonia below the level of the lesion, and damage to the basal ganglia, as seen in individuals with Parkinson's disease, results in rigidity.

Muscle Strength

Impaired muscle strength, or weakness, may impair patient function. Trunk or lower extremity weakness may adversely affect gait or balance. Limited strength in the scapulothoracic or rotator cuff musculature can alter normal upper extremity biomechanics, leading to pain and/or dysfunction. Muscle weakness can be the result of many causes. Weakness can occur from damage to areas of the CNS or peripheral nervous system. Damage at the neuromuscular junction, where the nerve connects to the muscle, can result in weakness in disorders such as myasthenia gravis. Damage to the lower motor neurons (peripheral nerves), which connect the CNS to the muscles, can result in weakness from compressive injuries such as carpal tunnel syndrome or diseases including diabetes mellitus; viruses that attack the nerve tissues, including herpes varicella zoster (shingles) or Epstein-Barr; and an acute inflammatory demyelinating neuropathy, Guillain-Barré syndrome, which damages motor, sensory, and autonomic nerve fibers. Damage to an upper motor neuron (eg, the brain or within the spinal cord) may also result in weakness depending on the area and extent of damage in the brain or spinal cord. Finally, lack of activity during the recovery process may lead to disuse weakness.[2]

Several methods of examining muscle strength are available: formal manual muscle testing, dynamometry, and functional testing. Several grading systems are used for manual muscle testing. Daniels and Worthingham describe a scale from 0 to 5. Grades 1 and 2 indicate the patient's ability either to achieve a voluntary muscle contraction or to move a body segment in a gravity minimized plane. Grades 3 through 5 indicate the patient's ability to move against gravity with increasing amounts of manual resistance.[39] Kendall et al[40] rely on a scale of 0 to 10. Grades of 1 to 3 indicate the patient's ability to move with gravity minimized, and grades of 4 to 10 indicate the patient's ability to move against gravity with increasing amounts of manual resistance. A hand-held dynamometer,[41] which measures the force applied at the point of application, can also be used to measure grip strength.

Performing manual muscle tests on a patient recovering from a neurological disorder can be difficult, and, in general, the interrater reliability of manual muscle testing against gravity with manual resistance is variable.[42,43]

Table 6-2
Terms Used for Motor Examination

Term	Definition and Comments
Muscle tone	The tension in the muscle fibers of a resting muscle. Muscle tone is tested by passively moving the limb through its ROM and feeling for the amount of tension that is present. Muscle tone is not directly correlated with the patient's ability to move. Once the rigidity is relaxed, the muscles are often simultaneously weak and thus may show a decreased response to a quick stretch.
Spasticity	Velocity-dependent resistance to movement as a result of neuromuscular overactivity with resistance to movement increasing as the speed and amplitude of the movement increases.
Hyperreflexia	Excessive reflex response to muscle stretch. Hyperreflexia usually does not interfere with active movement. Often identified during testing of deep tendon reflexes.
Hypertonia	Excessive resistance to active or passive stretch.
Rigidity	A state of severe hypertonia. Both the agonist and antagonist are hyperactive, causing rigidity around the joint, although there is not necessarily an increase in response of the muscle to quick stretch.
Hypotonia	Decrease resistance to active and passive stretch. Hypotonia can be an insult in parts of the brain, but indicates that the lower motor neuron is not functioning adequately to create normal muscle tone. Hypotonia can also be the result of disuse of a muscle over time, which is a severe problem with patients who have been bedridden or inactive.
Motor paralysis	Impaired ability to generate muscular force. This can be due to a problem within the muscle, the motor neuron leading to the muscle, or an insult at a higher level than the spinal cord.
Flaccidity	Absence of muscle tone. This also can be due to a problem within the muscle, the motor neuron leading to the muscle, or an insult at a higher level than the spinal cord, although flaccidity is considered more severe than paralysis.

Adapted from Lundy-Ekman L. *Neuroscience: Fundamentals for Rehabilitation.* St. Louis, MO: Elsevier; 2013.

Table 6-3
Modified Ashworth Scale

0	No increase in muscle tone.
1	Slight increase in muscle tone, manifested by a catch-and-release or minimal resistance at the end of the ROM when the affected part is moved in flexion or extension.
1+	Slight increase in muscle tone, manifested by a catch followed by minimal resistance throughout the remainder (less than half) of the ROM.
2	More marked increase in muscle tone through most of the ROM but affected part easily moved.
3	Considerable increase in muscle tone; passive movement difficult.
4	Affected parts rigid in flexion and extension.

Reprinted from Bohannon RW, Smith MB. Interrater reliability of a modified Ashworth scale of muscle spasticity. *Phys Ther.* 1987;67(2):206-207, with permission of the American Physical Therapy Association.

When formal muscle testing is not possible, the patient's functional movements can be observed for signs of weakness, such as difficulty transitioning from supine-to-sit positions, the inability to rise from a seated position without pushing with the arms, or difficulty stepping up a curb. A specific pattern of weakness may indicate the area of damage within the CNS or peripheral nervous system. For example, lower motor neuron (peripheral nerve) damage, such as a lesion to the deep peroneal nerve, could result in difficulty with ankle dorsiflexion and toe extension.

Such a condition may prevent an individual from dorsiflexing the foot while stepping up onto a curb or dorsiflexing the foot during the swing phase of the gait cycle. Additionally, damage to the L4-5 and S1 nerve roots that supply the deep peroneal nerve could also create weakness with ankle dorsiflexion and toe extension. A comparison of strength in muscles innervated by both the deep peroneal nerve and those innervated by the L4-5 and S1 nerve roots can help the clinician make determinations about the source of muscle weakness.

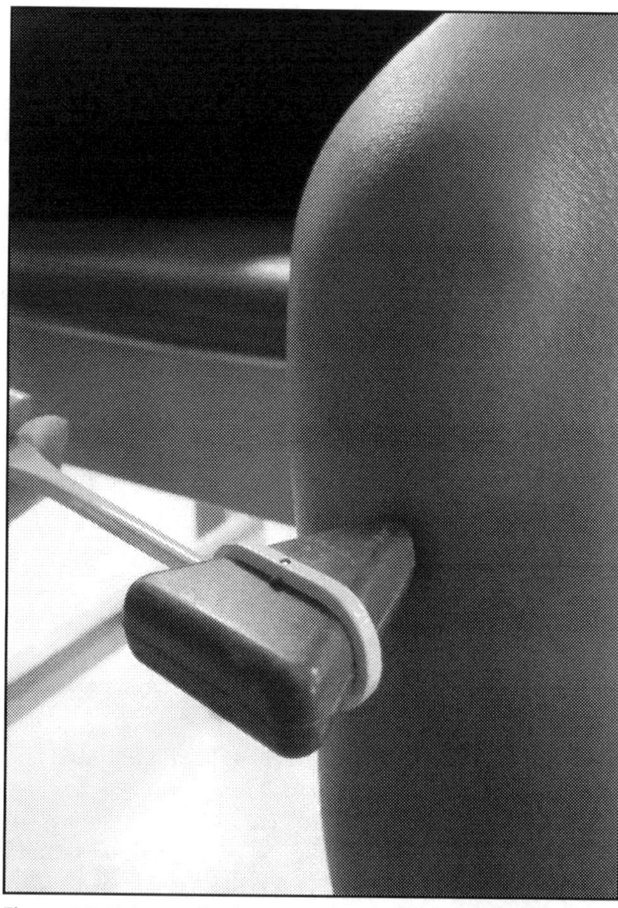

Figure 6-8. Using a reflex hammer to test phasic stretch reflex.

Phasic Stretch Reflexes

A *phasic stretch reflex* is a reflexive muscle contraction in response to a quick stretch.[44]

Myotatic reflex, muscle stretch reflex, and deep tendon reflex are interchangeable with the term phasic stretch reflex. Presence of a phasic stretch reflex indicates that the monosynaptic reflex arc from the tendon through the spinal cord to the muscle is intact. Phasic stretch reflexes are tested by striking the tendon with a reflex hammer (Figure 6-8) and should be compared bilaterally. Phasic stretch reflexes are graded as follows[26]:

- 0 = No response; always abnormal
- 1 + = A slight but definitely present response; may or may not be normal
- 2 + = A brisk response; normal
- 3 + = A very brisk response; may or may not be normal
- 4 + = A tap elicits a repeating reflex (*clonus*); always abnormal

An involuntary repetitive flexion and extension of the joint in response to a phasic stretch is known as clonus.[45] A clonus is examined by applying a quick stretch stimulus and then maintaining the stretch. A clonus that fades after a few beats is known as *unsustained*, whereas a clonus that continues is known as *sustained*. The presence of a sustained clonus is never normal.

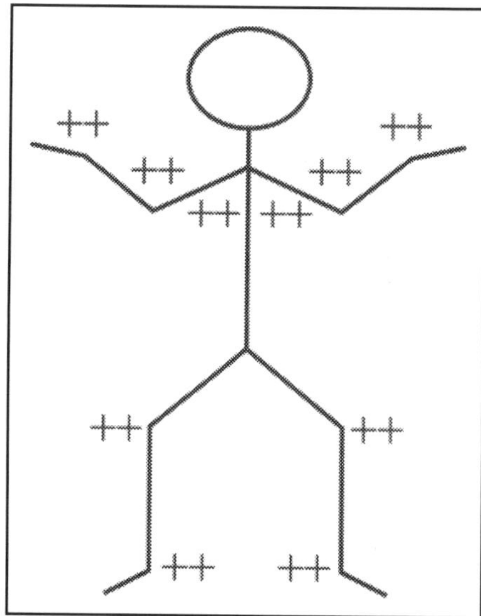

Figure 6-9. Normal results of testing phasic stretch reflexes.

The results are frequently documented on a stick figure (Figure 6-9) with the number of "+"s corresponding to the grade of the reflexive response.

Synergy

Muscles that normally work together to produce a movement are known as *synergists*.[46] An abnormal synergy occurs when stereotypic coactivation of muscles results in an abnormal coupling of movements at adjacent joints.[33] Refer to Table 6-4, which identifies the synergies commonly seen in patients with CNS insults.

For example, during a lower extremity flexor synergy, the affected limb will tend to move into a combination of hip flexion, abduction, and external ration, with knee flexion, and ankle dorsiflexion/inversion (Figure 6-10). A flexion synergy during gait may lead to the inability of a patient to effectively place the foot on the ground at initial contact, potentially resulting in a fall.

Assessment of synergies is part of a comprehensive motor evaluation. One method of assessing synergies is the motor function section of the Fugl-Meyer Assessment of Motor Recovery After Stroke.[47] The patient is first asked to demonstrate a complete synergy by demonstrating active hip flexion, abduction external rotation with knee flexion, and ankle dorsiflexion/inversion of the affected leg. The patient is then asked to demonstrate movements out of synergy. For example, while standing, the patient is asked to place the affected lower extremity in 90 degrees of knee flexion with the hip in 0 degrees of extension and the ankle in dorsiflexion. Each component of the movement is scored based on how the movement component is performed.

Table 6-4
Synergy Patterns of the Extremities

Limbs	*Flexion Synergy Components*	*Extension Synergy Components*
Upper	• Scapular retraction, elevation, hyperextension • Shoulder abduction, external rotation • Elbow flexion • Forearm supination • Wrist and finger flexion	• Scapular protraction • Shoulder adduction, internal rotation • Elbow extension • Forearm pronation • Wrist and finger flexion
Lower	• Hip flexion, abduction, external rotation • Knee flexion • Ankle dorsiflexion, inversion • Toe dorsiflexion	• Hip extension, adduction, internal rotation • Knee extension • Ankle plantar flexion, inversion • Toe plantar flexion
Reprinted with permission from O'Sullivan SB. Assessment of motor function. In: O'Sullivan SB, Schmitz TJ, eds. *Physical Rehabilitation: Assessment and Treatment.* 4th ed. Philadelphia, PA: FA Davis; 2001.		

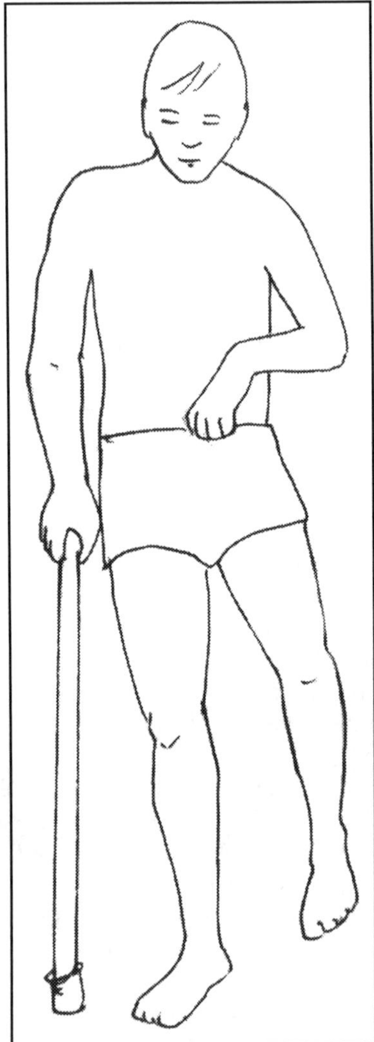

Figure 6-10. Patient attempting to ambulate with a lower extremity flexor synergy.

Developmental (Primitive) Reflexes and Reactions

Developmental or *primitive reflexes* are stereotypical patterns that occur in response to specific stimuli, and they represent basic survival patterns of function.[48] Individual reflexes appear at specific ages. Because of this, developmental reflexes can be used to determine a child's level of development.[49] The presence of primitive reflexes beyond certain ages of development may be a signal of neurological dysfunction.[49] Also, primitive reflexes may reappear in patients who have had CNS damage such as stroke or brain injury, or may appear when an adult is tired or under stress.[48] The presence of these reflexes may interfere with the patient's functional ability.[49]

The physical therapist assistant must be able to identify the influence of developmental reflexes because the abnormal presence or absence of these reflexes may interfere with movement. For example, the patient may have difficulty rolling if there is a strong asymmetrical tonic neck reflex present.

Righting reactions are important in establishing and maintaining the relationship and alignment of the head, trunk, and extremities, and in controlling the vertical/upright posture against gravity. *Equilibrium responses* are patterns of movement that dynamically maintain balance of the whole body as the BOS changes and the center of gravity (COS) moves in space.[48] *Protective reactions* serve to help safeguard a person if equilibrium reactions fail. All of these reactions begin to develop after 6 months, and persist throughout life.[48] Failure to develop these reactions or responses in infancy or loss of them later in life may indicate CNS damage, which can be detrimental to the individual's function and safety.[49]

The developmental reflexes, righting reactions, equilibrium responses, and protective responses are described, along with testing, in Table 6-5.

Coordination

Coordination involves the sequencing, timing, and grading of multiple muscle groups, resulting in movement that is smooth, efficient, and accurate with the activation of joints and muscles at the correct time with the correct amount of force.[50] Impaired coordination results in multiple disorders. The following are common tests used to examine coordination:

- Nose-finger-nose (Figure 6-11) is a test for *dysmetria* (the inability to make a movement of the appropriate distance). Dysmetria is tested by asking the patient to use the index finger to touch the nose then the therapist's finger. The therapist observes whether the patient is accurate or undershoots the target (*hypometria*) or overshoots the target (*hypermetria*).[50]
- *Dysdiadochokinesia* is the inability to make rapid alternating movements. It is tested by examining the patient's ability to produce rapid forearm supination-pronation or heel-toe movement smoothly with the correct force.[33]
- Heel-to-shin is a test for *ataxia* (a decreased coordination of muscle movements). The patient is placed in the supine position and requested to run the heel of one leg down the shin of the opposite leg.[50]
- The Fregly-Graybiel Ataxia Test Battery[51] is a combination test for both coordination and balance. The test is composed of the following components: sharpened Romberg (standing heel-to-toe) with the eyes closed, walk 5 steps on a rail with the eyes open, stand on rail with eyes open, stand on a rail with eyes closed, stand on right leg with eyes closed, stand on left leg with eyes closed, and walk on the floor with eyes closed.
- Running and skipping may be used to identify impaired coordination in high-functioning patients who are ambulating without apparent deficits.

Cranial Nerve Examination

Cranial nerves are peripheral nerves that originate from different structures in the brain.[33] There are 12 cranial nerves, which are designated using Roman numerals I through XII. Cranial nerve I is the olfactory nerve and originates in the telencephalon. Cranial nerve II is the optic nerve and originates in the diencephalon. Cranial nerve III (oculomotor) and IV (trochlear) originate in the midbrain. Cranial nerves V (trigeminal), VI (abducens), and VII (facial) arise from the pons. The remaining cranial nerves, VIII (vestibulocochlear), IX (glossopharyngeal), X (vagus), XI (accessory), and XII (hypoglossal), arise from the medulla. The cranial nerves have 4 major functions[33]:

1. Innervation of the muscles of the face, eyes, tongue, tongue, jaw, and 2 neck muscles, the sternocleidomastoid and the trapezius.
2. Transmittal of somatosensory information from the skin and muscles of the face and temporal mandibular joint.
3. Transmittal of special sensory information related to vision, hearing vestibular, taste, smell, and visceral sensation.
4. Parasympathetic regulation of heart rate, blood pressure, breathing, digestion, and control of pupil size and the curvature of the lens of the eye.

Examining the cranial nerves provides information about the integrity of the parts of the brain where the nerves originate and about the functional loss caused by damage to the nerves.[33]

- Cranial nerve I (olfactory) controls the sense of smell and is tested by presenting familiar, nonirritating odors such as citrus, coffee, or cloves to each nostril. Damage to cranial nerve I may result in the inability to identify the substance (*anosmia*), a heightened sense of smell (*hyperosmia*), an altered sense of smell (*parosmia*), or the perception that a normal smell is unpleasant (*carosmia*).
- Cranial nerve II (optic) controls vision and is tested by examining the patient's visual acuity and the ability to perceive objects in different areas of the visual fields, acuity of vision, and pupillary response, in conjunction with cranial nerve III, to a bright light. Damage to cranial nerve II may result in complete loss of vision (*anopsia*), loss of half the field of vision of both eyes (*hemianopsia*), or loss of a quarter of the field of vision (*quadranopsia*).
- Cranial III (oculomotor) controls several of the muscles of the eyes and is tested by examining the patient's ability to look up, down, inward toward the nose (*adduction*), and combined up and in (a diagonal movement). Damage to cranial nerve III results in difficulty performing those specified eye movements.
- Cranial nerve IV controls the inferior oblique muscle, which causes the eyes to move down and in (*adduction*) and is tested by examining the patient's ability to move the eye down and in (a diagonal movement) concurrently. Damage to cranial nerve IV results in difficulty performing the specified eye movements.
- Cranial nerve V (trigeminal nerve) includes 3 divisions: the mandibular, maxillary, and ophthalmic divisions. It controls facial sensation and the muscles of mastication (masseter, temporal, pterygoid, mylohyoid, and digastric) and is tested by using a pinprick to examine sensation of the face and manual muscle testing of the muscles of mastication. Damage to cranial nerve V results in impaired sensation to the face, weakness of the muscle of mastication, and impaired ability to chew.
- Cranial nerve VI (abducens nerve) innervates the lateral rectus muscle of the eye, which controls eye

Table 6-5

Developmental Reflexes and Reaction Assessment

Reflex	*Testing Position and Stimulus*	*Response*
Flexor withdrawal	• Supine or sitting position • Noxious stimulus (pinprick) to sole of foot	• Toes extend, foot dorsiflexes, entire leg flexes uncontrollably
Crossed extension	• Supine position • One leg fixed in extension • Noxious stimulus to ball of foot of the leg fixed in extension	• Opposite leg flexes, then adducts and extends
Traction	• Start in supine position • Grasp forearm and pull up from supine into sitting position	• Flexion of the shoulders, elbows, wrists, and fingers
Moro	• Sitting position • Sudden change in position of head in relation to trunk • Drop patient backward from sitting position	• Extension, abduction of arms, hand opening, and crying followed by flexion, adduction of arms across chest
Startle	• Any position • Sudden loud or harsh noise	• Sudden extension or abduction of arms; crying
Palmar grasp	• Any position • Maintained pressure to palm of hand	• Maintained flexion of fingers
Plantar grasp	• Supine or sitting position • Maintained pressure to ball of foot under toes	• Maintained flexion of toes
Asymmetrical tonic neck	• Any position (commonly tested in supine) • Rotation of the head to one side	• Flexion of arms and legs on skull side, extension of arms and legs on chin side ("bow and arrow" or "fencing posture") • Response may be stronger in the arms than legs
Symmetrical tonic neck	• Any position (commonly tested in supine) • Flexion or extension of the head.	• With head flexion: flexion of arms, extension of legs • With head extension: extension of arms, flexion of legs
Symmetrical tonic labyrinthine	• Prone or supine position	• With prone position: increased flexor tone or flexion of all limbs • With supine position: increased tone or extension of all limbs
Positive supporting	• Upright standing position • Contact to the ball of the foot	• Rigid extension (co-contraction) of the legs
Associated movements or reactions	• Any position • Resisted voluntary movement in any part of the body	• Involuntary movement in a resting extremity or increase in tonic muscle tension
Neck righting acting on the body	• Supine position • Passively turn head to one side	• Body rotates as a whole (logrolls) to align the body with the head
Body righting acting on the body	• Supine position • Passively rotate upper or lower trunk segment	• Body segment not rotated follows to align the body segments
Labyrinthine head-righting	• Upright position (standing or sitting) • Blindfold eyes; alter body position by tipping body in all directions	• Head orients to vertical position with mouth horizontal

(continued)

Table 6-5 (continued)

Developmental Reflexes and Reaction Assessment

Reflex	*Testing Position and Stimulus*	*Response*
Optical righting	• Upright position (standing or sitting) • Alter body position by tipping body in all directions	• Head orients to vertical position with mouth horizontal
Upper extremities; protective extension forward, sideward, and backward	• Sitting, kneeling, or standing position • Displace the COS outside of the BOS	• Forward: Fingers and elbows extend, shoulders flex to support and to protect the body from falling • Sideward: Fingers and elbows extend, shoulders abduct • Backward: Fingers and elbows and shoulders extend
Lower extremities; protective staggering forward, backward, and sideward	• Standing • Displace the COS outside of the BOS.	• Forward: Subject steps forward when balance displaced forward • Backward: Subject steps backward when balance displaced backward
Equilibrium reactions: tilting	• Supine, sitting, or standing position on a movable object such as a balance board or ball • Displace the COS by tilting or moving the support surface	• Curvature of the trunk toward the upward side along with extension and abduction of the extremities on that side; protective extension on the downward side
Equilibrium reactions: postural fixation	• Sitting or standing position • Displace the COS in relation to the BOS but not outside of BOS • Can also be observed during voluntary activity	• Sideward force: Curvature of the trunk toward the external force with extension and abduction of the extremities on the side to which the force was applied • Backward force: Trunk flexion, extension of elbows with flexion of shoulders, and in standing plantar flexion of ankles • Forward force: Trunk extension, extension of arms, and in standing, dorsiflexion of ankles

Adapted from Barnes MR. *The Neurophysiological Basis of Patient Treatment. Vol II: Reflexes in Motor Development.* Atlanta, GA: Stokesville Publishing; 1978.

abduction and is tested by having the patient move the eye laterally. Damage to cranial nerve VI results in the inability to move the eye laterally.

- Cranial nerve VII (facial nerve) innervates the muscles of facial expression (eg, the orbicularis oris, nasalis, and orbicularis occuli) and is tested by manually muscle testing the muscles of facial expression. Damage to cranial nerve VII results in paralysis of the muscles of facial expression.
- Cranial nerve VIII (vestibulocochlear) controls hearing and vestibular function (balance).
- The hearing component (cochlear division) of the vestibulocochlear nerve is examined by formal auditory testing or having the examiner rub his or her fingers close to the patient's ear, then determining whether the patient is able to hear the sound. The vestibular component is tested through formal vestibular testing

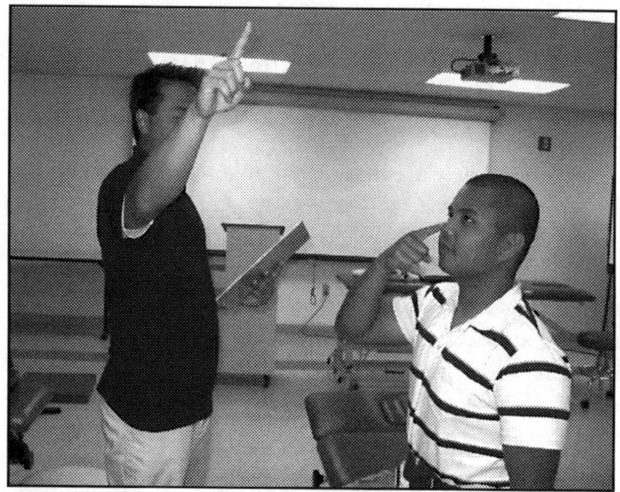

Figure 6-11. Nose-finger-nose coordination test.

or a basic screening test for balance. Damage to cranial nerve VIII results in impaired hearing and/or balance.

- Cranial nerve IX (glossopharyngeal nerve) controls swallowing and, in conjunction with cranial nerve X, the sensation on the posterior third of the tongue and pharynx, as well as the gag reflex. Cranial nerve IX is examined by testing the gag reflex by touching a tongue depressor to the posterior portion of the tongue or pharynx to determine whether a gag reflex is elicited. Damage to cranial nerve IX may adversely affect the patient's ability to swallow.
- Cranial nerve X (vagus nerve) provides innervation of the larynx (in conjunction with cranial nerve IX), pharynx, and viscera. Cranial nerve X is tested by looking for symmetrical elevation of the soft palate while the patient says, "Ahhh." Damage to cranial nerve X affects the patient's ability to swallow and speak. Digestive functions may also be adversely affected, and patients may stop eating because of the fear of choking.
- Cranial nerve XI (accessory nerve) innervates the trapezius and the sternocleidomastoid muscles and is tested by manually muscle testing the trapezius and sternocleidomastoid muscles. Damage to cranial nerve XI results in ipsilateral paralysis of the affected muscles.
- Cranial nerve XII (hypoglossal nerve) innervates the intrinsic muscles of the tongue. Cranial nerve XII is examined by having the patient protrude the tongue and observing the tongue for deviation or atrophy. The patient may also be requested to push the tongue into the cheek. The examiner tests the strength of the tongue by pushing against the tongue from the outside of the cheek. Damage to cranial nerve XII results in deviation of the tongue to the side of the lesion and may affect speech and swallowing.

Examinations for Balance

Balance is based on input from the somatosensory, visual, and vestibular systems and includes several important components:

- COG: "The place in a system or body where the weight is evenly dispersed, and all sides are in balance."[52]
- BOS: "The area of the body that is in contact with the support surface."[50] The BOS may include the contact area of an assistive device such as a walker or crutches.
- Equilibrium: Allows the body as a whole to adapt to changes or perturbations in the relationship of the COG over the BOS.[48]
- Protective reactions (parachute reactions): Extensor responses in the extremities, which occur when the COG is moved beyond the BOS as protection during a fall by either placing the hand out to regain equilibrium, or stepping with the leg opposite to the perturbation.[53]
- Limits of stability: How far an individual in the upright position can lean in any direction without external support, such as taking a step, reaching with the arm(s), or falling.[54] The specific limits of stability vary depending on height, weight, and body composition such as leg length, foot size, and ROM of the hips, knees, ankles, and forefoot of the individual being tested.

The major automatic postural responses (Figure 6-12) include the ankle, hip, stepping, and suspensory strategies, also known as *balance synergies*.[54]

- The ankle strategy/synergy occurs to counteract small displacements from the COG. The body moves as a unit over the feet, with the muscles contracting from distal to proximal. The head and hips move in the same direction, at the same time, as a unit. This synergy elicits muscle response at the ankles first.
- The hip strategy/synergy is used in specific situations such as a narrow surface or the edge of a surface where the individual does not want to step forward. The hip strategy is more complex than the ankle strategy because the head and hips move in opposite directions, occurring when sway is large, fast, and nearing the limits of stability. The hip strategy elicits muscle contractions from proximal to distal.
- The suspensory strategy/synergy also occurs in response to large displacements and results in a squatting response to lower the COG.
- The stepping strategy/synergy occurs in response to large displacements and results in the realignment of the BOS under the center of mass. Normal walking is an example of the use of the stepping strategy or synergy as the individual moves forward beyond the normal BOS and then replaces the foot under the BOS at heel strike.

Examination of balance includes the examination of automatic postural responses to both fast and slow perturbations, anticipatory postural responses, and volitional postural response as seen in normal activities of daily living, such as rising from a chair or walking on uneven surfaces.

There are 2 tests for examining automatic postural responses. The first test is the Sensory Organization Test, in which the patient is positioned on a computerized movable force plate with a movable visual surround[54] (Figure 6-13). The force plate tests the somatosensory component of balance and body sway, and the movable surround and blindfold test the visual component of balance. The force plate and the visual surround are changed to alter the surface and visual environment. By combining configurations of the force plate, movable surround, and blindfold, the examiner is able to isolate components of the balance system. The test is divided into 6 conditions:

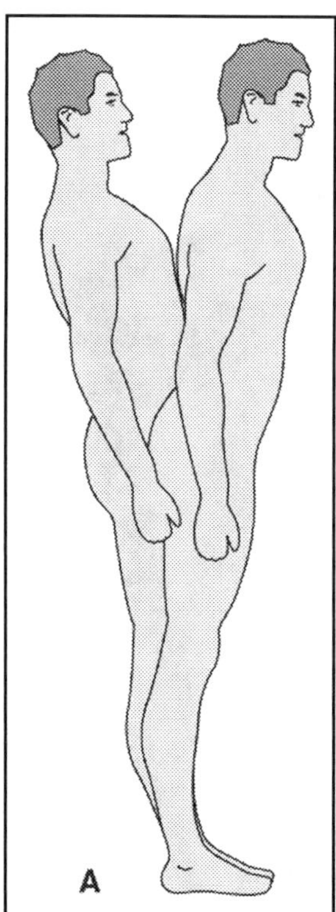

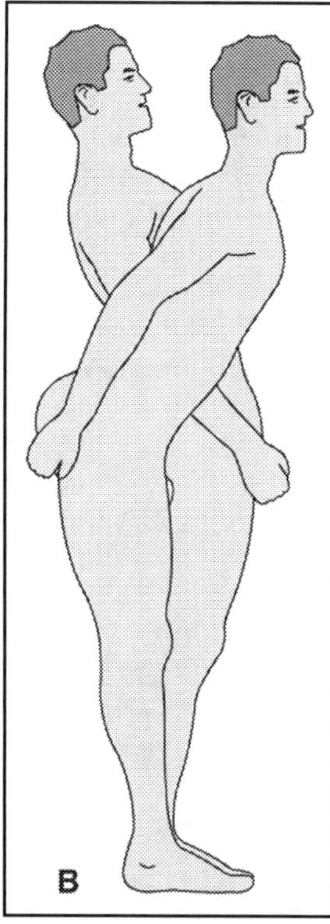

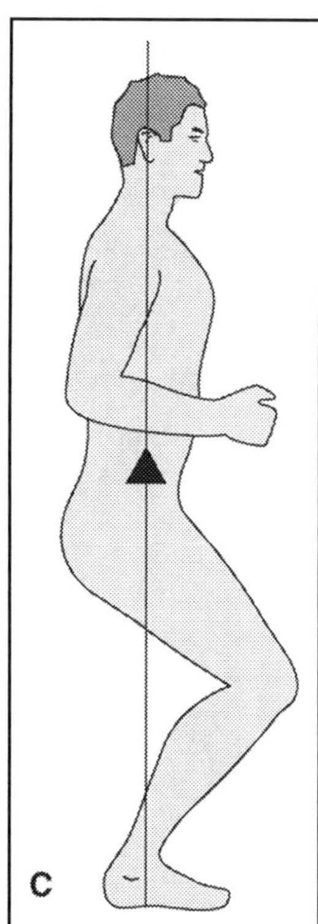

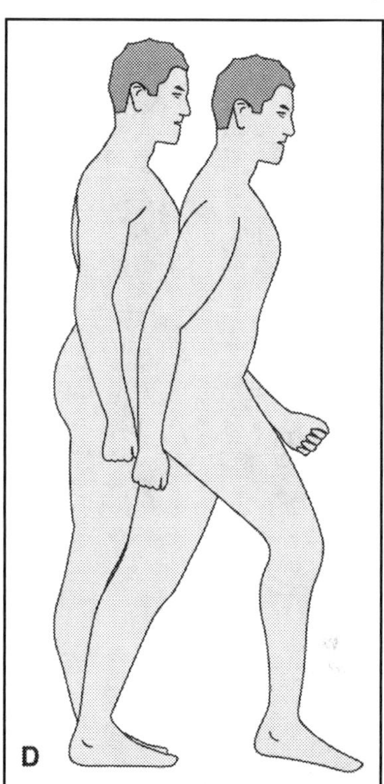

Figure 6-12. Automatic postural strategies. (A) Ankle strategy. (B) Hip strategy. (C) Suspensory strategy. (D) Stepping strategy. (Adapted from Allison L, Fuller K. Balance and vestibular dysfunction. In: Umphred DA, Lazaro RT, Roller ML, Burton GU, eds. *Umphred's Neurological Rehabilitation.* 6th ed. St. Louis, MO: Elsevier; 2013: 654.)

1. In condition 1, the patient is receiving correct information from all 3 senses (vision, vestibular, and somatosensory); this acts as a baseline test.
2. In condition 2, the eyes are obscured with a blindfold so that the patient is not receiving visual input, and only somatosensory and vestibular input remain.
3. In condition 3, the visual surround moves in conjunction with the patient's sway, providing inaccurate visual input that the patient must ignore. Somatosensory and vestibular inputs remain available.
4. In condition 4, the support surface adjusts to the patient's sway, giving inaccurate somatosensory input while visual and vestibular inputs are still available.
5. In condition 5, vision is absent, and the support surface is sway referenced, resulting in no visual input and inaccurate somatosensory input. Only vestibular input is available.
6. In condition 6, the force plate and visual surround are sway referenced, and again, the only accurate input is vestibular input.

The Sensory Organization Test examines which inputs are available to the patient and whether the patient can compensate for missing or distorted input. For example, if the patient demonstrates difficulty with condition 2, in which vision is obscured but somatosensory and vestibular inputs are unaffected, the patient might have difficulty in low-light situations, such as going to the bathroom at night. If the patient demonstrates difficulty with condition 4, in which somatosensory input is distorted by the sway-referenced force plate, but visual and vestibular input are not affected, the patient may have difficulty walking on compliant surfaces, such as thick carpeting. Input may also be distorted by physiologic or body system issues that have little to do with the neurological medical diagnosis in CNS insults. Examples might be impaired vision from diabetes, cataracts, macular degeneration, or Ménière's disease, or decreased sensation as found in peripheral neuropathies. Computer-based equipment, such as the NeuroCom SMART EquiTest (Natus Medical Incorporated)[55] (Figure 6-14) and the Biodex Balance System (Biodex)[56] (Figure 6-15), can be used for examining and treating balance deficits and incorporate many of these factors into the programming.

The Clinical Test for Sensory Integration on Balance (CTSIB) was developed for use in the clinic and does not rely on computerized technology.[54] This test mimics the conditions of the Sensory Organization Test by using dense foam to replicate the movable force plate, a blindfold to obscure vision, and a modified Japanese lantern to replicate the movable surround (Figure 6-16). Note that research has not supported the use of the modified Japanese lantern as an adequate substitute for the sway-referenced, movable surround.

Further tests assess both static balance and dynamic balance. *Static balance* refers to the patient's ability to maintain an upright position. Although the word "static" is used to describe this component of balance, "quiet" may

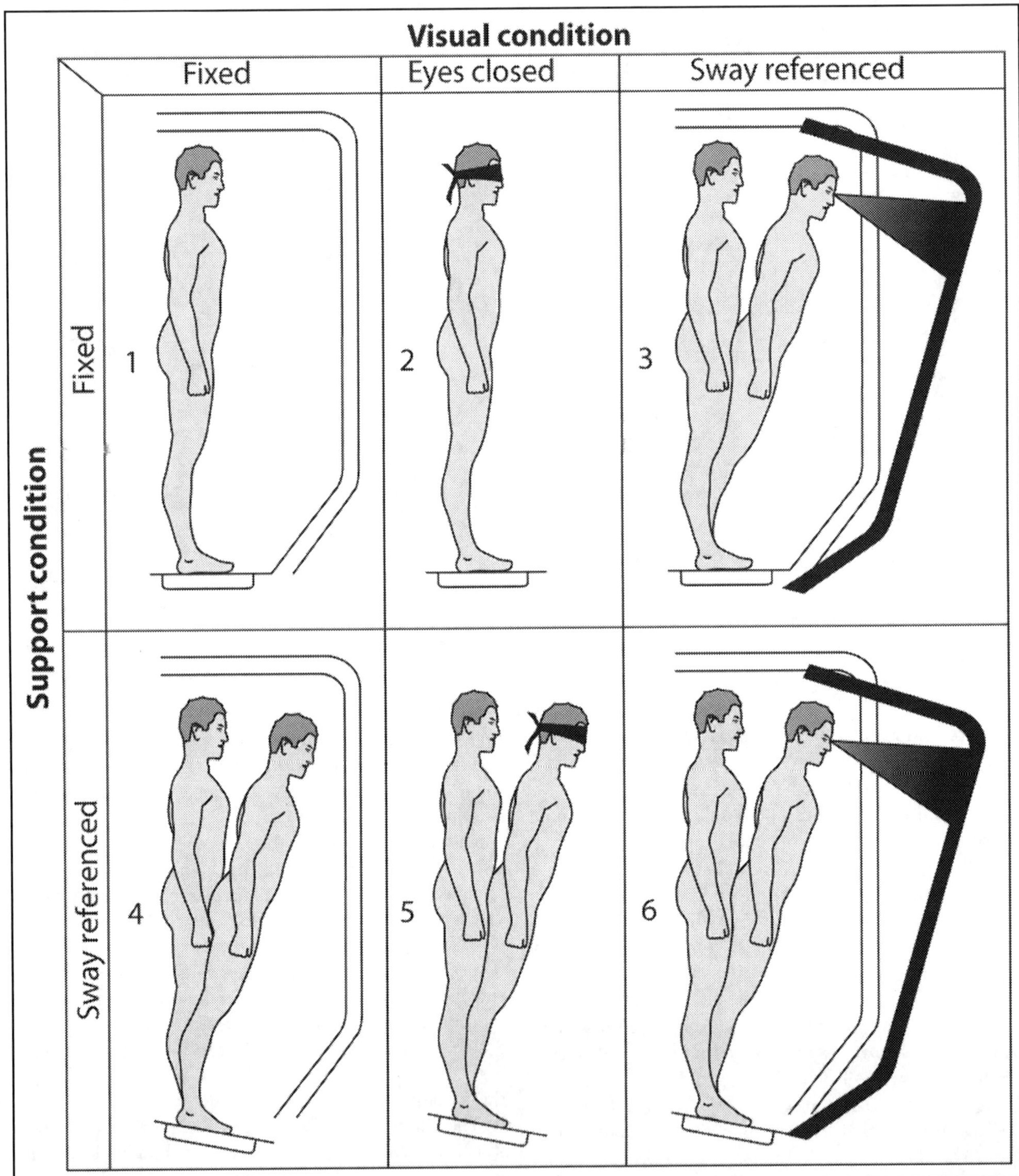

Figure 6-13. The 6 Sensory Organization Test conditions. The Sensory Organization Test determines the relative reliance on visual, vestibular, and somatosensory inputs for postural control using computerized dynamic posturography. (Adapted from Allison L, Fuller K. Balance and vestibular dysfunction. In: Umphred DA, Lazaro RT, Roller ML, Burton GU, eds. *Umphred's Neurological Rehabilitation*. 6th ed. St. Louis, MO: Elsevier; 2013: 658.)

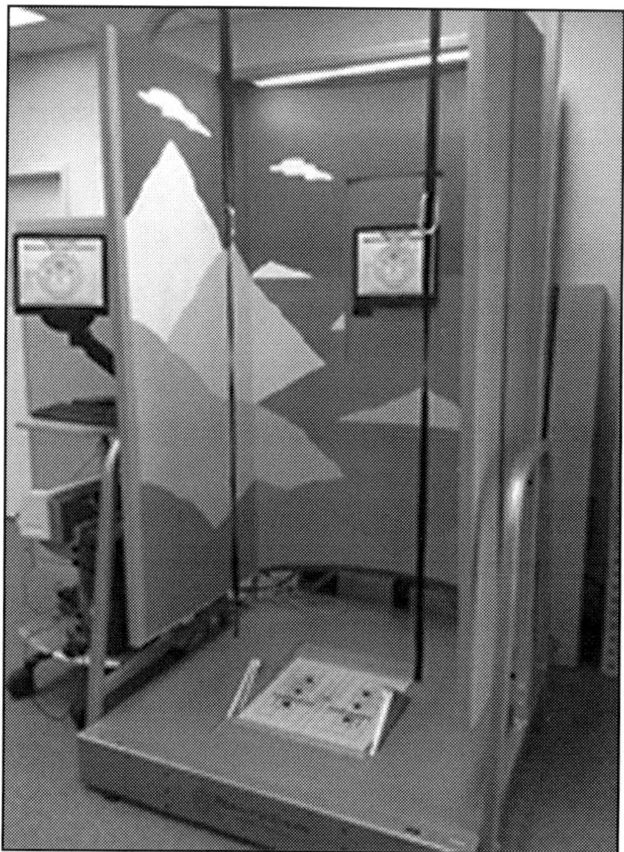

Figure 6-14. NeuroCom SMART EquiTest.

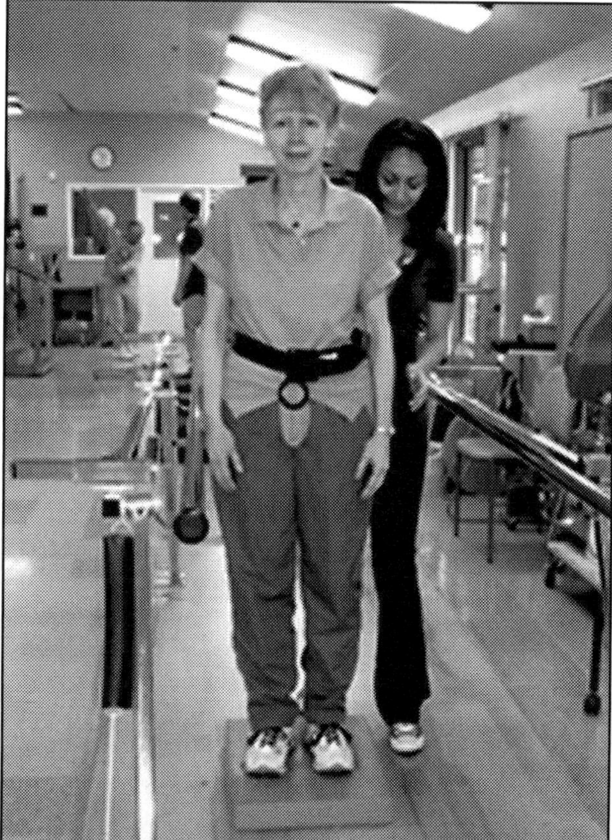

Figure 6-15. Biodex Balance System.

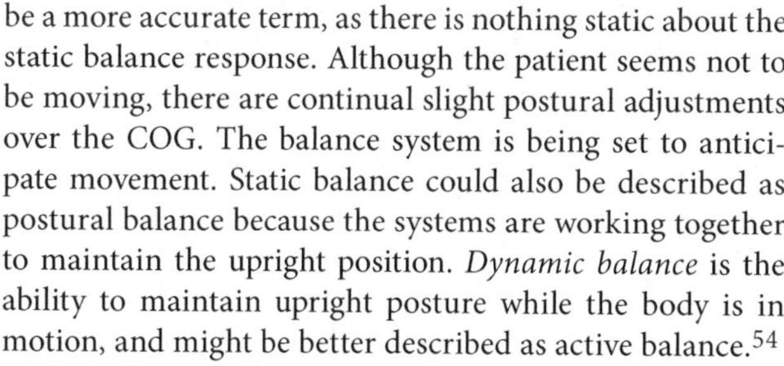

be a more accurate term, as there is nothing static about the static balance response. Although the patient seems not to be moving, there are continual slight postural adjustments over the COG. The balance system is being set to anticipate movement. Static balance could also be described as postural balance because the systems are working together to maintain the upright position. *Dynamic balance* is the ability to maintain upright posture while the body is in motion, and might be better described as active balance.[54]

Quiet (static) balance is tested by observing the patient's ability to maintain a sitting and standing position.[54] To test active (dynamic) balance, the patient's ability to maintain an upright position while moving the COG within or outside of the BOS is evaluated (Table 6-6). The Rehabilitation Measures Database provides a comprehensive collection of balance assessment instruments available in the public domain. The database can be accessed by visiting https://www.sralab.org/rehabilitation-measures.

Functional Activities

Functional activities refer to the client's ability to perform functional skills and activities of daily living. The therapist first identifies the functional activities that the patient is able and not able to do, hypothesizes the possible impairments causing the limitations, and then tests the body systems and subsystems to identify the nature and extent of the impairment. What can the patient do, and

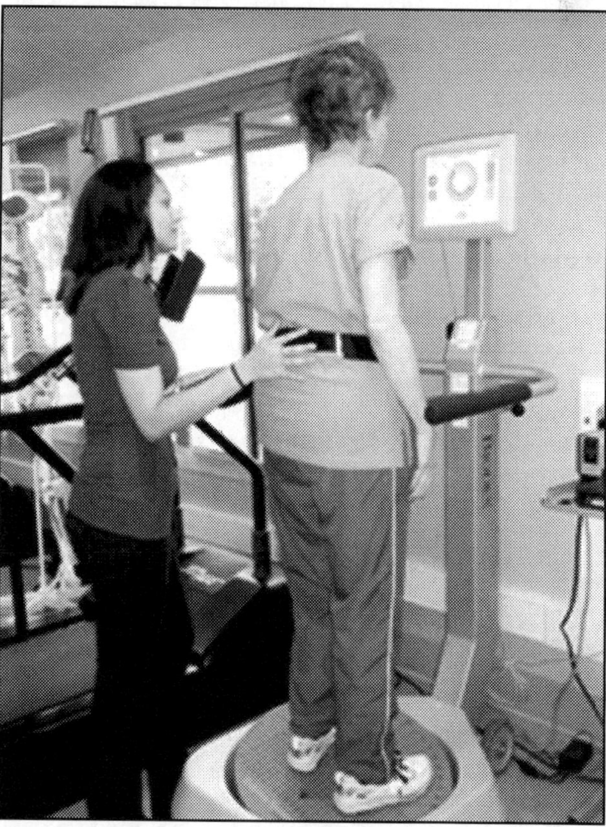

Figure 6-16. The Clinical Test for Sensory Integration on Balance using dense foam to mimic condition 4 of the Sensory Organization Test.

Table 6-6
Functional Balance Grades

Normal	• Quiet/Static: The patient maintains steady balance without hand-hold support. • Active/Dynamic: The patient accepts maximal challenge and easily shifts his or her weight (full ROM in all directions).
Good	• Quiet/Static: The patient maintains balance without hand-hold support, and there is limited postural sway. • Active/Dynamic: The patient accepts moderate challenge, and he or she maintains balance when picking up an item from the floor.
Fair	• Quiet/Static: The patient maintains balance with hand-hold support; however, he or she may need minimal assistance occasionally. • Active/Dynamic: The patient accepts minimal challenge, and he or she maintains balance when turning his or her head or trunk.
Poor	• Quiet/Static: The patient needs hand-hold support plus moderate to maximal assistance to maintain his or her position. • Active/Dynamic: The patient cannot accept challenge or move without losing his or her balance.

Adapted from O'Sullivan SB, Schmitz TJ. *Physical Rehabilitation: Assessment and Treatment.* 5th ed. Philadelphia, PA: FA Davis; 2007 and Allison LK, Fuller K. Balance and vestibular dysfunction. In: *Umphred's Neurological Rehabilitation.* 6th ed. St. Louis, MO: Elsevier; 2013.

how? What can the patient not do, and why? The approach is proactive and collaborative, capitalizing on the patient's potential and goals and promoting the therapist/patient partnership. It is important for the physical therapist or physical therapist assistant examining the patient's functional activity status to be receptive to the patient's view of these functional abilities. It is useful to initially examine tasks where the patient may fail, as this can demonstrate an unexpected ability for the patient to perform the task successfully. However, there is no need to examine a functional skill repeatedly if there is a high likelihood of failure for the patient. This is extremely important, because asking the patient to fail over and over is discouraging, decreases motivation to continue trying, and can create a negative treatment environment. On the other hand, when the physical therapist assistant has a patient who is confident in the ability to perform a task, it is important to let the patient realize the limitations. The patient's awareness of an inability to perform a task may act to motivate the patient's participation in physical therapy to work toward performing the task with less assistance and decreased risk of injury.

Multiple functional activities are assessed during the examination. These activities may include the patient's ability to roll, perform supine-to-sit, transfer (eg, to bed, chair, or car), perform sit-to-stand, and walk or propel a w/c. In pediatric patients, developmental positions such as prone on elbows, quadruped, kneeling, and half-kneeling are examined.[2]

Accurate documentation of patient functional ability must include the amount of assistance, if any, required to perform a skill or task, as well as the amount of time required for completion of that task. Table 6-7 lists the terminology derived from the Functional Independence Measure (FIM; Uniform Data System for Medical Rehabilitation)[57] describing assistance levels required by the patient. When selecting the appropriate descriptive term for the amount of assistance that the patient requires, the clinician must accurately assess the amount of effort put forth by the patient for the task, as opposed to the amount of effort put forth by the clinician.

Standardized tests provide an objective assessment of a patient's impairments or functional performance. Physical therapist assistants must understand the components of these tests as they execute and progress patient interventions. Components of the tests may be retested during interventions, revealing information regarding a patient's functional improvement and progression toward goals to be communicated to the patient and physical therapist. Many tests are available to the physical therapy community, and it is important for the physical therapist to identify those tests that are appropriate, valid, and reliable based on the patient's diagnosis and presentation. Examples of these tests are discussed next. Many of the tests discussed are available for personal use at the Rehabilitation Measures Database website.[57,58]

Standardized Impairment and Functional Tests

Berg Balance Scale

The Berg Balance Scale[59] measures static and dynamic balance abilities. The test takes 15 to 20 minutes to complete. It involves 14 tasks, including sitting-to-standing, standing unsupported, reaching forward with outstretched arm while standing, retrieving an object from the floor, and turning 360 degrees. The patient's ability to perform these tasks is given a score of 0, 1, 2, 3, or 4. The higher the score on a measure indicates greater independence. The

Table 6-7

Terminology and Definitions of Assistance Levels

Independent	Patient consistently performs the skill safely with no one present and in a timely manner. If an assistive device is needed, include the name of the device.
Supervision or Setup	Patient performs 100% of the task but requires verbal cueing, someone standing by, or someone must set up needed items.
Contact Guarding	Patient performs 100% of the task but person assisting gives full attention to patient and has hands on patient for possible assistance or possible loss of balance.
Minimal Assistance	Patient expends 75% or more of the effort for the task.
Moderate Assistance	Patient expends 50% to 75% of the effort for the task.
Maximum Assistance	Patient expends 25% to 50% of the effort for the task.
Dependent	Patient expends less than 25% of the effort for the task.

Adapted from Guide for the Uniform Data Set for Medical Rehabilitation. *(Including the Adult FIM Instrument).* Version 4.0. Buffalo, NY: State University of New York at Buffalo; 1993.

total possible score is 56. A score of less than 45 indicates an increased risk of falling. A modified version of the test includes only the advanced balance items (items 6 through 14) and is used for testing higher functioning individuals. (The video for Chapter 6 shows an individual performing the Berg Balance Scale.)

Functional Reach

The Functional Reach Test[60] was developed as a quick screening for balance deficits in older individuals. The Functional Reach Test measures a patient's ability to reach forward beyond arm's length while standing without falling and maintaining a fixed BOS. A Modified Functional Reach Test was developed for patients who are unable to stand and is performed sitting. Newton developed the Multidirectional Reach Test, which, in addition to forward reach, also examines the patient's ability to reach sideways and backward. Normative values are affected by age and height. This test takes approximately 5 minutes to complete.

Tinetti Performance Oriented Mobility Assessment

The Tinetti Performance Oriented Mobility Assessment test[61] was developed for use with an elderly population. The test is composed of 2 sections. The first section assesses balance and is composed of 9 items, including coming to standing, initial standing balance, and turning. The second section assesses gait and comprises 7 items, including initiating gait, step symmetry, and sway of trunk during gait. A score of 0 to 2 is used in most categories, with a maximum score of 16 for balance and 12 for gait, and a maximum combined score of 28. A score of less than 18 out of 28 indicates a high risk for falling. The test takes 10 to 15 minutes to complete.

Timed Up and Go

The Timed Up and Go (TUG)[62] measures the time it takes for an individual seated in a firm chair with arms and a back rest to stand up, walk 3 meters, turn around, and return to the chair. Cut-off scores indicating increased fall risk are available in Table 6-8.[63] The test typically takes 5 minutes or less to complete. Variations of the TUG include the addition of cognitive and motor challenges, which has been found to increase the time for completion of the TUG, but had no effect on the ability to predict fall risk. (The video for Chapter 6 shows an individual performing the TUG.)

Motor Assessment Scale

The Motor Assessment Scale[64] assesses motor recovery over time. The scale is composed of 8 items examining motor function (ie, supine-to-side-lying, supine-to-sit, sit-to-stand, balanced sitting, walking, upper-arm function, hand movements, and advanced hand function) and one item examining muscle tone. The items are scored on a scale of 0 to 10, with 0 indicating that the patient is unable to perform the task, and 6 indicating optimal performance. The item examining muscle tone is difficult to use because of a lack of concise criteria for scoring, and as a result, this item may be omitted.[65,66]

Barthel Index

The Barthel Index[67] assesses the amount of assistance needed by a patient. The scale is composed of 10 items (ie, feeding, bathing, personal toilet, dressing, bowel, bladder, toilet transfers, transfers to chair and bed, ambulation, and stair climbing). Each item is scored as 0, 5, 10, or 15, with 0 indicating that the patient is unable to perform the task, and higher scores, which vary from 5 to 15 depending on the item, indicating that the patient is independent. The total score will indicate the patient's dependence, level of care, and number of hours of assistance needed.

Functional Independence Measure

FIM[58,67] is used to supply data to the Uniform Data System for Medical Rehabilitation from participating facili-

Table 6-8

Timed Up and Go Cut-Off Scores

	Cut-Off Score(s)	*Sensitivity (% Fallers)*	*Specificity (% Nonfallers)*	*Overall Prediction*	*Predicted Probability*
TUG	≥ 13.5	80%	100%	90%	.77
***TUG**manual*	≥ 14.5	86.7%	93.3%	90%	.5
***TUG**cognitive*	≥ 15	80%	93.3%	86.7%	.5

Reprinted from Shumway-Cook A, Brauer S, Woollacott M. Predicting the probability for falls in community-dwelling older adults using the Timed Up and Go Test. *Phys Ther.* 2000;80(9):896-903 with permission from the American Physical Therapy Association.

ties. The data are used to develop summary reports for the facility. The FIM consists of 18 items in 3 domains that are examined at admission and discharge. Self-care examines the patient's ability in eating, grooming, bathing, dressing upper and lower extremities, and toileting. Sphincter control examines bladder and bowel control. The transfer section examines the patient's ability to perform bed/chair/w/c transfers and toilet/shower transfers. The locomotion section examines the patient's ability to walk or propel a w/c and manage stairs. The communication section examines the patient's comprehension and expression. Finally, the social comprehension section examines the patient's social interaction, problem-solving skills, and memory. The items are scored on a scale of 1 through 7, with 1 indicating total assistance or not testable, and 7 indicating complete independence. The FIM is a proprietary scale, and the examiner should be certified in the FIM System before entering the results into the medical record.

A version of this test, called the weeFIM, is available for use in the pediatric setting.

Participation

Participation in the International Classification of Function, Disability and Health terminology as developed by the World Health Organization is defined as an individual's involvement in a life situation.[68] Some examples of aspects of participation that can be examined for each individual include domestic life, interpersonal relationships, and community, social, and civic life. The term used to denote problems that individuals may experience in involvement in life situations is *participation restriction.* It is always important to obtain the patient's perception of how any medical conditions, impairments, and activity limitations affect involvement in life and community. Many of the tests for participation and self-efficacy available for the physical therapist to administer are in self-report format. Examples of tests used to collect data about participation are the Activities-Specific Balance Confidence Scale,[69] Short Form 36,[70] and Dizziness Handicap Confidence Inventory.[71]

Conclusion

The American Physical Therapy Association (APTA) has developed a model (Figure 6-17), based on a series of assumptions (Table 6-9), for supervision of the physical therapist assistant by the physical therapist.

After the initial examination, establishment of goals, and plan of care established by the physical therapist, the physical therapist assistant algorithm (see Figure 6-17) should help the physical therapist assistant determine progression within the plan of care, when a repeat of the initial tests and measures are needed, and/or when the patient's functional behavior needs to be discussed with the physical therapist. The physical therapist assistant needs to always remember that drawing conclusions from the tests and measures that change the plan of care is the responsibility of the physical therapist and should not be placed within the scope of work of the physical therapist assistant.

This chapter provides an overview of the physical therapy examination process initially performed by the physical therapist during the evaluation of the neurologically impaired patient, including the protocols for administration of more common tests and measures. The physical therapist assistant must understand the reasoning behind the examination and administered tools specific to the patient diagnosis and presentation. This knowledge, including the use of standard tests, assists the physical therapist assistant in contributing to the measurement of "the patient's progress with gait, locomotion, balance, and mobility."[72] The physical therapist assistant serves a key role in functioning as the clinician who, during patient encounters and administration of interventions, measures progress and adjusts interventions within the plan of care based on reexamination of the test and measure outcomes obtained during the initial physical therapist's evaluation. This information further enhances the decision-making process between the physical therapist and the physical therapist assistant, which allows for the optimal level of care and improved outcomes. As the physical therapist assistant's educational level increases and the roles and responsibilities change, examination skills and analytical reasoning will become an even more critical aspect of the responsibilities of the physical therapist assistant.

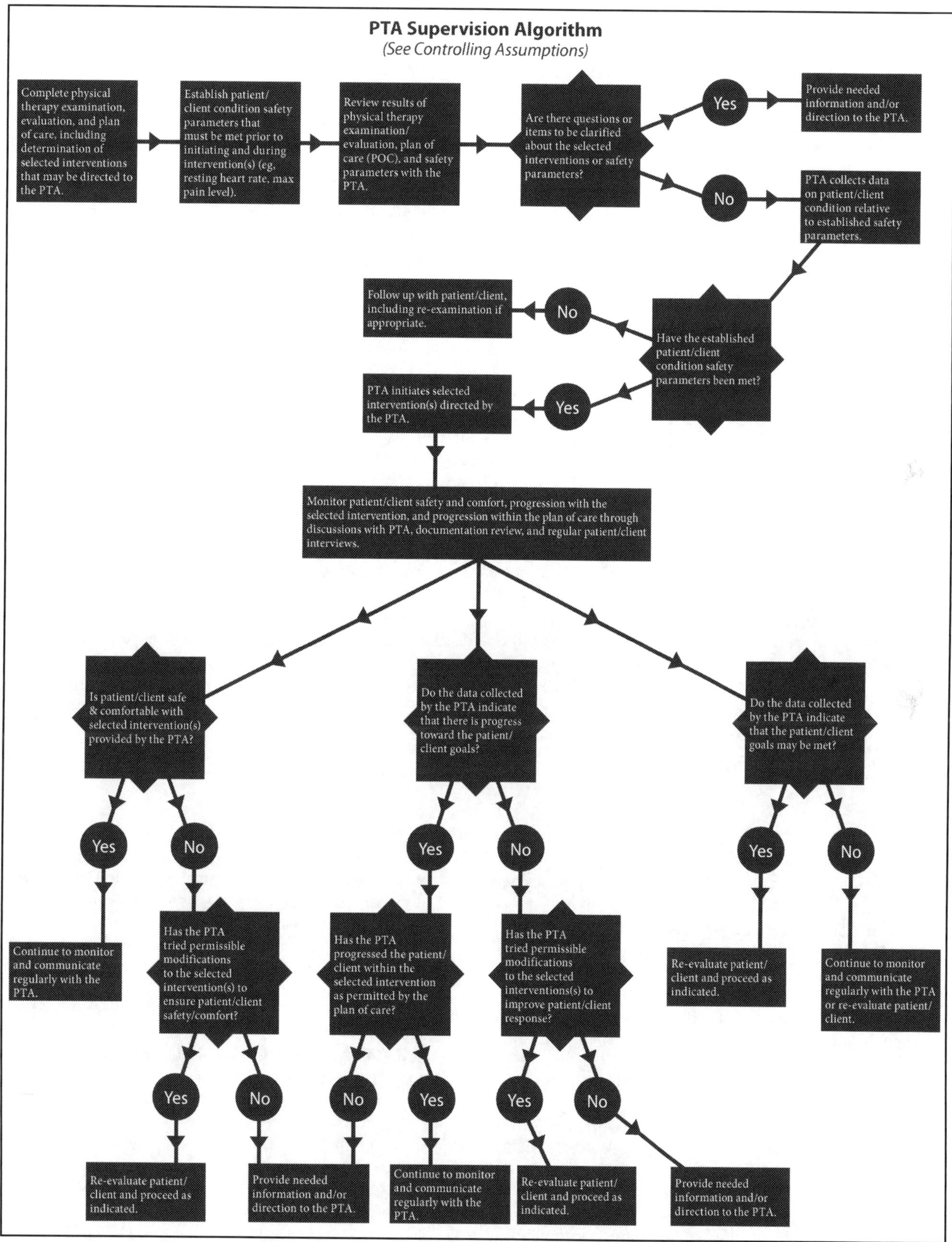

Figure 6-17. Physical therapist assistant supervision algorithm. (Reprinted from www.apta.org/PTinMotion/2010/9/PTAsToday, with permission of the American Physical Therapy Association. Copyright © 2010 American Physical Therapy Association.)

Table 6-9

Controlling Assumptions for Physical Therapist Assistant Supervision

• The physical therapist integrates the 5 elements of patient/client management—examination, evaluation, diagnosis, prognosis, and intervention—in a manner designed to optimize outcomes. Responsibility for completion of the examination, evaluation, diagnosis, and prognosis is borne solely by the physical therapist. The physical therapist's plan of care may involve the physical therapist assistant assisting with selected interventions.
• The physical therapist assistant has the knowledge, skills, and value-based behaviors needed to help the physical therapist provide selected interventions as described in the plan of care. Physical therapist assistants are clinical problem-solvers who ensure patient/client safety and comfort and complete interventions selected to achieve desired outcomes. Other than physical therapists, physical therapist assistants are the only valid providers of physical therapy services.
• The physical therapist directs and supervises the physical therapist assistant consistent with APTA House of Delegates positions, including Direction and Supervision of the Physical Therapist Assistant; APTA core documents, including Standards of Ethical Conduct for the Physical Therapist Assistant; federal and state legal practice standards; and institutional regulations.
• All selected interventions are directed and supervised by the physical therapist. The physical therapist assistant does not perform interventions that require immediate and continuous examination and evaluation throughout, as described in APTA House of Delegates position Procedural Interventions Exclusively Performed by Physical Therapists. Procedural interventions within the scope of physical therapy practice that are performed exclusively by the physical therapist include, but are not limited to, spinal and peripheral joint mobilization/manipulation (which are components of manual therapy) and sharp selective debridement (which is a component of wound management). The physical therapist is also responsible for ensuring the physical therapist assistant has the knowledge and skills required to safely and effectively complete the intervention.
• The physical therapist remains responsible for physical therapy services provided when the physical therapist's plan of care involves the physical therapist assistant assisting with selected interventions.
• Selected intervention(s) include the procedural intervention, associated data collection, and communication—including written documentation associated with the safe, effective, and efficient completion of the task.
• The algorithm may represent decision processes employed for either a patient/client interaction or an episode of care.
• Communication between the physical therapist and physical therapist assistant regarding patient/client care is ongoing. The algorithm does not intend to imply a limitation or restriction on communication between the physical therapist and physical therapist assistant.
Adapted from http://www.apta.org/SupervisionTeamwork/PTAProblemSolvingAlgorithm/. Accessed June 3, 2018.

References

1. *Guide to Physical Therapist Practice 3.0.* Alexandria, VA: American Physical Therapy Association; 2015.
2. Lazaro RT. Examination procedures. In: Umphred D, Carlson C, eds. *Neurorehabilitation for the Physical Therapist Assistant.* Thorofare, NJ: SLACK Incorporated; 2006.
3. Johns Hopkins Medicine. Vital Signs (Body Temperature, Pulse Rate, Respiration Rate, Blood Pressure). https://www.hopkinsmedicine.org/healthlibrary/conditions/cardiovascular_diseases/vital_signs_body_temperature_pulse_rate_respiration_rate_blood_pressure_85,P00866. Accessed January 25, 2018.
4. Schmitz T. Vital signs. In: O'Sullivan SB, Schmitz TJ, eds. *Physical Rehabilitation.* 6th ed. Philadelphia, PA: FA Davis; 2014.
5. Fairchild SL, O'Shea RK, Washington R. *Pierson and Fairchild's Principles & Techniques of Patient Care.* 6th ed. St. Louis, MO: Saunders; 2018.
6. PT Direct. Measuring Heart Rate. https://www.ptdirect.com/training-delivery/client-assessment/taking-heart-rate-measurements. Accessed January 25, 2018.
7. Ashley EA, Niebauer J. Cardiovascular Examination. In: *Cardiology Explained.* Remedica; 2004.
8. Kai T, Kuzumoto Y. Effects of a dual L/N-type calcium channel blocker cilnidipine on blood pressure, pulse rate, and autonomic functions in patients with mild to moderate hypertension. *Clin Exp Hypertens.* 2009;31(7):595-604. doi:10.3109/10641960902929453
9. Shugushev HH, Gurizeva MV, Vasileknko VM. Effect of bronchodilators on heart rate variability in patients with chronic obstructive pulmonary disease. *Rational Pharmacotherapy in Cardiology.* 2007;3(4):51-54. doi:10.20996/1819-6446-2007-3-4-51-54
10. Mayo Clinic. The most commonly prescribed type of antidepressant. https://www.mayoclinic.org/diseases-conditions/depression/in-depth/ssris/art-20044825?pg=2. Published September 17, 2019. Accessed January 29, 2018.
11. Cleveland Clinic. Vital Signs. https://my.clevelandclinic.org/health/articles/10881-vital-signs. Accessed January 29, 2018.
12. Walker J. Assessing respiratory rate and function in the community. *J Community Nurs.* 2016;30(5):50-54.
13. American College of Sports Medicine. *ACSM's Guidelines for Exercise Testing and Prescription.* 9th ed. Philadelphia, PA: Wolters Kluwer Health/Lippincott, Williams and Wilkins; 2014.

14. American College of Cardiology. New ACC/AHA High Blood Pressure Guidelines Lower Definition of Hypertension. http://www.acc.org/latest-in-cardiology/articles/2017/11/08/11/47/mon-5pm-bp-guideline-aha-2017. Published November 13, 2017. Accessed January 29, 2018.
15. McCallum L, Higgins D. Measuring body temperature. *Nurs Times.* 2012;108(45):20-22.
16. Pocock G, Richards CD, Richards DA. *Human Physiology.* 5th ed. Oxford, England: Oxford University Press; 2017.
17. Marieb EN, Hoehn K. *Human Anatomy & Physiology.* 10th ed. New York, NY: Pearson; 2016.
18. Commission on Accreditation in Physical Therapy Education. PTA Standards & Required Elements. http://www.capteonline.org/uploadedFiles/CAPTEorg/About_CAPTE/Resources/Accreditation_Handbook/CAPTE_PTAStandardsEvidence.pdf. Accessed January 25, 2018.
19. Williamson A, Hoggart B. Pain: a review of three commonly used pain rating scales. *J Clin Nurs.* 2005;14(7):798-804. doi:10.1111/j.1365-2702.2005.01121.x
20. Scherder EJ, Bouma A. Visual analogue scales for pain assessment in Alzheimer's disease. *Gerontology.* 2000;46(1):47-53. doi:10.1159/000022133
21. Melzack R. The McGill Pain Questionnaire: major properties and scoring methods. *Pain.* 1975;1(3):277-299. doi:10.1016/0304-3959(75)90044-5
22. Wong D, Baker C. Wong-Baker FACES Pain Rating Scale. http://www.wongbakerfaces.org/. Accessed January 25, 2018. doi:10.1037/t05330-000
23. Feldt KS. The checklist of nonverbal pain indicators (CNPI). *Pain Manag Nurs.* 2000;1(1):13-21. doi:10.1053/jpmn.2000.5831
24. Warden V, Hurley AC, Volicer L. Development and psychometric evaluation of the Pain Assessment in Advanced Dementia (PAINAD) scale. *J Am Med Dir Assoc.* 2003;4(1):9-15. doi:10.1097/01.JAM.0000043422.31640.F7
25. Srouji R, Ratnapalan S, Schneeweiss S. Pain in children: assessment and nonpharmacological management. *Int J Pediatr.* 2010;2010:474838. doi:10.1155/2010/474838
26. O'Sullivan SB. Examination of motor function: motor control and motor learning. In: O'Sullivan SB, Schmitz TJ, eds. *Physical Rehabilitation.* 6th ed. Philadelphia, PA: FA Davis; 2014.
27. Folstein MF, Folstein SE, McHugh PR. "Mini-mental state". A practical method for grading the cognitive state of patients for the clinician. *J Psychiatr Res.* 1975;12(3):189-198. doi:10.1016/0022-3956(75)90026-6
28. Mini-Mental State Examination Second Edition: MMSE-2. http://www4.parinc.com/Products/Product.aspx?ProductID=MMSE-2. Accessed January 31, 2018.
29. Cullen B, O'Neill B, Evans JJ, Coen RF, Lawlor BA. A review of screening tests for cognitive impairment. *J Neurol Neurosurg Psychiatry.* 2007;78(8):790-799. doi:10.1136/jnnp.2006.095414
30. Bigley GK. Sensation. In: Walker HK, Hall WD, Hurst JW, eds. *Clinical Methods: The History, Physical, and Laboratory Examinations.* 3rd ed. Boston, MA: Butterworths; 1990.
31. Bhattacharya S, Mishra RK. Pressure ulcers: current understanding and newer modalities of treatment. *Indian J Plast Surg.* 2015;48(1):4-16. doi:10.4103/0970-0358.155260
32. Schmitz TJ. Examination of sensory function. In: O'Sullivan SB, Schmitz TJ, eds. *Physical Rehabilitation.* 6th ed. Philadelphia, PA: FA Davis; 2014.
33. Lundy-Ekman L. *Neuroscience: Fundamentals for Rehabilitation.* 4th ed. St. Louis, MO: Saunders; 2013.
34. Shirley Ryan AbilityLab. Nottingham Assessment of Somato-Sensations. https://www.sralab.org/rehabilitation-measures/nottingham-assessment-somato-sensations. Accessed January 29, 2018.
35. Reese NB. *Muscle and Sensory Testing.* 3rd ed. St. Louis, MO: Saunders; 2012.
36. Gilman S, Newman SW. *Manter and Gatz's Essentials of Clinical Neuroanatomy and Neurophysiology.* 10th ed. Philadelphia, PA: FA Davis; 2003.
37. Haugh AB, Pandyan AD, Johnson GR. A systematic review of the Tardieu Scale for the measurement of spasticity. *Disabil Rehabil.* 2006;28(15):899-907. doi:10.1080/09638280500404305
38. Bohannon RW, Smith MB. Interrater reliability of a modified Ashworth scale of muscle spasticity. *Phys Ther.* 1987;67(2):206-207. doi:10.1093/ptj/67.2.206
39. Hislop HJ, Montgomery J. *Daniels and Worthingham's Muscle Testing: Techniques of Manual Examination.* 9th ed. Philadelphia, PA: WB Saunders; 2013.
40. Kendall FP, McCreary EK, Provance PG, Rodgers MM, Romani WA. *Muscles: Testing and Function, with Posture and Pain.* 5th ed. Philadelphia, PA: Lippincott Williams & Wilkins; 2005.
41. White DJ. Musculoskeletal examination. In: O'Sullivan SB, Schmitz TJ, eds. *Physical Rehabilitation.* 6th ed. Philadelphia, PA: FA Davis; 2014.
42. Clark R, Locke M, Hill B, Wells C, Bialocerkowski A. Clinimetric properties of lower limb neurological impairment tests for children and young people with a neurological condition: A systematic review. *PLoS One.* 2017;12(7):e0180031. doi:10.1371/journal.pone.0180031
43. Lescher PL. *Pathology for the Physical Therapist Assistant.* Philadelphia, PA: FA Davis; 2011.
44. Posner JB, Saper CB, Schiff N, Plum F. *Plum and Posner's Diagnosis of Stupor and Coma.* New York, NY: Oxford University Press; 2007.
45. Campbell WW, DeJong RN. *DeJong's The Neurologic Examination.* 7th ed. Philadelphia, PA: Lippincott Williams & Wilkins; 2013.
46. Lippert LS. *Clinical Kinesiology and Anatomy (Clinical Kinesiology for Physical Therapist Assistants).* 6th ed. Philadelphia, PA: FA Davis; 2017.
47. Gladstone DJ, Danells CJ, Black SE. The fugl-meyer assessment of motor recovery after stroke: a critical review of its measurement properties. *Neurorehabil Neural Repair.* 2002;16(3):232-240. doi:10.1177/154596802401105171
48. Martin ST, Kessler M. *Neurologic Interventions for Physical Therapy.* 3rd ed. St. Louis, MO: Saunders; 2016.
49. Zafeiriou DI. Primitive reflexes and postural reactions in the neurodevelopmental examination. *Pediatr Neurol.* 2004;31(1):1-8. doi:10.1016/j.pediatrneurol.2004.01.012
50. Shumway-Cook A, Woollacott MH. *Motor Control: Translating Research into Clinical Practice.* 5th ed. Philadelphia, PA: Wolters Kluwer; 2017.
51. Graybiel A, Fregly AR. A new quantitative ataxia test battery. *Acta Otolaryngol.* 1966;61(4):292-312. doi:10.3109/00016486609127066
52. Center of gravity. http://www.yourdictionary.com/center-of-gravity. Accessed January 6, 2013.

53. Ryerson SD. Movement dysfunction associated with hemiplegia. In: *Umphred's Neurological Rehabilitation*. 6th ed. St. Louis, MO: Elsevier; 2013. doi:10.1016/B978-0-323-07586-2.00032-7
54. Allison LK, Fuller K. Balance and vestibular dysfunction. In: *Umphred's Neurological Rehabilitation*. 6th ed. St. Louis, MO: Elsevier; 2013. doi:10.1016/B978-0-323-07586-2.00031-5
55. Natus Medical Incorporation. NeuroCom Balance Master Systems. http://www.natus.com/index.cfm?page=products_1&crid=271&contentid=397. Accessed January 25, 2018.
56. Biodex. Physical Medicine and Rehabilitation, Nuclear Medicine Supplies and Accessories, Medical Imaging Tables and Accessories. http://www.biodex.com/. Accessed January 25, 2018.
57. *Guide for the Uniform Data Set for Medical Rehabilitation. (Including the Adult FIM Instrument)*. Version 4.0. Buffalo, NY: State University of New York at Buffalo; 1993.
58. Shirley Ryan AbilityLab. Rehabilitation Measures. https://www.sralab.org/rehabilitation-measures. Accessed January 25, 2018.
59. Berg K, Wood-Dauphinee S, Williams JI, Gayton D. Measuring balance in the elderly: preliminary development of an instrument. *Physiother Can*. 1989;41(6):304-311. doi:10.3138/ptc.41.6.304
60. Duncan PW, Weiner DK, Chandler J, Studenski S. Functional reach: a new clinical measure of balance. *J Gerontol*. 1990;45(6):M192-M197. doi:10.1093/geronj/45.6.M192
61. Tinetti ME. Performance-oriented assessment of mobility problems in elderly patients. *J Am Geriatr Soc*. 1986;34(2):119-126. doi:10.1111/j.1532-5415.1986.tb05480.x
62. Podsiadlo D, Richardson S. The timed "Up & Go": a test of basic functional mobility for frail elderly persons. *J Am Geriatr Soc*. 1991;39(2):142-148. doi:10.1111/j.1532-5415.1991.tb01616.x
63. Shumway-Cook A, Brauer S, Woollacott M. Predicting the probability for falls in community-dwelling older adults using the Timed Up & Go Test. *Phys Ther*. 2000;80(9):896-903. doi:10.1093/ptj/80.9.896
64. Carr JH, Shepherd RB, Nordholm L, Lynne D. Investigation of a new motor assessment scale for stroke patients. *Phys Ther*. 1985;65(2):175-180. doi:10.1093/ptj/65.2.175
65. Loewen SC, Anderson BA. Predictors of stroke outcome using objective measurement scales. *Stroke*. 1990;21(1):78-81. doi:10.1161/01.STR.21.1.78
66. Malouin F, Pichard L, Bonneau C, Durand A, Corriveau D. Evaluating motor recovery early after stroke: comparison of the Fugl-Meyer Assessment and the Motor Assessment Scale. *Arch Phys Med Rehabil*. 1994;75(11):1206-1212. doi:10.1016/0003-9993(94)90006-X
67. Guccione AA, Scalzitti DA. Examination of functional status and activity level. In: O'Sullivan SB, Schmitz TJ, eds. *Physical Rehabilitation*. 6th ed. Philadelphia, PA: FA Davis; 2014.
68. Lazaro RT, Roller ML, Umphred DA. Differential diagnosis phase 2: examination and evaluation of functional movement activities, body functions and structures, and participation. In: *Umphred's Neurological Rehabilitation*. 6th ed. St. Louis, MO: Elsevier; 2013. doi:10.1016/B978-0-323-07586-2.00017-0
69. Powell LE, Myers AM. The Activities-specific Balance Confidence (ABC) Scale. *J Gerontol A Biol Sci Med Sci*. 1995;50A(1):M28-M34. doi:10.1093/gerona/50A.1.M28
70. Anderson C, Laubscher S, Burns R. Validation of the Short Form 36 (SF-36) health survey questionnaire among stroke patients. *Stroke*. 1996;27(10):1812-1816. doi:10.1161/01.STR.27.10.1812
71. Jacobson GP, Newman CW. The development of the Dizziness Handicap Inventory. *Arch Otolaryngol Head Neck Surg*. 1990;116(4):424-427. doi:10.1001/archotol.1990.01870040046011
72. American Physical Therapy Association. Minimum required skills of physical therapist assistant graduates at entry-level. http://www.apta.org/uploadedFiles/APTAorg/About_Us/Policies/BOD/Education/MinReqSkillsPTAGrad.pdf#search=%22minimum%20required%20skills%20physical%20therapist%20assistant%22. Accessed January 25, 2018.

Chapter 7

Psychosocial and Cognitive Issues Affecting Therapy

Elizabeth Ching, OTD, MEd, BSOT, OTR/L and Gordon U. Burton, OTR/L, PhD

KEY WORDS Adjustment | Anger | Anxiety | Denial | Depression | Disengagement | Engagement | Hope | Hostility | Shock | Spirituality

Chapter Objectives

- Identify the 6 stages of adjustment.
- Discuss the difference between engagement and disengagement.
- Realize that all people, not just clients, are in a state of adjustment.
- Recognize that each client is unique and needs to have individualized treatment.

This chapter discusses the role of psychosocial and cognitive factors that may affect the rehabilitation management of patients and clients with movement disorders secondary to neuromuscular dysfunctions. As we focus on evidence-based practice, it is important to remember that the client's values and preferences and important aspects of an evidence-based practice. Cognitive and psychosocial factors may have a significant influence on the clients' progress (or lack thereof) in rehabilitation and should always be considered to achieve optimal outcomes. Why do any of us do the things we do? Why do we get up and go through the trials and tribulations that we experience each day? How do we deal with our bodies changing year to year? How do we deal with the fact that we will all die someday? How do we deal with all the changes in our lives? How do we deal with changes in our activity and participation in life? How do we deal when confronted with disease and pathology, whether it be ourselves, our family, or our clients?

These are some of the questions that clients may be dealing with on a daily basis, but with a bit of a different slant. We are all trying to discover our unique purposes and how we are to identify and play roles that match this uniqueness that results in our attainment of the highest quality in life possible. Just like therapists, clients try to adjust to life. Clients have challenges; some of the challenges are unexpected, and some are challenges for which they are not prepared. Most of us do not think about having an accident and severing our spinal cord, losing some of our brain functions, developing a tumor, or all of the above, but when it happens to us, we have to deal with its reality. In this chapter, "dealing with it" will be called *adjusting* or *adapting* to a disability. Some people adjust or adapt well, while others do not, although most people adjust well enough to get by in society. In this chapter, we will discuss some of the highlights of this process, what it means to therapy, and your role as the physical therapist assistant clinician in the process.

Adjustment is an ongoing process. We are not suddenly adjusted to something. Adjustment is a fluid process that does not flow in just one direction. Family and loved ones often do not go through this process at the same speed or in the same way. Thus, the therapist must always be aware of where each client and each support person is at all times within this adjustment process to create the best environment and to provide the best intervention. The physical

Lazaro RT, Umphred DA, eds.
Umphred's Neurorehabilitation for the Physical Therapist Assistant, Third Edition (pp 155-165).

therapist assistant's role is to make the therapy process progress as smoothly and efficiently as possible.

Each day, you must adjust to successes, failures, accomplishments, and inadequacies. Some are consistent failures, while others are consistent accomplishments. A client is no different. Adjustment and adaptation are how you get through life. We all have limitations to which we must adjust—you may never be that celebrity that you would like to be—but we will adjust, adapt, and move on with the process of living and aging. You may have had friends that never did adjust to not being what they wanted to be and are now angry or dysfunctional because of it. If we do not adapt, we become dysfunctional even if we have more life or therapeutic skill potential than others around us do. This may explain why some successful people in high school did not stay successful later in life. They did not adapt to changing life demands.

Some of the keys to facilitating adaptation in the client are to know how that client is unique and to learn each client's adaptation process. Do not try to make each client the same as every other client, and do not force your ways of coping on them. Two case studies in this chapter will help the reader develop both sensitivity to and the cognitive understanding of this adjustment process and how it changes as the client goes through life. One case involves a person who is growing up with a disability, and the other involves a person who acquired the disability after reaching adulthood.

In this chapter, Elena is a client who was born with cerebral palsy. She has had to adjust to being "different" all her life, and her "different" is normal for her, so it is within defined limits.[1] She has had to adjust to a society that often does not identify a role for her or has either a negative or an overly positive role that her medical diagnosis has forced on her. Elena can be emotionally damaged by either overly positive or overly negative stereotypes. An example of how an overly positive stereotype may cause problems is when a person is told he or she must give to society because of a gift of great intelligence. The person may have no need to be overly productive and is criticized or rejected because this potential is not being actualized to society's satisfaction. A negative stereotype may have the same damaging effect by limiting concepts of what could be accomplished, thus preventing individuals from growing and adapting to "be all that they could be."

Elena must find her place and use her talents to accomplish what she would like to in life. This goal is difficult for every individual to accomplish, but for a client such as Elena, it may be even more difficult because she will have some perceived and real motor limitations that may prevent her from accomplishing this goal. Elena may have impairments in her upper and lower limbs resulting in activity limitations, even with the best therapy. She has to find ways to accommodate for these limitations to prevent them from hampering her love of life. Elena needs to learn how to deal with others and to deal with her physical body in a way that will allow her to adapt to what is needed physically, emotionally, and spiritually. Elena's case study is mentioned throughout this chapter to apply components of adjustment and adaptation to her life process.

The second case study used in this chapter involves a young adult male, Kai. Kai acquired a spinal cord injury (SCI) in his 20s. Following the traumatic injury, he is adapting his goals and dreams to fit with his new capabilities and limitations. A therapist must always be aware of the attitudes of clients toward life activities preceding and following an injury. This event is not all negative, because Kai was not goal-directed or focused before the accident. In that respect, Kai may benefit from the structure and guidance he will receive as part of this rehabilitation. He now must deal with the stereotypes and prejudices of others, as well as some of the stereotypes and prejudices that he had regarding individuals he considered disabled before he was injured. He will have to discard some of his old goals or ways of dealing with life activities and challenges but will have an opportunity to focus on what he values as important. This focus can lead to a better life for Kai. Some clients have said that they did not like who they were before their accident or where they were going with their lives, and that the disability was a "Godsend" to them. (It should be noted that these words were never spoken from a client with a new acute injury, but from clients years after their injury.) Similarly, clients have communicated that "I had 10,000 opportunities before my injury and I only have 5,000 now, but in either case, I could only accomplish 1,000 of them."

Roles are the patterns of operating that we go through each day without even thinking. They are how people go through most of life. There are roles for a child, a spouse or partner, a worker, a student, or any other stage or component of life. These roles allow adults to respond as if they were still children interacting with parents. Roles allow each of us to function as a sibling in one situation and a parent in another. Individuals are not aware of these roles, but these roles control individual behavior unless each person thinks about those behaviors and decides to change them. Roles are useful because, as individuals, none of us have the time or energy to treat each situation as a new and novel one. In the case of a new impairments, activity limitations, and the restrictions to participating in life activities that we valued before the injury or disease, all our roles must be rethought and reexamined. This process takes time, energy, and a lot of emotional turmoil. Often, the person cannot define the problem.

In the case of a person with an early or congenital impairments and activity limitations, as in our case study of Elena, that person must reexamine the current roles and beliefs in light of changes in function following therapy, deterioration of movement function following a surgery, or simply because role expectations were unrealistic in the first place. With an acquired disability, such as in the case study of Kai, the person is forced to reexamine all standard roles and change them where appropriate. He not only has to face impairments that affect his performance of activities, but he is also forced to deal with complex and primarily social phenomena. If individuals do not yet know their own new abilities and limitations, they may have challenges finding and developing appropriate new roles. The physical therapist assistant must be aware of how hard it is for Kai and Elena to reexamine all that they hold as true and, at the same time, deal with the cognitive and physical demands of the medical system and rehabilitation. If Elena were improving in therapy, she might wonder why this therapy was not offered earlier, and wonder how many ways her life would have been improved if this had happened when she was younger. She might also feel threatened by her newfound abilities, since she may have always used the lack of these abilities as a reason for not engaging in other threatening activities or roles (eg, dating, interacting socially with friends, or assuming gainful employment).

Kai may be experiencing similar emotional reactions as Elena, but from another perspective. He may feel that all his abilities are slipping away. He may feel that all he has sacrificed for or delayed gratification for has been wasted. Individuals who have delayed having sex may feel that, following an accident such as a spinal injury, they will never know this aspect of life and feel angry about this great loss. Kai may need help in the redirection of his life roles and goals.

Performance is the main goal of therapy and is the main way that a person demonstrates capability. When performance or participation is impaired, the person may be threatened emotionally. When emotionally threatened, performance may be impaired. This is why it is important for the physical therapist and physical therapist assistant to always be aware of the client and the client's support system's unique perspectives on the ramifications of the functional loss and the body systems creating that loss. The emotional system can assist or hinder therapy. Interaction with the staff may be the key to facilitating the client's growth and development with regard to emotional stability and security. The following are some key points for the reader to keep in mind.

Growth and Adaptation

The therapist must keep in mind the context from which the client is coming. The client may have been walking around with no major problems just a few days ago, and has now suddenly entered the physical therapy setting. The trauma may be multifaceted: the physical trauma that may have occurred to the client, the emotional trauma occurring to the client and the client's support system, and the trauma of each of these bodily systems trying to protect the others. The interaction of these multifaceted components with one's life may lead to post-traumatic stress syndrome. This syndrome usually occurs within the first 6 months following the injury. This syndrome is observed more often in women,[2-4] but because of cultural barriers, can be hidden with men. The client may blame others, try to protect others, or be so self-absorbed that little else in the world is seen or heard. It may be helpful to get psychological aid for the client early in therapy if this syndrome is preventing optimal outcomes or creating obstacles in therapy.[5-9]

It is the physical therapist assistant's job to develop a trusting relationship with the client. Through this relationship, the client can be supported to focus on the goals of therapy and work on a positive perspective. Some facilities consider clients' past histories of trauma and use a trauma-informed care approach to assist clients overcome challenges to successful health outcomes.[10] One error of the medical system is focusing on the disability and pathology, and not on the person and the positive capabilities still within the client's grasp.[11] This focus on the negative may cause the client to see only the injury, disease, or pathology and nothing else. In a US Department of Veterans Affairs hospital, spouses of people with SCIs formed a group focusing on why the partners were married in the first place, and never looked at the disability as disabling. After a short while, people concluded that they did not marry their spouses for their legs, and the fact that the legs no longer worked was not a major issue after all. This started the decentering from the medical disability model, and the focus began being placed on the people and their future, which is the International Classification of Functioning, Disability and Health[12] model today. If we can help clients focus on their function and not their dysfunction, which is a goal of cognitive behavioral therapy,[13] the effect of therapy following treatment will be much better. More work needs to be performed to help clients realize their existing potential and to live their lives with the highest quality.[14-20]

Focusing on how to live, move, and function is one of the keys to helping the client and the family work toward the future.[21,22] The physical therapist assistant, under the direction of the physical therapist, must help the client focus on the direction of treatment objectives and demonstrate how therapy translates into meeting the client's goals.[11] To discover the client's true goals, the therapist must gain the trust of the client and establish sound lines of communication. Distrusting health professionals may obstruct the adjustment process and lead to negative consequences.[23-26] Whenever possible, the client's support system should be enlisted to help establish realistic support for the client and establish goals. It has been found that if the client trusts the health professional, the client will be more adherent and will seek assistance when it is needed.[27,28]

In the case of Elena, the physical therapist and physical therapist assistant may work with Elena and her family to see what goals would be realistic and within the domain of physical therapy. In the case of Kai, the goals may include the accomplishment of previous goals, if they are realistic, or may involve modifying his previous goals with adaptations. This is an issue in therapy for many reasons, but most crucially, when people feel unworthy or disempowered, they tend to perform poorly and have problems with adherence. This reaction may slow or stop the progress of therapy. Helping the client adapt to the new body will help achieve the goals in therapy. Helping clients realize what they can accomplish, and empowering them with the concept that they can find a way around many barriers and negative situations, will be a critical aspect of every therapeutic intervention.

Body Image

Body image is an all-encompassing concept that involves how the person and, to some extent, the support system, views the person, and roles that are expected to be assumed by that person. Many clients experience negative feelings about their bodies and generally negative psychological experiences after injury.[29-32] Even when clients do not have readily observable disfigurements, they often still report changes in body image and negative feelings of self-worth. One issue that may arise relating to body image is sexuality. This concept may take many behavioral forms: flirting, harassment, questions about fertility, or questions regarding whether the client is capable of performing the sex act at all. Flirting may be a sign that clients have had an assault on their sexuality. By flirting, clients are often trying to determine if they are still seen as a sensual being. In this case, a physical therapist assistant may establish therapeutic boundaries gently by explaining that dating or flirting with clients is not allowed. This is to ensure that clients do not think that the refusal is about their body system problems, functional limitations, and inability to participate. Sensitivity should be used, because a client could think, "If a health professional finds me repulsive, then no one will ever see me as attractive." It is important for the therapist to try to ascertain the intent behind the behavior. Usually, this can be accomplished by evaluating feelings about the interaction. It is not within the scope of a physical therapist assistant's duties to determine the stage of adjustment that may be directing client behavior. However, it is within the scope of a physical therapist assistant's duties to develop caring sensitivity and be able to report to the physical therapist or other health care professionals what has been observed in the client's behavior. If you, as the physical therapist assistant, do not feel threatened or demeaned when the client is flirting, you still must report this to the physical therapist to record. If you feel defensive, demeaned, or very uncomfortable, then you may be experiencing harassment. A clinician should never be harassed on the job, and this client's behavior should be stopped immediately; a physical therapist assistant must tell the client that the behavior is making him or her feel uncomfortable, and that it should stop now. Again, a therapist should mention this behavior to the supervisor and/or team. If the staff considers the behavior chronic, a treatment plan should be designed to stop this behavior. This plan is not the responsibility of the physical therapist assistant, but carrying out appropriate responsive behaviors to the patient's inappropriate actions is within that scope. It is important, however, to remember that sexual health should not be a neglected area of client treatment. It may take time for the client to ask the appropriate questions.[33,34]

Questions about any physical performance are within the domain of physical therapy. If the client is asking for information regarding positioning during sex, then this may be brought to the attention of a therapist. If the questions are regarding fertility, these should also be referred to an appropriate health professional. None of these questions should be discouraged or neglected, because this area is important for the client's motivation and sexual health.[35-39] It is important for the physical therapist assistant to know that in SCI, fertility will generally not be impaired for women and non-binary people,[40] but issues of lubrication before sex should be addressed by the appropriate person. Men and non-binary people may have erection problems and ejaculation issues, but this can also be addressed by the appropriate person. It is now thought that male and non-binary fertility issues resulting from an SCI may be dealt with and should not be ignored.[41-45]

Elena may need to work on body image problems that have resulted from the misperceptions she gained from other people and the media. She may also have learned not to enjoy her body and to deny positive sensations because she has been clinically touched most of her life without regard to her need for privacy.

Kai, on the other hand, may need to talk to other people who have been disabled for a while to explore acquired misconceptions and negative stereotypes regarding the impact of disabilities and, specifically, his functional limitations. He may also benefit from practical information that people with similar medical diagnoses can provide.

Family and Client Adjustment

The role of the family must never be forgotten. Partner relationships have been found to be negatively affected by a member being disabled in conditions such as pediatric SCI and other disabilities,[46-49] but is being questioned in conditions such as adult-onset SCI.[50] It has been shown that adjustment and quality of life can be adversely affected by an inadequate physical environment, thus making the person more dependent, which can result in poor relationships.[46-55] This can also be seen with the families in which a member has had a brain injury.[56] In studies on muscular dystrophy, it was found that physical dependence is not the only variable that needs to be considered; psychological issues need to be identified and considered as part of intervention.[57,58] According to Turner and Cox, the client and the family need help to work on a number of elements: "to develop new views of vulnerability and strength, make changes in relationships, and facilitate philosophical, physical and spiritual growth."[58] Turner and Cox also felt that the medical staff could facilitate the following: "recognizing the worth of each individual, helping them to envision a future that is full of promise and potential, actively involving each person in their own care trajectory, and celebrating changes to each person's sense of self."[58] Man observed that each family copes differently in relation to a family member with a brain injury, and that the family's structure should be explored to develop intervention guidelines.[59] It has also been noted that health care professionals should view the situation from the family's perspective to approach and support the family's adaptation.[60] This should be performed to help the client and the family accept the disability but, at the same time, to help them keep the negative views of society in perspective.[61] In general, it has also been found that family support is a significant factor in the client's subjective functioning,[62] and that social engagement is productive.[63]

When dealing with children, it is important to realize that they often feel responsible for almost anything that happens in life (eg, divorce, siblings getting hurt, or general arguments between parents). The therapist must help the client and the siblings realize that they are not responsible for the client's condition. Part of this magical thinking that often appears is the concept that bad things happen to bad people; thus, the child is bad because a bad thing has happened. It is important to be sensitive to this ideation and help dispel this maladaptive thought pattern, since it is not true or productive for the client or the siblings and may cause further adjustment problems later in treatment. Siblings of the client should be helped to see their roles as supportive siblings, and should not be placed in the role of caretakers of the sibling with body system and functional limitations. In this way, all children can grow naturally without any one of the children being the recipient of all the family's undivided attention. At the same time, children with functional limitations will probably need physical assistance, therapy, increased medical care, and thus, more time devoted to them; this is reality.

The medical establishment should always note that having body system and functional problems is expensive in ways in which they are often not aware. There are the obvious medical costs of therapy, surgery, a wheelchair (w/c), or orthoses, but there are also other costs such as the possibility of extra transportation, catheters for urination, w/c maintenance, adaptive clothing, and other ongoing costs not covered by most insurance plans. These costs add up and contribute to the emotional costs and demands on the family. Significant others may feel the need to work more to earn the money to cover such expenses, but then that person will not be around to help. This is only one of the many dilemmas that must be dealt with for the support system of the person confronted with body system and functional problems. The family may be encouraged to contact such groups as the Family Caregiver Support Network (www.caregiversupportnetwork.org) to get information and assistance with diverse topics such as being a caregiver, legal and financial aid, and communications (this group tends to focus on the adult, but may still be a wonderful aid). Such groups will give information to all who need it and help empower the family. This takes the focus off the medical condition and may help the family gain a better and more balanced perspective on the condition.

Elena may have to work on skills that will encourage assertiveness and better decision-making. She may need to help her family allow her to be more independent and become more of a risk-taker in all aspects of her life.

Kai may need to work on coping skills and strategies that will help him deal with crises. He may have preconceived ideas of the limitations of someone with his medical diagnosis that will need to be changed.

Stress, Crisis, Loss, and Grief

The adaptation process has been much theorized and much speculated upon, and it would appear that the human being is so complex that no 2 individuals react in exactly the same way. This is a comforting fact, because it means each of us is a truly unique individual. This also means that when you deal with clients, each is unique and is not a diagnosis or a routine entity. To do a good job, you have to listen to their stories, know the context of their lives, know their values, and understand their goals. This is a major undertaking in the context of a treatment session, but it should be your ideal goal for each client. This section will examine some thoughts on how clients adapt to a disability.

After an injury or disabling condition that limits function, the client and the family may go through an episode of depression that may interfere with the progress of therapy.[64-67] Depression and other inadequate coping modes will impede progress of therapy and decrease levels of life satisfaction for all involved.[3,68] Attempting to help the client and family members avoid depression by keeping them involved in functional and meaningful therapeutic activities is the challenge.[52] The longer the client is in a forced helplessness situation, the more likely it is that the client will feel depressed. Focusing on a positive goal that is relevant to the client and the family may help keep the client directed toward the future and away from the negative aspects of the situation. If focusing on the client's goals is not enough, other treatment may be needed, and psychiatric assistance may be requested.[37,69,70] Acceptance of the disability without surrendering to the condition has been found to be associated with less anger, less hostility, and higher self-efficacy in the individual.[71,72] Denial may work for the very early stages of the disability, but if it lasts, it will hamper the client's progress. A client once explained that when he could not do anything, denial was very helpful, but as soon as he could start doing things for himself and others, denial was not at all helpful. Thus, the therapist's job is to help the client defocus from the physical impairment and disability by focusing on function and the client's goals. If this is performed and the focus is on adaptive activities that have meaning to the client, the client will not experience the role of helplessness and dependence, and quality of life will be maximized.[73-78]

Livneh and Antonak presented a primer for counselors that can be adapted to assist the therapist in dealing with clients' adjustment to disability.[79] There is no normal or right way for a person to go through the adjustment process, and often, we will not see clients long enough to observe all of the stages of adjustment. Remember, people don't reach and remain in a static state of "adjustment." We are all in states of adjustment to life, and clients are no different.

Some of the observed mechanisms that have been noted are shock, anxiety, denial, depression, anger/hostility, and adjustment. All of these can be seen at some point in the client's life. These aspects of adjustment may be seen at any point of rehabilitation. Although the client may appear adjusted to one aspect of the functional limitations, the same client may be greeted with some new aspect of those limitations not previously experienced. The client may then go into shock and start adjusting to this aspect of the problem anew. Adjustment is a process, not a place. Clients who have been adjusted to their disability for many years will lose or even gain function over time and must adjust to these changes. This is not a static process.

One aspect that the therapist must watch out for is a form of coping called *disengagement*. This may be denial or avoidance behavior, which can take many forms. It can result in substance abuse, blame, or refusal to interact. Research regarding people with brain injuries has demonstrated that if a client's premorbid coping style was to drink or use other drugs, the client may revert to these same styles of coping, which can result in poor rehabilitation outcomes.[80-83] It is important to help the client out of this negative loop. The skills of a therapist may not be enough to perform this in the short time that the client is in treatment, so a referral to social work or psychiatry may be in order. It is still the therapist's job to help promote engagement activities—these behaviors are goal-oriented, problem-solving, information-seeking, and doing things to positively overcome obstacles and demonstrate independence.

Livneh and Antonak[79] promote activities for the health professional such as:

- Assisting clients to explore the personal meaning of the disability. A way of doing this would be to help the client not demonstrate emotional outbursts or to look at emotions and put them into perspective. The intent is to train the clients to "master" control over their emotions.
- Assisting clients to obtain relevant and accurate medical information regarding their condition, including the description, prognosis, anticipated functional problems, and implications related to vocation and occupation.[43] This may be performed by helping the client and family access online resources or helping them find medical references in the library.[43]
- Providing clients with experiences that they can share with their families and groups. These strategies permit clients (usually with similar disabilities or common life experiences) and, if applicable, their family members or significant others, to share common fears, concerns, needs, and wishes."[43] This can be performed in rather unobtrusive ways. For example, scheduling clients with the same disability at the same time so that they meet in the waiting room or while conducting group mat activities organically cultivates interaction. Another example would be to hire individuals with disabilities who are health care professionals who can discuss and model positive behaviors and answer relevant questions from the client's perspective. Remember that all clients are potential teachers for you as well as other clients.[43]
- Teaching clients adaptive coping skills for successful community functioning. Examples include assertiveness, interpersonal relations, decision-making, problem-solving, stigma management, and time management.[79] This can be in the form of role-playing situations. For example, an able-bodied person asking why the client is in a w/c; that person preaching to the w/c user because he must have offended God in some way, otherwise he would not be in a w/c; or telling the client that it is such a shame that she is disabled because she is so good-looking and could have found a man if it were not for the disability. Role-playing can also be used to help a person deal with the possibly awkward experience of going to bed with a new partner and having to explain how to be undressed, what those tubes coming out of the body are for, or what positions are best for someone with this condition.[79]

Elena may work on role-playing to develop the skill to ask someone out on a date or to learn to be assertive at the bank or store. Kai may need to work on how to ask for assistance without feeling dependent or how to physically defend himself in the w/c.

Hope and Spiritual Aspects

The process of hope can be a generalized and positive force to reduce depression, the sense of powerlessness, and grief.[84-87] Clients need a realistic sense of hope. The question of what is realistic is always open to interpretation. For example, a client with quadriplegia who was a deer hunter swore he would go back to the mountains in the fall and shoot a deer. All the staff believed that he was not being realistic, but he came in with venison in the fall from the deer he shot. Another client with quadriplegia lived on the East Coast and said that when he left the hospital, he would drive to the West Coast to live. The staff laughed about this, but sure enough, he was discharged and drove to the West Coast to live. Having hope keeps most of us going in life.

Hope is not always realistic. How many people really believe that they will win the lottery, if not this time, then maybe the next? Sometimes it is this hope that saves us from being overwhelmed by the other realities of life. Try not to take all of the client's hopes and dreams away. That client may win the lottery, shoot a deer, or drive to another part of the country.

Spirituality is something that can provide hope, connection with others, and the reason for or meaning of existence. It is amazing that the medical community has been slow to accept the power of spirituality, since this area gives meaning to so many people's lives. Spirituality has been linked to health perception, a sense of connection with others, and well-being.[88-93] Anything that helps the client put the disability into perspective and move on with life in a healthy way is good. The Western medical system is based on pathology and focuses on that. Physical therapy focuses on function, movement activities, and behavioral change that is productive. One of the dangers of the medical system is the entrapment in pathology to the point that the client may not see anything but pathology. Spirituality may help the client and the family to see that there is more to life than pathology, stimulate interaction with others, put the disability in perspective, give meaning to life (and the disability), and give the person hope and a sense of well-being.[89] This is what we all want for the client and the family.

Elena may benefit from talking to other people with cerebral palsy who have families, are chief executive officers of businesses, or are doing whatever they would like to do.

Kai may tap into what his new goals and dreams really are to see ways to accomplish those dreams.

Cultural Aspects

The therapist must attend to the culture, subculture, and beliefs of the client's family.[94-99] This concept includes beliefs about the world, and maybe a belief about the cause of the disability or at least how the client is viewing the disability. Asking "Why do you think this happened to you?" can lead to a very enlightening experience. "Causes" may range from: "God is punishing me," "I deserved it," or "Life is against me." The answer may frame the way that treatment is presented to the client. Using the client's frame of reference may promote trust, mutual acceptance of values, greater adherence with treatment, and a broadening of the therapist's view of the world. One of the great things about therapy is that clients teach us so much about life. Recognizing why a client does something that looks different to us may lead to a key to what that client may need in treatment. It may also help the physical therapist assistant see the world from a different perspective. Do not hesitate to let the client know that he or she helped you. Helping others is empowering to the client as well as the therapist.

As a health professional, you need to reflect on your own world view. We all have existing personal, social, and cultural beliefs and biases. Rather than denying implicit bias, what is most important is to acknowledge one's own implicit bias to challenge those stereotypes when they arise in the delivery of health care. Delivering culturally competent care is integral to the physical therapist assistant accreditation standards, and culturally responsive care is critical to providing the best interventions for the clients we serve. You may have heard of the Golden Rule: Treat others like you would like to be treated. But have you heard of the Platinum Rule: Treat others how they would like to be treated?[100] For example, you can ask clients (especially older adults) how they would like to be addressed. They may prefer to be called "Mr.", "Mrs.", or "Ms." which may be dependent on when, how, and where they were raised. As a physical therapist assistant, you want to be as client-centered as possible by respecting how clients prefer to be identified.

One example of how the client's perspective can be different from the therapist's is if, during treatment, a client says that she is going to die. When presented with the fact that she is in rehabilitation, is not going to die, and is about to be discharged, she falls silent. It is not until the client gets home that the therapist realizes the client was going back to a dangerous neighborhood, and that the client's fears of death have merit. Someone who is a vulnerable older adult and very disabled in this area of town is in a life-threatening situation, and she probably is going to die (unless other arrangements are quickly made for her discharge). If the therapist had listened better and knew the client's living situation, this incident could have been avoided. It should be noted that the therapist did try to find out what the client meant. The client thought that it was so obvious (in the client's world) that the therapist's lack of knowledge was a lack of caring for the client's well-being. We should try to avoid this kind of miscommunication.

If you guessed that the older adult in the example above was a person of color, you would probably be correct. Race is a social determinant of health; that is, race determines access to quality health care. Structural forces in our society impact health outcomes beyond individual patient encounters.[101] Controlling for income, people of color have poorer health outcomes. Health disparities disproportionately affect people of color. The vulnerable older adult in the example above lived in a dangerous neighborhood because of inequities of wealth and other socioeconomic power imbalances that impact quality of life and other health issues such as stress and ultimately mortality rates. Health professionals have codes of ethics, and some of those codes mandate reducing health disparities and advocating for social justice.[102] We want to effect changes in societal structures to reach health equity for all.

Beliefs and values of cultures and families can play a profound role in the course of treatment. Such things as physical difficulties that can be seen are usually better accepted than problems that cannot be seen, such as brain damage that changes an individual's personality.[103-105] A person with a back injury may be seen as lazy, whereas a person with a double amputation will be perceived as needing help. At the same time, a person who has lost a body part may be seen as "not all there" in some cultures and is avoided socially. Thus, being attuned to the culture and beliefs of the client is imperative in therapy.

Elena will have some of her beliefs challenged. She will need to examine how she thinks about her possible future roles. She may want to examine whether she would like to have children, be a professional woman, or both. She will have to develop skills that will promote her goals, and she may look to role models who can demonstrate the positive behaviors that are necessary to accomplish these goals.

Kai was very unfocused in his life before the injury and will need help clarifying some of the behaviors that did not work for him before. In doing so, he will have to dispel some of the myths about people with disabilities that he was taught in his culture. With help, he may be able to see this event as a new beginning that will help him have a fresh start.

Adjustment to disability opens individuals to a unique situation and allows them to adapt to a changing environment in a productive way. If the person is not able to alter *maladaptive* behaviors and grow in a productive way, the best physical therapy in the world will not be able to make significant progress. We may get a client to perform all the correct exercises and movement patterns, but not be a productive person who enjoys life. The physical therapist assistant needs to be aware of ways to promote productive behavior that results in a more functional person. It is not the physical therapist assistant's job to be a psychologist, an occupational therapist, or a social worker, but it is important to assist the team and to promote productive behavior and function. The role of psychosocial function is intricately linked to quality of life issues. Movement not only expresses the motor system, but is also an avenue that clients can use to express emotions, interact with other individuals, be empowered to bodily functions, and feel good about themselves. Physical therapist assistants, as team members and colleagues who are delegated the responsibility of physical therapy interventions, need to identify their own personal beliefs, safety issues, biases, and learning styles, and respect each patient's uniqueness. With this comprehension incorporated into a physical therapist assistant's behavior, that physical therapist assistant will become a much better therapist, have better adherence from patients, and feel more satisfied as a provider of health care.

References

1. Collins S, Couture B, Kang MJ, et al. Quantifying and visualizing nursing flowsheet documentation burden in acute and critical care. *AMIA Annu Symp Proc.* 2018;2018:348-357.
2. Women, Trauma and PTSD. US Department of Veterans Affairs. Accessed May 25, 2018. https://www.ptsd.va.gov/professional/treat/specific/ptsd_research_women.asp
3. Bruffaerts R, Vilagut G, Demyttenaere K, et al. Role of common mental and physical disorders in partial disability around the world. *Br J Psychiatry.* 2012;200(6):454-461. doi:10.1192/bjp.bp.111.097519
4. Richards T, Garvert DW, McDade E, Carlson E, Curtin C. Chronic psychological and functional sequelae after emergent hand surgery. *J Hand Surg Am.* 2011;36(10):1663-1668. doi:10.1016/j.jhsa.2011.06.028
5. Shalev AY, Ankri Y, Gilad M, et al. Long-term outcome of early interventions to prevent posttraumatic stress disorder. *J Clin Psychiatry.* 2016;77(5):e580-e587. doi:10.4088/JCP.15m09932
6. Hannah SD. Psychosocial issues after a traumatic hand injury: facilitating adjustment. *J Hand Ther.* 2011;24(2):95-102. doi:10.1016/j.jht.2010.11.001
7. Brewin CR, Garnett R, Andrews B. Trauma, identity and mental health in UK military veterans. *Psychol Med.* 2011;41(8):1733-1740. doi:10.1017/S003329171000231X
8. Haagsma JA, Polinder S, Toet H, et al. Beyond the neglect of psychological consequences: post-traumatic stress disorder increases the non-fatal burden of injury by more than 50%. *Inj Prev.* 2011;17(1):21-26. doi:10.1136/ip.2010.026419
9. Freedy JR, Magruder KM, Mainous AG, Frueh BC, Geesey ME, Carnemolla M. Gender differences in traumatic event exposure and mental health among veteran primary care patients. *Mil Med.* 2010;175(10):750-758. doi:10.7205/MILMED-D-10-00123
10. SAMHSA's Concept of Trauma and Guidance for a Trauma-Informed Approach. https://store.samhsa.gov/system/files/sma14-4884.pdf. Accessed May, 10 2018.
11. Mazaux JM, Croze P, Quintard B, et al. Satisfaction of life and late psycho-social outcome after severe brain injury: a nine-year follow-up study in Aquitaine. *Acta Neurochir Suppl (Wien).* 2002;79:49-51. doi:10.1007/978-3-7091-6105-0_11
12. International Classification of Functioning, Disability and Health (ICF). World Health Organization. http://www.who.int/classifications/icf/icf_more/en/. Accessed May 25, 2018.
13. Psychology Today. Cognitive Behavioral Therapy. https://www.psychologytoday.com/us/therapy-types/cognitive-behavioral-therapy. Accessed May 10, 2018.
14. Ayyangar R. Health maintenance and management in childhood disability. *Phys Med Rehabil Clin N Am.* 2002;13(4):793-821. doi:10.1016/S1047-9651(02)00046-3
15. Fusco O, Ferrini A, Santoro M, Lo Monaco MR, Gambassi G, Cesari M. Physical function and perceived quality of life in older persons. *Aging Clin Exp Res.* 2012;24(1):68-73. doi:10.1007/BF03325356
16. King J, Yourman L, Ahalt C, et al. Quality of life in late-life disability: "I don't feel bitter because I am in a wheelchair". *J Am Geriatr Soc.* 2012;60(3):569-576. doi:10.1111/j.1532-5415.2011.03844.x
17. Dahan-Oliel N, Shikako-Thomas K, Majnemer A. Quality of life and leisure participation in children with neurodevelopmental disabilities: a thematic analysis of the literature. *Qual Life Res.* 2012;21(3):427-439. doi:10.1007/s11136-011-0063-9
18. Rosenbaum P, Gorter JW. The 'F-words' in childhood disability: I swear this is how we should think! *Child Care Health Dev.* 2012;38(4):457-463. doi:10.1111/j.1365-2214.2011.01338.x
19. Bossaert G, Colpin H, Pijl SJ, Petry K. The attitudes of Belgian adolescents towards peers with disabilities. *Res Dev Disabil.* 2011;32(2):504-509. doi:10.1016/j.ridd.2010.12.033

20. "Strengths-Based Approaches for Working with Individuals." Iriss. https://www.iriss.org.uk/resources/insights/strengths-based-approaches-working-individuals. Accessed May 25, 2018.
21. Woods K, Bond C, Humphrey N, Symes W, Green L. *Systematic review of Solution Focused Brief Therapy (SFBT) with children and families.* Nottingham, England: DFE Publications; 2011.
22. Jalayondeja C, Kaewkungwal J, Sullivan PE, Nidhinandana S, Pichaiyongwongdee S, Jareinpituk S. Factors related to community participation by stroke victims six month post-stroke. *Southeast Asian J Trop Med Public Health.* 2011;42(4):1005-1013.
23. LaVeist TA, Isaac LA, Williams KP. Mistrust of health care organizations is associated with underutilization of health services. *Health Serv Res.* 2009;44(6):2093-2105. doi:10.1111/j.1475-6773.2009.01017.x
24. Pinto RZ, Ferreira ML, Oliveira VC, et al. Patient-centred communication is associated with positive therapeutic alliance: a systematic review. *J Physiother.* 2012;58(2):77-87. doi:10.1016/S1836-9553(12)70087-5
25. Lee YY, Lin JL. How much does trust really matter? A study of the longitudinal effects of trust and decision-making preferences on diabetic patient outcomes. *Patient Educ Couns.* 2011;85(3):406-412. doi:10.1016/j.pec.2010.12.005
26. Sloots M, Dekker JH, Pont M, Bartels EA, Geertzen JH, Dekker J. Reasons of drop-out from rehabilitation in patients of Turkish and Moroccan origin with chronic low back pain in The Netherlands: a qualitative study. *J Rehabil Med.* 2010;42(6):566-573. doi:10.2340/16501977-0536
27. Brennan N, Barnes R, Calnan M, Corrigan O, Dieppe P, Entwistle V. Trust in the health-care provider-patient relationship: a systematic mapping review of the evidence base. *Int J Qual Health Care.* 2013;25(6):682-688. doi:10.1093/intqhc/mzt063
28. Kuipers K, Rassafiani M, Ashburner J, et al. Do clients with acquired brain injury use the splints prescribed by occupational therapists? A descriptive study. *NeuroRehabilitation.* 2009;24(4):365-375. doi:10.3233/NRE-2009-0491
29. Linton SJ, Shaw WS. Impact of psychological factors in the experience of pain. *Phys Ther.* 2011;91(5):700-711. doi:10.2522/ptj.20100330
30. Deans S, Burns D, McGarry A, Murray K, Mutrie N. Motivations and barriers to prosthesis users participation in physical activity, exercise and sport: a review of the literature. *Prosthet Orthot Int.* 2012;36(3):260-269. doi:10.1177/0309364612437905
31. Bombardier CH, Fann JR, Tate DG, et al; PRISMS Investigators. An exploration of modifiable risk factors for depression after spinal cord injury: which factors should we target? *Arch Phys Med Rehabil.* 2012;93(5):775-781. doi:10.1016/j.apmr.2011.12.020
32. Sylliaas H, Thingstad P, Wyller TB, Helbostad J, Sletvold O, Bergland A. Prognostic factors for self-rated function and perceived health in patient living at home three months after a hip fracture. *Disabil Rehabil.* 2012;34(14):1225-1231. doi:10.3109/09638288.2011.643333
33. Field N, Prah P, Mercer CH, et al. Are depression and poor sexual health neglected comorbidities? Evidence from a population sample. *BMJ Open.* 2016;6(3):e010521. doi:10.1136/bmjopen-2015-010521
34. Sander AM, Maestas KL, Pappadis MR, Sherer M, Hammond FM, Hanks R; NIDRR Traumatic Brain Injury Model Systems Module Project on Sexuality After TBI. Sexual functioning 1 year after traumatic brain injury: findings from a prospective traumatic brain injury model systems collaborative study. *Arch Phys Med Rehabil.* 2012;93(8):1331-1337. doi:10.1016/j.apmr.2012.03.037
35. Centers for Disease Control (CDC). Taking a Sexual History. https://www.cdc.gov/std/treatment/sexualhistory.pdf. Accessed May 25, 2018.
36. Kreuter M, Taft C, Siösteen A, Biering-Sørensen F. Women's sexual functioning and sex life after spinal cord injury. *Spinal Cord.* 2011;49(1):154-160. doi:10.1038/sc.2010.51
37. Nortvedt MW, Riise T, Myhr KM, Landtblom AM, Bakke A, Nyland HI. Reduced quality of life among multiple sclerosis patients with sexual disturbance and bladder dysfunction. *Mult Scler.* 2001;7(4):231-235. doi:10.1177/135245850100700404
38. Cardoso FL, Savall AC, Mendes AK. Self-awareness of the male sexual response after spinal cord injury. *Int J Rehabil Res.* 2009;32(4):294-300. doi:10.1097/MRR.0b013e3283106ab7
39. Alriksson-Schmidt AI, Armour BS, Thibadeau JK. Are adolescent girls with a physical disability at increased risk for sexual violence? *J Sch Health.* 2010;80(7):361-367. doi:10.1111/j.1746-1561.2010.00514.x
40. "Understanding non-binary people: A guide for the media." http://transmediawatch.org/Documents/non_binary.pdf. Accessed May 10, 2018.
41. Love L, Bombardier CH, Linsenmeyer TA, et al; Consortium for Spinal Cord Medicine. Sexuality and reproductive health in adults with spinal cord injury: a clinical practice guideline for health-care professionals. *J Spinal Cord Med.* 2010;33(3):281-336. doi:10.1080/10790268.2010.11689709
42. Iremashvili V, Brackett NL, Ibrahim E, Aballa TC, Lynne CM. Semen quality remains stable during the chronic phase of spinal cord injury: a longitudinal study. *J Urol.* 2010;184(5):2073-2077. doi:10.1016/j.juro.2010.06.112
43. Hirsch IH. Optimizing fertility potential in spinal cord injured men. *Can J Urol.* 2012;19(5):6437.
44. SpinalCord.com. Fertility after SCI. https://www.spinalcord.com/fertility-after-paralysis-spinal-cord-injury. Accessed May 25, 2018.
45. Trofimenko V, Hotaling JM. Fertility treatment in spinal cord injury and other neurologic disease. *Transl Androl Urol.* 2016;5(1):102-116.
46. Vogel LC, Krajci KA, Anderson CJ. Adults with pediatric-onset spinal cord injuries: part 3: impact of medical complications. *J Spinal Cord Med.* 2002;25(4):297-305. doi:10.1080/10790268.2002.11753632
47. Majnemer A, Shevell M, Law M, Poulin C, Rosenbaum P. Indicators of distress in families of children with cerebral palsy. *Disabil Rehabil.* 2012;34(14):1202-1207. doi:10.3109/09638288.2011.638035
48. Evans SA, Airey MC, Chell SM, Connelly JB, Rigby AS, Tennant A. Disability in young adults following major trauma: 5 year follow up of survivors. *BMC Public Health.* 2003;3(1):8. doi:10.1186/1471-2458-3-8
49. Roscigno CI, Swanson KM. Parents' experiences following children's moderate to severe traumatic brain injury: a clash of cultures. *Qual Health Res.* 2011;21(10):1413-1426. doi:10.1177/1049732311410988

50. Kreuter M. Spinal cord injury and partner relationships. *Spinal Cord.* 2000;38(1):2-6. doi:10.1038/sj.sc.3100933
51. Botticello AL, Rohrbach T, Cobbold N. Differences in the community built environment influence poor perceived health among persons with spinal cord injury. *Arch Phys Med Rehabil.* 2015;96(9):1583-1590. doi:10.1016/j.apmr.2015.04.025
52. Jaracz K, Grabowska-Fudala B, Kozubski W. Caregiver burden after stroke: towards a structural model. *Neurol Neurochir Pol.* 2012;46(3):224-232. doi:10.5114/ninp.2012.29130
53. Carod-Artal FJ, Egido JA. Quality of life after stroke: the importance of a good recovery. *Cerebrovasc Dis.* 2009;27(suppl 1):204-214. doi:10.1159/000200461
54. Raina P, O'Donnell M, Rosenbaum P, et al. The health and well-being of caregivers of children with cerebral palsy. *Pediatrics.* 2005;115(6):e626-e636. doi:10.1542/peds.2004-1689
55. Tramonti F, Gerini A, Stampacchia G. Individualised and health-related quality of life of persons with spinal cord injury. *Spinal Cord.* 2014;52(3):231-235. doi:10.1038/sc.2013.156
56. DeBaillie AM. The Effects of Traumatic Brain Injury on Families. OpenSIUC. http://opensiuc.lib.siu.edu/gs_rp/552. Accessed May 18, 2018.
57. Nätterlund B, Ahlström G. Activities of daily living and quality of life in persons with muscular dystrophy. *J Rehabil Med.* 2001;33(5):206-211. doi:10.1080/165019701750419590
58. Turner S, Cox H. Facilitating post traumatic growth. *Health Qual Life Outcomes.* 2004;2(1):34. doi:10.1186/1477-7525-2-34
59. Man DW. Hong Kong family caregivers' stress and coping for people with brain injury. *Int J Rehabil Res.* 2002;25(4):287-295. doi:10.1097/00004356-200212000-00006
60. Taanila A, Syrjälä L, Kokkonen J, Järvelin MR. Coping of parents with physically and/or intellectually disabled children. *Child Care Health Dev.* 2002;28(1):73-86. doi:10.1046/j.1365-2214.2002.00244.x
61. de Klerk HM, Ampousah L. The physically disabled woman's experience of self. *Disabil Rehabil.* 2003;25(19):1132-1139. doi:10.1080/09638280310001596199
62. Koukouli S, Vlachonikolis IG, Philalithis A. Socio-demographic factors and self-reported functional status: the significance of social support. *BMC Health Serv Res.* 2002;2(1):20. doi:10.1186/1472-6963-2-20
63. Kimura M, Yamazaki S, Haga H, Yasumura S. The prevalence of social engagement in the disabled elderly and related factors. *ISRN Geriatr.* 2013;2013:1-8. doi:10.1155/2013/709823
64. Martz E, Livneh H, Priebe M, Wuermser LA, Ottomanelli L. Predictors of psychosocial adaptation among people with spinal cord injury or disorder. *Arch Phys Med Rehabil.* 2005;86(6):1182-1192. doi:10.1016/j.apmr.2004.11.036
65. Pakenham KI, Cox S. Test of a model of the effects of parental illness on youth and family functioning. *Health Psychol.* 2012;31(5):580-590. doi:10.1037/a0026530
66. Bombardier CH, Richards JS, Krause JS, Tulsky D, Tate DG. Symptoms of major depression in people with spinal cord injury: implications for screening. *Arch Phys Med Rehabil.* 2004;85(11):1749-1756. doi:10.1016/j.apmr.2004.07.348
67. Pakenham KI, Cox S. Test of a model of the effects of parental illness on youth and family functioning. *Health Psychol.* 2012;31(5):580-590. doi:10.1037/a0026530
68. Chan RC. Stress and coping in spouses of persons with spinal cord injuries. *Clin Rehabil.* 2000;14(2):137-144. doi:10.1191/026921500675826560
69. Kishi Y, Robinson RG, Kosier JT. Suicidal ideation among patients during the rehabilitation period after life-threatening physical illness. *J Nerv Ment Dis.* 2001;189(9):623-628. doi:10.1097/00005053-200109000-00009
70. Andelic N, Sigurdardottir S, Schanke AK, Sandvik L, Sveen U, Roe C. Disability, physical health and mental health 1 year after traumatic brain injury. *Disabil Rehabil.* 2010;32(13):1122-1131. doi:10.3109/09638280903410722
71. Treharne GJ, Lyons AC, Booth DA, Mason SR, Kitas GD. Reactions to disability in patients with early versus established rheumatoid arthritis. *Scand J Rheumatol.* 2004;33(1):30-38. doi:10.1080/03009740310004685
72. Hoffman M. Bodies completed: on the physical rehabilitation of lower limb amputees. *Health (London).* 2013;17(3):229-245. doi:10.1177/1363459312451177
73. Holmbeck GN, Westhoven VC, Phillips WS, et al. A multimethod, multi-informant, and multidimensional perspective on psychosocial adjustment in preadolescents with spina bifida. *J Consult Clin Psychol.* 2003;71(4):782-796. doi:10.1037/0022-006X.71.4.782
74. Sofi F, Molino Lova R, Nucida V, et al. Adaptive physical activity and back pain: a non-randomised community-based intervention trial. *Eur J Phys Rehabil Med.* 2011;47(4):543-549.
75. Voll R. Aspects of the quality of life of chronically ill and handicapped children and adolescents in outpatient and inpatient rehabilitation. *Int J Rehabil Res.* 2001;24(1):43-49. doi:10.1097/00004356-200103000-00006
76. Chiarello LA, Palisano RJ, Bartlett DJ, McCoy SW. A multivariate model of determinants of change in gross-motor abilities and engagement in self-care and play of young children with cerebral palsy. *Phys Occup Ther Pediatr.* 2011;31(2):150-168. doi:10.3109/01942638.2010.525601
77. Ville I, Ravaud JF, Group T; Tetrafigap Group. Subjective well-being and severe motor impairments: the Tetrafigap survey on the long-term outcome of tetraplegic spinal cord injured persons. *Soc Sci Med.* 2001;52(3):369-384. doi:10.1016/S0277-9536(00)00140-4
78. Majnemer A, Shevell M, Law M, Poulin C, Rosenbaum P. Level of motivation in mastering challenging tasks in children with cerebral palsy. *Dev Med Child Neurol.* 2010;52(12):1120-1126. doi:10.1111/j.1469-8749.2010.03732.x
79. Livneh H, Antonak RF. Psychosocial adaptation to chronic illness and disability: a primer for counselors. *J Couns Dev.* 2005;83(1):12-20. doi:10.1002/j.1556-6678.2005.tb00575.x
80. MacMillan PJ, Hart RP, Martelli MF, Zasler ND. Pre-injury status and adaptation following traumatic brain injury. *Brain Inj.* 2002;16(1):41-49. doi:10.1080/0269905011008812
81. Center for Substance Abuse Treatment. SAMHSA/CSAT Treatment Improvement Protocols. Substance Use Disorder Treatment for People With Physical and Cognitive Disabilities. Rockville, MD: US Substance Abuse and Mental Health Services Administration; 1998. Report No: (SMA) 98-3249.
82. West SL. Substance use among persons with traumatic brain injury: a review. *NeuroRehabilitation.* 2011;29(1):1-8. doi:10.3233/NRE-2011-0671

83. DeLambo DA, Chandras KV, Homa D, Chandras SV. Spinal cord injury and substance abuse: implications for rehabilitation professionals. http://counselingoutfitters.com/vistas/vistas10/Article_83.pdf. Accessed September 5, 2013.
84. Lohne V. Hope in patients with spinal cord injury: a literature review related to nursing. *J Neurosci Nurs.* 2001;33(6):317-325. doi:10.1097/01376517-200112000-00006
85. Shiri S, Wexler ID, Feintuch U, Meiner Z, Schwartz I. Post-polio syndrome: impact of hope on quality of life. *Disabil Rehabil.* 2012;34(10):824-830. doi:10.3109/09638288.2011.623755
86. Nunnerley JL, Hay-Smith EJ, Dean SG. Leaving a spinal unit and returning to the wider community: an interpretative phenomenological analysis. *Disabil Rehabil.* 2013;35(14):1164-1173. doi:10.3109/09638288.2012.723789
87. Kortte KB, Stevenson JE, Hosey MM, Castillo R, Wegener ST. Hope predicts positive functional role outcomes in acute rehabilitation populations. *Rehabil Psychol.* 2012;57(3):248-255. doi:10.1037/a0029004
88. Delgado C. A discussion of the concept of spirituality. *Nurs Sci Q.* 2005;18(2):157-162. doi:10.1177/0894318405274828
89. Maggi L, Ferrara PE, Aprile I, et al. Role of spiritual beliefs on disability and health-related quality of life in acute inpatient rehabilitation unit. *Eur J Phys Rehabil Med.* 2012;48(3):467-473.
90. Lucchetti G, Lucchetti AG, Badan-Neto AM, et al. Religiousness affects mental health, pain and quality of life in older people in an outpatient rehabilitation setting. *J Rehabil Med.* 2011;43(4):316-322. doi:10.2340/16501977-0784
91. Potter ML, Zauszniewski JA. Spirituality, resourcefulness, and arthritis impact on health perception of elders with rheumatoid arthritis. *J Holist Nurs.* 2000;18(4):311-331; discussions 332-336.
92. Svalina SS, Webb JR. Forgiveness and health among people in outpatient physical therapy. *Disabil Rehabil.* 2012;34(5):383-392. doi:10.3109/09638288.2011.607216
93. Waldron-Perrine B, Rapport LJ, Hanks RA, Lumley M, Meachen SJ, Hubbarth P. Religion and spirituality in rehabilitation outcomes among individuals with traumatic brain injury. *Rehabil Psychol.* 2011;56(2):107-116. doi:10.1037/a0023552
94. Treloar LL. Disability, spiritual beliefs and the church: the experiences of adults with disabilities and family members. *J Adv Nurs.* 2002;40(5):594-603. doi:10.1046/j.1365-2648.2002.02417.x
95. Saravanan B, Manigandan C, Macaden A, Tharion G, Bhattacharji S. Re-examining the psychology of spinal cord injury: a meaning centered approach from a cultural perspective. *Spinal Cord.* 2001;39(6):323-326. doi:10.1038/sj.sc.3101149
96. Jull JE, Giles AR. Health equity, aboriginal peoples and occupational therapy. *Can J Occup Ther.* 2012;79(2):70-76. doi:10.2182/cjot.2012.79.2.2
97. Look MA, Kaholokula JK, Carvhalo A, Seto T, de Silva M. Developing a culturally based cardiac rehabilitation program: the HELA study. *Prog Community Health Partnersh.* 2012;6(1):103-110. doi:10.1353/cpr.2012.0012
98. Kwong K, Chung H, Cheal K, Chou JC, Chen T. Disability beliefs and help-seeking behavior of depressed Chinese-American patients in a primary care setting. *J Soc Work Disabil Rehabil.* 2012;11(2):81-99. doi:10.1080/1536710X.2012.677602
99. Liu F, Williams RM, Liu HE, Chien NH. The lived experience of persons with lower extremity amputation. *J Clin Nurs.* 2010;19(15-16):2152-2161. doi:10.1111/j.1365-2702.2010.03256.x
100. Nagayama Hall GC. The Platinum Rule. Psychology Today. https://www.psychologytoday.com/us/blog/life-in-the-intersection/201702/the-platinum-rule. Accessed October 2, 2018.
101. Wallace SP. Equity and social determinants of health among older adults. *J Am Soc Aging.* 2015;38(4):6-11.
102. American Nurses Association. Code of Ethics for Nurses 2016. https://anacalif.memberclicks.net/assets/Events/RNDay/2016%20code%20of%20ethics%20for%20nurses%20-%209%20provisions.pdf. Accessed May 15, 2018.
103. Brown SA, McCauley SR, Levin HS, Contant C, Boake C. Perception of health and quality of life in minorities after mild-to-moderate traumatic brain injury. *Appl Neuropsychol.* 2004;11(1):54-64. doi:10.1207/s15324826an1101_7
104. Lindsay S, King G, Klassen AF, Esses V, Stachel M. Working with immigrant families raising a child with a disability: challenges and recommendations for healthcare and community service providers. *Disabil Rehabil.* 2012;34(23):2007-2017. doi:10.3109/09638288.2012.667192
105. Clarke P, Smith J. Aging in a cultural context: cross-national differences in disability and the moderating role of personal control among older adults in the United States and England. *J Gerontol B Psychol Sci Soc Sci.* 2011;66(4):457-467. doi:10.1093/geronb/gbr054

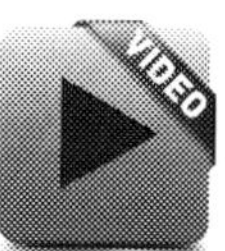

Chapter 8
Roles of the Physical Therapist Assistant in Neurocritical Care

Rodiel Kirby Baloy, PT, DPT, EdS, MS and Lauren Eberhardt, PT, DPT, NCS

KEY WORDS Fowler's position | Intensive care unit | Neurocritical care unit

Chapter Objectives

- Describe the roles of the physical therapist assistant in the management of patients in the neurocritical care unit (NCU).
- Identify neurologic conditions where admission to a critical care unit may be needed.
- Discuss monitoring devices that are typically used in neurocritical units.
- Describe principles on optimal positioning for neurocritical patients.
- Discuss considerations regarding early mobility in patients in the NCU.

Today's critical care units are environments where groups of professionals work together in the specialized care of the high-risk patient. Physical therapists and physical therapist assistants work with teams of individual specialties based on set practice guidelines. The common foundations of critical care among these personnel include the application of complex equipment, the use of close monitoring devices, and nursing surveillance interventions to prevent the deterioration of the patient's condition.[1]

In the United States, an increased incidence of acute hospitalizations and emergency room visits has been brought about by increasing sedentary lifestyles, lack of access to regular quality health care, and activity-related trauma. In a study by the Academy of Emergency Medicine, the country saw an increase in intensive care unit (ICU) admissions from 2.79 million in 2002/2003 to 4.14 million in 2008/2009.[2] This represents an increase of 48.8% and a mean biennial increase of 14.2%. By comparison, overall emergency department visits within the same time frame increased by a mean of 5.8%/biennial period.[2]

Similar trends are noted in NCUs. Between 2000 and 2008, the total number of NCU admissions at the Columbia University Medical Center, for example, increased by 49.9%. The demographics of such admissions include a patient average age of 54 to 56 years, with almost equal distribution among male and female patients.[3] As neurocritical care advances and bigger and larger facilities are being built, these numbers may continue to change.

Communication

Physical therapist assistants encounter patients referred to the NCU who are referred for neurologic conditions and also for the management of pain, airway maintenance, ventilation, cardiovascular stabilization, anticoagulation, and an increase in intracranial pressure (ICP), among other reasons. Common among these conditions are patients whose consciousness may be affected, or whose neuromuscular weakness is severe enough to make communication difficult. The physical therapist assistant may then consult the nursing team, the referring physician, and other health care professionals to establish the best method of communicating with the client. The patient's family is also a source

Lazaro RT, Umphred DA, eds.
Umphred's Neurorehabilitation for the Physical Therapist Assistant, Third Edition (pp 167-183).

Box 8-1

General Criteria for Admission to Neurocritical Care Units

- Impaired level of consciousness
- Impaired airway protection
- Progressive respiratory impairment or the need for mechanical ventilation
- Seizures
- Clinical or computed tomographic evidence of raised ICP caused by a space-occupying lesion, cerebral edema, or hemorrhagic conversion of a cerebral infarct
- General medical complications (eg, hyper/hypotension, aspiration pneumonia, sepsis, cardiac arrhythmias, or pulmonary emboli)
- Monitoring (eg, level of consciousness, respiratory function, continuous intracortical electroencephalography)
- Specific treatments (eg, neurosurgical intervention, or Intravenous or arterial thrombolysis)

Source: Howard, Kullmann, Hirsch, 2003.

Box 8-2

General Principles of Assessment and Resuscitation from Acute Stroke

- Airway management
    - Tracheal intubation is indicated when there is:
        - Impaired level of consciousness (eg, Glasgow Coma Score less than 9)
        - Progressive respiratory impairment or respiratory failure
        - Impaired cough and airway clearance
        - Pulmonary edema/aspiration
        - Seizure activity
        - Intubation may also be required before diagnostic or therapeutic procedures such as magnetic resonance imaging or thrombolysis
- Maintenance of adequate arterial blood pressure/cerebral perfusion pressure
- Intravenous fluid management
- Temperature control
- Seizure control
- Institution of enteral nutrition
- ICP management
- Medical treatment of complications (eg, sepsis)
- Other management related to the underlying cause (eg, anticoagulation, thrombolysis, evacuation of hematoma, or clipping and coiling of intracerebral aneurysms)

Source: Howard, Kullmann, Hirsch, 2003.

of information. It is helpful to have the immediate family members be familiar with the current clinical picture and the management of the patient's health.[4]

Indications for Neurologic Intensive Care Admission

Among emergency department visits, the general criteria for admission into the NCU can be found in Box 8-1.[4]

Patients with certain neurological diseases such as stroke, Guillain-Barré syndrome (GBS), myasthenia gravis, and central nervous system infections have overall better outcomes than patients with secondary neurological diseases seen within general ICUs.[4] These conditions, however, require that the patients use some form of ICU support for extended durations. Prolonged stays in the ICU place a psychological drain not just on the patients, but also on their caregivers, nurses, physicians, and other health care professionals.

Spinal Cord Lesions

High cord lesions lead to acute respiratory distress and will require ventilatory support. Patients with a long history of spinal cord injury (SCI) may develop skeletal anomalies at the foramen magnum or may be admitted after accidents or traumatic events.

Stroke

Patients diagnosed with a stroke are normally admitted into a NCU during the acute phase. These patients may require resuscitation followed by continued monitoring and observation for neurologic deterioration.

The principles of assessment and resuscitation from acute stroke are similar regardless of the underlying cause (Box 8-2).

Middle Cerebral Artery Occlusion

Patients with middle cerebral artery occlusion may suffer from quick deterioration associated with brain edema. This leads to poor prognosis toward functional recovery. After a patient with a middle cerebral artery stroke is stabilized, early thrombolysis maybe administered. The edema and brain infarction requires ICP measurement. The effect of the edema, however, is not always seen in ICP measurements.[5] This requires bedside monitoring of other symptoms such as cardiac arrhythmias, pulmonary emboli, and the development of seizures.

Cerebellar Infarcts

Cerebellar infarcts are characterized by slow deterioration in the brainstem and late cerebellar signs. The insult to the brainstem may arise from compression due to brain edema. This compression may also lead to an obstruction of the cerebrospinal fluid causing the development of hydrocephaly. ICP measurements are then closely monitored in cerebellar infarct patients.[4]

Status Epilepticus

In *status epilepticus*, seizures lasting about 5 minutes happen in succession, and the patient does not recover consciousness between episodes. This condition may arise from traumatic events, encephalitis, the presence of brain tumors or cerebrovascular disease, or an effect of medication.[6] Patients with status epilepticus and other severe epilepsies require admission into the ICU. The goal of admission into neurocritical care involves managing the seizure, preventing its recurrence, managing the cause, and preventing complications including cardiopulmonary problems such as aspiration pneumonia or cardiac arrhythmia. Due to the nature of possible organ affectations, patient respiratory and cardiac function are monitored, including patient vital signs and ventilation status. An electroencephalography monitor is also necessary. Continued electroencephalography monitoring will identify any deterioration of a convulsive status.

Multiple Sclerosis

Multiple sclerosis is associated with the development of respiratory decline due to weakness of the respiratory musculature and affectation of breathing regulatory centers. Acute multiple sclerosis flareups with plaque formation in the brainstem will severely affect respiration, requiring admission to neurocritical care. The patient will require continued ventilatory and respiratory support.

Movement Disorders

Patients with movement disorders, such as those with Parkinsonian-type syndromes, may develop respiratory distress related to impairment of breathing control and weakness of the vocal cords. Severe affectation of breathing and respiration will require admission to neurocritical care for airway support.

Guillain-Barré Syndrome

Patients with GBS may develop several symptoms. GBS may present with both motor and sensory axonal neuropathy, where paralysis may rapidly develop over the course a few hours requiring tracheal intubation and ventilation assistance. Further bulbar deterioration and phrenic neuropathy will require continued airway support. Respiratory failure takes place in approximately 30% of patients with GBS.[7]

Autonomic impairments in GBS may cause cardiac conditions such as tachycardia or arrhythmia. This may require electrocardiogram and cardiac monitoring. Other adverse symptoms may include *hyponatremia* (low blood sodium levels), gastrointestinal tract affectation, and confusion.[4]

Critical Care Monitoring

Patient admission into the NCU is based upon the need to manage acute neurological and life-threatening emergencies. In the NCU, control of breathing (eg, airway and respiration), brain edema, and hemodynamic issues are monitored and controlled. In such a scenario, medical doctors, nurses, and other health care professionals observe the patient and intervene when necessary. Physical therapists and physical therapist assistants play a role in managing secondary effects and complications.

In the neurocritical care environment, the close monitoring of patients is performed with the goal of early intervention. When the critically ill patient is presenting with signs of organ deterioration or further cellular damage, the use of equipment to optimize tissue recovery is then initiated. An example of this is oxygen supplementation to supply depleted tissues. When vigilant and precise monitoring is practiced, the chance of patient mortality is decreased.[8] Because organs may be affected in a neurologic event, several methods exist in which systems may be monitored.[4]

Vital Signs

Physical therapist assistants must be well-versed in the measurement of vital signs. Continued monitoring of these signs over the course of therapy is essential for safe treatment and exercise. The vital signs a physical therapist assistant must be familiar with include pulse rate, respiratory rate, blood pressure, temperature, and pain levels (see Chapter 5). It is recommended that physical therapist assistants measure these signs before, during, and after treatment. In the NCU, the physical therapist assistant has access to the bedside monitor where the pulse rate and blood pressure are displayed. A therapist must, however, also have access to the tools for the monitoring of vital signs including a sphygmomanometer and a stethoscope. Careful monitoring allows the therapist to determine the patient's ability to tolerate exercise.

Pulse Oximetry

Pulse oximetry is a measure of oxygen saturation in the blood. In the NCU, it is measured using the bedside monitor or a pulse oximeter (Figure 8-1). Normal oxygen saturation level is between 92% to 100%.[9] A low number, such as a reading of below 60%, indicates *hypoxemia*, which may be due to a circulation or respiration issue and may cause shortness of breath. In these situations, supplemental oxygen may be needed.

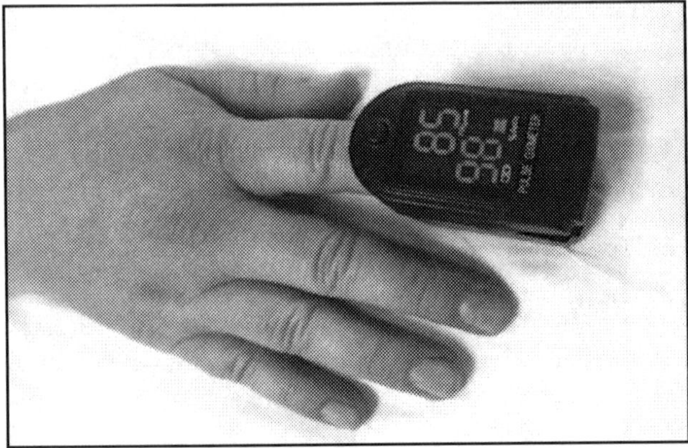

Figure 8-1. Measurement of oxygen saturation via a pulse oximeter.

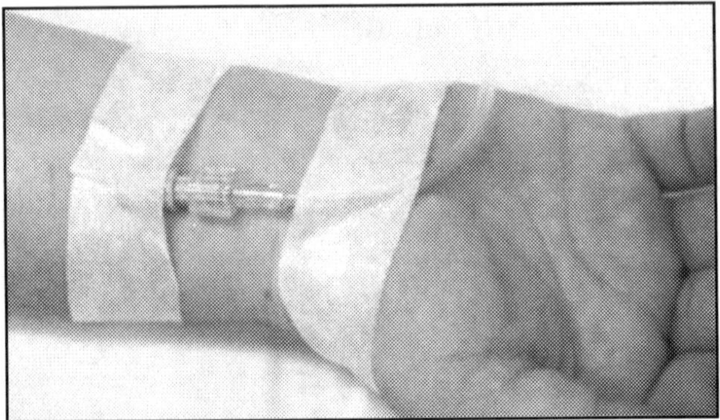

Figure 8-2. An arterial line or art-line is a convenient way to take blood samples for the laboratory.

Monitors, Lines, and Tubes

Bedside Monitor

A *bedside monitor* uses a computer screen to monitor essential patient functions such as the pulse rate, blood pressure, ICP, and oxygen saturation. It may also display the electrocardiogram output, cardiac output, and other measurements. Wires or leads from the patients head, arms, trunk, and legs are attached to sensing devices that send information to a processing unit and displayed on screen. This machine is usually found near the head or beside the patient.[10]

Alarms are triggered when certain vital functions fall below or rise above the normal or preset range. Dislodging one of the leads or wires may also trigger an alarm. Nursing is immediately informed, and medical staff aid the patient to reattach a dislodged lead or to attend to the patient in a medical emergency.

Central Venous Pressure Line, or Central Line, or Triple Lumen

A *central venous pressure line* is a large catheter placed through a vein in the shoulder or neck into the right atrium of the heart. The pressure at the end of heart diastole is then recorded by the catheter, and interpreted by a manometer which provides a central venous pressure reading.[11] The catheter's large size also allows for the administration of fluids and medication.

Arterial Line or Art-Line

The *arterial line* is a catheter placed into an artery in the wrist (Figure 8-2). This measures blood pressure readings and is a convenient way for nursing to take blood samples.

Intravenous Line

An *intravenous (IV) line* is a catheter inserted in a vein (Figure 8-3). An IV line is a way to administer fluids and medications to the patient. It also allows access to the veins to pull blood. It is recommended that IV lines be placed in a comfortable location for the client.

Intravenous Pumps

An *IV pump* is a small machine perched on a pole on the patient's bedside. There may be several of these poles that have bags of fluids. These types of pumps work with the IV line to administer medications or fluids for hydration to the patient.

Endotracheal Tubes

Endotracheal tubes are flexible tubes inserted into the oral or nasal cavity and into the trachea. This allows patients to breathe through the tube, especially in situations when they have no consciousness or have neurological conditions that make breathing difficult. These tubes can control the patient's airway or provide mechanical ventilation. Physical therapist assistants must be aware that an endotracheal tube maybe a sign that the patient is not fully awake and needs help breathing. Physical therapist assistants must also note that since the tube passes through the larynx and vocal cord, the patient is not able to talk until the tube is removed.

Nasogastric or Orogastric Tube

A *nasogastric* or *orogastric tube* (NGT) is a flexible tube inserted through the nose or mouth and into the patient's stomach. It is used to prevent the patient from vomiting and is normally used 48 to 72 hours post-surgery. When used to remove stomach contents, a physical therapist assistant may notice that the NGT is attached to a suction bottle bedside. If the patient will stay in the NCU, the NGT may be used to provide the patient with nutrition.

Feeding Tubes

Nutrition administration to a patient staying in neurocritical care may begin with the use of the IV line. In the event of a prolonged stay in neurocritical care, the patient may then be administered nutrition through the NGT. However, NGTs carry the risk of fluid aspiration and are easily pulled. A gastrostomy tube may then be used to reduce such risk. A gastrostomy tube is a flexible tube surgically inserted directly into the stomach. This allows the patient to continue to receive valuable nutrients essential for recovery and healing.

A conscious neurologic patient who is able to speak and swallow must be referred to the speech pathologist, who will prepare the patient for safe eating. A swallow test or a barium test will be administered to determine any difficulties or issues with swallowing, including pain or bloodstained vomiting.

Cervical Brace or Neck Brace

Patients with a traumatic brain injury (TBI) or patients admitted for severe head and neck trauma are usually seen in the NCU wearing a hard or soft neck brace. An example of a hard cervical brace is the Philadelphia collar. This immobilizes the neck to prevent further damage. Most head traumas may have associated neck issues that will require healing and stability.

Swan-Ganz Catheter

The *Swan-Ganz catheter* is used to measure hemodynamic function such as blood flow pressure and fluid status. This thin, specialized catheter is used to obtain measures of pressure and fluid status. The catheter is inserted directly into the right side of the heart and pulmonary artery with a balloon at the end to prevent displacement.

Restraints

Restraints are soft leather or cloth devices used on patients who may knowingly or unknowingly harm others or pull and displace tubes by mistake. Small children, difficult patients, and agitated patients are restrained after all other methods have been exhausted. The Joint Commission on Accreditation of Healthcare Organizations and the Center for Medicare and Medicaid have guidelines for restraining. Most patients with restraints are closely monitored and evaluated. Physical therapist assistants must alert nursing if they notice that the restraints have caused peripheral circulation issues, skin breakdown, or infections, or have become loosened by biting, kicking, or pulling.

Sequential Compression Devices

Sequential compression devices are plastic tubes wrapped in sleeves placed around the legs. They are connected under the bed to a machine that blows air into the tubes. The pressure on the legs helps blood flow better to prevent blood clots.

Traction

Sometimes bones may not heal well in a cast. They may need to have a small amount of tension or weight placed at the fracture site. This *traction* helps the bones heal in the best position. The tension is created by a series of cords, bars, and weights.

Ventilator

A *ventilator* is a machine used to help the patient breathe and keep enough oxygen in the blood. A tube is inserted through the mouth or nose into the trachea, or wind pipe, and is attached to the ventilator. The patient will not be able to talk until the tube is removed.

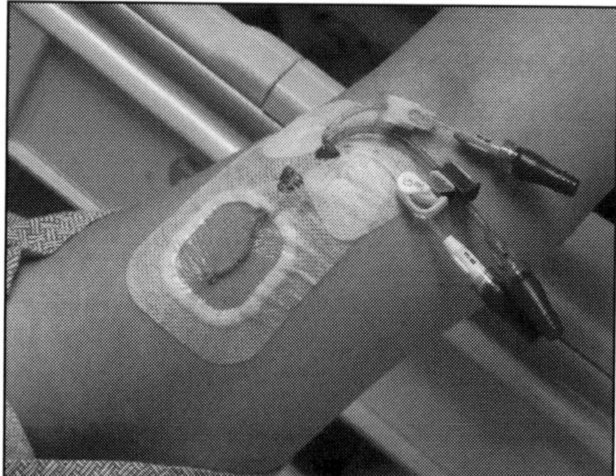

Figure 8-3. An IV line can be used to administer fluids to the patient.

Shunt

A *shunt* is a thin plastic tube placed into the fluid spaces of the brain. The shunt keeps cerebrospinal fluid from draining from the brain down into the abdominal cavity. It may be needed to treat *hydrocephalus*, which occurs when cerebrospinal fluid builds up instead of being absorbed, and causes pressure on the brain.

Chest Tubes

Chest tubes are inserted into the pleural space between the ribs and the lungs. They drain fluid, air, or blood that can collect in this space. This tube will be attached to a drainage system. Sometimes suction is used to help it drain better. The suction causes the bubbling noise heard at the end of the bed.

Intracranial Pressure Monitoring in Brain Edema

Intracranial Pressure Monitor

This small pressure sensor is placed surgically beneath the skull. It attaches to the ICP monitor at the top of the bed, allowing staff to continuously watch the ICP.

Specialized Critical Care Equipment for Neonates

The physical therapist assistant may also encounter specialized equipment used in the critical care of neonates. Following is basic information regarding this equipment.[12]

Oxygen Hood

Usually made of plastic or plexiglass, the oxygen hood provides oxygen in a controlled and closed environment, usually on the head of an infant.

Extracorporeal Membrane Oxygenator

The extracorporeal membrane oxygenator[13] uses a filter to supplement an infant's blood with oxygen. This device is normally used for infants with severe respiratory distress. An infant using this device is usually not stable for physical therapy.

Positioning in the extracorporeal membrane oxygenator requires the infant's head to be rotated to a side. This will require therapy following stabilization to encourage better movement patterns.

Radiant Warmer

A flat bed to allow for tubes and lines for an infant, a radiant warmer also has an adjustable surface with a radiant heat source.

Isolette

Formerly referred to as an incubator, the isolette is an enclosed plastic or plexiglass area creating a humidified environment in a controlled temperature. Portholes and doors allow nurses, therapists, and caregivers access to the infant. Neonates are kept in an isolette until temperature homeostasis is observed.

Positioning in the Intensive Care Unit

Positioning is crucial in the early stages of an injury to prevent further secondary complications such as contractures, pressure sores, edema, and deep vein thrombosis. Early intervention in the acute phases can begin once the patient is medically stable.

Cerebrovascular Accident

A patient who has experienced an acute cerebrovascular accident will need positioning by the physical therapist assistant immediately after the initial physical therapy evaluation. Patients should be positioned out of abnormal postures that are typically assumed to prevent contractures due to soft tissue shortening. While this is discussed under cerebrovascular accidents, the principles are also applicable to patients with abnormal tonal problems following central nervous system insults.

Typical Abnormal Posturing

The patient may present with an upper extremity flexion synergy and lower extremity extension synergy. The scapula will be in a downward rotated position and may have winging present when the patient is weight-bearing. The upper extremity is held in internal rotation with adduction of the shoulder, elbow flexion, forearm pronation, wrist flexion, ulnar deviation, and finger flexion (Figure 8-4). The glenohumeral joint is typically depressed and, along with the downward rotation of the scapula, may cause shoulder subluxation. The lower extremity is typically extended at the hip and the knee with the hip in adduction, internal rotation, and ankle plantar flexion.

Supine

Proper positioning is important to prevent development of abnormal postures and secondary impairments such as contractures or bedsores. For the affected upper extremity, the scapula should be protracted, and slightly abducted with flexion at the shoulder so the arm can rest on a pillow when in supine. The elbow should be extended with the wrist in neutral, fingers extended, and the thumb abducted. The hand and wrist may be positioned in a resting splint in this position to prevent contractures, or may be placed on a pillow for support. One common mistake in positioning a patient who has hypertonia in the upper extremity is to place a soft object like a towel roll in the hand to open the hand and extend the fingers. Due to the presence of increased tone, a soft and pliable object such as a towel can create a trigger for the patient to squeeze the hand into a fist. This is why a resting splint that is much less pliable is recommended. (Figure 8-5) For the affected lower extremity, the pelvis should be protracted, and a small towel roll should be placed under the knee to prevent hyperextension. If the patient has excessive plantar flexion, a resting splint can be useful to correct the abnormal posture and bring the ankle to a more neutral position (Figure 8-6).

Another common mistake when positioning a patient who has hypertonia in the lower extremity is to place a firm object against the soles of the feet to prevent plantar flexion. Due to the presence of increased tone, the patients will typically press against the firm surface with the forefoot, going into further plantar flexion.

Side-Lying on the Hemiplegic Side

The affected upper extremity should be placed in scapular protraction so the patient is not lying directly on the affected shoulder. This will also prevent spasticity in the scapular retractors, which will drastically reduce scapulohumeral motion. The affected upper limb should be placed in slight shoulder abduction and external rotation with the elbow extended. The forearm should be placed in supination with the wrist neutral, fingers extended, and thumb abducted. Often, a pillow placed in front of the patient along the trunk will provide stability and comfort to the unaffected upper extremity. The lower extremity should be placed in 1 of 2 positions. The first is to have the hip extended and the knee flexed. The second is to have the pelvis protracted with the hip and knee slightly flexed (Figure 8-7).

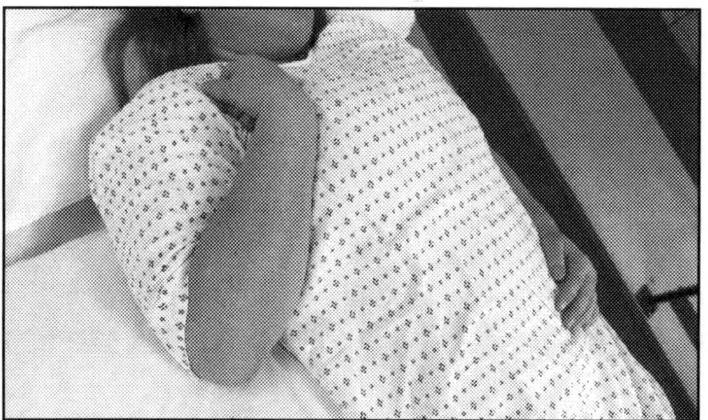

Figure 8-4. Typical abnormal posturing of the upper limb in a patient with a cerebrovascular accident.

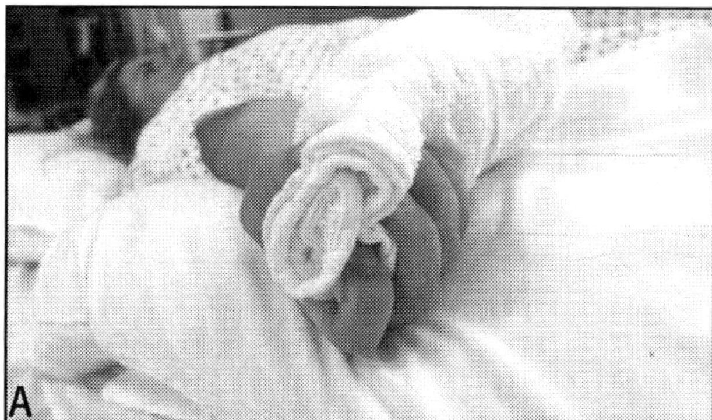

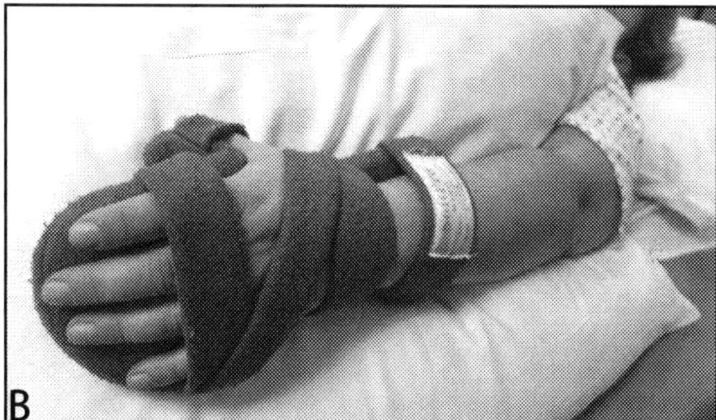

Figure 8-5. (A) Towel roll placement vs (B) resting hand splint on a patient with a cerebrovascular accident.

Side-Lying on the Non-Hemiplegic Side

The affected upper extremity should be placed in scapular protraction by placing the arm onto a pillow in front of the patient. The elbow should be extended with the wrist in neutral, the fingers extended, and the thumb abducted. The affected lower extremity should be placed with the hip and knee flexed forward in front of the unaffected leg and supported on a pillow (Figure 8-8).

Traumatic Brain Injury

A patient with a TBI can follow general positioning standards as those who are post-cerebrovascular accident. In addition, the patient should be positioned in bed or in the wheelchair with the head in neutral. This positioning can reduce the effects of tonic neck reflexes, which may be present in the early stages after a TBI. Gravity affects the vestibular system, especially when supine, and turning of the head affects the proprioceptors of the neck. Both have the potential of triggering reflex activity from the brainstem that often is called *tonic neck reflexes*. The patient who is confined in bed should be turned every 2 hours to prevent skin breakdown and contractures. Splints, such as Multi Podus (Restorative Care of America) boots, may also be used to prevent further contractures while the patient is immobile (Figure 8-9).

Positioning for a patient post-TBI will also influence interaction with the environment. This includes sensory integration and attention or cognition. For example, a patient who is positioned properly in the Fowler's position with the head in neutral can be introduced to charts or graphs that serve as memory aides. Physical therapist assistants can incorporate cognitive training with repetition of names, photo charts, routine activities, and other basic recall information into their treatment with these patients. Having the head of the bed elevated in the Fowler's position is also beneficial to manage increased ICP in patient's after a TBI. When the patient is lying flat, the effects of gravity can increase ICP.

The physical therapist assistant should expect to provide continual reminders and cues to person, place, and time. Carryover of a task is unlikely in the acute states of a severe injury. Another strategy to improve attention is to work in a closed environment. Having little distraction—such as people, television, and bright lights—helps patients focus on the task at hand. Patients may experience mental and physical fatigue during treatment and need frequent rest breaks. Signs of mental fatigue include increased irritability, decreased concentration, decreased performance of a task, and delayed initiation of movement (see Chapter 12).

Feedback is also important to improve learning and attention. In the early stages, the therapist immediately provides feedback in an extrinsic manner. However, as the patient progresses, feedback will be more beneficial if it is intrinsic in nature. The physical therapist assistant should remember that a patient who has decreased attention will likely become overwhelmed with too much feedback. Using concise and simple verbal cues will create a better learning environment.

Spinal Cord Injury

For patients who have experienced a SCI, the development of pressure sores is the primary concern. Patients in the ICU must be turned every 2 hours by staff. If an area of the patient's body develops redness, the position of the patient must be altered immediately to reduce the pressure. Skin condition will initially be monitored 24 hours a day by nursing staff, family members, and therapists. The goal

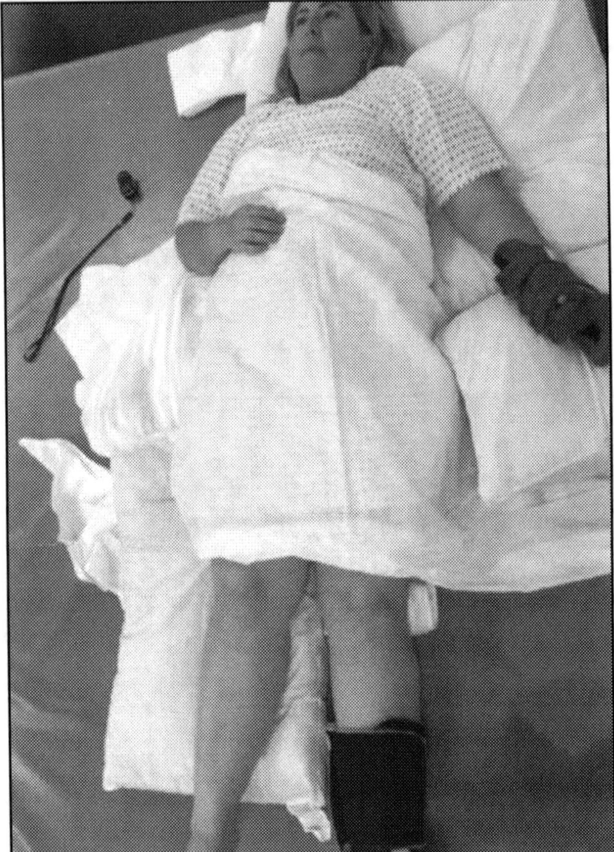

Figure 8-6. Optimal positioning in the supine position.

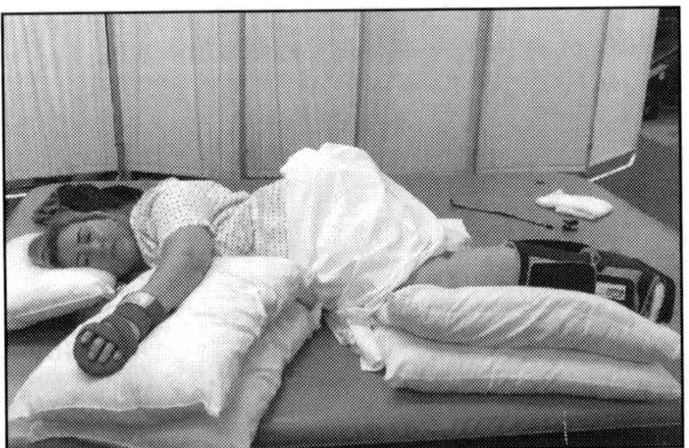

Figure 8-8. Optimal positioning in the side-lying position on the unaffected side.

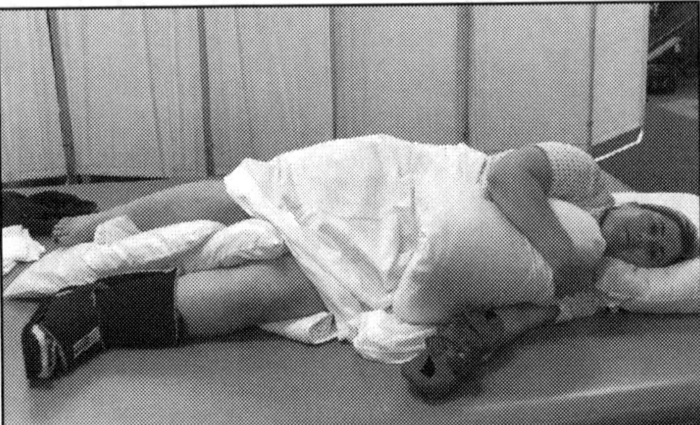

Figure 8-7. Optimal positioning in the side-lying position on the affected side.

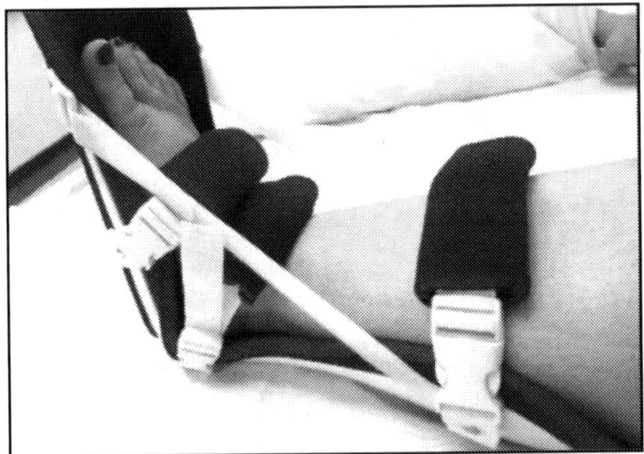

Figure 8-9. Night splint to prevent contractures.

for the patient is to be independent at skin checks once returning home.

Another concern among patients with an SCI is that of poor venous return. This may cause increased risk of deep vein thrombosis development. The loss of the ability of the muscles to create a "pump" in the lower extremities will decrease the amount of venous return and therefore increase the risk of developing blood clots. Also, vessel walls deteriorate with prolonged pressure and lead to deep vein thrombosis development. This will be true for any individual whose circulatory system is in stasis. Elastic support stockings, such as thromboembolism-deterrent hose, can assist with providing pressure upward from the distal limb toward the heart. Turning the patients every 2 hours will diminish the amount of pressure that is placed on the large vessels. Also, frequent passive range of motion programs can reduce the risk of blood pooling and assist with venous return. The physical therapist assistant should focus on elevating the lower extremities above the heart while the patient is in supine to improve venous return.

Patients with an SCI have an increased risk of developing contractures due to the lack of optimal movement and the muscle imbalance that develops over time. To prevent contractures, the physical therapist assistant must be diligent in positioning the patient. The hip joints will likely develop hip flexion, internal rotation, and adduction contractures. The contracture risk will decrease if the patient is positioned out of these postures, ideally spending time in prone each day.

In the upper extremity, patients develop either flexion or extension contractures along with internal rotation and adduction of the shoulder. The physical therapist assistant should provide positioning strategies out of these abnormal postures. If necessary, the patient may use splints to prevent contracture development. Some joints, however, will benefit from slight contractures to maintain functional ability. For example, a therapist should avoid overstretching the finger flexors because of the benefit that tightness in the finger flexor tendons may have on maintaining a hand that can form a grip when the wrist is extended, otherwise known as the process of *tenodesis*. Also, in patients with tetraplegia, tightness of the muscles in the lower trunk can improve sitting posture and increase stability of the trunk.

Pediatrics

When not properly positioned during recovery, critically ill neonates are prone to developing postural abnormality as well as developmental problems. Some positions that cause deformities include[14]:

- "W" positioning of the upper extremities (shoulder is abducted and externally rotated, and elbows are flexed).
- "Frog-Leg" posturing of the lower extremities (hip is abducted and externally rotated, and knees are flexed).
- Spine hyperextension with scapular retraction and elevation.

Physical therapist assistants also encounter infants who need splinting or who are undergoing splinting of the extremities for improving range of motion, to support limbs, to provide immobilization, and to prevent deformities. The physical therapist assistant must consider the fragile nature of the neonate's integumentary system.[14]

Early Mobility

In recent years, the need for early mobility in patients in the ICU has gained more support and evidence. Patients receiving early mobility have been found to have better outcomes and have shorter stays in the ICU compared to patients who do not receive early mobility.[15] In addition, patients who received physical therapy within the first 48 hours after intubation had no complications, compared to those who did not receive physical therapy. Careful monitoring of vital signs is important to determine if a patient is medically stable enough to participate in early mobility activities (Box 8-3). Patients who meet these criteria can participate in physical therapy 3 to 5 times a week with continual monitoring by the interdisciplinary team.

The Safe Prescription of Mobilizing Patients in Acute Care Settings task force[17] created criteria for safe mobilization of patients in the ICU who have shown hemodynamic stability (Tables 8-1 and 8-2).

Moving in Bed

A major barrier to beginning bed mobility with patients in the ICU is the presence of hemodynamic instability.[18] *Hemodynamic instability* is characterized by bradycardia, tachycardia, blood pressure lability, hypoxia, and/or hypoperfusion (Table 8-3). Hemodynamic instability, however, is not clearly defined in the literature. It has been suggested that when turning a patient in small increments (15 degrees at a time), hemodynamic changes may occur but are considered stable if they return to the patient's baseline within 10 minutes of the activity (Table 8-4).[18] A physical therapist assistant in the ICU should begin by having adequate help to secure all lines and tubes, and to safely turn the patient. The therapist should then begin with small movements and monitor all hemodynamic changes (see Table 8-4). If changes occur to heart rate, respiratory rate, blood pressure and/or oxygen saturation, the therapy should not be immediately stopped. The physical therapist assistant should give the patient time to see if baseline values return. If the patient does not return to baseline, nursing staff and the supervising physical therapist must be notified immediately.

Another strategy to begin movement in the bed is to assist the patient into the chair position in supine. By elevating the head of the bed and flexing the hips and knees to be at 90 degrees, the patient can mimic the sitting position in a completely supported position.

When moving patients who have sustained a SCI, spinal stabilization is crucial. The physical therapist assistant must use the logroll technique to maintain optimal spinal alignment. The physical therapist assistant may place pillows between the patient's legs to prevent twisting of the lower body and pelvis on the spine. If a patient has a cervical spine injury, the patient should be wearing a cervical collar during all mobility activities.

Supine-to-Sit

When going from supine-to-sitting with patients in the ICU, monitoring of the blood pressure and heart rate is very important. Many individuals will experience orthostatic hypotension as a result of intolerance to the upright position after prolonged immobility in the supine position. Specifically, individuals with neurological injuries may be at increased risk due to the lack of optimal muscle pump

Box 8-3

Recommended Criteria for Early Mobility

- Heart rate of 40 to 130 beats/minute
- Systolic blood pressure of less than 180 mm Hg
- Mean arterial pressure greater than 65 mm Hg
- Mechanical ventilation less than 100 mm Hg
- Pulse oximetry greater than 88% to 90%
- Respiratory rate less than 40 breaths/minute
- Mechanical ventilation settings of fraction of inspired oxygen less than 0.60 and positive end-expiratory pressure less than 10
- Alert, able to follow commands and no agitation

Source: Harris, Shahid, 2014.

Table 8-1

Safe Mobilization of Patients in the Intensive Care Unit

	Stage I	***Stage II***	***Stage III***	***Stage IV***
Target Level of Consciousness	• RASS -5 to -2	• RASS -2 to -1	• RASS -1 to +1	• RASS -1 to +1
Strength Criteria to Enter Level			• Arm movement against gravity	• Arm and leg movement against gravity
Turning and Bed Mobility	• Every 2 hours, patient to assist as able	• Every 2 hours, same as level 1 plus: scooting/bridging, supine-sit, sit-supine	• Every 2 hours, gradual withdrawal of assistance. Initiation of training to promote independence.	• Every 2 hours, focus on training to promote independence
Positioning and Devices	• Keep head of bed greater than 30 degrees • Apply splints and other positioning devices per physical therapist/occupational therapist • Prevent pressure ulcers, especially on feet and sacrum	• Same as level 1	• Same as level 1; assess for seating needs	• Same as level 3
Exercise Program	• Passive range of motion	• Active assisted range of motion • Breathing exercises • Stretching • Balance/coordination for head, neck, and trunk	• Same as level 2 with more active involvement. Consider adding arm ergometry.	• Same as level 3. Consider weight-bearing and weight-shifting activities.
Mobilization	• Head of bed greater than 45 degrees for 30 to 60 minutes twice a day; midline head/neck position	• High Fowler's or cardiac chair position for 30 to 60 minutes 3 times a day* • May include tilt table or transfer to chair using mechanical lift*	• Dangle legs off side of bed (patient in sitting; may use ceiling lift for heavy patients) • Start with 5 to 10 minutes sitting balance (initially once a day, and progress to twice a day) • If appropriate strength, sit-to-stand with and without a walker	• If level 3 activities are successful, add weight-shifting and transfers • Initially 30 minutes in a chair (initially once a day and progressing to twice a day) • If transfer is successful, begin ambulation per patient tolerance with and without an assistive device

*Precautions for patients with hypotension. Abbreviation: RASS; Richmond Agitation Sedation Scale. Adapted from Howard RS, Kullmann DM, Hirsch NP. Admission to neurological intensive care: who, when, and why? *J Neurol Neurosurg Psychiatry*. 2003;74(suppl 3):iii2-iii9. doi:10.1136/jnnp.74.suppl_3.iii2.

Table 8-2

Richmond Agitation Sedation Scale (RASS)

Description	Score
Combative, violent and immediate danger to staff	4+
Very agitated, pulls tubes and lines, aggressive	3+
Agitated, frequent non-purposeful movement, fights ventilator	2+
Restless, anxious but not aggressive or vigorous	1+
Alert and calm	0
Drowsy, not fully alert, sustained wakening (eye-opening/contact) to voice greater than 10 seconds	1-
Light sedation, briefly awakens with eye contact to voice less than 10 seconds	2-
Moderate sedation, movement or eye-opening, but no eye contact	3-
Deep sedation, no response to voice, but movement or eye opening to physical stimulation	4-
Unarousable, no response to voice or physical stimulation	5-

Reprinted with permission from Sessler CN, Gosnell MS, Grap MJ, et al. The Richmond Agitation-Sedation Scale: validity and reliability in adult intensive care unit patients. *Am J Respir Crit Care Med*. 2002;166(10):1338-1344. doi:10.1164/rccm.2107138.

Table 8-3

Managing Turning With Patients Who Have Hemodynamic Instability

Hemodynamic Instability: Signs that Prevent Turning

- Life-threatening arrhythmia with symptomatic response (ventricular fibrillation, ventricular tachycardia, supraventricular tachycardia)
- Active fluid resuscitation (no fluid in = no systemic blood pressure)
- Active hemorrhaging: cardiac surgery/active tampenade, gastrointestinal bleed with use of Blakemore tube, active hemorrhaging following trauma
- Change in baseline hemodynamic parameters (eg, blood pressure, heart rate, oxygen saturation, and respiratory rate) that does not return to baseline within 10 minutes of position change (and is not an expected result based on diagnosis)

Recommendations for the Hemodynamic Unstable Patient (If the Patient Has Any of the Signs That Prevent Turning)

A trial should be attempted at least every 8 hours to determine if ability to return to turning every 2 hours is possible

- Provide mini-turns (serial small turning) for hygiene and linen changes
- Weight-shift every 30 minutes and elevate heels off bed
- Reposition the patient's body every hour and consider passive range of motion
- Consider continuous lateral rotation therapy, with slow and low angles of rotation, and gauge response

Unstable Fractures

- Patients with unstable pelvic injuries, logroll patient only, with approval of medical doctor
- Place pillows and wedges between legs to maintain optimal alignment
- Do not use continuous lateral rotation therapy with unstable spinal fractures
- Cervical fractures/unstable: only logroll patient once properly fitted cervical collar is in place

Adapted from Brindle CT, Malhotra R, O'Rourke S, et al. Turning and repositioning the critically ill patient with hemodynamic instability: a literature review and consensus recommendations. *J Wound Ostomy Continence Nurs.* 2013;40(3):254-267. doi:10.1097/WON.0b013e318290448f.

function in the lower extremities that bring blood back up to the heart through the venous system. The physical therapist assistant may start acclimating the patient to the upright position by bringing the head of the bed gradually upright and monitoring vitals at intervals. Allowing the patient to rest with every elevation change will allow time to adapt to the new upright position.

Individuals who have hemiplegia will have a more difficult time moving from supine-to-sit over the unaffected side. However, both directions should be practiced. When moving the patient who has a hemiparetic upper extremity, the physical therapist assistant must ensure that the glenohumeral joint is protected due to its high risk of subluxation. The affected upper extremity should be crossed over the body when rolling toward the unaffected side. During supine-to-sit, the physical therapist assistant should promote weight-bearing through the affected upper extremity through the bed whenever possible. Weight-bearing will encourage muscle activation, co-contraction for stability around the joint, and reduction in tone. The physical therapist assistant can also place the patient in a side-lying position on the affected elbow to promote weight-bearing. This can be done in part through practice of supine-to-sit. The patient will have a more difficult time pushing off the bed from side-lying on the affected side, so this task should be practiced. The therapist may have to support the lower extremities on and off the bed while the patient pushes to the sitting position. The reverse direction should also be practiced to improve controlled lowering of the upper body onto the bed. In patients who have sustained an SCI, the lower extremities must be lowered or raised on and off the bed at the same time as the upper body is moving to prevent side-bending of the trunk, which would bring the spine out of optimal alignment.

Sitting Balance and Tolerance

A patient needs to be able to attend to the following tasks in supine to be able to progress to sitting at the edge of the bed: passive, active assisted, active, and resisted range of motion to all extremities.[19] Once the patient is able to achieve sitting at the edge of the bed, the physical therapist assistant will focus on trunk control, reaching, and sitting tolerance for cardiovascular and respiratory endurance. In patients with hemiparesis, focus will be on weight-bearing through the affected extremity, reaching across midline to minimize neglect, and trunk control.

Patients with SCI who have been prescribed a spinal brace will likely have orders to don the brace once sitting to maintain an optimally aligned spine. Patients who have paraplegia with active control of their triceps should be instructed in externally rotating and hyperextending the shoulders with the elbow and wrist in extension (fingers maintained in flexion to prevent overstretching of tenodesis mechanism; Figure 8-10). Patients without triceps function can be taught to use the shoulder musculature to mechanically achieve extension of the arm. Patients are taught to hyperextend their shoulders with the forearm supinated and toss their hand onto the bed. When the hand comes into contact with the mat, the humerus is flexed to cause the elbow to extend, since the arm is in a closed chain position. To maintain this position, the patient must quickly depress the scapula and stabilize the arm.

During early sitting activities, mirrors can be used to provide visual feedback to the patient (Figure 8-11). The physical therapist assistant can use a vertical line or a piece of tape placed vertically on the mirror as orientation to the upright and vertical position. The physical therapist assistant should provide manual approximation to the shoulders to promote co-contraction of musculature around the shoulder joint. Weight-shifting and scooting can then begin at the edge of the bed to prepare the patient for transfers.

Often a co-treatment may need to be performed in patients who are very low level. For example, patients with a TBI with a Rancho Los Amigos Scale level of 1 to 4[20] will typically need to have 2-person assistance to move to an upright position at the edge of the bed. Tilt tables provide early weight-bearing through the lower extremities and acclimation to the upright position, and may improve overall levels of alertness in these patients. Vital signs should be carefully monitored on a consistent basis whenever adjusting the tilt table to a new degree of elevation. If any vital signs do not return to baseline, the patient should be brought back to the previous degree of tilt where vitals remained stable.

Transfers

Once the patient has demonstrated an ability to maintain a stable sitting position with good trunk control and stable vitals, the patient can begin sit-to-stand training at the edge of the bed. Patients with SCI will initiate transfers by learning lateral squat transfers or sliding board transfers from the bed to the chair and back. Patients who are able to stand may start by using a specialized ICU platform walker (Figure 8-12). This will allow patients to stand and take steps with a stable platform to support the upper body. For safety, the physical therapist assistant must always place a gait belt on the patient during early transfer and ambulation activities.

Initially when performing transfers with patients, the physical therapist assistant can begin with the bed elevated slightly so standing becomes easier for the patient. If the patient is stronger on one side of the body, the wheelchair is typically placed on that stronger side so the patient can transfer to the stronger side. This is a good compensatory strategy initially to make transfers more successful. Eventually, however, the patient should be instructed in moving to both the affected and unaffected side. During the transfer, the therapist should assist at either the trunk or the pelvis.

Table 8-4

Strategies to Prevent Hemodynamic Changes in Response to Turning

- Secure lines
- Have adequate staff present to provide turn
- Turn patient 10 to 15 degrees and pause for 15 seconds, watching monitor
- Continue turning incrementally to achieve full lateral position for skin care
- Slowly return to 30-degree turning position using wedges and pillows to position
- Monitor response to turn over the next 10 minutes
- Individualize turning schedule based on changes in Braden Score (risk for pressure ulcers) and patient condition

Adapted from Brindle CT, Malhotra R, O'rourke S, et al. Turning and repositioning the critically ill patient with hemodynamic instability: a literature review and consensus recommendations. *J Wound Ostomy Continence Nurs.* 2013;40(3):254-267. doi:10.1097/WON.0b013e318290448f.

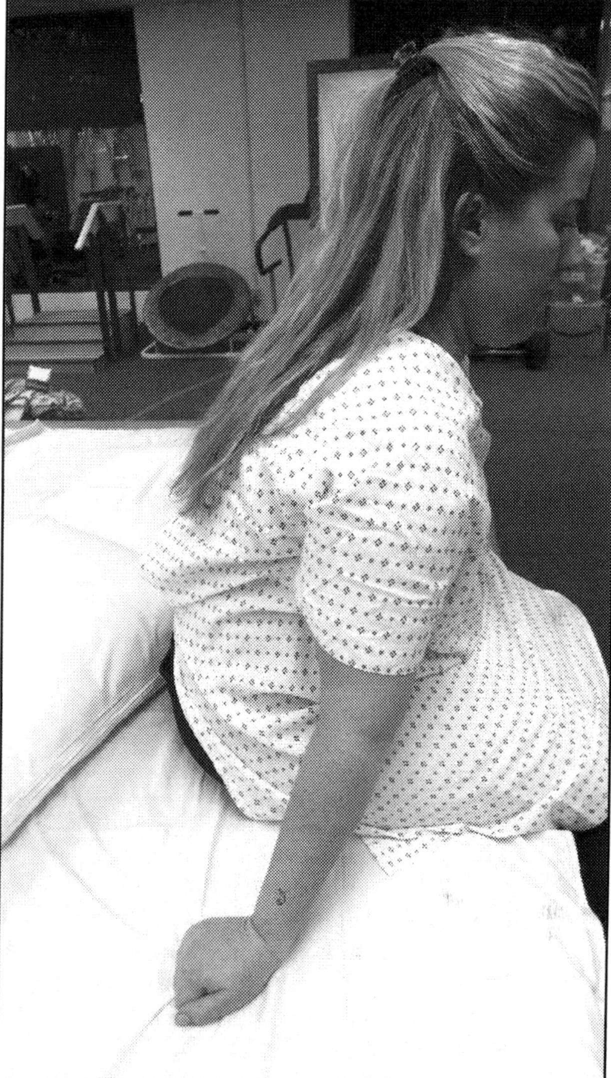

Figure 8-10. Upper extremity positioning and stabilization in sitting, SCI.

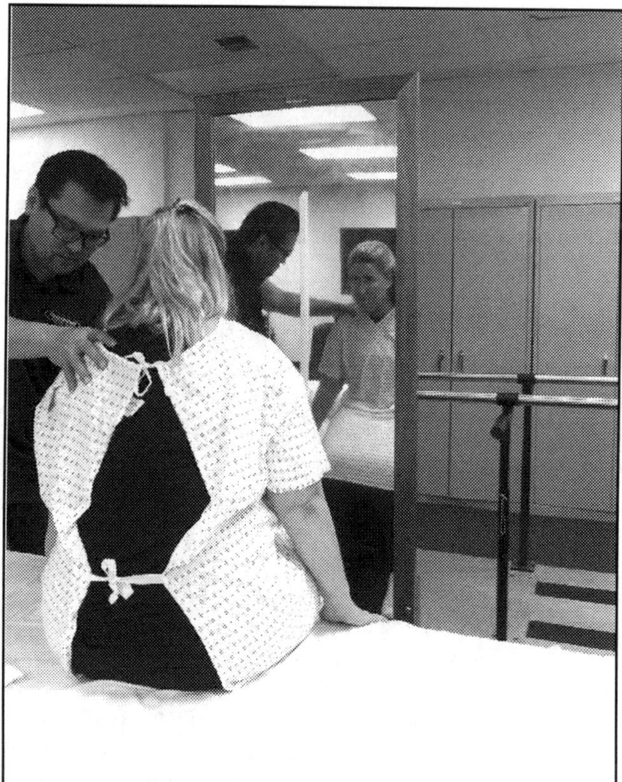

Figure 8-11. Using a mirror as a visual feedback upper extremity stabilization in sitting, SCI.

Special Equipment

The ICU is home to innovative technology and equipment that allow patients to be more successful in their rehabilitation. The supine exercise bike is used with patients who are primarily receiving physical therapy in bed. This bike rolls up to the patient's bed and allows the patient to perform a bicycle exercise to strength the lower extremities in the supine position (Figure 8-13).

If patients are unable to be lifted manually out of the bed, therapists use ceiling lifts to move the patient from the bed to the chair or the bathroom. This allows patients to achieve a sitting position to improve alertness and cardiorespiratory endurance while maintaining safety for the therapist and the patient. A ceiling lift works similar to a Hoyer lift, but is attached to a track in the ceiling of the hospital room (Figure 8-14). This track moves from the bed to positions around the room for easy transport of the patient. The patient is placed in a sling attached to a central moving mechanism similar to that of a Hoyer lift. The benefit of a ceiling lift is that no bulky equipment has to be maneuvered around the room, specifically avoiding connections of lines and tubes (Figure 8-15).

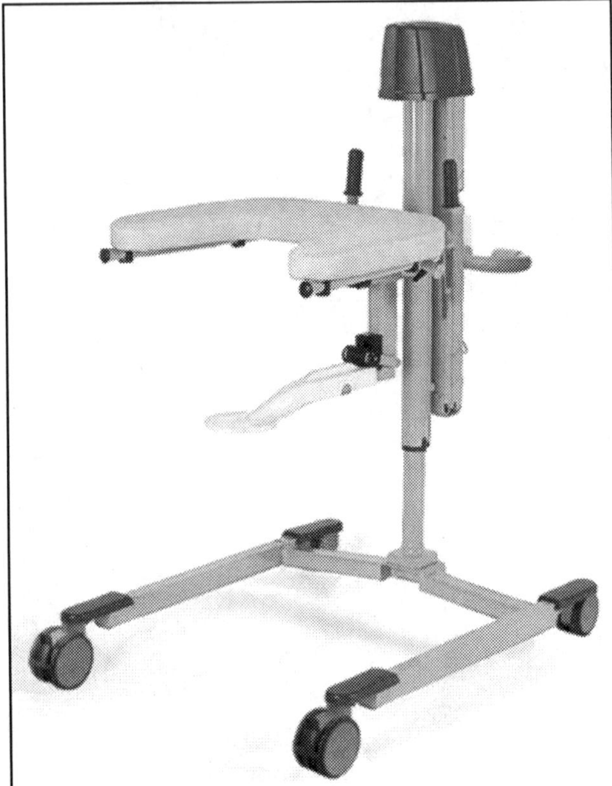

Figure 8-12. Arjo Walker. (Reprinted with permission from Arjo.)

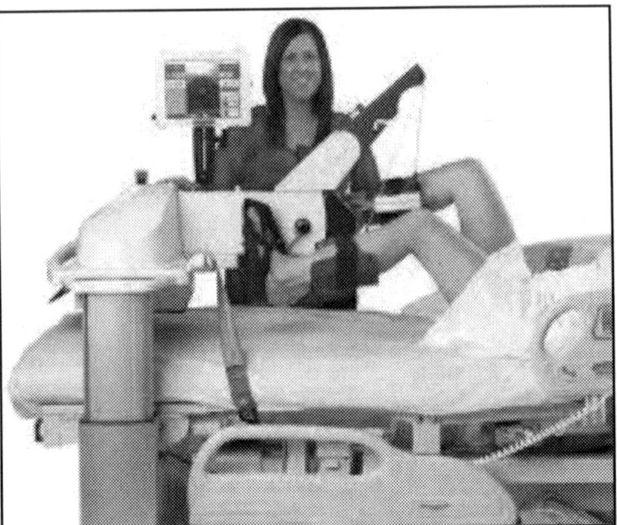

Figure 8-13. Restorative Therapies RT 300 Supine Bike. (Reprinted with permission from Restorative Therapies.)

Another valuable piece of equipment in the ICU is the portable ventilator. This allows patients who are on ventilation the opportunity to be involved in early mobility programs. The ventilator is able to roll along with the patient during movement (Figure 8-16). The therapist will likely require another person to manage the ventilator while the therapist is handling the patient.

Communicating Response to Care

Physical therapist assistants must work closely with the supervising physical therapist in the management of patients in acute care. These patients can be medically unstable and are at high risk of secondary injury. The physical therapist assistant is responsible for communicating to the physical therapist whenever there is a change in status of a patient, a decline in function, unstable vital signs, or adverse reaction to treatment. The supervising physical therapist will need to see patients who require continual changes to their plan of care.

The physical therapist assistant will also need to be in constant communication with the nurses, physicians, and respiratory therapists. If the patient is on a ventilator, the physical therapist assistant will often need to coordinate therapy when the respiratory therapist is present. The nursing staff will need continual reports of vitals and changes in baseline values during therapy. The physician may be contacted once the supervising physical therapist is notified of any change in status or adverse responses to treatment.

Interdisciplinary Team

In the ICU, the physical therapist assistant is a part of a very complex interdisciplinary team including intensive care nurses, physicians, respiratory therapists, occupational therapists, speech therapists, patients, and their families. To optimally care for a patient, clear and consistent communication must occur among the members of the team.

Perceived barriers to early mobilization include fear of pulling out tubes and lines, scheduling therapy with nurses and respiratory therapists for a patient who is on a ventilator, staff shortages, amount of time to mobilize a patient on multiple lines, and safety concerns.[16] To reduce the incidence of perceived barriers inhibiting a patient's ability to receive early mobility, the therapy team must educate and communicate with the other staff members about what will be involved in the treatment and collaborate on safety concerns that may arise.

Family and Staff Training

The physical therapist assistant plays a role in family and staff training to ensure safe and efficient recovery of patients in the ICU. Patients who have upper extremity hemiplegia are at higher risk of subluxation of the affected glenohumeral joint. Staff members and family must be educated in proper handling of the patient during positioning and turning activities. Emphasis should focus on avoiding pulling or traction to the affected upper extremity. While positioned in the bed or in sitting, the patient's affected arm must be adequately supported at all times to prevent the weight of the arm with gravity pulling the joint out of place (Figure 8-17).

If the patient has unilateral neglect, the family should be educated on drawing attention toward the neglected side. Family members can stand on the affected side, place the television or radio on the affected side, and even turn on lights only on the affected side. These activities will promote recognition of the neglected side. Items such as the call bell and water (if applicable) should always be placed on the side that the patient is aware of, to ensure the patient can alert staff if needed.

Patients who have experienced a TBI may exhibit some behavioral impairments. The family should be introduced to the Rancho Los Amigos Level of Cognitive Functioning Scale[20] for information about their family member's current state of cognition.[21] If the patient is entering into a stage of cognition that includes agitation and confusion, educate the family about what to expect. Family members and staff should model calm behavior despite patient outbursts. Egocentric behavior should be expected, and patients will typically have difficulty understanding other points of view. Also, the patient will have difficulty maintaining focus and attention during many phases after a brain injury. The family members and staff should be educated about preventing overstimulation by only allowing 1 or 2 individuals in the room at once, keeping voices relatively quiet, and minimizing loud noises and lights in the patient's room.

Among patients with SCI, family members should be educated about routine skin checks. This will be done by the nursing staff in the ICU, but the family will have to help with this once the patient is home and until the patient is independent. Family and staff should be educated on log-rolling and on appropriately donning and doffing spinal braces and orthotics if applicable. Patients with high-level SCI's (eg, T6 and above) will be at risk of autonomic dysreflexia, a medical emergency. *Autonomic dysreflexia* is reflex sympathetic outburst that may present with seizures, retinal hemorrhage, pulmonary edema, renal insufficiency, myocardial infarction, cerebral hemorrhage, and in some cases, death. Family members should be educated about the signs of autonomic dysreflexia as well as the most common causes. If unable to identify and remove the noxious stimuli immediately, the family needs to be educated to notify the nursing staff immediately.

No matter what diagnosis the patient has, the family should always have a clear line of communication with the therapist. The physical therapist assistant should provide the family with realistic expectations of the patient's capabilities and limitations as set forth by the prognosis in the plan of care. Families can take part in passive range of motion exercises to prevent joint contractures and simple bed exercises if applicable. Family members who will perform these activities must be trained and evaluated on their accuracy with a therapist present. Giving a family member a task will allow the family members to feel more helpful as they take an active part in the patient's recovery.

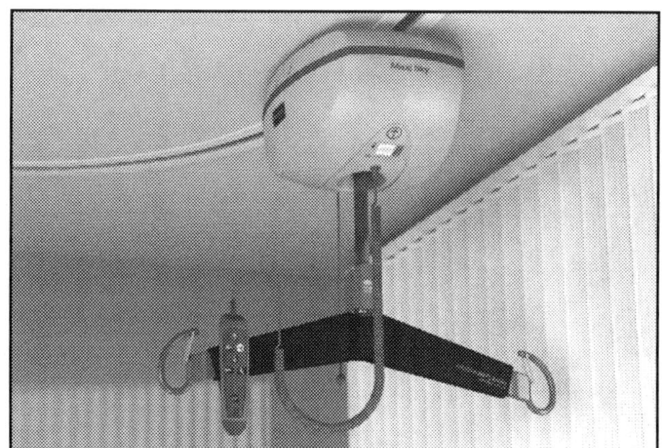

Figure 8-14. Arjo Ceiling Lift. (Reprinted with permission from Arjo.)

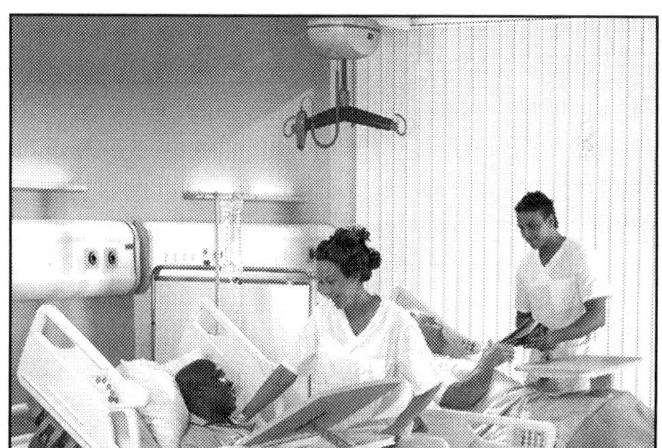

Figure 8-15. Arjo Maxi Sky 2 Ceiling Lift. (Reprinted with permission from Arjo.)

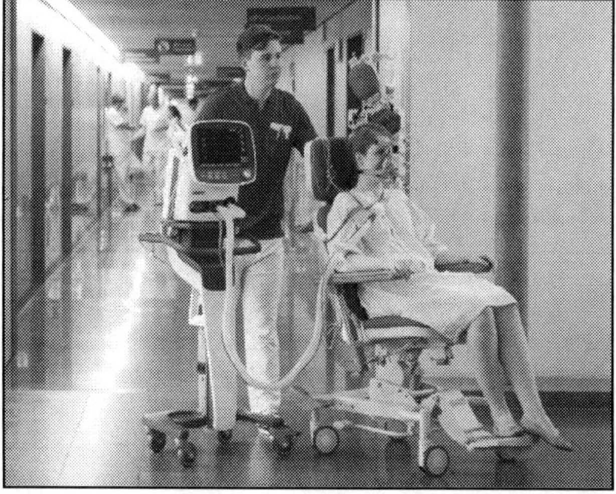

Figure 8-16. Hamilton Medical Hamilton-C3 Transport Ventilator. (Reprinted with permission from Hamilton Medical.)

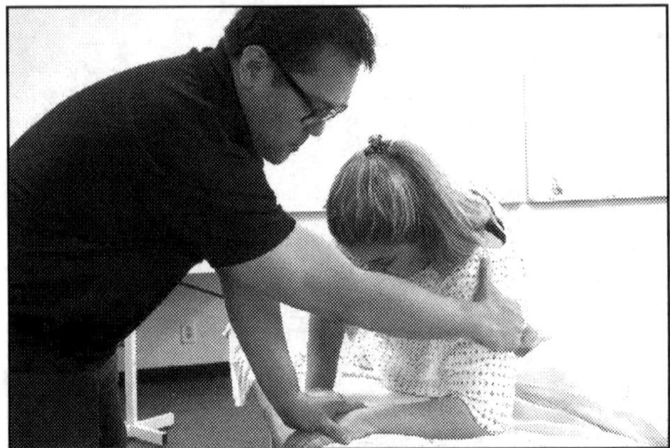

Figure 8-17. Supporting the affected extremity to prevent subluxation.

Conclusion

This chapter provided an overview of the roles of the physical therapist assistant in NCUs, as delegated by the physical therapist. The complex nature of the interventions, the presence of specialized equipment, and the fragility of the patients' conditions necessitate a highly specialized and closely coordinated patient care to optimize outcomes. Physical therapy plays an important role in this setting, and a physical therapist/physical therapist assistant team provides critical interventions aimed at optimizing the patient's mobility and function.

Case Study

Mr. Fin is a 72-year-old man who recently was admitted to the ICU after sustaining a fall causing a right (R) intracranial hemorrhage. He has a history of diabetes mellitus type 2, hypertension, and atrial fibrillation. X-rays revealed that during the fall, Mr. Fin sustained a fracture to his (R) femoral neck. He underwent surgery and placement of an open reduction and internal fixation on the (R) femur 1 day ago. Mr. Fin has the following lines/tubes in place: A-line (R) arm, IV (L) ventral forearm, oxygen 2L/min, and an endotracheal tube. The physical therapist has evaluated the patient and determined that his Richmond Agitation Sedation Scale level is -1. The patient is stable in all hemodynamic parameters but will need constant monitoring during therapy. The physical therapist has given the physical therapist assistant the following instructions:

1. Perform passive range of motion and active assisted range of motion in supine. The range of motion in the right lower extremity is adjusted accordingly according to pain tolerance.
2. Elevate the head of the bed to 45 degrees, and instruct the patient in breathing exercises.
3. Transfer to the cardiac chair.
4. Instruct the patient in balance exercises, maintaining trunk and head in midline in the cardiac chair position.

Questions

1. What vital signs need to be monitored throughout the treatment?
2. What are signs of hemodynamic instability during activity?
3. Assuming the patient has a significant drop in blood pressure during the balance activities, what would the physical therapist assistant's next step be? Whom would the physical therapist assistant need to communicate with regarding the patient's vital signs?

References

1. Booker KT. *Critical Care Nursing: Monitoring and Treatment for Advanced Nursing Practice.* Ames, IA: John Wiley & Sons, Inc; 2015.
2. Mullins PM, Goyal M, Pines JM. National growth in intensive care unit admissions from emergency departments in the United States from 2002 to 2009. *Acad Emerg Med.* 2013;20(5):479-486. doi:10.1111/acem.12134
3. Zacharia BE, Vaughan KA, Bruce SS, et al. Epidemiological trends in the neurological intensive care unit from 2000 to 2008. *J Clin Neurosci.* 2012;19(12):1668-1672. doi:10.1016/j.jocn.2012.04.011
4. Howard RS, Kullmann DM, Hirsch NP. Admission to neurological intensive care: who, when, and why? *J Neurol Neurosurg Psychiatry.* 2003;74(suppl 3):iii2-iii9. doi:10.1136/jnnp.74.suppl_3.iii2
5. Dunn LT. Raised intracranial pressure. *J Neurol Neurosurg Psychiatry.* 2002;73(suppl 1):i23-i27. doi:10.1136/jnnp.73.suppl_1.i23
6. Cherian A, Thomas SV. Status epilepticus. *Ann Indian Acad Neurol.* 2009;12(3):140-153. doi:10.4103/0972-2327.56312
7. Ng KK, Howard RS, Fish DR, et al. Management and outcome of severe Guillain-Barré syndrome. *QJM.* 1995;88(4):243-250.
8. Andrews FJ, Nolan JP. Critical care in the emergency department: monitoring the critically ill patient. *Emerg Med J.* 2006;23(7):561-564. doi:10.1136/emj.2005.029926
9. Vold ML, Aasebø U, Wilsgaard T, Melbye H. Low oxygen saturation and mortality in an adult cohort: the Tromsø study. *BMC Pulm Med.* 2015;15(1):9. doi:10.1186/s12890-015-0003-5
10. Chatterjee S, Miller A. *Biomedical Instrumentation Systems.* Clifton Park, NY: Delmar Cengage Learning; 2011.
11. Holmes N, Schilling-McCann J. *Lippincott's Nursing Procedures.* 5th ed. Philadelphia, PA: Lippincott, Williams, & Wilkins; 2009.
12. March of Dimes. Common NICU Equipment. https://www.marchofdimes.org/complications/common-nicu-equipment.aspx. Accessed October 2, 2018.
13. Stanford Children's Health. Procedures and Equipment in the NICU. https://www.stanfordchildrens.org/en/topic/default?id=procedures-and-equipment-in-nicu-90-P02358. Accessed October 2, 2018.
14. O'Shea R. Pediatrics for the Physical Therapist Assistant. St. Louis, MO: Saunders Elsevier; 2009.

15. Morris PE, Goad A, Thompson C, et al. Early intensive care unit mobility therapy in the treatment of acute respiratory failure. *Crit Care Med.* 2008;36(8):2238-2243. doi:10.1097/CCM.0b013e318180b90e
16. Harris CL, Shahid S. Physical therapy-driven quality improvement to promote early mobility in the intensive care unit. *Proc Bayl Univ Med Cent.* 2014;27(3):203-207. doi:10.1080/08998280.2014.11929108
17. Dean E, Reid D, Chung F, et al. Safe prescription of mobilizing patients in acute care settings: What to assess, what to monitor, when not to mobilize, and how to mobilize and progress. SAFEMOB Task Force. http://med-fom-clone-pt.sites.olt.ubc.ca/files/2012/05/SAFEMOB_Final18673.pdf. Accessed October 2, 2018.
18. Brindle CT, Malhotra R, O'rourke S, et al. Turning and repositioning the critically ill patient with hemodynamic instability: a literature review and consensus recommendations. *J Wound Ostomy Continence Nurs.* 2013;40(3):254-267. doi:10.1097/WON.0b013e318290448f
19. Engel HJ, Needham DM, Morris PE, Gropper MA. ICU early mobilization: from recommendation to implementation at three medical centers. *Crit Care Med.* 2013;41(9)(suppl 1):S69-S80. doi:10.1097/CCM.0b013e3182a240d5
20. Hagen C, Malkmus D, Durham P. *Levels of Cognitive Functioning.* Downey, CA: Rancho Los Amigos Hospital; 1972.
21. Rancho Los Amigos Level of Cognitive Functioning Scale. https://www.neuroskills.com/resources/rancho-los-amigos-revised.php. Accessed October 2, 2018.

Please visit www.routledge.com/9781630915650 to access additional material.

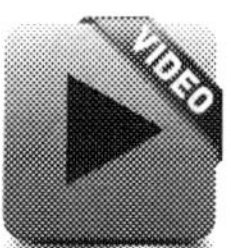

Chapter 9

Children With Central Nervous System Insult

Kristine N. Corn, PT, MS, DPT and Darcy A. Umphred, PT, PhD, FAPTA

KEY WORDS Anoxic brain injury | Athetosis | Cerebral palsy | Diplegia | Facilitation | Handling techniques | Hemiplegia | Hypoxic brain injury | Inhibition | Quadriplegia | Triplegia

Chapter Objectives

- Introduce the more frequently treated pediatric medical neurological diagnoses from insults that occur in utero, at birth, or shortly after birth.
- Differentiate between trauma to the central nervous system (CNS) in the neonate and acquired trauma after 2 years of age that primarily affects the motor system.
- Introduce some of the more common characteristics observed in the pediatric patient with the medical neurological diagnosis of cerebral palsy (CP).
- Introduce handling and treatment ideas for the child with neurological impairment.

Physical therapist assistants working in the pediatric neurological clinic or hospital will treat a wide and varied population of children who will continually challenge their critical thinking and creativity. When a child's CNS is damaged, 1 or more systems can be affected, depending on the location and cause of the insult. Physical therapists and physical therapist assistants treat children with movement dysfunction and/or sensory processing disorders to prevent skeletal deformities and encourage normal development of motor, perceptual, and cognitive skills. Often, insults to the CNS affect postural core/axial muscle tone as well as distal muscle tone, strength, and sensory processing. The postural tone and motor control will influence and be influenced by feedback and feedforward information from all the sensory systems (see Chapter 4). Some of the more common CNS diagnoses treated in a pediatric physical therapy department are CP, genetic disorders, autism spectrum disorders, sensory processing dysfunction, anoxic/hypoxic, and traumatic brain injury (TBI).

For some of these disorders, the causation is clear, whereas in other CNS dysfunctions, the causation is not well understood or is unknown. It is always helpful to have a clear medical diagnosis, but this is not always possible. As the profession of physical therapy deals with movement dysfunctions resulting from CNS insults and not the pathology itself, the patient's clinical signs and symptoms (ie, functional limitations) guide the physical therapist to determine the appropriate treatment program for each individual. The physical therapist will then determine what portion of the treatment program will be delegated to the physical therapist assistant, and whether it is appropriate for the physical therapist assistant to perform follow-up examinations that identify whether the intervention is meeting expected goals. In some of these medical diagnoses, such as CP and TBI, the specific therapy movement diagnosis and movement disorder depend on muscle tone, controlled patterns of movement, and the areas or segments of the body involved, which often reflect the anatomy involvement that led to the medical diagnosis.

Lazaro RT, Umphred DA, eds.
Umphred's Neurorehabilitation for the Physical Therapist Assistant, Third Edition (pp 185-210).

Table 9-1
Areas of Motor Involvement

Area of Central Nervous System Involvement Due to Bleeds or Anoxia		
Area of Insult	**Cause**	**Involvement**
Periventricular	Central bleed	Diplegic
Parietal lobe	Hemispheric bleed	Hemiplegic
Frontal motor	Global ischemia	Quadriplegic
Distal cortical		Spastic/multisystem
Cerebellar	Anoxia	Quadriplegic athetoid
Diencephalon	Total asphyxia	Ataxic
Classification by Muscle Tone		
Pathology	**Tone Quality**	**Impairment**
Hypertonic	High tone	Decreased joint mobility and motor control problems
Hypotonic	Low tone	Increased joint mobility and motor control problems
Mixed programming	Low to high tone	Increased joint mobility of trunk and neck. Decreased joint mobility of the extremities and motor control problems.
Fluctuating programming	Athetoid	Decreased grading of strength/joint range of motion, poor stabilization, often normal mobility
Regulatory inconsistencies in programming	Ataxic	Trunk instability, increased joint mobility, and gait disturbances in force, rate, timing

Although physical therapy always considers that medical diagnosis, the physical therapist's responsibility and focus are to treat movement disorders associated with the functional limitation of the child. As classification of muscle tone often identified with a medical diagnosis, it is beneficial when evaluating and analyzing motor dysfunction and determining appropriate treatment (Table 9-1).

Table 9-2 describes the area or areas of the body involved in motor dysfunction.

Cerebral Palsy

CP is the most common medical diagnosis and resulting physical disability of childhood. Children with CP are generally seen as having motor control problems; however, they may demonstrate sensory deficits that affect the CNS's normal maturation of motor control, and ultimately their general development and function. The individual with CP incurred damage to the CNS during gestation (ie, prenatal), at the time of birth (ie, natal), or within the first few weeks of life (ie, postnatal). Basic patterns of motor behavior have not been established at the time of the insult. These basic components of movement are essential in developing normal postural alignment, equilibrium, and protective responses. As the child begins to move, more automatic behaviors or stereotypical motor behaviors are repetitively demonstrated and elicited by sensory input or intention. These motor behaviors may become the dominant movement patterns as the child develops, because of the limitations in available motor control. These patterns are considered abnormal and interfere with normal skill acquisition and motor control, ultimately limit their motor learning, and often restrict the more complicated motor behaviors seen in children considered their age match (see Chapter 4). Depending on the child's age when the insult occurred and the extent of the involvement, a wide variety of dysfunction in postural control and skill development will be observed.

With or without a formal medical diagnosis of CP, a neonate who has suffered a CNS insult will, within the first few weeks of life, present subtle signs of motor involvement, unless the damage has been fairly severe. The infant's tone may be initially low or hypotonic, causing decreased head and trunk control. Reflexive movement patterns are present and may be appropriate based on the infant's age (or corrected age for those born prematurely). The physical therapist must be well appraised of normal neonatal development. It is more common that a child of 12 months or older who is diagnosed with CP is referred for physical therapy because the child has not achieved the normal milestones and appropriate developmental skills (eg, coming to sit or sitting if placed in that position, and moving independently from the sitting position). Children who are 12 months old should be crawling, pulling to stand, practicing standing balance, or even beginning to take their first steps (see Chapter 3).[1,2] Once the physical therapist has evaluated the

Table 9-2

Classification by Areas of Involvement

Medical Classification	***Movement Dysfunction***
Hemiplegic	More significant involvement of either left or right extremities with often lesser involvement of opposite extremities
Diplegic	The trunk and lower extremities have greater involvement than the upper extremities
Triplegic	The trunk and 3 extremities
Quadriplegic	The trunk and all 4 extremities

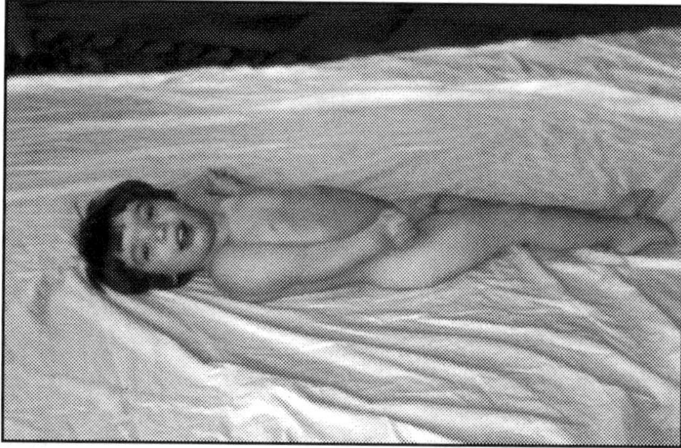

Figure 9-1. A child with severe tonal abnormality will often demonstrate involvement in all 4 extremities. This child would be considered to have spastic quadriplegia.

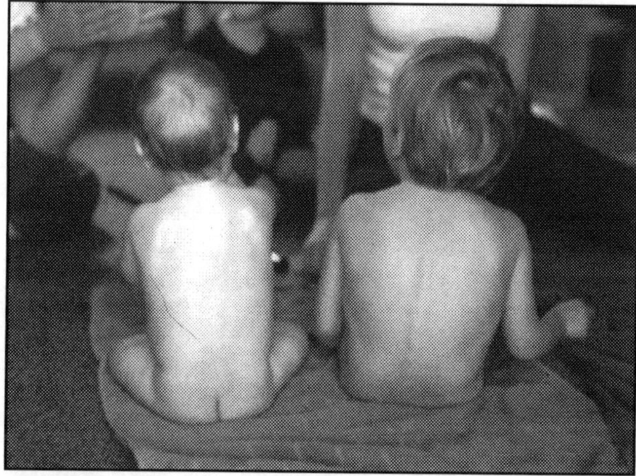

Figure 9-2. Comparison of sitting postures of a normal 6-month-old child to his 2-year-old brother with the diagnosis of spastic athetosis: Posterior view.

child and determined what abnormal motor patterns are limiting function and normal progression of movement, what normal motor behaviors need to be practiced, what sensory systems need to be heightened, and which ones require dampening, a plan of care can be established. This plan of care often incorporates the need to eliminate reflexive patterns that are limiting the development of normal movement while integrating protective responses, postural control, and improving motor responses that will lead to better motor control. From that plan of care, the physical therapist should be able to delegate activities that are within the physical therapist assistant's competencies.

The older child, between 18 months and 4 years, may have developed compensatory patterns of movement that the physical therapist assistant will be able to recognize as abnormal movement patterns that limit functional movement and the child's progression in motor control. The movement maybe labored as the child attempts to overcome hypertonicity, asymmetric muscle tone, and decreased postural stability. Repetitive abnormal posturing that accompanies increased muscle tone will eventually cause contractual deformities of the soft tissues and can create more permanent joint deformities. When this occurs, there is poor alignment of the joints in relation to each other, interfering with positioning, handling, and care. Encouraging the child to continue to practice these abnormal patterns does not reflect motor learning concepts, even though repetitive practice leads to learning. The physical therapist needs to determine whether those specific patterns will lead to greater function or limit the progress of the child to future function. If just practicing leads to limitation, that plan of care will not empower the child to the flexibility to engage in future social activities requiring more complex motor function and will limit that child's potential quality of life.

Generally, these musculoskeletal problems are first observed in the more involved extremities (Figure 9-1). Without therapy and parental involvement, these soft tissue deformities may cause bony changes, skeletal deformities, and eventual dislocations. Although the hypotonic child does not have to work against increased muscle tone, the child needs to develop sufficient muscle strength and postural control to overcome gravity and be able to come to sit and stand. The hypotonic child generally presents with poor to fair head and trunk control (Figures 9-2 and 9-3). Low tone often causes deformities of the spine due to lack of sufficient symmetric postural control. With either hypertonia or hypotonia, a complex interaction interferes with selective motor control.[3] Selective motor control is defined as the ability to independently move a joint voluntarily. The inability to isolate a movement without activating or using other parts of a limb is thought to be correlated with the severity of the CNS lesion. Selective motor control is important for the motor control needed for normal functional activities. The physical therapist will differentiate these motor dysfunctions as part of the initial assessment. The physical therapist may continue to evaluate the inter-

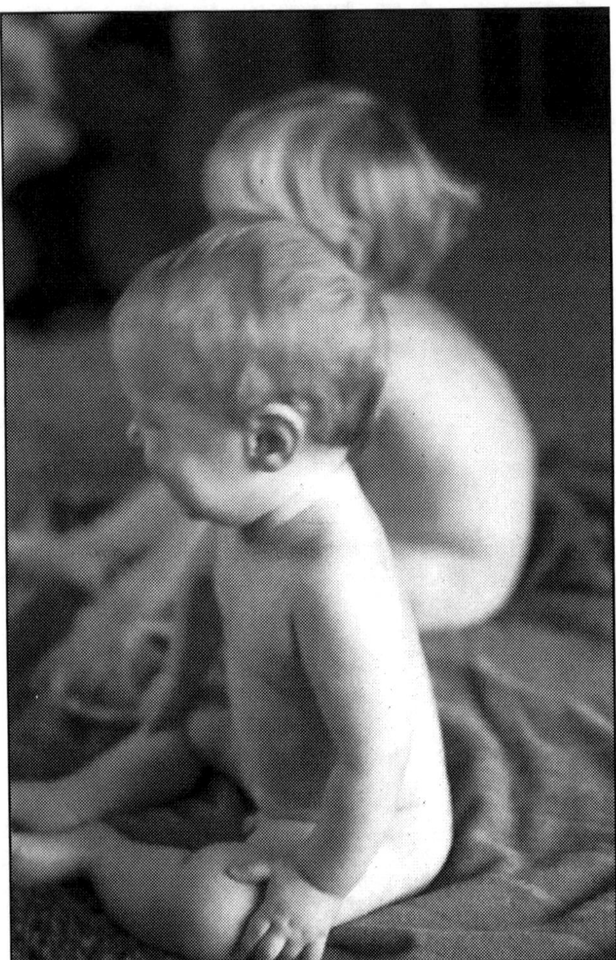

Figure 9-3. A 6-month-old child to his 2-year-old brother with the diagnosis of spastic athetosis: Lateral view.

ventions used and the progress made during each treatment session, or delegate some of examination responsibilities to the physical therapist assistant. The physical therapist assistant may be the primary professional responsible for the intervention, but the physical therapist should always be informed about changes in the child, including positive and negative responses to that intervention. The delegation of intervention to the physical therapist assistant depends on the stability of the child's CNS, the degree of movement dysfunction, the involvement of the body systems of the child, and the skill level of the physical therapist assistant.

The severity of the insult has a significant role in determining the results of habilitation and is extremely important in prescribing the intensity, duration, and type of therapeutic intervention. Children diagnosed with CP are often classified as mild, moderate, or severe. Generally, with appropriate, intensive treatment initiated by 4 to 6 months of age, a mildly involved child will develop sufficient motor control to allow for normal movement patterns, and a moderately involved child will have mild deficits in movement development after physical therapy. A severely involved child can often change, becoming a child with moderate to moderately severe involvement. Although the medical diagnosis of CP is static, the growing and maturing CNS has plasticity (see Chapter 4), and, if the environment nurtures those movements, the motor system will express these motor changes by increased fluidity of movement and skill development. In turn, the opposite can occur without appropriate and intensive treatment at an early age: the mildly involved child often develops moderate disabilities, the moderately involved child develops severe disabilities, and the child who was initially severe often becomes even more involved.

Traumatic and Anoxic/Hypoxic Injury

This medical diagnosis is generally applied to children over the age of 2 years. Children with TBI and near-drowning have one aspect of their CNS involvement in common: both patients have sustained trauma to a nervous system that has already established normal patterns of movement and postural control. Thus, the child will have some knowledge of how to move based on motor memory and motor learning or control up to the age of the insult. This prior learning is often helpful in treatment, as opposed to the child with CP, who has had minimal to no experience developing normal patterns of movement and postural control.

CNS contusions and lacerations of the patient with a TBI can occur with or without skull fracture. Damage can affect any area of the brain, or laceration of the blood vessels supplying the brain can reduce the supply of oxygen to the area of brain. Cranial nerves may be injured, and diffuse axonal injury is the most common cause of primary lesions (see Chapter 12).[3,4] These injuries may result in coma or a persistent vegetative state secondary to damage as the result of lack of oxygen. These lesions can cause increased intracranial pressure, cerebral hypoxia or ischemia, intracranial hemorrhage, electrolyte imbalance from swelling, secondary infection, and seizures.[5] After a brain injury, there are often physiological, cognitive, and behavioral changes along with movement dysfunction. As the child's CNS is adjusting to the insult and changes, the family and their CNSs are also reacting to changes to their family member. The family's input to the child with CNS damage can dramatically affect the outcome of therapy.[6,7]

Physical Therapy Prognosis and Outcome

Many of the treatment interventions used for children with CP can be applied to the patient with either contusions or anoxia; however, the outcome may be different based on the neural plasticity and/or prior learning. Although many authors have found that patients younger than age 20 usually recover,[8,9] this is not always the case. Van der Naalt et al[8] report a positive correlation between outcomes of patients with mild to moderate brain injury, lesions seen on computed tomography, and patients with cerebral edema. The Glasgow Coma Scale is a consistent outcome predictor that is used with head trauma and near-drowning (see Chapter 12).

Outcomes for children with CP will vary based on the area of insult, severity, and when treatment is initiated.[10,11] Hoon et al[12] studied sensory motor deficits in CP children born preterm and used diffusion tensor imaging studies to determine that the fibers in the cortico-spinal and posterior thalamic tracks were significantly lower than those in children in the control groups. With early intervention, it is generally possible to improve the functional outcome in mildly and moderately involved children. The child's severe movement limitations may become less severe, and the child may even be able to achieve some functional movement goals. In all cases, physical therapy can make a significant difference in the lives of the child and the family by empowering them regarding what the child can do, and may progress to being able to do, even if the functional outcomes will never be considered normal.

Evaluation of the Child With Neurological Impairments

Many tests and assessments can be used to determine a child's functional status (see Chapter 10, Appendix A: Core Assessment Tools). Some are used to determine the developmental age, others to establish motor control and function, and still others to determine the child's neurological status. Some evaluations are administered by neurologists, whereas others are performed in the clinic by the physical therapist and occupational therapist. The physical therapist assistant may be asked to perform and record some of the data collection, but the physical therapist will interpret the findings.

Initially, the physical therapist takes a thorough history of the pregnancy, labor, and delivery, and the child's medical history. It is essential to assess impairments of all systems. These would include musculoskeletal, cardiopulmonary, neurological (sensory and motor), and integumentary systems. Specifically, the physical therapist should assess muscle tone, muscle strength, joint range of motion (ROM), brainstem reflexes, sensory processing of the sensory organs, patterns of posture and movement, and functional activities of daily living of the child based on age-appropriate skills and play. General cognitive and social skills must be noted and considered when assessing the child's overall development.

When evaluating a very young child, it is important for the physical therapist to recognize how rapidly the immature nervous system changes. These children must be reevaluated on an ongoing basis. The physical therapist may ask the physical therapist assistant to identify changes to determine when reassessment is required, irrespective of who does the examination. Handling and positioning of the child, effectively or ineffectively performed, can dramatically affect the child's sensory motor system and positively or negatively alter motor abilities and skills. Consequently, the physical therapist assistant must be able to identify the effects of handling, positioning, sensory processing, and other interventions during a treatment session and report to the physical therapist. Feedback from the physical therapist assistant is essential in determining and identifying the necessary changes needed in the treatment program. Thus, the physical therapist assistant must be able to differentiate changes in muscle tone and ROM, the quality and quantity of the movement being facilitated, and the state of the sensory systems,[3] and identify the development of or automatic repetition of practice of functional skills during a treatment session, as well as identify what error-corrects have occurred.

During assessment of an older child, the physical therapist must examine the same systems as with the infant; however, contractures, deformities, and diminished motor development will affect motor function at a more complex level of development. From motor control theory,[4] it is important to determine whether the basic motor patterns are available to the child and appropriately used, the appropriate movement patterns are selected or modified, anticipatory reactions are present if internal feedback is to be used correctly, sensory systems are able to perceive information from the environment and respond appropriately, and the patient is able to use a variety of motor patterns that match appropriate performance and desired outcomes (see Chapter 4).

Therapists use a large variety of tests to evaluate the motor development and functional skills of children with CP (see Chapter 10, Appendix A: Core Assessment Tools). The instruments the physical therapist selects to evaluate the child with CP have differences. The physical therapist assistant needs to be aware of what the exam results mean in relation to the plan of care. The physical therapist assistant will not initially evaluate the child or choose the instrument to be used, but follow-up examinations may fall into the practice of the physical therapist assistant. If the physical therapist assistant is unfamiliar with the instrument selected by the physical therapist and is asked to perform follow-up examinations, it is the physical therapist assistant's responsibility to either make sure the physical therapist teaches the physical therapist assistant how to use the examination tool and then cross-checks for reliability of the test result between the physical therapist and the physical therapist assistant, or to obtain additional education to administer the specific test with reliability. No instrument tells the therapist everything regarding what body systems have deficits and how that affects functional movement. Specific tests that examine specific systems like reflex testing do not tell the therapist how those results affect the child's ability to functionally move in all spatial positions, nor will a functional test inform the therapist of specific body systems that are causing the movement problems. For that reason, it is the therapist's responsibility to interpret the results and analyze the relationships between body system problems and how they affect functional movement and thus limit the child's developmental progression. Some therapists have a difficult time making those analyses, and some find it very easy. Similarly, some physical therapist assistants quickly see the links among specific system tests such as balance, muscle power, reflexes, and core postural system problems, and how the results of those tests affect movement. For these reasons, it is very important that the physical therapist and physical therapist assistant communicate their thoughts, and that both, as professionals, help each other grow, learn, and become better clinicians.

Treatment of the Child With Neurological Impairments

Children with neurological impairment from birth trauma, TBI, or near-drowning have or may develop abnormal postural tone that can lead to the development of musculoskeletal complications. The long-term effect of inappropriate movement patterns can lead to catastrophic orthopedic problems. These musculoskeletal impairments generally mean that the sensory motor system should be assessed and treated early in the child's development. Whatever the cause, children with CNS insults will present with postural tone that is outside the range of normal: either too high (hypertonic) or too low (hypotonic), or asymmetrical between the 2 sides of the trunk. Tone can also be mixed or fluctuating (*athetoid*) or ataxic depending on the area of involvement within the CNS.

Postural tone and control are established by the CNS and respond to the child's environment (see Chapters 3 and 4). The postural tone controlled from the CNS is influenced by the sensory motor feedback from the sensory organs and receptors. The environment in which a child is treated will also influence a treatment session. For example, if a child has high extensor muscle tone, often due to poor postural muscle control or joint stability, and the therapy treatment area is noisy and distracting, the sensory input itself can be overwhelming and will often increase that tone. Given that increase in tone, the child's CNS will have greater difficulty regulating muscle function and postural control. This problem can often be eliminated by decreasing the sensory input to the child that is coming from the environment. Eliminating the excessive noise, dimming the lights, lowering the volume and pitch of the therapist's voice, and making sure the touch itself is deep pressure vs light touch are all aspects of the intervention strategies that can be beneficial to the child. Reintroducing those types of inputs at a later date is an important aspect of the plan of care to ensure the child has control of the motor system in spite of the environmental influences.

In the case of generalized low tone, it may be beneficial to have a more stimulating environment to arouse the CNS. The sensory systems are often not given sufficient importance when treating children and need to be better regulated by the therapist and recognized for the impact they can have on treatment.[11] The same is also true for the respiratory and oral motor components that are often overlooked and undertreated in this population of children. Therapists may not realize the significant impact breathing and oral motor function have on specific motor behaviors, the general motor control system, and ultimately the development of the child.

Gravity cannot be eliminated from life, but the influence can be reduced by the child's position in space or unloading the weight using support systems. By placing a child in side-lying as opposed to prone or supine positions, the influence of the cervical reflexes is reduced. In side-lying, slow, rhythmical, rotational movement of the trunk can further decrease hypertonicity of the extensor muscles both functionally for postural control through coactivation as well as control of truncal movement in functional activities. It is important to note that using rotation through the body axis will often alter the tone created by abnormal synergy patterns that limit the child's function. This activity can be delegated to a physical therapist assistant. As high tone is reduced, it is then possible to work toward passive ROM of the trunk as well as the extremities to maintain functional range to support normal movement development. Sitting or standing vertical positions can also help eliminate gravitational effects on the postural system and decrease the coactivation demands placed on the motor control system, and often fall within the child's initial functional control.

When the skeletal structures are vertical and properly aligned, this posture promotes vertebral stacking, appropriate muscle firing, generally causing a decrease in high muscle tone in the hypertonic muscles and an increase in muscle tone in the low-toned child through the normal postural responses of the CNS. The reason for this change is that a vertical posture requires less muscle power to hold a head or trunk upright when the center of gravity (COG) is over the base of support (BOS) than when the child is off vertical and the COG is outside the BOS. Gravitational pull and biomechanics cause these differences. Once there is sufficient increase in strength or normal muscle power, this technique may be used effectively by moving the COG slightly outside or beyond the established BOS, activating the firing of desired muscle synergies and facilitating the development of greater postural strength (ie, coactivation) and control.

In this pediatric CP population, stereotypical posturing and repetitive patterns of movement can be observed in the trunk and extremities. These patterns are often due to hypertonicity accompanied by weakness and the lack of normal postural patterns or motor programs. Initially, the child may present with general hypotonus (referred to as a *floppy baby*), but commonly hypertonus develops, particularly in the extremities, as gravity demands stabilization of the joints to develop ways to respond to the activity. As the child does not have the strength to meet the demands of gravity or the functional activity, the CNS will try to increase the tone of muscles to meet those requirements.

In a normally developing newborn, flexor tone has already developed during fetal maturation. This child at birth begins to increase the firing of the extensor muscles as well as the ROM, but after contraction the child will rebound back into a more flexed posture. In a premature infant or a child suffering an insult at birth, generalized low tone predominates without this flexor bias. Extensor tone is generally the first to develop in these children, partially influenced by the CNS and partially by environmental demands such as gravity, positioning, and motivation. If the extensor muscles prevail without the balance of the flexor muscles, the child will be unable to establish midline head control and will become asymmetric, often causing shortening of cervical and thoracic spine on one side (see Figure 9-1). This ipsilateral asymmetry generally occurs on the side of the body with higher tone. The child with increased extension will usually present with the lower extremities (LEs) in extension, adduction, and eventually internal rotation with the feet in plantar flexion. The upper extremities (UEs) are more variable in their posturing but are generally dominated by flexion at the shoulder, elbow, wrist, and hand, along with ulnar deviation. These patterns of movement are seen in all postures and often intensify as the child elicits intentional responses and is motivated to stabilize the body against gravity. As children repetitively use these patterns for postural control and movement, the patterns are learned and become stronger, and it is then more difficult to alter or normalize function. These behaviors are consistent with present theories of motor learning and control (see Chapter 4). Older children not receiving early intervention will have practiced and learned any available patterns of movement, which may be very limited, making it more difficult to intervene and promote or facilitate normal movement and good postural control.

In the hypotonic child, weakness and/or lack of postural control may also provoke posturing into abnormal patterns to provide stability. This helps the child stabilize vision but can dramatically affect normal development of the motor system. Without intervention, these children will most likely develop contractures and deformities of the joints, as well as spinal curves that will limit functional activities such as independent sitting, coming to stand, and walking.[13] Limitation in those early functional activities lead to more limitations in future functional activities that an adolescent or adult sees as everyday motor skills.

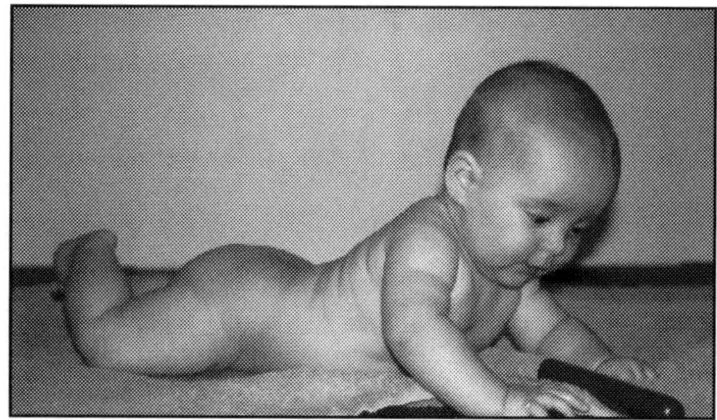

Figure 9-4. Normal postural development of a 3- to 4-month-old child.

Treatment Strategies

Treatment must be designed to improve functional movement and postural control over the proximal (ie, trunk and axial joints of shoulders and hips) and distal joints, minimize and/or prevent contractures and deformities, maintain or improve the respiratory function, improve oral motor function for feeding and pre-speech activities, organize and integrate the sensory systems, develop attachment to caregivers, and promote social interaction and appropriate responses. No therapist can cognitively think through all these components as the child is being treated, so recognizing normal responses to handling the child is the best way to summarize whether all these components are being integrated. The more the movement looks and feels normal, the more the therapist can assume the child is integrating many of these aspects of normal sensory and motor development. If the child is enjoying the movement and eager to continue to practice as part of play, then the potential for motor learning increases. To achieve higher functional levels of motor skills, a child must develop levels of competency working against gravity. In the initial stages of normal development, the child works on head control and shoulder girdle development while prone (Figure 9-4) or supine (Figure 9-5), bringing head, hands, and trunk to midline and thereby establishing the basis for postural control against gravity in sitting, standing, and ambulation. When this does not occur and there is insufficient tone (Figure 9-6) or increased tone (Figure 9-7), then normal development does not occur. As normal trunk and hip strength increase, at approximately 6 months old, the child can be placed in the sitting position. The infant without insult should sit with an erect spine, gradually gaining strength and stability for postural control and balance (Figure 9-8). The normal infant will spend a lot of waking hours practicing the development of postural control and balance while increasing in strength, endurance, range, and confidence over motor programs during play. This progres-

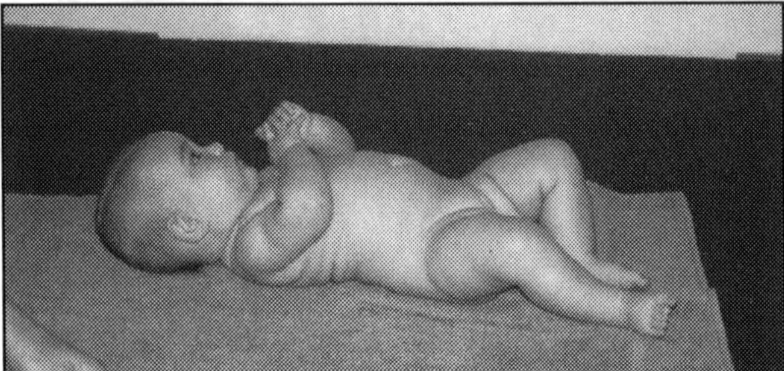

Figure 9-5. Normal development and tonal characteristics of the supine posture of a 3- to 4-month-old child.

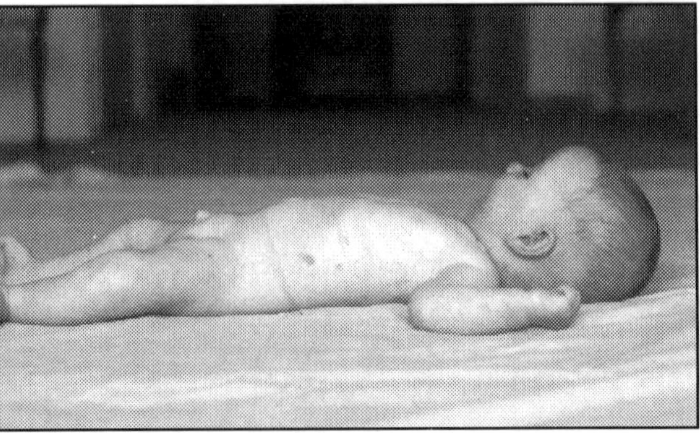

Figure 9-6. A child presented with extreme hypotonia at 6 months old. Although all 4 extremities were hypotonic at this age, he later developed and was diagnosed as a child with spastic diplegia.

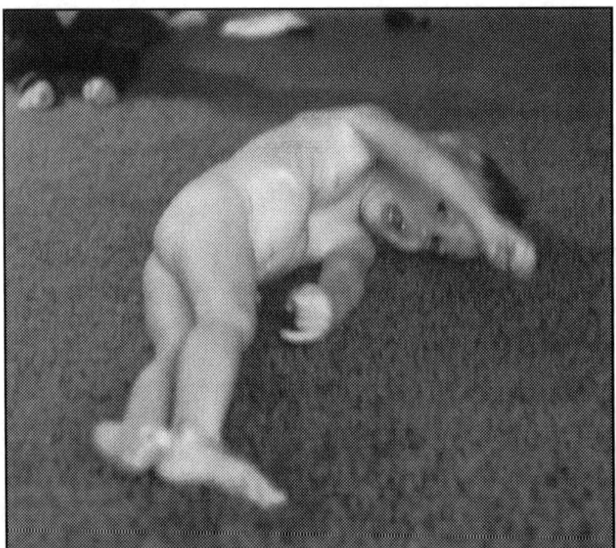

Figure 9-7. Child is diagnosed with spastic athetosis at age 2. Take focus on the rib cage; note the flaring of the rib cage with the retracted sternum.

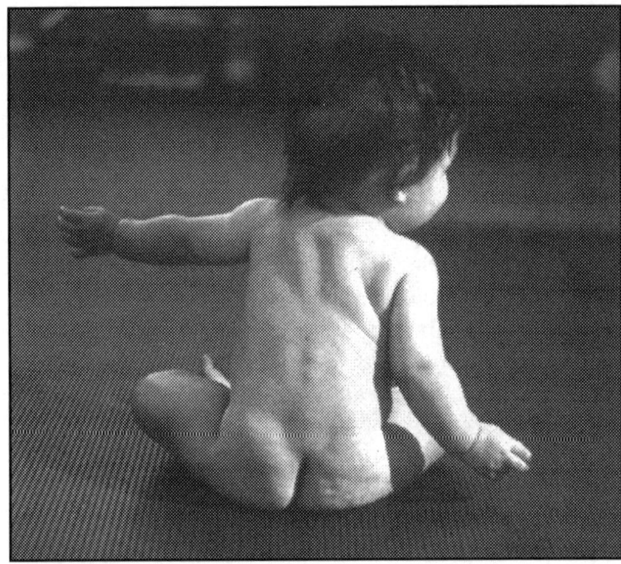

Figure 9-8. Child with normal development by age 7 to 8 months has adequate postural coactivation to allow for balance while her body is in motion. Function requires control of posture, equilibrium, protective responses, rotational forces, and perturbations against gravity while in motion.

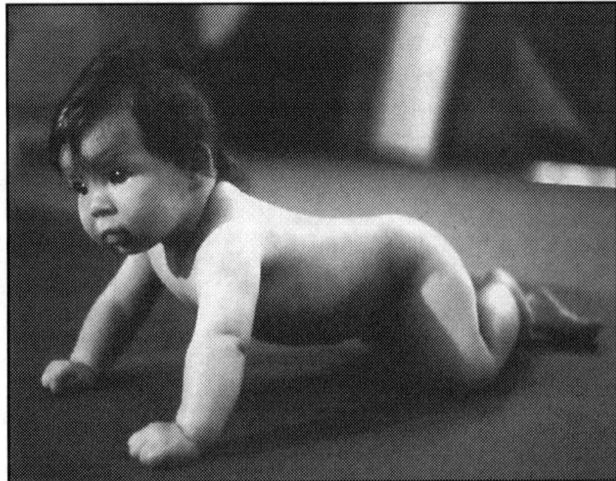

Figure 9-9. Child is 7 to 8 months old. The child has the motor skill to come to all fours and remain in that position. Note that the hands are fists, which is normal when children first get up into this posture. In time, the hands will open and weight-bear through the palmar surface with fingers and wrist extended.

sive development allows the child without CNS deficits to control and practice more difficult programs and challenges presented within the environment. A child with CP will also spend that time trying to control the motor system to gain greater independence in function. Unfortunately, the programs available are often limited (ie, stereotypic) and thus will limit the child's control over the environment.

Between 7 and 8 months old, the able-bodied child develops sufficient strength in the lower trunk musculature and pelvic girdle to allow coming to all fours (Figure 9-9); eventually, the child will develop the ability to weight-shift and crawl. Ultimately, the goal for all children is the ability to ambulate with a good-to-normal efficient gait pattern; use both hands for playing and learning; and have the postural stability of the trunk, neck, and back of the tongue to communicate verbally. Because of the need for the motor system

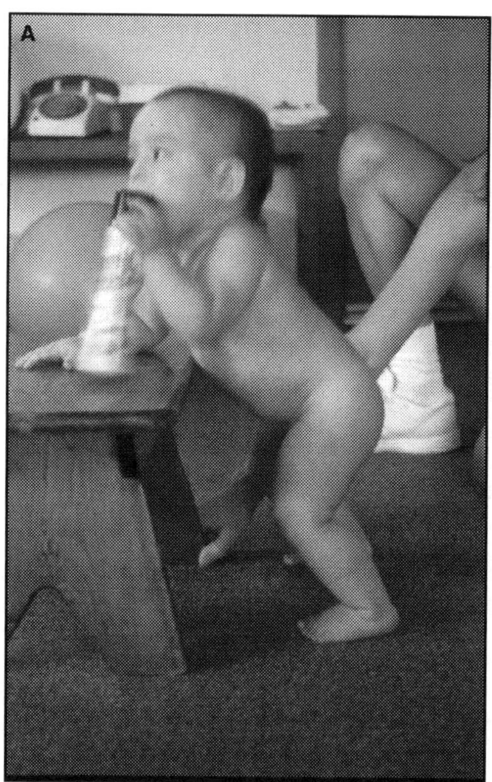

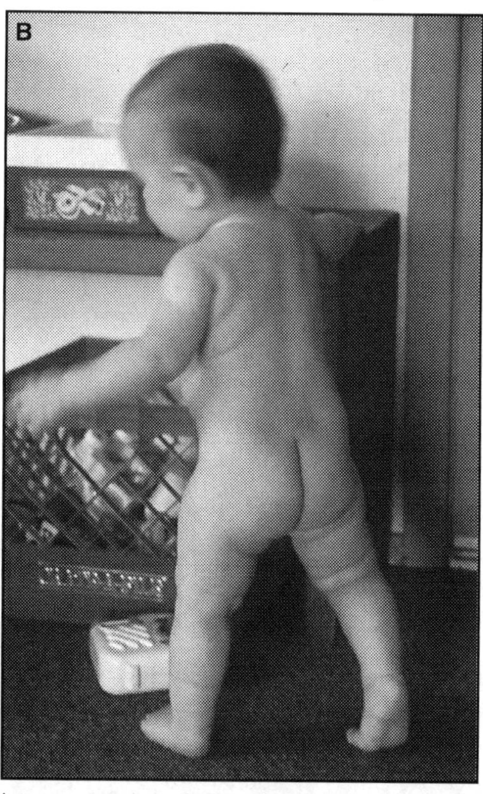

Figure 9-10. (A) Normal child early standing and cruising between 9 and 12 months old. Side view: Child standing using a hip synergy COG forward requiring upper body support. (B) Posterior view: Same child with weight distributed between lower limbs, but balance strategies still require upper body support: Early cruising.

to control walking, balance, and posture simultaneously, early ambulation requires the child to often use 1 UE to assist (Figure 9-10). Once those programs become more automatic, and the variance within all of them is under more control by the CNS, the child will shift to 2 points of support, leaving the UEs free to explore during ambulation. Children with normal functioning motor systems achieve these motor milestones, and these milestones are the basis for establishing developmental norms or developmental tests. These normally developing children have had adequate normal sensory input that gives the CNS the opportunity to organize and integrate the information. This in turn gives these children the ability to produce normal, appropriate motor responses, such as correcting their balance and/or catching themselves with protective responses. Unfortunately, in children with CP, many of these functional abilities are not possible. The severity and area of trauma to the CNS will be an important factor in the child's motor and cognitive abilities. It has been found, however, that by initiating treatment early, before abnormal patterns of posture and movement become well-established and the skeletal system has been adversely affected, children can gain functional control. Neuroplasticity can be achieved by a child with appropriate interventions. Treatment can be effective through handling and positioning, eliminating gravity, increasing or decreasing sensory perception, and changing postural tone while teaching new and more functional patterns of postural control and movement. The following are some basic concepts that can help promote improved postural control and movement:

- *Positioning*: To promote symmetry and midline control throughout the body while preventing neck hyperextension, elevated shoulders with adducted scapulae, trunk hyperextension, anterior pelvic tilt, and LE adduction with internal rotation.
- *Therapeutic handling*: To improve tactile, vestibular, proprioceptive, visual, and auditory processing[4-6,14-17]; assist in normalizing postural tone; develop righting and protective responses; and integrate sensory processing. When using techniques to encourage normal movement, it is extremely important for both the physical therapist and physical therapist assistant to use appropriate hand placement to stimulate and enhance the intended sensory motor responses. These techniques, often called *handling techniques*, allow the child to practice normal programming and correction of error while the therapist prevents the child from using stereotypic or abnormal patterns. The vestibular system may likely be the most dominant sensory stimuli and, when used effectively, can either dampen the effects of hypertonus or heighten tone in the depressed postural system.[7,14,17]
- *Inhibition and facilitation*: To promote more normal postural tone and encourage better ROM. Generally,

the movement used by the therapist will first be inhibitory to decrease the high tone, followed by facilitation into normal patterns of function and movement.[17]

- *Water therapy*: To alter muscle tone abnormalities, decrease the gravitational demands on postural muscles, and decrease resistance of movement of the extremities (eg, bathtub or pool).
- *Oral motor therapy*: To alter the muscle tone (hyper or hypo) of the oral motor structures to promote use of the cheek, lips, and tongue for feeding skills and prespeech and speech function.
- If therapy is not done in the home, then home exercise programs to augment clinic-based therapy and empower the family, caregivers, and/or patient are vital. Home programs encourage repetitive practice of normal movement patterns to further guarantee motor learning and encourage neuroplasticity. As discussed in Chapter 3, the child needs this repetitive practice to gain permanent motor control. Because the physical therapist or physical therapist assistant cannot spend the needed time with the child to guarantee function, active participation by family and caregivers needs to be integrated into the plan of care.

No matter what a child's functional level, it is critical to teach movement that can lead to function. Thus, it becomes important to know and understand normal movement patterns and how they develop. The physical therapist and physical therapist assistant are responsible for helping the child produce normal movement to gain or regain functional control over the demands of life. Life is about movement. There is great joy in being able to move and, ultimately, to move effortlessly, effectively, and efficiently. During treatment, it is important that the physical therapist and physical therapist assistant strive to reach functional goals. To attain a functional goal, specific techniques may be used to promote more normal movement and function for ADL. Refer to Bly's book[18] for examples of how to assist a child in rolling, crawling, and coming to sit or stand, and for a discussion of the importance of the therapist's handling skills, as it is beyond the scope of this chapter to discuss all these movement patterns. Also refer to the videos that accompany this book to visually recognize how a therapist might facilitate normal movement, whether that movement is elicited in an infant, child, or adult. As the child matures, adjunct therapies, such as horseback riding (hippotherapy), swimming, skiing, and dancing are wonderful activities that will help transfer therapy into function along with creating a normal, healthy environment that is fun and encourages social interactions. Many of these activities can be community-based and help provide both socialization and group participation.

Treatment Strategies That May Be Delegated to a Physical Therapist Assistant

Children with CNS motor dysfunction have postural tone that is either too high or too low, creating functional limitations in the child's ability to control the environment. To maximize therapeutic techniques, it is important to first dampen or heighten the postural tone to bring it closer to normal, ultimately leading to coactivation around joints of the body important to the specific movement. These techniques should maximize the effects of the interventions on functional motor control over appropriate environmental activities. The following are some of the recommended treatment techniques or positions used by the physical therapist or physical therapist assistant. If a technique does not bring about the desired outcome, then try something else vs staying with something that is not working to bring about the desired response at the moment. If the physical therapist assistant thinks the plan of care should be changed, then it is always appropriate to discuss those changes with the physical therapist.

Decreasing Postural Tone

- *Side-lying, sitting, or standing postures.* Encourage some internal postural tone or control without a demand that causes the CNS to compensate with abnormal tone.
- *Slow, gentle rocking with rotation* while in side-lying, sitting, kneeling, or standing, and with specific emphasis on rotation within the trunk axis. Rapid spinning in short bursts and changing directions can decrease spasticity with the understanding that one must be aware of the response needed for the individual child.
- *Rhythmic bouncing* on the therapist's knee or using a ball.
- *Slow movement in anterior-posterior, horizontal, vertical, and inverted postures.* The child may be suspended in the physical therapist assistant's arms while swinging or using a hammock, swing, or scooter board.
- *Firm, consistent touch,* avoiding intermittent touch. Firm or maintained touch causes the CNS to adapt, whereas intermittent/light touch provokes a withdrawal or a protective reaction.
- *Deep pressure through joint structures* (especially the axial trunk). This pressure is not very hard, although not light, but is maintained and has a calming effect on the CNS and develops postural tone or coactivation. The exact amount of maintained pressure depends upon the response of the child. This can be performed manually, using a neoprene vest, or using a weighted blanket. It is very important when using deep pressure

through joint structures that the joints themselves are in proper alignment. If the physical therapist assistant is unsure of that alignment, the physical therapist should be consulted.

- *Inhibition of abnormal patterns of posture using antagonist pattern with rotation.* If the child holds the arm in internal rotation, shoulder and elbow flexion with forearm pronation, wrist flexion, and finger flexion, then shoulder abduction with external rotation, elbow extension, and forearm supination with wrist and finger extension would inhibit that static posture. The rotation (ie, external vs internal, supination vs pronation) is a pivotal component of the child's CNS motor function and release of the abnormal posture. The therapist should never try to elicit a release through a quick motion or by use of extreme force because the quick motion elicits a stretch reaction and facilitates the abnormal pattern. In addition, a quick or powerful force elicited by the therapist has the potential of injuring and tearing the child's striated muscle fibers. The type of stretch should be slow and consistent. As the child's CNS begins to relax the tone, the physical therapist assistant can increase the range without causing any pain or discomfort. The physical therapist assistant always needs to remember that just static positioning of a child outside of abnormal patterns will not teach the child's CNS how to move in and out of that pattern. Thus, facilitating active motion should always be a focus of intervention either as part of the movement moving away from the abnormal positioning or pattern, or as active contraction once range has been achieved.
- *Enhancement of normal patterns of movement* in all spatial postures once postural tone is closer to normal. These movement patterns must be easy for the child to assist if the therapeutic goal is to have the child's CNS gain control over the movement. It is essential to develop sufficient trunk strength for postural control during both quiet coactivation in sitting and standing and in all other planes of movement. Initially the child should be placed in and out of positions that ask the trunk to maintain postural control within and off vertical. The intervention might begin within a small (eg, approximately 5 to 10 degrees off vertical in all directions) ROM that the child's CNS can function with control, and then increase the range as the responses become more automatic. If the child begins to lose control, the intervention should be changed. The cause for the loss of control may be fatigue, lack of endurance, or boredom. Regardless, if the response continues to elicit an inappropriate movement pattern, the specific activity needs to be changed. Once the child can control postural function in vertical, moving to more horizontal postural patterns can be introduced, such as on elbows or a 4-point (ie, hands and knees) position.
- *Using rotation to decrease tone within the trunk muscles.* Placing a child in side-lying and working on rotation within the body axis will often decrease the strong extensor tone within the trunk itself. It is recommended that the physical therapist assistant use 1 LE to begin the movement pattern by flexing and externally rotating the hip with knee flexion. Once the child's motor system begins to respond with a body-on-body rotation followed by the head, the abnormal extensor tone will become more normal, and the physical therapist assistant should feel an effortless response by the child.

Increasing Extensor Tone and Strengthening Muscles for Postural Control

- *Rapid movement using anterior-posterior, horizontal, or angular movement while in prone.* The physical therapist assistant can hold the child in his or her arms, over a ball, in a hammock swing, or on a scooter board using a slight incline to facilitate automatic postural extension of the head, trunk, and extremities. Again, it is important to remember that any movement performed quickly and creating a change in direction must be monitored and appropriate to the child's motor skills. The therapist must make sure the child has adequate control in the neck muscles to respond to the weight of the head and to avoid a whiplash injury.
- *Facilitation of a biomechanically aligned, upright posture.* This is accomplished by increasing proprioception input through joint compression down through the trunk with small perturbations. Emphasis must be placed on accurate alignment of the trunk. If the alignment is abnormal, the child will learn that pattern of movement, which has the potential of creating lordosis, kyphosis, or scoliosis. These spinal curvatures are often seen in children with CP and create secondary problems in the coronary and pulmonary systems.
- *Rapid and irregular bouncing and movement.* While holding the child in the arms, on the lap, on a ball, or in a hammock swing, the physical therapist assistant can quickly bounce the child and elicit postural or extensor responses while the child feels safe and secure, thus facilitating normal movement responses without creating fear.
- *Weight-shifting of the child.* Initially weight-shift the child on a noncompliant surface, such as a hardwood or linoleum floor, while sitting or standing.
- *Weight-shift* in sitting or standing *on a compliant surface* (eg, dense foam or tilt board). This intervention enhances visual and vestibular balance reactions along with postural control. These surfaces take away the normal proprioceptive input from the legs and trunk, and force the child's CNS to interrupt the visual and vestibular sensory information to respond appropriately to the perturbation. In that way, the therapist is

demanding the CNS respond with normal movement given less sensory information, or with some conflict between sensory input from visual/vestibular and proprioception.

- *Spinning.* This rapid acceleration increases vestibular stimulation and improves postural control. It can be performed by using a hammock or net swing, regular swing, or Sit 'n Spin (Playskool). **Caution:** Overstimulating a child's system may cause autonomic responses, such as vomiting and headaches. Thus, the intervention needs to be highly monitored and the rate/speed of the spinning gauged to the child's responses. If a child does not tolerate any spinning activity, vestibular input can begin symmetrically by having a child on a scooter board that can go down a small incline while the child is prone, and then moving to sitting. Once the child can tolerate symmetrical input, moving to asymmetrical input or slow spinning can help organize and process vestibular input.
- *Intervention must be balanced with sufficient flexor tone.* After increasing postural extensor tone (ie, short extensor muscles of the trunk and axial joints) and muscle strength in a treatment session, flexor tone must be balanced to provide stability around the joints and promote movement that is smooth, fluid, and controlled.

Increasing Trunk Flexor Tone and Muscle Strength for Postural Control and Mobility

- In supine: Bring the child's hands to midline or bring the child's hands to knees and/or feet into flexion. Initially, the child may need assistance, especially when taking shoulder protraction to neutral and the humerus into external rotation. This flexor pattern encourages development of flexor tone within a spatial position that biases the extensor muscles because of gravity's pull on the vestibular mechanism within the ears, and the tactile input to the extensor surface of the skin. While in this position, the child can be rocked back and forth, which will decrease hypertonicity of the extensor muscles while encouraging flexor bias.
- Breast- or bottle-feeding: With the child having proper alignment, work toward midline head control with hands to midline.
- Rolling: Facilitate from supine to side-lying to prone, with an emphasis on trunk rotation and head control. As the neck begins to flex and rotate, the arm on the non–weight-bearing side may retract, influenced by the asymmetrical tonic neck reflex. If the therapist assists the arm into protraction as the neck rotates, often the child will demonstrate some functional reach and/or protective extension.
- Crawling: Reciprocal hands and knees or hands and feet, making sure the trunk flexors are active. The child may be placed on a scooter board to take away a proportion of demands on the postural system while encouraging reciprocal movement of limb patterns.
- Bouncing the child on the physical therapist assistant's knee or on a ball with the child's trunk slightly off vertical in a posterior direction. This encourages head-righting toward vertical while facilitating neck flexion. Taking the child's trunk slightly off vertical in an anterior direction or toward the therapist will encourage neck extension. Working back and forth over vertical increases ROM of the neck and helps establish fluid coactivation of neck flexors and extensors. This head control is critical as the child moves in and out of more complex functional patterns during the development of motor control. Without that normal head control, the child will compensate with abnormal tonal patterns to try to establish stability.[13]
- Swinging: Maintain flexion and extension for postural control with movement (ie, coactivation) using a hammock or regular swing. Once the child has the ability to functionally control the trunk through postural coactivation of both flexors and extensors, play activities become fun, and the child will often laugh and smile. It will also decrease the frustration often seen in children who lack that postural coactivation.
- Spinning: Use postures in greater flexion while maintaining extension for postural control (ie, coactivation; eg, swing, Sit 'n Spin, rotating chair, or in physical therapist assistant's arms). Again, it must be stressed that the child should respond with normal motor reactions that are emotionally positive to the child. If the child is scared, then reduce the speed and observe the reactions; as the child tolerates the movement, again increase the speed using the child's reactions to determine the rate of the movement.

Inhibition and Facilitation Techniques

Techniques that are considered either inhibitory or facilitatory are specific movements or positioning of the child, performed by the therapist, to decrease or increase the child's sensory motor system's responses to gravity, position in space, and movement. These treatment approaches may be used with the techniques already described. When there is an increase in muscle tone, in either a synergy pattern pulling in multiple muscles or a specific muscle response, treatment techniques that decrease tone will be required.

Before presenting a discussion of intervention techniques for a child with the medical diagnosis of either quadriplegia or diplegia, a description of typical postures of the trunk, UEs, and LEs is presented here. During therapy, these children will present with many of the following postures, but each child presents variations based on the specific damage to the CNS and the environmental influences.

Typical Patterns Seen in Children With Cerebral Palsy and Diplegia or Quadriplegia

Upper Thorax and Upper Extremities

The upper thoracic spine is often extended, causing the scapulae to adduct. The shoulder girdle is elevated and protracted, the humerus adducted and internally rotated, the elbow flexed, the forearm pronated, the wrist flexed with ulnar deviation, and the fingers flexed.

Lower Thorax and Lower Extremities

The lower thoracic and lumbar spine will often be extended with the pelvis rotated forward; hips are extended, adducted, and internally rotated; knees are extended; and feet are plantarflexed.

Techniques to Correct These Typical Postures

- Place child in side-lying and gently rock forward and backward, adding passive rotation around the axis of the trunk. Be sure to do this activity to the right and the left side.
- When in the supine position, tone permitting, bring the LEs into flexion and the UEs into extension, and hold until there is further decrease in tone. Then, begin to add small weight-shifts, working toward postural control and balance in midline. These movement are not forceful, but rather are done slowly as the abnormal muscle tone begins to release.
- Gradually bring the child into the supine position with the neck and trunk in flexion and the LEs flexed and abducted, and bring the arms into adduction to abduct or release the scapulae.
- The LEs are in hip flexion and may be brought out into some abduction and external rotation. Again, this is done slowly and under a relaxed gentle movement by the therapist. The child must experience *no pain*.
- Once the child is able to initiate and more easily attain these positions and hold them with less assistance, then it may be possible to gradually assist the child's movement toward sitting, over into prone, or into postures requiring the head to come up with support on the forearms (on elbows). Do not prevent the child from using normal movement. The child may be able to control part of the range while needing help with other parts. During the time the child can control, that control should be allowed. When an abnormal tonal response begins to develop, then the therapist should dampen that response, usually using rotation away from the stereotypic pattern, and help assist the child's CNS ability to dampen the abnormal and use or run the normal motor pattern.

Presenting the many inhibition and facilitation techniques are far beyond the scope of this chapter. For a more thorough discussion of specific techniques, refer to Bly.[16,17]

Many specific techniques will be taught while in a clinical setting or at continued education courses. Colleagues find solutions to problems and often very willing to share. The therapist needs to be open to listening and watching other therapists who are using techniques that are working. Observation can be a wonderful way to gain additional skills. The answer to every patient problem can be found within the patient. The physical therapist assistant will often inadvertently find solutions to problems, as will the physical therapist. The key is communication with each other. The patient wants only to be empowered to gain or regain independence in movement or function taken away by some pathology or accident. The role of the physical therapist and physical therapist assistant is to help the patient along that path of learning and not become the obstacle to the patient. With the help of the physical therapist/physical therapist assistant, the child will have a much better opportunity to develop normal movement responses to the demands of the environment and more independent motor control to participate in life. Both the physical therapist and physical therapist assistant must remember that functional movement should not force a child to use tremendous effort or the movement, even if practiced, will not lead to function but only to frustration and limitations in movement as the child progresses.

Therapeutic Use of Toys

Play and the interaction of toys serve many purposes during therapy. Play is an important and integral part of physical therapy and needs to be an important aspect of a physical therapist assistant's repertoire of clinical skills. Play promotes development of motor, cognitive, and social skills through fun and function, and may help distract the child during a therapy session to accomplish the necessary functional outcome. Toys are a key element to the success or failure of play during a treatment session.

Consider the following when selecting toys to be used during therapy or when suggesting toys to facilitate therapy at home:

- The child's capabilities
- The child's needs
- The cost of the toy
- Toys/equipment that can be inexpensively replicated

- What cognitive and motor skill(s) the toy can develop or expand

Children with gross motor delays may benefit from toys or activities requiring sitting balance to build postural tone. Examples of toys that encourage the use of these specific motor programs are exercise balls, Bilibo (MOLUK), Sit 'n Spin, ride-on push toys, swings, prone scooter boards, slides, climbing gyms, and trampolines. For fine motor delays, choose toys that encourage movement and are repetitive, such as shape sorters, peg boards, simple puzzles, blocks, and activities to assist with processing sensory information, such as beans, sand, and crazy foam. Always remember that repetitive practice is necessary for motor learning. Thus, repetitive play during therapy and with family/caretakers will only enhance that learning as long as the play is enjoyable and effortless. Chose mediums within which a toy can be hidden that encourage exploration and nonspecific results, such as corn meal, beans, and modeling compound. Playing with cars, trucks, or any rolling toy while prone, 4-point, sitting, or in another spatial position can encourage the development of trunk stability as well as UE mobility and gross grasp patterns. Using a toy, such as an airplane that is flying in space, puts even greater demand on the limb holding the toy, requiring more stability of the trunk and axial joint.

Children like to explore new textures and objects. Containers with everyday household items, such as wooden spoons, measuring cups, plastic scrubbers, and measuring spoons, can motivate the child to play and imitate caregivers' normal activities. Activities that encourage manipulation help to build strength and endurance in postural function of the trunk and supporting axial joints as well as the distal segment engaged in the manipulation. Throwing and catching balls of different sizes, throwing balls into baskets, bowling a ball toward a target, using a bat and t-ball, playing musical instruments, and encouraging arts and crafts are all play activities that can have meaning to the child. As long as the child is enjoying the activity and is successful at the task, these toys can augment any therapeutic environment.

For children to work on fine motor skills and problem-solving, consider puzzles, blocks of different weights and sizes, nesting blocks, and textured blocks that can help with tactile sensitivities and are fun. When children get a little older and toys are not necessarily the answer, telling stories and making up games with counting or rhyming are often sufficient to keep the child engaged and working with you.

Children with reduced or limited lung capacity along with low-tone facial muscles can be encouraged to blow using as deep a breath as possible. Initially, the physical therapist assistant should have the child blowing items that require minimum effort, such as cotton balls, ping pong balls, and whistles or into something that elicits bubbles. Later, the physical therapist assistant can encourage blowing against greater resistance, such as playing musical instruments. How the therapist presents any of these items and interacts with the child in play will determine to some extent the child's willingness to make play his or her occupation.

Technology Today

Today, the use of technology has become common practice within the clinical setting of a physical therapist. Computer gaming systems, such as the Wii (Nintendo; Figure 9-11) provide the physical therapist and the physical therapist assistant a tool to motivate children and adults to engage in specific interactive activities that can enhance balance, strength, endurance, and functional body movement as well as challenge memory and problem-solving skills in a fun and functional way. These types of interactive activities are becoming more easily available and cost-effective, and can be used within the home environment as part of a home program.[19,20]

Similarly, the use of robotic technology either as an exoskeleton or as a body weight–support system is found in many physical therapy clinics. A variety of systems can assist the patient to move UEs or LEs. Because of the cost, robotic exoskeletons have not yet been adapted for easy use with most children and are seldom being used outside of a large clinical and research environment, but some are now available for specific reasons.[21-23] The available body weight–support systems provide 2 variations in how to decrease body weight. A few systems decrease the weight of the body by inflating a large lower trunk and body suit that the client is fitted into. Once the air inflates and the suit begins to fill, the therapist can determine just how much of the body weight needs to be reduced. These systems can be placed above a treadmill so the therapist can elicit walking once the treadmill is turned on. The second type of body weight–support system uses a harness.[24,25] The legs fit though the harness, and then the harness is fitted to a suspension arm that lifts the body vertically to decrease the individual's body weight. The therapist can adjust the harness system to align the trunk vertically. Again, many of these systems are suspended over a treadmill. Once the treadmill is turned on and the patient's body weight is reduced, the physical therapist/physical therapist assistant team can trigger a forward-stepping reaction in both legs. If those reactions cannot be elicited, then one or both LEs can be moved by therapy team members to try to enhance the learning or relearning of the motor program for normal walking. As is true of all motor learning, repetition of practice is needed for learning of the motor program and for providing an opportunity for the CNS to gain motor control. Many times, the program is present, but the power needed to walk is insufficient, so using body weight–supported treadmill training (BWSTT) allows the patient to build up strength while practicing walking.[19]

Many of the body weight–support systems have not yet been adapted for use with children. One system that has been designed and used effectively with children is the

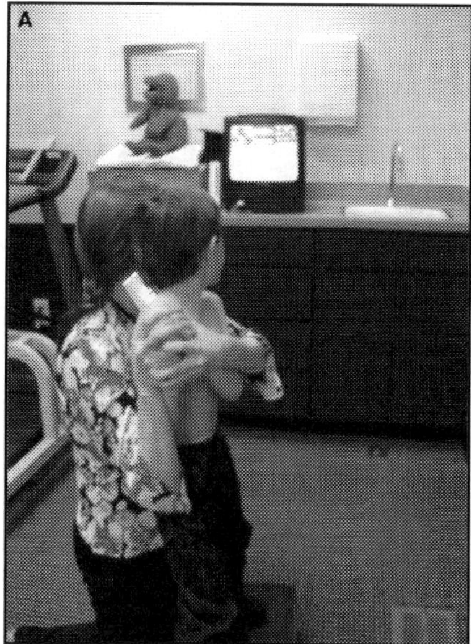
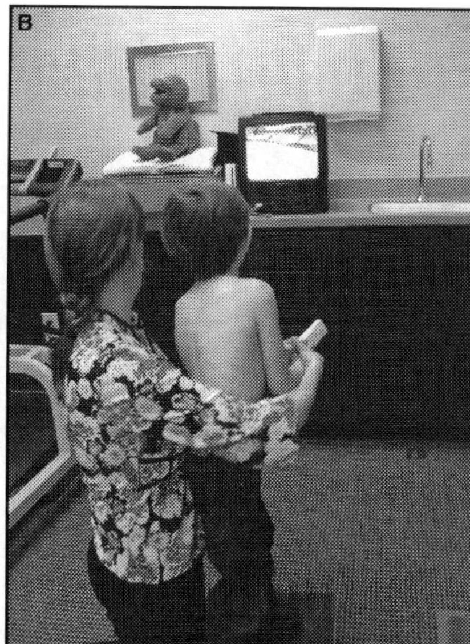
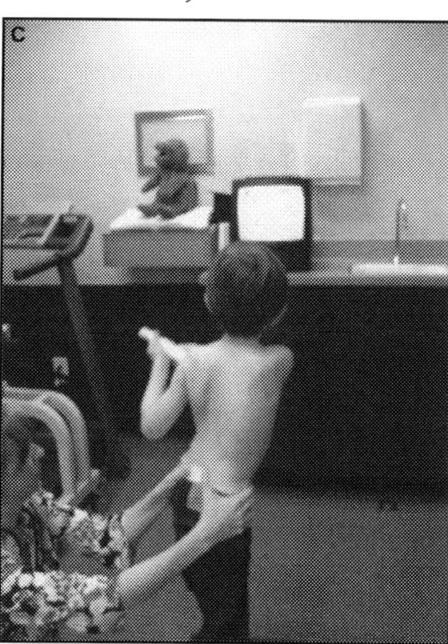

Figure 9-11. Use of the Wii as a therapeutic tool. (A) Initiating swing using controller as if he was swinging at target on Wii. (B) Midswing at target on Wii. (C) Ending swing.

LiteGait (Mobility Research).[26] This system can be used in initial learning or retraining for adults as well as children. BWSTT has been shown to cause activation on the somatosensory cortices of children with CP and thus increase the potential for normal interaction between sensory and motor function.[27] Similar to all BWSTTs, the LiteGait provides the physical therapist and physical therapist assistant the possibility of promoting improved weight-bearing and gait patterns by controlling postural alignment through an adjustable harness that supports the trunk and the amount of body weight the child's motor system needs to control the movement. Obviously, with the ability to unload the LEs, the opportunity to facilitate improved patterns of movement is possible. The therapist must always be aware of the child's COG and that weight needs to be forward over the foot to enhance that weight-shifting and stepping pattern. The physical therapist or physical therapist assistant is able to manually assist limb placement and improve the motor programs while working to increase strength and endurance. Watch the foot, and make sure when you are assisting that you have push-off from the forefoot and heel strike as the foot comes down after swing phase. As the patient improves, the physical therapist needs to determine when the patient should attempt greater weight-bearing into the LEs while maintaining proper alignment and control throughout the entire gait cycle. A patient may be placed initially on a treadmill for consistence of surface and repetition of practice. Once the child can run the programs of gait, the plan of care should move to practicing walking on uneven or compliant surfaces. The LiteGait (Figure 9-12), similar to other BWSTT systems, can be adapted to overground walking depending on the needs of the child. When placing a pediatric patient on a treadmill, it is often necessary to reduce the treadmill speed to 0.5 miles per hour or less. Many of these patients do not have the ability to reciprocally move at greater speeds. Unfortunately, this piece of equipment may be too costly for small, independent pediatric therapy clinics. Very few families have the funds available to purchase a piece of equipment that provides this type of practice in a home program setting, but this may change as the demand for these types of products increases and production becomes more automated. Refer to Chapter 19 for additional information regarding BWSTT as well as other devices to enhance motor learning.

Therapeutic Horseback Riding

Individuals have enjoyed riding horses as far back as humans were aware of horses. Horses have provided a means of expedited travel as well as assisting in the labor of transportation and farming. It has been only within the past few decades that horses have provided a new role. They have become a therapeutic tool used by physical, occupational, and speech therapists[28] when working with individuals with movement disorders. *Hippotherapy,* also called therapeutic horseback riding, provides a dynamic BOS, making it an excellent method for improving neck and trunk tone and strength, postural control, balance, and motor planning.

The dynamic, three-dimensional movement of a horse's gait simulate normal pelvic movements of the rider, allowing the rider to respond with upright head and trunk control and appropriate postural reactions imposed by the horse during riding. Hippotherapy has been used for years with children with CNS insults such as those diagnosed with CP. Some facilities have an experienced therapist/back rider who will support a child who has insufficient tone and postural control by riding behind and providing the needed control, support, and therapeutic interventions

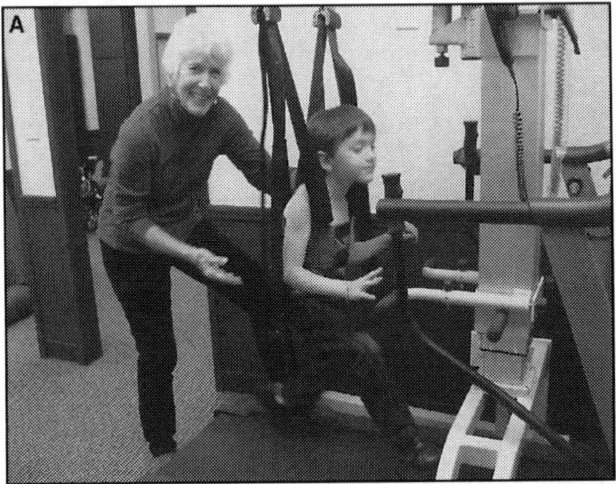

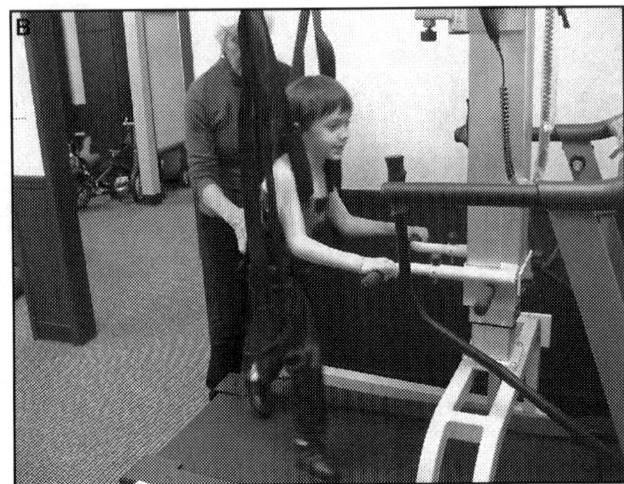

Figure 9-12. (A) Use of a body weight–support system. Ambulation on the LiteGait. (B) Running on the LiteGait.

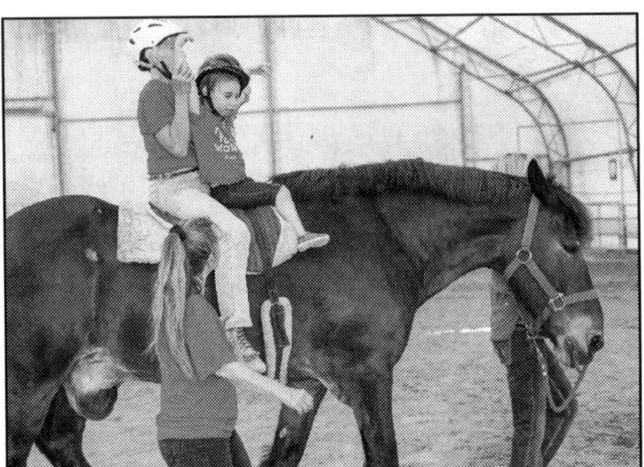

Figure 9-13. EC is a child with CP, spastic athetoid quadriplegic, being supported and facilitated by a therapist/back rider to increase spinal extension and postural control of head and neck.

(Figure 9-13). As the rider improves in motor control, a back rider is no longer needed. Side walkers then provide safety and encouragement for the child. The rider on the horse is receiving information from multiple input systems that provide information both internally from the body's feedback as well as from the external surroundings.[29-31]

Each session for a child is different, and each child has different challenges. As can be seen in at the beginning of the ride, EV lacked sufficient postural tone (Figure 9-14A).[29-31] As the rider EV progressed through the session, she gained better motor control and could sit astride the horse, using only side walkers (Figure 9-14B). She could support herself with handles attached to the pads she was sitting on independently. By the end of the riding session, the movement of the horse had increased her core muscle tone, and she was able to weight-shift and rotate while sitting with improved postural alignment (Figure 9-14C).[32]

As a child's postural control becomes closer to normal, the specific postural pattern a child is asked to assume will increase the difficulty.[33] KW was born with CNS damage causing a residual hemiplegia, but he now has the strength and stability in his hips and shoulder joints to maintain control in all fours on the horse at a walk (Figure 9-15).[33] KW progressed further by being challenged in knee standing (Figure 9-16). First, he maintained the position while the horse was standing, and then he progressed to walking. Ultimately, the rider was motivated and had sufficient balance to progress to an even more difficult position. He moved to standing on the back of the horse while the horse was stationary and, if appropriate, progressed to the horse walking (Figure 9-17).[30]

To achieve these motor skills, children earlier on in the program may be placed in positions including prone, supine, and backward-sitting (Figures 9-14 through 9-17). Once the rider has stability and control, games can be introduced for distraction and enjoyment. This takes the attention off of riding and into a feedforward motor program while the focus of the child is placed on to a cognitive function and increasing the play activity. Many different challenges will help push the rider to greater success; these include having the horse walk over poles at different heights, up onto and over a bridge, and/or up and down degrees of inclines; and/or increasing the speed and direction of movement of the horse.[34]

Safety is a major concern in a horseback riding program; hence, the horses must have a calm temperament and be extremely well-trained. They must have good conformation and a normal gait pattern to provide maximum quality movement while challenging the rider. To ensure safety, a horse leader and 2 side walkers accompany each child. The side walker assists with the rider's exercise program while maintaining the COG over the BOS and asking for repetition of specific movements that will eventually allow the rider to automatically adjust with the horse's movement. Three systematic reviews[29,30,35] targeting lower limb function in children with CP identified hippotherapy as an

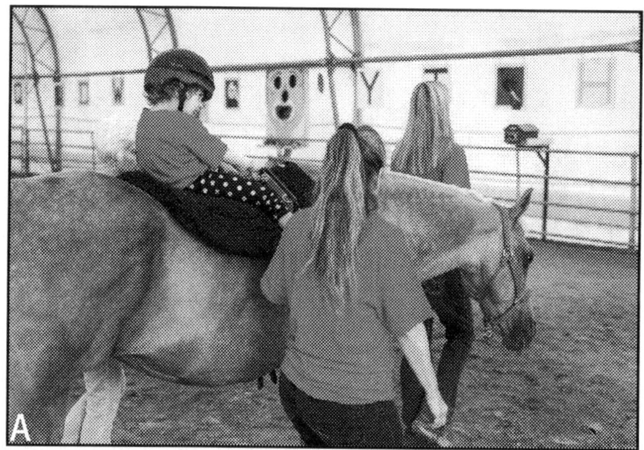

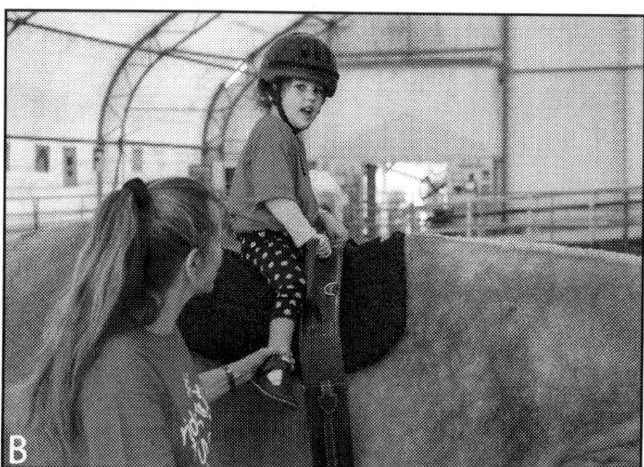

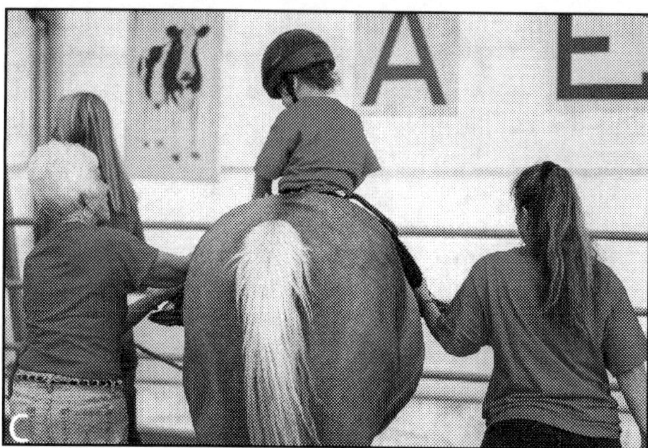

Figure 9-14. (A) EV is diagnosed as having CP, athetoid quadriplegic. She has advanced from requiring a back rider but lacks sufficient postural tone at beginning of ride and sits with poor posture. (B) EV is diagnosed as having CP, athetoid quadriplegic. She responds to the perturbations of the horse making appropriate adjustments for balance once sufficient postural tone has been achieved during the riding session. (C) EV at end of ride has improved postural control and attains good sitting posture as a result of the horse's movement allowing her to weight-shift.

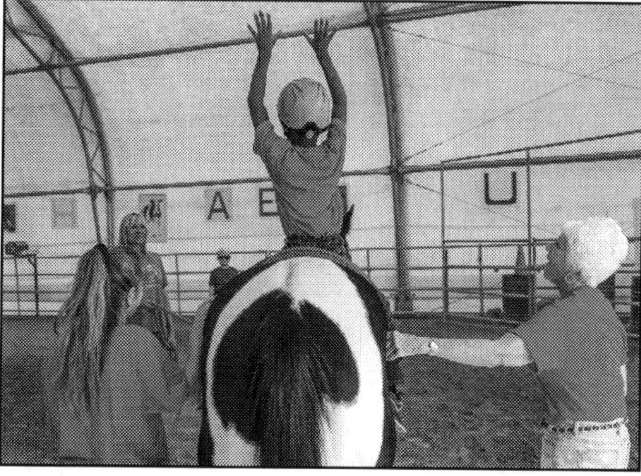

Figure 9-15. KW had a brain bleed at birth causing CP, right hemiplegia, and sensory processing dysfunction. He has been riding for 5 years and now has normal postural control with greatly improved stability at hips and shoulders. He can sustain stability in all fours with perturbations from the horse's gait.

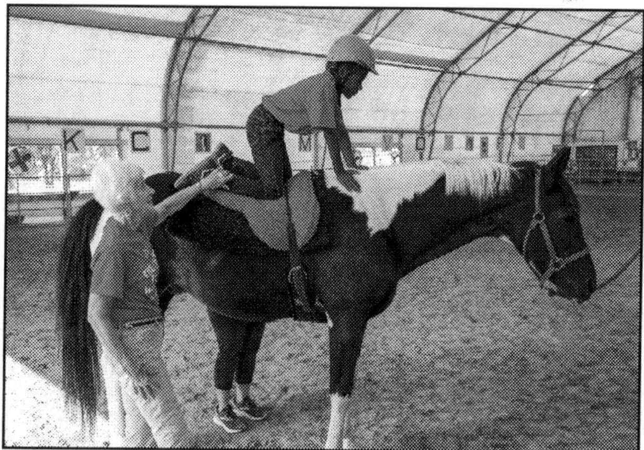

Figure 9-16. KW in knee standing increasing hip and trunk strength and stability through weight-bearing and weight-shifting.

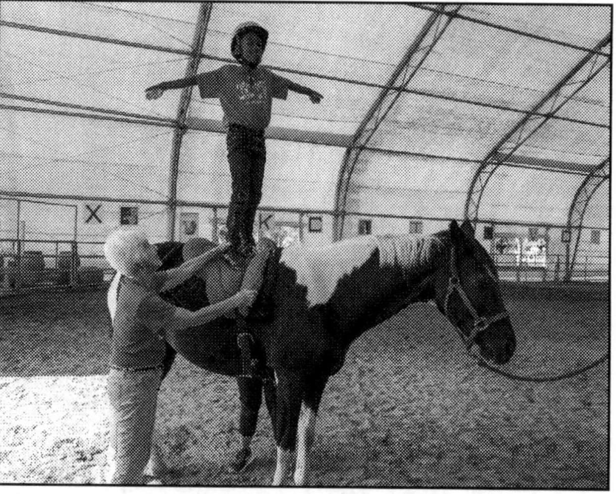

Figure 9-17. KW recently achieved standing posture and balance using all sensory systems, feeling safe and secure, and loving every moment.

intervention that can be very beneficial. Researchers[36-38] also found that hippotherapy had a positive effect on gross motor function in children with CP, as well as having a positive effective in treating postural symmetry and reactions within the trunk and hips. Children with the specific diagnosis of spastic diplegia also showed significant positive result in motor function following hippotherapy.[28,39]

Hippotherapy is not limited to the treatment of children and has been found to be very effective in treating adults with medical diagnoses resulting in CNS damage.[40-43] More recently, hippotherapy has been used to treat veterans with head trauma, amputations, and post-traumatic stress disorders. This type of therapeutic intervention can be directly correlated to the International Classification of Functioning, Disability and Health model and its focus on normal activities and active participation in life. There are certainly major costs to this type of intervention, such as the boarding and medical costs of maintaining these animals. The horses that provide the best interventions are often older and calmer and thus will face normal aging. But, to most therapists, the benefit provided to children with CP far outweighs any cost that it might take to maintain the health and longevity of these animals. For additional information regarding hippotherapy, visit a site such as www.ridetowalk.org. Refer to online videos for additional information on the use of hippotherapy.

Questions for Today, Research of Tomorrow

Many questions or problems posed by physical therapists today will affect the role of the physical therapist assistants in the future. As children age, their needs and environments also change, along with how the medical system may treat their medical body system problems. All these aspects of life will affect the children as they age toward adulthood and into their adult life.

School-Aged Child: Kindergarten to Middle School

Many children in the United States no longer receive physical therapy either in their homes or a clinic-based environment once they reach school age. Instead, physical therapy is offered in many schools through the Individuals with Disabilities Education Act (IDEA) of 1987, which was reauthorized in 2004 and amended through Public Law 114-95 in December 2015.[44] The core team (ie, family, teachers, therapists) at school determine what the educational goals, including functional activities for the year, should be in an individual instructional plan. The therapist may be required to strictly address only activities that are needed for the student to access the school curriculum. This precludes the therapist from working on the components of movement strategies needed for a functional activity at home or in the community. In other settings, the therapist may only be allowed to request appropriate equipment or adjust table and chair heights. How to bridge the gap and maintain ROM, core and extremity strength, balance and progression of movement function, are yet to be answered, and thus many students may not receive the necessary therapy to allow the child to continue learning motor function and participating in activities as he grows. Research is now becoming available as school-based colleagues are studying the effectiveness of school-based therapy programs.[45] Physical therapists and physical therapist assistants are educated to help patients minimize their functional limitations; hence, therapists need to promote the best care possible. Standing up for these individuals to support their growth, development, and the ability to reach their highest potential should be the goals for the profession of physical therapy and the role the physical therapist assistant will play.

Adolescence to Adulthood

Improved movement and sensory organization in a child's early years of therapy is crucial in reaching functional goals in adulthood. Many children diagnosed with CP or TBI as infants and small children now walk, talk, have become professionals, and live independently. However, many may continue to struggle with some of the same problems in their childhood and face difficulties resulting from their original concerns, such as cervical, shoulder, hip, knee or back pain due to the inability to move and/or walk with completely normal parameters of movement. Others may continue to have difficulty regulating their body temperature, have less energy, and fatigue more easily. As their bodies grow, so does the physical demand placed upon them. If individuals have been independent ambulators but walked with gait deviations, they may have increased the biomechanical demands placed on their joints, causing them to require a wheelchair or ambulatory assist as they age to conserve energy as well as preserve their joints. The role of the physical therapist assistant may become critical to activities and life participation of those individuals.[46,47]

Therapy Approaches

Many approaches exist for treating CP and TBI. Research has not clearly identified which approaches are best.[48,49] Functional outcomes depend on variables such as the severity of damage to the CNS, the age of the child, parental commitment, frequency of treatment, availability of treatment, and finances. However, research has shown that the frequency of functionally related treatment is a major factor in positive functional outcomes.[45,50] Which of these approaches will become the skill set of the physical therapist assistant will depend upon the direction and responsibility the profession of physical therapy takes. Complementary therapy (see Chapter 18) approaches may be more integrated into the practice of the physical therapist assistant along with the new and creative treatments that develop from clinicians and researchers.

Conclusion

Today, most of the children who were traumatized in utero or at birth or who had an insult early in their life will reach adulthood and progress into aging. Searching Medline or the internet, information regarding chronic problems within this population of individuals can be found under the heading "adults with development disabilities." Many of these individuals have or will develop movement problems or associated organ system dysfunction as they age, due to the stress and abnormality of movement and its force on the bones, muscles, nerves, peripheral vascular system, and internal organs. How the physical therapist will approach these new challenges and what will be delegated to the physical therapist assistant is not known today, but will certainly be part of their evolving roles in the health care delivery system. This should involve a clear classification of problems based not on a medical or pathological diagnosis, but rather on a movement diagnosis made by physical therapists and occupational therapists, who, as the movement specialists, relate function not to a medical diagnosis but rather to a movement limitation that takes away function and quality of life.[51]

Case Studies

Case #1

TC was born 2 months premature. During labor, his mother experienced a drop in blood pressure. At birth, TC was diagnosed with kidney dysfunction, and at 9 months of age, he underwent surgery to correct the problem. At 16 months of age, he was diagnosed with CP, only after his mother repeatedly asked the pediatrician about her concerns. He was first diagnosed with diplegia; however, the physical therapist determined that this child's motor deficits included his trunk, both legs, and one arm (ie, triplegia). At 18 months of age, he began physical therapy. At the time of evaluation, he lacked adequate head control, had no trunk control, and could not bear weight on his LEs. When placed in the standing position, his LEs pushed into the support surface with the ball of his forefoot, which stimulated the positive support reflex, thereby producing extension, adduction, and internal rotation of the LEs with the feet plantarflexed and inverted. The left UE was held in flexion, and the neck was hyperextended. Following 6 months of treatment, once weekly, and a home exercise program performed daily, he was able to be placed in sitting and maintain this position independently while perturbing his COG during play. He began rolling over in both directions, creeping on all fours, pulling up onto his knees, and attempting to pull to stand. When he began therapy, there were minimal vocalizations. Following 6 months of intervention, he had multiple vocalizations and a vocabulary of 30 words because of improved posture and motor control of his head/neck and trunk as well as the postural control of the back of the tongue. That postural control directly affected respiration, phonation, and articulation.

Physical therapy interventions included the following:

- Altering and decreasing abnormal postural tone to reflect coactivation.
- Increasing trunk extensor power for postural control.
- Increasing trunk flexor function for stability and mobility.
- Repeating newly acquired motor skills is necessary to develop function or motor learning.

If the child requires immediate intervention and experienced handling control, the physical therapist may choose not to delegate treatment to the physical therapist assistant. Once the child begins to demonstrate internal motor learning and control, the physical therapist assistant could work on all of these within that skill, working to the outer limits to allow the child the opportunity to practice, self-correct, and develop normal patterns of movement.

Questions

1. What positions or postures could the physical therapist assistant consider using with TC? Consider that his trunk tone is low, whereas his 3 extremities demonstrate high muscle tone.
2. Once postural tone is closer to normal and facilitated movement can be freer and easier, why would the physical therapist ask the physical therapist assistant to incorporate an activity where gravity is resisted?
3. Trunk extension must be balanced by trunk flexion. List 3 ways that you would develop trunk flexion strength.
4. Determine one functional posture in which you would place TC, and explain what activity you would use to encourage repetition to get motor learning and eventually motor control.
5. When is it appropriate for the physical therapist assistant to change or advance the child into new movement patterns?

Update on TC, Second Edition

TC is now 10 years old. He was receiving physical therapy twice weekly and then did not receive services for 9 months. When he returned, he had lost many of the skills he had achieved. Since that time, he has received therapy twice weekly, focused on reducing his hypertonicity, maintaining and improving his ROM, and building strength to increase good functional alignment. His main modes of mobility are crawling and a motorized wheelchair that has been pursued and supported by his family. However, he has the ability to achieve ambulation with the use of a walker. He has progressed to being able to walk with moderate assistance for balance. TC has increased gross motor control of his left UE, allowing him to use it for assistance or support. There has been little to no follow-through of the therapist's suggested home programs, which has hampered his progress and motor learning. TC attends a regular classroom with an instruction aide but does not participate in extracurricular activities, limiting his social growth, self-confidence, and self-esteem. It is important to note that gains through therapy can still be made that will help him both medically and educationally.

Question

1. What has been the major reason for TC's slow, or lack of, progression?

Update on TC, Third Edition

TC, now 15 years old, has grown tremendously. His stature is short, and he has developed good musculature of his trunk and right UE, rivaling able-bodied 15- to 16-year-old males. His left UE and both LEs continue to be less functional. His left arm has become a fairly efficient assistant while the LEs have developed strong hip adductors and internal rotators due to a consistent flexor pattern used when transferring or attempts to ambulate. As is common in children with CP, TC is experiencing an increase in spasticity as he is growing. As his bones grow and the muscles are put on stretch, they become tighter and more spastic. In TC's case, when he was younger it was possible to intervene, improve his postural tone and ROM, and facilitate better patterns of movement. As he grew, his size and strength became more difficult to manage, and, unfortunately, his therapy sessions were reduced from twice weekly to once weekly. Thus, his functional mobility in gait was not retained. A year ago, TC was happy with his abilities and did not mind being restricted to his wheelchair, because it moved much faster than his 2 legs. However, TC has decided he wants to be able to walk. He has the potential, the motivation, and drive to achieve this function. Unfortunately, it will require orthopedic surgery to lengthen muscles in his LEs and initially intensive physical therapy to achieve this goal.

Case #2

JS and his twin sister were born 1 month prematurely, delivered by emergency caesarean section because his heart rate dropped during his mother's nonstress test. At birth, he weighed 3 pounds, 5 ounces, and he sustained an anoxic/ischemic event. He remained in the neonatal unit for 1 month, going home 1 week later than his twin, who had no complications. At 12 months of age, he was diagnosed with CP, and initially received therapy. At 2.5 years, his family moved to another state, where he received physical and speech therapy for 2.5 years. At the time of evaluation in their new location, he presented with severe motor involvement as well as sensory dysfunction. All sensory systems were involved, which negatively influenced the motor system and caused a severe increase in muscle tone, irritability, and fear of movement. Increased muscle tone interfered with all movements of the extremities as well as the oral and facial muscles, affecting eating and sound production for speech. He did not have head or trunk control and could not be placed sitting or standing. He had no speech but communicated with crying.

He received intensive therapy consisting of physical therapy 3 times weekly and speech therapy 1 time weekly in a private clinic. Emphasis was placed on decreasing his extensor tone, increasing or maintaining his ROM, developing postural tone and control, increasing strength, and facilitating normal movement patterns. He had demonstrated potential for motor learning by showing significant improvement after 2.5 years of therapy. He was independent in sitting on the floor and in an appropriately fitting chair. He could pull himself to standing and maintain the upright posture to play. He could communicate verbally but lacked sufficient respiratory support for loud sound production. His left UE was used for playing, manipulating toys and objects, and feeding himself, while the right UE minimally assisted. He attended a regular kindergarten with the assistance of an aide. He rode in a therapeutic horseback riding program once a week, where he gained further strength and postural control. JS's therapy has continued and will be ongoing until he is no longer making progress toward his goals both within the therapeutic setting and educationally. As children grow and mature, it is essential that they receive therapy to help them achieve their full potential.

Questions

1. Following the evaluation and during JS's initial therapy sessions, the physical therapist delegated to the physical therapist assistant sensory integration activities as part of intervention and functional skills such as swinging, spinning in a hammock, and bouncing on a ball in prone or sitting.
   What motor behaviors would a physical therapist assistant be looking for during therapy that would indicate the child is improving?
2. How can the physical therapist assistant work on increasing flexor and extensor postural tone to facilitate head and trunk strength and control? How would the physical therapist assistant use therapeutic tools such as a ball, bolster, a swing, or a knee to facilitate this control?
3. How would a physical therapist assistant progress the child within an identified activity for the child to have greater internal control?
4. Between 2 and 6 months of initial treatment, JS's increased tolerance for processing sensory information permitted better organization of the motor system. He was less irritable, less fearful of movement, and he began to develop some head control in vertical. He was able to hold his head upright with neck elongation for 30 to 60 seconds. He began reaching for objects with his right UE that previously was held in flexion at the shoulder, elbow, and wrist. At this point in his therapy, the physical therapist assistant was respon-

sible through play for developing strength in the cervical and shoulder girdle musculature to promote good head control. This was done by placing the child in a mechanically aligned sitting posture both on hard and compliant surfaces. With support of his trunk, the physical therapist assistant weight-shifted him slowly, causing his COG to shift outside of his BOS (anterior and posterior and lateral). She then applied compression down through the shoulders, and then move to the hips. Then she used the hips as the pivotal point to cause perturbations. She was instructed to only perturb the BOS to the limit of the child's ability to allow him to practice successfully.

How would the physical therapist assistant know if the perturbations were too hard? What would the physical therapist assistant look for in the child's behavior that would suggest the perturbations were creating appropriate learning?

5. During this same time, the physical therapist assistant was also responsible for developing head control in vertical as well as off vertical in sitting. She was taught how to support the trunk appropriately using control from the shoulders, mid-trunk, and hips. She learned to weight-shift him in all planes. The LEs were inhibited from moving into flexion, adduction, and internal rotation during these activities by controlling the legs at the hips and thighs.

   What motor behavior by the child would the physical therapist assistant use to know that the intervention was progressing in a positive direction? Why might noise or sudden movements by other individuals cause the child to lose control?

6. During this phase, the physical therapist assistant was given responsibility for developing strength and stability of the child's UEs. She was instructed to place the child in prone in weight-bearing, weight-shift him initially on forearms, and then progress to extended arms as strength permitted. Initially, work on noncompliant surfaces on an angle off vertical, and work toward horizontal. As the child's strength and stability improve, the child was moved to compliant surfaces.

   What 2 motor behaviors exhibited by the child would help the physical therapist assistant know the goals of strength and stability of the UEs were being met?

7. During this phase, the physical therapist increased the respiratory capacity through manual trunk mobilization, and the physical therapist assistant was responsible for maintaining the mobility through side-lying and gentle rocking. Then, the physical therapist assistant was instructed to follow with functional activities requiring blowing, sucking, and voicing.

   What techniques might the physical therapist assistant use to increase respiratory capacity?

8. Between 6 and 12 months of physical therapy, JS's head-righting had emerged, and head control was developing. The physical therapist assistant was given responsibility for developing trunk rotation. She was shown how to rotate the shoulder girdle and/or the pelvic girdle around the vertical axis in side-lying, prone, supine, and sitting postures. She used an activity that required rotating first to one direction and then to the other. The body would follow the head in a righting reaction, which allows the child to move more freely. Creating an environment where the child is playing will motivate greater self-control and motor learning. For example, the physical therapist assistant could place a toy on one side of the child so that he has to reach to pick it up, and then rotate to the other side to complete the activity.

   What motor behaviors by the child would clue the physical therapist assistant that the physical therapist needs to reassess and potentially change the program?

9. During this phase, the physical therapist assistant was given the responsibility for developing transition skills from supine to prone to sitting as well as transition through the sitting postures available to him. Postural tone close to normal with proper alignment is necessary for movement to occur as fluidly and normally as possible. The physical therapist assistant was instructed to guide him with as little or as much assistance as is necessary to help him achieve the movement successfully. As the child improved, the physical therapist assistant was to slowly reduce the assistance while having the child still succeed at the activity.

   Why is this last guidance a clear indication that motor learning and control are in progress?

10. During this phase, the physical therapist assistant was given the responsibility for developing strength and stability of the shoulder and pelvic girdle muscles by positioning in prone on forearms or in weight-bearing on all fours or on hands and feet. Initially, the child was placed on elbows in prone and weight-shifted from side-to-side. The child's head was stabilized as if a turtle was poking his head out of a shell. The physical therapist assistant had to ensure the child was not simply biomechanically resting on his joint structures instead of using his own muscle power. When a child only uses positioning to remain on elbows, he will look as if his head was down in a shell and little postural control will be seen within the shoulder girdle. Once the child can hold with perturbations and begin to weight-shift on his elbows, the physical therapist assistant can use a toy to encourage reaching with 1 arm while supporting on the other. This activity can also be done on extended elbows or on all fours.

    What would the physical therapist assistant look for to make sure the child is gaining strength and greater stability?

Progression of Physical Therapist Assistant Intervention

Once most of these activities were developing, and there was increased strength and mobility, the following activities were also delegated to the physical therapist assistant:

- Increase cervical and upper thoracic muscle strength by placing him:
  - In prone position, on forearms, while playing and weight-shifting.
  - On extended arms while reaching and playing.
  - In prone position on a scooter board or platform swing or suspended in the physical therapist assistant's arms while moving him through space.
- Develop trunk responses to correcting or righting itself between the lower and upper trunk so that the trunk goes into a symmetrical pattern or proper alinement by:
  - Rolling in a horizontal position.
  - Sitting on a lap, ball, or roll as a quiet sitting activity or during play.
  - Swinging with trunk support. Use an appropriate swing that provides adequate support or, while the child is sitting on the lap of the therapist during the swinging activity, support the child at the pelvis and allow the child to respond to the imposed movements.
  - Carry him facing away from the caregiver and with his hips on the caregiver's hip, thus encouraging the child to sit up using postural extension and socially interact with the environment for extended periods of time.
- Develop active trunk rotation around the vertical axis in sitting by having the child:
  - Swing a bat or racket.
  - Sit or straddle a roll while reaching and touching his feet or picking up objects off the floor with both hands to 1 side and then to the other.
- Teach transitional movements (eg, supine-to-sit, rolling, all fours, knee-standing-to-half-kneel, coming to standing from the floor or a chair, and facilitating gait by handling at the hips or shoulders):
  - Supine-to-sit using diagonal movement patterns, which would be considered a partial rotation pattern from supine-to-sit.
  - Moving the child from prone to all fours, handling from the hip. From prone, handling should guide the pelvic girdle back over the knees while encouraging the arms to weight-bear.
  - From side-sit, either have the child come up to or pull to knee standing, weight-shift in kneeling. Then rotate the pelvis to encourage 1 leg to come into a half-kneeling position. Work or play in half-kneeling so the child weight-shifts onto 1 leg and off the other. Then, have the child come to stand off the half-kneeling leg. Guidance can come from either the back at the hips or the front at the shoulder girdles, arms, or trunk.
- Increase standing balance while engaging the UEs in play by:
  - Cruising on the furniture or wall.
  - Standing while drawing.
  - Catching and throwing a ball or Frisbee (Wham-O).
  - Riding a bike.

Questions

1. Are any of the previously mentioned interventions activities inappropriate to delegate to the physical therapist assistant?
2. At what time, if ever, should the physical therapist assistant go back to the PT to discuss the interventions?

Update on JS, Second Edition

JS is now almost 14 years old. He has continued to receive physical therapy several times per week. Therapy has continued to focus on decreasing tone, maintaining and improving ROM, and building strength to increase good functional alignment as he progresses in his motor learning. In 2008, a pump was surgically implanted to deliver a continuous low dose of baclofen, which has significantly decreased his hypertonicity and his ability to build strength and function. Unfortunately, JS has needed 2 subsequent surgeries to repair and then replace the pump. Prior to these surgeries, JS was not receiving the baclofen, and thus tone increased, again limiting progress of his LEs. His mobility is limited to a motorized wheelchair that he can drive with either hand. He has consistently good head and trunk control in his chair. As his body has improved and he has developed better motor control, there has been good improvement in social interactions with his peers and others, allowing him to participate fully in scouting activities and hippotherapy. His family has been very involved and supportive of therapy and makes sure he is included in as many normal activities as possible. He has further potential, such as gaining sufficient LE control to be able to perform an independent transfer. It would be important for him to continue to have therapy to help him achieve both his medical and educational goals, particularly as he is still a child who will continue to grow and develop.

Update on JS, Third Edition

JS, now 19 years old, continues to be seen for physical therapy 2 to 3 times weekly to help him retain spinal ROM and alignment, and build additional strength in his trunk, shoulder, and pelvic girdle muscles. The baclofen, which is delivered through a pump he received 5 years ago to decrease spasticity in his LEs, tends to go systemic, decreasing strength in his extremities as intended. However, this medication has also decreased strength in the neck and trunk musculature, where postural tone has always been hypotonic. The baclofen has caused his spinal to severely collapse laterally to the right with associated spinal rotation. His only upright posture is in sitting, and he spends most of his day in his power chair. The hip flexors and adductors became shortened, surgery was performed to release the hamstrings bilaterally. Unfortunately, this weakened his ability to bear weight on his LEs, and the contractures of the hip flexors remained the same, resulting in an increased lumbar lordosis, pelvic rotation, and hip flexion contractures. He received a sit-to-stand power wheelchair a year ago that can be driven in the standing position. It was not fitted correctly, and the insurance company would not provide funds to have the chair properly fitted until a year later. Consequently, standing to maintain bone density and the many other positives provided by being upright where not achieved. His trunk continues to be very weak, although slow and gradual gains are being achieved through repetitive practice and demands placed on the postural system through mobilizing his spine and pelvis, strengthening his trunk and extremities, monitoring his alignment and making adjustments as is needed. He continues to be involved in once-weekly hippotherapy, which is his favorite outing of the week. This life activity further helps him develop neck and trunk strength.

References

1. Ghassabian A, Sundaram R, Bell E, Bello SC, Kus C, Yeung E. Gross motor milestones and subsequent development. *Pediatrics.* 2016;138(1):e20154372. doi:10.1542/peds.2015-4372
2. Scalise-Smith D, Umphred DA. Movement Analysis Across the Life Span. In: Lazaro RT, ed. Reina-Guerra SG, Quiben M. *Umphred's Neurological Rehabilitation.* 7th ed. St. Louis, MO: Elsevier; 2019.
3. Gaebler-Spira D. Overview of sensorimotor dysfunction in cerebral palsy. *Top Spinal Cord Inj Rehabil.* 2011;17(1):50-53. doi:10.1310/sci1701-50
4. Umphred DA, Lazaro R, Roller M, Burton G, eds. *Umphred's Neurological Rehabilitation.* 6th ed. St. Louis, MO: Mosby; 2013.
5. Leahy BJ, Lam CS. Neuropsychological testing and functional outcome for individuals with traumatic brain injury. *Brain Inj.* 1998;12(12):1025-1035. doi:10.1080/026990598121936
6. Hanks RA, Jackson AM, Crisanti LK. Predictive validity of a brief outpatient neuropsychological battery in individuals 1-25 years post traumatic brain injury. *Clin Neuropsychol.* 2016;30(7):1074-1086. doi:10.1080/13854046.2016.1194479
7. Ownsworth T, Fleming J, Tate R, et al. Do people with severe traumatic brain injury benefit from making errors? A randomized controlled trial of error-based and errorless learning. *Neurorehabil Neural Repair.* 2017;31(12):1072-1082. doi:10.1177/1545968317740635
8. van der Naalt J, Hew JM, van Zomeren AH, Sluiter WJ, Minderhoud JM. Computed tomography and magnetic resonance imaging in mild to moderate head injury: early and late imaging related to outcome. *Ann Neurol.* 1999;46(1):70-78. doi:10.1002/1531-8249(199907)46:1<70::AID-ANA11>3.0.CO;2-L
9. Williams MW, Rapport LJ, Hanks RA, Millis SR, Greene HA. Incremental validity of neuropsychological evaluations to computed tomography in predicting long-term outcomes after traumatic brain injury. *Clin Neuropsychol.* 2013;27(3):356-375. doi:10.1080/13854046.2013.765507
10. Hanks RA, Rapport LJ, Waldron-Perrine B, Millis SR. Role of character strengths in outcome after mild complicated to severe traumatic brain injury: a positive psychology study. *Arch Phys Med Rehabil.* 2014;95(11):2096-2102. doi:10.1016/j.apmr.2014.06.017
11. Kahn-D'Angelo L. The neonatal intensive care unit. In: Palisano RJ, Orlin M, Joseph Schreiber J, eds. *Campbell's Physical Therapy for Children Expert Consult.* 5th ed. Philadelphia, PA: WB Saunders; 2018.
12. Hoon AH Jr, Stashinko EE, Nagae LM, et al. Sensory and motor deficits in children with cerebral palsy born preterm correlate with diffusion tensor imaging abnormalities in thalamocortical pathways. *Dev Med Child Neurol.* 2009;51(9):697-704. doi:10.1111/j.1469-8749.2009.03306.x
13. Lee HM, Galloway JC. Early intensive postural and movement training advances head control in very young infants. *Phys Ther.* 2012;92(7):935-947. doi:10.2522/ptj.20110196
14. Reid LB, Rose SE, Boyd RN. Rehabilitation and neuroplasticity in children with unilateral cerebral palsy. *Nat Rev Neurol.* 2015;11(7):390-400. doi:10.1038/nrneurol.2015.97
15. White-Traut RC, Nelson MN, Silvestri JM, Cunningham N, Patel M. Responses of preterm infants to unimodal and multimodal sensory intervention. *Pediatr Nurs.* 1997;23(2):169-175.
16. Bly L, Whiteside A. *Facilitation Techniques Based on NDT Principles.* San Antonio, TX: Therapy Skill Builders; 1998.
17. Bierman JC, Franjoine MR, Hazzard CM, Howle J, Marcia Stamer M. *Neuro-Developmental Treatment: A Guide to NDT Clinical Practice.* New York, NY: Theime Medical Publisher, Inc; 2016.
18. Bly L. *Motor Skills Acquisition in the First Year.* 2nd ed. San Antonio, TX: Therapy SkillBuilders; 2010.
19. Byl K, Byl N, Byl M, et al. Integrating technology into clinical practice in neurological rehabilitation. In: Umphred D, Lazaro R, Roller M, Burton G, eds. *Umphred's Neurological Rehabilitation.* 6th ed. St. Louis, MO: Mosby; 2013:1113-1172. doi:10.1016/B978-0-323-07586-2.00047-9
20. Visser A, Westman M, Otieno S, Kenyon L. Home-based body weight-supported treadmill program for children with cerebral palsy: a pilot study. *Pediatr Phys Ther.* 2017;29(3):223-229. doi:10.1097/PEP.0000000000000406
21. Aubin PM, Sallum H, Walsh C, Stirling L, Correia A. A pediatric robotic thumb exoskeleton for at-home rehabilitation: the Isolated Orthosis for Thumb Actuation (IOTA). *IEEE Int Conf Rehabil Robot.* 2013;2013:6650500. doi:10.1109/ICORR.2013.6650500
22. Bayón C, Lerma S, Ramírez O, et al. Locomotor training through a novel robotic platform for gait rehabilitation in pediatric population: short report. *J Neuroeng Rehabil.* 2016;13(1):98. doi:10.1186/s12984-016-0206-x

23. Samadi B, Achiche S, Parent A, Ballaz L, Chouinard U, Raison M. Custom sizing of lower limb exoskeleton actuators using gait dynamic modelling of children with cerebral palsy. *Comput Methods Biomech Biomed Engin.* 2016;19(14):1519-1524. doi:10.1080/10255842.2016.1159678
24. Emara HA, El-Gohary TM, Al-Johany AA. Effect of body-weight suspension training versus treadmill training on gross motor abilities of children with spastic diplegic cerebral palsy. *Eur J Phys Rehabil Med*. 2016;52(3):356-363.
25. DiBiasio PA, Lewis CL. Exercise training utilizing body weight-supported treadmill walking with a young adult with cerebral palsy who was non-ambulatory. *Physiother Theory Pract.* 2012;28(8):641-652. doi:10.3109/09593985.2012.665983
26. Mobility Research. LiteGait. http://www.litegait.com/. Accessed: September 2, 2018.
27. Kurz MJ, Wilson TW, Corr B, Volkman KG. Neuromagnetic activity of the somatosensory cortices associated with body weight-supported treadmill training in children with cerebral palsy. *J Neurol Phys Ther.* 2012;36(4):166-172. doi:10.1097/NPT.0b013e318251776a
28. Sylvester L, Ogletree BT, Lunnen K. Cotreatment as a vehicle for interprofessional collaborative practice: physical therapists and speech-language pathologists collaborating in the care of children with severe disabilities. *Am J Speech Lang Pathol.* 2017;26(2):206-216. doi:10.1044/2017_AJSLP-15-0179
29. Franki I, Desloovere K, De Cat J, et al. The evidence-base for conceptual approaches and additional therapies targeting lower limb function in children with cerebral palsy: a systematic review using the ICF as a framework. *J Rehabil Med.* 2012;44(5):396-405. doi:10.2340/16501977-0984
30. Zadnikar M, Kastrin A. Effects of hippotherapy and therapeutic horseback riding on postural control or balance in children with cerebral palsy: a meta-analysis. *Dev Med Child Neurol.* 2011;53(8):684-691. doi:10.1111/j.1469-8749.2011.03951.x
31. Kwon JY, Chang HJ, Yi SH, Lee JY, Shin HY, Kim YH. Effect of hippotherapy on gross motor function in children with cerebral palsy: a randomized controlled trial. *J Altern Complement Med.* 2015;21(1):15-21. doi:10.1089/acm.2014.0021
32. Hamill D, Washington KA, White OR. The effect of hippotherapy on postural control in sitting for children with cerebral palsy. *Phys Occup Ther Pediatr.* 2007;27(4):23-42. doi:10.1080/J006v27n04_03
33. Kwon JY, Chang HJ, Lee JY, Ha Y, Lee PK, Kim YH. Effects of hippotherapy on gait parameters in children with bilateral spastic cerebral palsy. *Arch Phys Med Rehabil.* 2011;92(5):774-779. doi:10.1016/j.apmr.2010.11.031
34. Davis E, Davies B, Wolfe R, et al. A randomized controlled trial of the impact of therapeutic horse riding on the quality of life, health, and function of children with cerebral palsy. *Dev Med Child Neurol.* 2009;51(2):111-119. doi:10.1111/j.1469-8749.2008.03245.x
35. Franki I, Desloovere K, De Cat J, et al. The evidence-base for basic physical therapy techniques targeting lower limb function in children with cerebral palsy: a systematic review using the International Classification of Functioning, Disability and Health as a conceptual framework. *J Rehabil Med.* 2012;44(5):385-395. doi:10.2340/16501977-0983
36. Snider L, Korner-Bitensky N, Kammann C, Warner S, Saleh M. Horseback riding as therapy for children with cerebral palsy: is there evidence of its effectiveness? *Phys Occup Ther Pediatr.* 2007;27(2):5-23. doi:10.1080/J006v27n02_02
37. Whalen CN, Case-Smith J. Therapeutic effects of horseback riding therapy on gross motor function in children with cerebral palsy: a systematic review. *Phys Occup Ther Pediatr.* 2012;32(3):229-242. doi:10.3109/01942638.2011.619251
38. Bertoti DB. Effect of therapeutic horseback riding on posture in children with cerebral palsy. *Phys Ther.* 1988;68(10):1505-1512.
39. McGibbon NH, Benda W, Duncan BR, Silkwood-Sherer D. Immediate and long-term effects of hippotherapy on symmetry of adductor muscle activity and functional ability in children with spastic cerebral palsy. *Arch Phys Med Rehabil.* 2009;90(6):966-974. doi:10.1016/j.apmr.2009.01.011
40. Beinotti F, Correia N, Christofoletti G, Borges G. Use of hippotherapy in gait training for hemiparetic post-stroke. *Arq Neuropsiquiatr.* 2010;68(6):908-913. doi:10.1590/S0004-282X2010000600015
41. Bronson C, Brewerton K, Ong J, Palanca C, Sullivan SJ. Does hippotherapy improve balance in persons with multiple sclerosis: a systematic review. *Eur J Phys Rehabil Med.* 2010;46(3):347-353.
42. Keren O, Reznik J, Groswasser Z. Combined motor disturbances following severe traumatic brain injury: an integrative long-term treatment approach. *Brain Inj.* 2001;15(7):633-638. doi:10.1080/02699050010009568
43. Silkwood-Sherer D, Warmbier H. Effects of hippotherapy on postural stability, in persons with multiple sclerosis: a pilot study. *J Neurol Phys Ther.* 2007;31(2):77-84. doi:10.1097/NPT.0b013e31806769f7
44. About IDEA. Individuals with Disabilities Education Act. https://sites.ed.gov/idea/about-idea/ Accessed September 10, 2018.
45. Effgen SK, McCoy SW, Chiarello LA, Jeffries LM, Bush H. Physical therapy related child outcomes in school: an example of practice-based evidence methodology. *Pediatr Phys Ther.* 2016;28(1):47-56. doi:10.1097/PEP.0000000000000197
46. Shen EYC. Adults with Cerebral Palsy: Independent Community Living Factors and Perceived Quality of Life. Doctoral Dissertation. Salt Lake City, UT: Rocky Mountain University of Health Professions; 2012.
47. Adults with Cerebral Palsy: Factors Influencing Independent Living and Perceived Quality of Life. IV STEP 2016. https://u.osu.edu/ivstep/poster/abstracts/014_shen-et-al/. Published July 10, 2016. Accessed June, 15 2018.
48. Park EY, Kim WH. Effect of neurodevelopmental treatment-based physical therapy on the change of muscle strength, spasticity, and gross motor function in children with spastic cerebral palsy. *J Phys Ther Sci.* 2017;29(6):966-969. doi:10.1589/jpts.29.966
49. Kashuba V, Bukhovets B. The indicators of physical development of children with cerebral palsy as the basis of differential approach to implementation of the physical rehabilitation program of using Bobath-therapy method. *J Educ Health Sport.* 2017;7(3):835-849.
50. Akhbari Ziegler S, Dirks T, Reinders-Messelink HA, Meichtry A, Hadders-Algra M. Changes in therapist actions during a novel pediatric physical therapy program: successes and challenges. *Pediatr Phys Ther.* 2018;30(3):223-230. doi:10.1097/PEP.0000000000000509
51. American Physical Therapy Association. "Physical Therapist Practice and the Movement System." https://www.apta.org/MovementSystem/WhitePaper/. Published November 2016. Accessed July 23, 2018.

Recommended Readings

Alberta Infant Motor Scale (AIMS)

Liao PJ, Campbell SK. Examination of the item structure of the Alberta infant motor scale. *Pediatr Phys Ther.* 2004;16(1):31-38. doi:10.1097/01.PEP.0000114843.92102.98

Pagliarulo MA. *Introduction to Physical Therapy.* 4th ed. St. Louis, MO: Mosby; 2012.

Yıldırım ZH, Aydınlı N, Ekici B, Tatlı B, Calişkan M. Can Alberta infant motor scale and milani comparetti motor development screening test be rapid alternatives to bayley scales of infant development-II at high-risk infants. *Ann Indian Acad Neurol.* 2012;15(3):196-199. doi:10.4103/0972-2327.99714

Bonnier B, Eliasson AC, Krumlinde-Sundholm L. Effects of constraint-induced movement therapy in adolescents with hemiplegic cerebral palsy: a day camp model. *Scand J Occup Ther.* 2006;13(1):13-22. doi:10.1080/11038120510031833

Occupational Therapy Assessments. Center for Innovative OT Solutions. http://www.ampsintl.com/AMPS/. Accessed December 28, 2012.

Fisher AG, Bray JK. *Development, standardization, and administration manual.* 7th ed. Fort Collins, CO: Three Star Press; 2010.

Gol D, Jarus T. Effect of a social skills training group on everyday activities of children with attention-deficit-hyperactivity disorder. *Dev Med Child Neurol.* 2005;47(8):539-545. doi:10.1017/S0012162205001052

Payne S, Howell C. An evaluation of the clinical use of the assessment of motor and process skills with children. *Br J Occup Ther.* 2010;68(6):277-280. doi:10.1177/030802260506800606

Russo RN, Crotty M, Miller MD, Murchland S, Flett P, Haan E. Upper-limb botulinum toxin A injection and occupational therapy in children with hemiplegic cerebral palsy identified from a population register: a single-blind, randomized, controlled trial. *Pediatrics.* 2007;119(5):e1149-e1158. doi:10.1542/peds.2006-2425

Bayley Scale of Infant and Toddler Development (BSID-III)

Pearson. Assessment & Information. *Bayley Scales of Infant and Toddler Development.* 3rd ed. (Bayley-III). http://www.pearsonassessments.com/HAIWEB/Cultures/en-us/Productdetail.htm?Pid=015-8027-23X. Accessed December 5, 2012.

Brazelton Neonatal Behavioral Assessment Scale (NBAS)

Boston Children's Hospital. The Brazelton Institute. Understanding the Baby's Language. www.brazelton-institute.com/intro.html. Accessed December 28, 2012.

Brazelton TB, Nugent JK. *Neonatal Behavioral Assessment Scale.* 3rd ed. London, England: MacKeith Press; 1995.

Dubowitz Neurological Assessment of Preterm and Full-Term Babies

Dubowitz L, Dubowitz V, Mercuri E. *The Neurological Assessment of the Preterm and Full-Term Newborn Infant.* 2nd ed. London, England: MacKeith Press; 1999.

Dubowitz L, Ricciw D, Mercuri E. The Dubowitz neurological examination of the full-term newborn. *Ment Retard Dev Disabil Res Rev.* 2005;11(1):52-60. doi:10.1002/mrdd.20048

Lissauer T. Physical examination of the newborn. In: Martin RJ, Fanaroff AA, Walsh MC, eds. *Neonatal-Perinatal Medicine: Diseases of the Fetus and Infant.* Vol 1. 9th ed. St. Louis, MO: Elsevier Mosby; 2011:485. doi:10.1016/B978-0-323-06545-0.00036-4

Gross Motor Function Classification System (GMFCS)

Palisano RJ, Cameron D, Rosenbaum PL, Walter SD, Russell D. Stability of the gross motor function classification system. *Dev Med Child Neurol.* 2006;48(6):424-428. doi:10.1017/S0012162206000934

Palisano RJ, Rosenbaum P, Bartlett D, Livingston MH. Content validity of the expanded and revised gross motor function classification system. *Dev Med Child Neurol.* 2008;50(10):744-750. doi:10.1111/j.1469-8749.2008.03089.x

Piana AR, Viñals CL, Del Valle MC, et al. [Neuromotor assessment of patients with spastic cerebral palsy treated with orthopedic surgery at the National Rehabilitation Institute] [in Spanish]. *Acta Ortop Mex.* 2010;24(5):331-337.

Gross Motor Function Measure (GMFM-66)

Russell DJ, Avery LM, Walter SD, et al. Development and validation of item sets to improve efficiency of administration of the 66-item Gross Motor Function Measure in children with cerebral palsy. *Dev Med Child Neurol.* 2010;52(2):e48-e54. doi:10.1111/j.1469-8749.2009.03481.x

Russell DJ, Rosenbaum PL, Avery L, Lane M. *Gross Motor Function Measure (GMFM-66 & GMFM-88) User's Manual.* London, England: MacKeith Press; 2002.

Russell DJ, Rosenbaum PL, Cadman DT, Gowland C, Hardy S, Jarvis S. The gross motor function measure: a means to evaluate the effects of physical therapy. *Dev Med Child Neurol.* 1989;31(3):341-352. doi:10.1111/j.1469-8749.1989.tb04003.x

Milani Comparetti Motor Development Screening Test (MCMDST)

Stuberg WA, White PJ, Miedaner JA, Dehne PR. *The Milani-Comparetti Motor Development Screening Test: Test Manual.* 3rd ed. Omaha, NE: University of Nebraska Medical Center, Meyer Children's Rehabilitation Institute; 1992.

Yıldırım ZH, Aydınlı N, Ekici B, Tatlı B, Calişkan M. Can Alberta infant motor scale and milani comparetti motor development screening test be rapid alternatives to bayley scales of infant development-II at high-risk infants. *Ann Indian Acad Neurol.* 2012;15(3):196-199. doi:10.4103/0972-2327.99714

Motor Assessment Scale (MAS)

Sabari JS, Lim AL, Velozo CA, Lehman L, Kieran O, Lai JS. Assessing arm and hand function after stroke: a validity test of the hierarchical scoring system used in the motor assessment scale for stroke. *Arch Phys Med Rehabil.* 2005;86(8):1609-1615. doi:10.1016/j.apmr.2004.12.028

Movement Assessment of Infants (MIA)

Chandler LC. Neuromotor assessment. In: Gibbs ED, Teti DM, eds. *Interdisciplinary Assessment of Infants: A Guide for Early Intervention Professional.* Baltimore, MD: Brookes; 1990.

Chandler L, Andrews M, Swanson M. *The Movement Assessment of Infants: A Manual.* Rolling Bay, WA: Infant Movement Research; 1980.

Pediatric Evaluation of Disability Inventory (PEDI)

de Brito Brandão M, Gordon AM, Mancini MC. Functional impact of constraint therapy and bimanual training in children with cerebral palsy: a randomized controlled trial. *Am J Occup Ther.* 2012;66(6):672-681. doi:10.5014/ajot.2012.004622

Haley SM, Coster WJ, Ludlow LH, et al. *Pediatric Evaluation of Disability Inventory (PEDI): Development, Standardization and Administration Manual.* Boston, MA: New England Medical Center Hospitals and PEDI Research Group; 1992.

Kao YC, Kramer JM, Liljenquist K, Tian F, Coster WJ. Comparing the functional performance of children and youths with autism, developmental disabilities, and no disability using the revised pediatric evaluation of disability inventory item banks. *Am J Occup Ther.* 2012;66(5):607-616. doi:10.5014/ajot.2012.004218

Pearson. Clinical Assessment. Pediatric Evaluation of Disability Inventory (PEDI). www.pearsonassessments.com/HAIWEB/Cultures/en-us/Productdetail.htm?Pid=076-1617-647&Mode=summary. Accessed August 2, 2013.

Pediatric Functional Independence Measure (WeeFIM)

Davis MF. Measuring impairment and functional limitations in children with cerebral palsy. *Disabil Rehabil.* 2011;33(25-26):2416-2424. doi:10.3109/09638288.2011.573059

Granger CR. *Guide for the Use of the Functional Independence Measure (WeeFIM) of the Uniform Data Set for Medical Rehabilitation.* Buffalo, NY: Research Foundation, State University of New York; 2000.

New South Wales Government. Lifetime Care & Support Authority. FIM and WeeFIM. www.lifetimecare.nsw.gov.au/fim_weefim.aspx. Accessed December 28, 2012.

Park EY, Kim WH, Choi YI. Factor analysis of the WeeFIM in children with spastic cerebral palsy. *Disabil Rehabil.* 2013;35(17):1466-1471. doi:10.3109/09638288.2012.737082

Uniform Data System for Medical Rehabilitation. The WeeFIM II Advantage. www.udsmr.org/Documents/WeeFIM/WeeFIM_II_System.pdf. Accessed December 28, 2012.

Prechtl Neurological Examination of the Full-Term Newborn Infant

Prechtl H. *The Neurological Examination of the Full-Term Newborn Infant.* 2nd ed. Philadelphia, PA: JB Lippincott; 1977.

Additional Recommended Readings

Goble DJ, Hurvitz EA, Brown SH. Deficits in the ability to use proprioceptive feedback in children with hemiplegic cerebral palsy. *Int J Rehabil Res.* 2009;32(3):267-269. doi:10.1097/MRR.0b013e32832a62d5

Shamsoddini A. Comparison between the effect of neurodevelopmental treatment and sensory integration therapy on gross motor function in children with cerebral palsy. *Iran J Child Neurol.* 2010;4(1):31-38.

Yoshida S, Hayakawa K, Yamamoto A, et al. Quantitative diffusion tensor tractography of the motor and sensory tract in children with cerebral palsy. *Dev Med Child Neurol.* 2010;52(10):935-940. doi:10.1111/j.1469-8749.2010.03669.x

Please visit www.routledge.com/9781630915650 to access additional material.

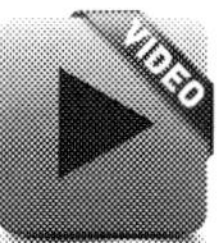

Chapter 10

Clients With Genetic and Developmental Problems

Eunice Shen, PT, PhD, DPT, PCS; Esmerita Roceles Rotor, PT, PhD; and Barbara H. Connolly, PT, DPT, EdD, C/NDT, FAPTA

Key Words Chromosomal disorders | Genetics | Mitochondrial disorders | Movement dysfunction | Multifactorial disorders | Neuro-developmental condition | Single-gene disorders

Chapter Objectives

- Describe genetic conditions with neuro-developmental concerns that are commonly referred to physical therapy.
- Identify and discuss children with developmental problems that may or may not be related to genetics.
- Describe clinical features that affect motor development and movement.
- Identify tests and measures that are used in examination.
- Identify physical therapy strategies to address motor and movement issues.
- Discuss essential features when working with children with genetic conditions and/or developmental problems, including early intervention and working in collaboration with other professionals and programs that work with these children through childhood.

The World Confederation for Physical Therapy[1] states that part of the scope of physical therapy practice includes providing services to individuals and groups of individuals to develop, maintain, and restore maximum movement and functional ability throughout the lifespan. This includes infants and children with neuro-developmental conditions brought about by genetic aberrations as well as other children who have developmental problems without specific genetic links. This chapter will present both areas of pediatric neurological conditions. No matter the cause, children with developmental delays have conditions that lead to long-term motor delays. These limit the child's ability to perform normal activities of daily living (ADL) and to participate in many areas of life. Specific genetic links to developmental problems will be presented first, followed by a more general discussion of medical diagnoses leading to development delays.

Genetic Conditions Leading to Neurological and Motor Development Concerns

Although numerous genetic conditions have been reported, this chapter is limited to genetic conditions that are diagnosed immediately after birth and those that have neurological features that affect development. The discussion in this chapter will involve infants, children, and adolescents with genetic conditions.

The Human Genome Project, which started in 1990 and completed in 2003, aimed to identify all the approximately 20,000 to 25,000 genes in human DNA.[2] This breakthrough has influenced health and medical practices. Currently, the

Lazaro RT, Umphred DA, eds.
Umphred's Neurorehabilitation for the Physical Therapist Assistant, Third Edition (pp 211-252).

importance of the role of genetics is being used in diagnosing, monitoring, and treating disease.[2] The United States started transitioning to the International Classification of Diseases, 10th Revision, Clinical Modification (ICD-10—CM) in 2015. Major birth defects surveillance in the United States will be affected due to the changes from the International Classification of Diseases, 9th Revision, Clinical Modification. This change will have implications in birth defects surveillance, prevalence estimates, and tracking birth defects trends, especially in the comparison of data in the 2 coding systems. The effects of the nomenclature changes can only be fully accessed once the implementation of the ICD-10-CM has taken place nationwide and worldwide.[3]

Physical therapists and other health care professionals may take on challenges brought about by strides made in genetics. Physical therapy professionals may find themselves in a position to suspect that a client has a genetic condition,[4] and the professional should therefore have the knowledge and skills to recommend that appropriate clients seek further help. There are 4 classifications of genetic disorders: single-gene disorders, mitochondrial disorders, chromosomal disorders, and multifactorial disorders.[5,6] Within these types, several conditions are diagnosed at birth or early childhood and will affect the neurological development of the child. Chromosome disorders may be due to numerical abnormalities or structural abnormalities.[5] Conditions such as Down syndrome (trisomy 21), Edwards' syndrome (trisomy 18), and Patau syndrome (trisomy 13) are due to numerical abnormalities; there may be a missing or an extra chromosome. In the case of DS or trisomy 21, there is an extra chromosome on the 21st pair of chromosomes.

Structural abnormalities of the chromosome also lead to chromosome disorders. Cri du chat syndrome and Prader-Willi syndrome are examples of this. In cri du chat syndrome, there is a deletion of the short arm of chromosome 5, whereas in Prader-Willi syndrome, there is a structural defect on chromosome 15. Single-gene disorders or Mendelian disorders are caused by an error in a single unit of genetic information.[6] These disorders can be classified as autosomal-dominant, autosomal-recessive, and X-linked disorders. In an *autosomal-dominant* condition, one parent will have a defective gene than can be passed on to the child. Examples include achondroplasia and osteogenesis imperfecta. In *autosomal-recessive* disorders, both parents are carriers of the defective gene. Parents are usually asymptomatic and may not know that they possess the defective gene until the child exhibits signs and symptoms. Examples of these are cystic fibrosis, sickle cell anemia, and Tay Sachs disease. In *X-linked* disorders, defective genes are on the X sex chromosome. Females are carriers of these genes and pass it on to their male offspring. Examples of these are Duchenne muscular dystrophy (DMD) and hemophilia.

Multifactorial genetic conditions are brought about by a complex interaction of genetics with environmental factors,[5] resulting in birth defects, such as cleft lip, cleft palate, and spina bifida.

Lastly, mitochondrial disorders are due to defects in the genes within the cytoplasm of the mitochondria. These are usually rare conditions associated with aging. Mitochondrial disorders can be inherited only from the mother.

A list of disorders according to type, characteristics, clinical features, and examples can be found in Table 10-1.

The genetic conditions that result in neurological problems that affect development will be discussed in detail as these are the most common medical diagnoses a physical therapist and physical therapist assistant will encounter.

Down Syndrome (Trisomy 21)

Down syndrome (DS), or trisomy 21, occurs in 1 in 700 live births.[7] This condition is the most frequent genetic cause of intellectual disability (ID). DS is brought about by a chromosomal genetic condition in which there is an extra chromosome in the 21st pair of chromosomes. Persons with DS are easily identified by their stereotypical appearance. Their heads are of a smaller size, with a flattened neck area, excess skin at the nape, flattened nose, small and lower placed ears, and slanting eyes. A simian crease at the palm of each hand is also typical, although that is also found in children and adults without genetic abnormalities. The Committee on Genetics in 2001 provided data and information on the health supervision for children with DS. The Committee reports that children with DS exhibit mental impairment in varying degrees, from mild (intelligence quotient [IQ] 50 to 70) to moderate (IQ 35 to 50) and occasionally severe deficits (IQ 20 to 35).[7] Medical conditions associated with this condition include congenital heart defects (50%), leukemia (less than 1%), hearing loss (75%), otitis media (50% to 70%), Hirschsprung's disease (less than 1%), gastrointestinal atresias (12%), eye diseases (60%), and thyroid disease (15%). It was found that children with DS had smaller cerebellar brain volume that could be responsible for motor coordination problems.[8] Children with DS have also been noted to have motor planning and execution problems (dyspraxia). Costa found that "individuals with DS had much diminished optokinetic and vestibular reflexes compared to typically developing individuals. As a consequence, it is likely that things may appear blurry when they ride a bike or play sports."[8]

Among the developmental genetic conditions, physical therapists and physical therapist assistants get to work most frequently with children with DS. Physical therapy concerns for this population include hypotonia, joint laxity, muscle weakness, poor coordination, and sensory perceptual problems. For infants and toddlers, physical therapists and physical therapist assistants work toward attaining gross and fine motor skills, such as rolling, sit-

Table 10-1

Overview of Genetic Disorders Affecting the Pediatric Age Group

Type of Disorder	*Characteristic of Disorder*	*Name of Disorder*	*Clinical Features*
Chromosome Abnormalities	Deviation in number of chromosomes, 47, XY, +21*	DS (trisomy 21)	Characteristic facial features, including flat occiput; flat face; upward slanting eyes; hypotonicity; broad, short feet and hands; protruding abdomen; intellectual disability; possible cardiac anomalies.
		Edwards' syndrome (trisomy 18)	Small stature; long, narrow skull; low-set ears; hypotonicity; rocker bottom feet; scoliosis; profound intellectual disability.
		Patau syndrome (trisomy 13)	Microcephaly; cleft lip and palate; polydactyly of hands and feet; severe to profound intellectual disability.
	Deviation in sex chromosomes	Turner syndrome (XO syndrome)	Congenitally webbed neck; growth retardation; ptosis of upper eyelids; lack of sexual development; congenital heart and kidney disease; scoliosis; low-normal intelligence.
		Klinefelter syndrome (XXY)	Long limbs; tall and slender build until adulthood when obesity becomes a problem (if testosterone replacement therapy is given); small penis and testes; low-average to mild intellectual disability; tremors; behavior problems.
	Partial deletion syndrome	Cri du chat syndrome (5p-)	High-pitched, catlike cry in infancy; microcephaly; low-set ears; hypotonicity; severe intellectual disability; scoliosis; clubfeet; dislocated hips.
		Prader-Willi syndrome (15q–)	Low tone with feeding disorder in infancy; insatiable appetite develops in toddlerhood; moderate intellectual disability; hyperflexibility; obesity; characteristic facial features, including almond-shaped eyes; and small stature, hands, feet, and penis.
		Williams syndrome (deletion near the elastin gene on chromosome 7)	Characteristic facial abnormalities, including prominent lips, medial eyebrow flare, and open mouth; mild microcephaly; mild growth retardation; short nails; mild to moderate intellectual disability; cardiovascular anomalies.
Specific Gene Defects	Autosomal dominant	Neurofibromatosis	Areas of hyperpigmentation or hypopigmentation of skin inducing café au lait spots or axillary freckling; tumors along nerves, in connective tissue, eyes, or meninges; macrocephaly; short stature. May have skeletal abnormalities, including scoliosis, bowing of long bones, and dislocations.
		Tuberous sclerosis	Brain lesions causing seizures and intellectual disability; skin lesions on cheeks around nose; café au lait spots; cyst-like areas in bones of fingers; kidney and teeth abnormalities.
		Osteogenesis imperfecta	Type I: Small stature; thin bones, bowing of the bones; fractures of long bones; hyperextensible joints; kyphoscoliosis; flat feet; thin skin; deafness in adult life; blue sclerae of eyes; blue or yellow teeth.

(continued)

Table 10-1 (continued)

Overview of Genetic Disorders Affecting the Pediatric Age Group

Type of Disorder	*Characteristic of Disorder*	*Name of Disorder*	*Clinical Features*
Specific Gene Defects	Autosomal dominant	Osteogenesis imperfecta	Type II: Prenatal growth deficiency; short limbs; multiple fractures; hypotonia; hydrocephalus; frequent early death.
			Type III: Short stature; bowing and angulation of long bones; multiple fractures; kyphoscoliosis.
			Type IV: Osteoporosis leading to fractures; variable mild deformity of long bones; normal sclerae of eyes; may have poor teeth.
	Autosomal recessive	Spinal muscular atrophy	Progressive muscle atrophy and weakness; normal intelligence; normal sensation: weakness may begin before birth, in early childhood, or in later childhood.
		Sickle cell disease	A group of diseases characterized by blood disorders related to hemoglobin defects. Mostly seen in people of African or, infrequently, of Mediterranean descent. Sickle-shaped red blood cells cause anemia and crises of blockages in veins, causing a variety of conditions. These include leg ulcers, arthritis, acute pain, and problems in major organ systems, including the spleen, liver, kidney, bones, heart, and central nervous system. Children may exhibit weakness, pain, or fever and may have growth retardation.
		Hurler syndrome	Normal or rapid growth during the first year with deterioration during the second year; coarse facial features characterized by full lips, flared nostrils, thick eyebrows, low nasal bridge, and prominent forehead; still joints; small stature; small teeth, enlarged tongue; kyphosis, short neck; clawhand; hip dislocation and other joint deformities; intellectual disability.
		Phenylketonuria (inability to metabolize phenylalanine)	Intellectual disability, growth retardation, hypertonicity, seizures, and pigment deficiency of hair or skin if left untreated. Can be successfully treated by limiting amount of phenylalanine in diet.
Sex-Linked Disorders (All Affected Are Boys, X-Linked)	Abnormal gene on X chromosome	Fragile X syndrome (one of the most common causes of intellectual disability in boys)	Elongated face, large ears, prominent jaw; enlarged testicles in adulthood; prolapse of the mitral valve in the heart. Intellectual disability usually severe, sometimes with aggressive behaviors. Some boys will have poor coordination and hypotonia.
		Duchenne Muscular Dystrophy (DMD)	Onset at 1 to 5 years. Progressive, rapid weakness at onset; characteristic gait disturbances including toe walking, abducted gait, lordosis, and waddling gait. In the past, loss of ability to walk by age 9 or 10 which can progress to weakness leading to wheel chair use, decrease independence in all areas and can lead to death by late teens through respiratory or cardiac failure. Fortunately today many of these children live into adulthood and remain engaged in life for a much longer period of time. Progressive weakness leads to wheelchair use, decrease independence in all areas and death through respiratory or cardiac failure sometime between late teens to middle age.

(continued)

Table 10-1 (continued)

Overview of Genetic Disorders Affecting the Pediatric Age Group

Type of Disorder	Characteristic of Disorder	Name of Disorder	Clinical Features
Sex-Linked Disorders (All Affected Are Boys, X-Linked)	Abnormal gene on X chromosome	Lowe syndrome	Progressive mental deterioration leading to moderate to severe intellectual disability; renal dysfunction; cortical cataracts with or without glaucoma leading to blindness later in life; hypotonicity; joint hyperextensibility; growth retardation; large, low-set ears; pale skin; blonde hair.
		Lesh-Nyhan syndrome	Moderate to severe intellectual disability; hypertonicity leading to dislocated hips; clubfoot; growth retardation; movement disorders, including chorea, ballistic movements, and tremor. Self-mutilating behaviors including lip-biting and fingertip-biting characterize this disease.

*The normal number of chromosomes is 46; 47 indicates an extra chromosome present. XY refers to genetic male.
+21 refers to the extra chromosome found on the #21 chromosome.
Reprinted with permission from Ratliffe KT. *Clinical Pediatric Physical Therapy*. Elsevier; 1998:219-274.

ting, crawling, standing, and walking. Current findings indicate that treadmill intervention may accelerate the development of independent walking in children with DS. Literature suggest that task-specific training, such as locomotor treadmill training, facilitates motor development.[9] As these basic skills are achieved, physical therapy could help young children master foundational movements and develop advanced motor abilities, such as running, throwing, catching, pedaling, and jumping. As children with DS grow older, obesity may also be an issue. It is important that these children engage in activities such as organized sports that promote mobility.

A study conducted by Shumway-Cook and Woollacott[10] on children with DS indicates that this group is functioning 18 to 24 months behind age level with a significant gradual decrease of performance in both static and dynamic balance tests. Functional balance issues normally seen in this group of children may be explained by problems in the postural control system.[10] This study found that DS children are able to respond to external perturbations in a manner similar to typically developing children, except that they have a delayed activation of these responses. As a result of slow responses, these children have problems reestablishing and maintaining stability. Further, the children showed poor development of their ability to organize their responses to changing environmental context.

The life expectancy for people with DS—50 years on average, with many living much longer—has increased more than fourfold since 1960.[11] Scientific advances have revealed links between DS and Alzheimer's disease. However, new investigations have identified promising new compounds that might be effective treatments for Alzheimer's disease and maybe ready for human testing in the near future.[12]

Prader-Willi Syndrome

Prader-Willi syndrome is brought about by a structural deformity of chromosome 15. It is relatively common, occurring in 1 of 15,000 to 1 of 30,000 births.[13] Like children with DS, these children also exhibit recognizable dysmorphic features such as a narrow bifrontal diameter, almond-shaped palpebral fissures, narrow nasal bridge, and thin upper lip. Hypopigmentation is notable with their fair hair, eyes, and skin color. Other clinical features include hypotonia and abnormal neurological functions, hypogonadism, developmental and cognitive delays, hyperphagia and obesity, short stature, and behavioral and psychiatric disturbances. Physical therapy is important in managing hypotonicity, motor delays, functional performance, and obesity.

Fragile X Syndrome

Fragile X syndrome is a single-gene X-linked disorder that leads to ID.[14] There is a silencing of the fragile X ID 1 gene that results to a reduction or absence of the fragile X ID protein needed for normal brain development.

Fragile X syndrome affects both males and females, although physical characteristics are mostly noted in males. The Centers for Disease Control and Prevention[15] estimates that 1 in every 4,000 to 5,000 males and 1 in 6,000 to 8,000 females is born with this condition. Most people with Fragile X syndrome have physical, developmental and behavioral skills limitations. (Box 10-1)[16]

Based on the list in Box 10-1, physical therapists and physical therapist assistants can contribute in the manage-

Box 10-1
Fragile X Syndrome Characteristics

- Physical characteristics:
  - Mild to moderate low muscle tone
  - Hyperextensible joints
  - Pes planus
  - High-arched palate
  - Mitral valve prolapse
  - Scoliosis
  - Pectus excavatum
  - Soft skin
- Behavioral characteristics:
  - Motor and speech delays
  - Short attention span
  - Hyperactive/hypoactive sensory responses
  - Hyperactivity
  - Dislike of change
  - Heightened anxiety
  - Poor auditory learning skills

ment of children with Fragile X syndrome by addressing physical symptoms of muscle tone, hyperextensible joints, motor delays, and impaired sensory responses. As children get older, issues of balance and coordination may arise, and these should also be addressed.[16]

Cri du Chat Syndrome

Cri du chat syndrome is a genetic disease that results from a deletion of the short arm of chromosome 5.[17] This rare disease occurs in 1 of 50,000 live-born infants.[11] Its distinct clinical feature is the infant's characteristic high-pitched cat-like cry from which the syndrome's name is taken. This is probably due to anomalies of the larynx, which is small, narrow, and diamond shaped. Infants have a distinct facial dysmorphism, microcephaly, and severe psychomotor and intellectual disability .[17] They initially present with hypotonia at birth, but this muscle tone is replaced by hypertonia as the child develops. A study on using the Denver Developmental Screening Test II established that half of the patients walk by themselves at 3 years old and all learn to walk by adulthood.[17] Of children with cri du chat syndrome, 25% are able to use short sentences at 4.5 years old, 50% at 5.5 years, and all at 10 years. They are also able to achieve some skills for ADL such as feeding at 3.5 years and dressing at 5 years. Despite severe cognitive and psychomotor delays, these children are able to learn and achieve many skills in childhood.

For children with cri du chat, magnetic resonance imaging reveals atrophy of the brainstem, which includes the pons, cerebellum, median cerebellar peduncles, and cerebellar white matter.[17] This helps to explain the motor dysfunctions that these children present.

Physical therapists may be called on to help improve suction and swallowing in infants diagnosed with cri du chat. Early rehabilitation can help them develop motor skills and prevent some psychomotor delays. Because the children may have sensory-neural deafness and speech delays, physical therapists may find that it is critical to collaborate with speech pathologists.

Individuals with cri du chat syndrome have a good prognosis for survival once they overcome medical difficulties in the first years of life.[17] Rehabilitative programs for children with cri du chat syndrome have led to improving psychomotor challenges that contribute to independent activities and social adaptation.

Rett Syndrome

Rett syndrome is a monogenic X-linked dominant disorder due to mutations in the methyl CpG binding protein 2, or *MECP2* gene. This gene is responsible for making the protein MECP2. The MECP2 protein is found all over the body but is most numerous in the brain.[18] It seems that this protein plays an important role in the function of nerve cells and maintenance of synapses. In Rett syndrome, mutations of the *MECP2* gene alter the structure or reduce the amount of the protein MECP2.[19]

Rett syndrome occurs in 1 out of 10,000 births and is seen in females. The *MECP2* gene is found in the X chromosome. Unlike females with 2 X chromosomes that allow them to survive on 1 normal X chromosome, the male child whose X chromosome is affected often does not survive in utero and results in miscarriage or stillbirth. If the males survive to birth, they usually have a very early death.[20]

A key characteristic of Rett syndrome is the neurological regression that severely affects motor, cognitive, and communication skills.[18] Parents will often recount that their daughter was born "normal" and was developing normally before they noticed her losing certain skills or abilities. Around the first year of life, a slowing down of development will be observed, followed by regression in psychomotor abilities such as movement and speech.[21]

Children with Rett syndrome exhibit severe ID, seizures, dystonia, incoordination, orthopedic deformities, muscle wasting with contractures, dyspraxia, agitation, and sleep disturbances. They may experience abnormal breathing patterns and display with cold and blue extremities.[18] A classic clinical feature of Rett syndrome is loss of hand function and the appearance of stereotypical hand movements further limiting function.[12] Girls demonstrate continuous repetitive midline movements with hand-wringing, hand-washing, and clapping.

Physical therapy for Rett syndrome is aimed at maintaining physical fitness and function and decreasing secondary complications of immobility.[21] Secondary complications may include kyphoscoliosis and foot deformities such as equinus, equinovalgus, or equinovarus.

Edwards' Syndrome

Trisomy 18, or Edwards' syndrome, is less common than DS but is the second most common autosomal trisomy. This chromosomal abnormality occurs in 1 in 3500 births.[7] Females are affected more than males at a 3:1 ratio.[22,23] This incidence may be higher if not for pregnancy termination and intrauterine fatal demise.[24] Only 5% to 10% of infants with trisomy 18 live beyond 1 year, and those who survive have profound neuro-development disabilities.[24,25] Although several abnormalities can manifest in this syndrome, the heart is affected 75% of the time, the gastrointestinal system 5% to 25% of the time, and less frequently, the central nervous system, craniofacial, eye, and limbs are affected. In addition, children with Edwards' syndrome have marked profound psychomotor and intellectual delays. Most are unable to achieve expressive language and independent ambulation.[23]

Physical therapists and physical therapist assistants address psychomotor and cognitive delays when working with infants with Edwards' syndrome. Symptoms to watch out for are listed in Box 10-2.

Box 10-2
Symptoms Related to Edwards' Syndrome

- Cardiovascular defects (eg, ventricular and atrial septal defects, and patent ductus arterioles)
- Respiratory problems (eg, upper airway obstruction and central apnea)
- Limb and spine malformations (eg, equinovarus, calcaneovalgus, overriding fingers, and scoliosis)
- Hypotonia in infancy, and hypertonia in older children
- Seizures in 25% to 50% of children
- Visual and auditory problems (eg, cataracts or corneal opacities, photophobia, sensorineural hearing loss)

Muscular Dystrophy

In 2014, a steering committee of experts from a wide range of disciplines was established to update the DMD care considerations. The committee identified 11 topics to be included in the care considerations. Eight of these topics were addressed in the original care considerations established in 2010: diagnosis, neuromuscular management, rehabilitation management, gastrointestinal and nutritional management, respiratory management, cardiac management, orthopedic and surgical management, and psychological management.[26] Three new topics have since been added: primary care and emergency management, endocrine management, and transition of care across the lifespan.[27,28] DMD will be discussed in more depth later in this chapter under special focus topics specific to selected conditions.

The 5 stages of DMD are pre-symptomatic, early ambulatory, late ambulatory, early non-ambulatory, and late non-ambulatory. In this chapter, the rehabilitation management for each of the 5 stages of DMD is shown in Appendix B: Five Stages of Duchenne Muscular Dystrophy and Rehabilitation Management. The key rehabilitation team member is usually a physical therapist. Other rehab personnel include the physicians, occupational therapist, physical therapist assistant, occupational therapy assistant, speech-language pathologist, orthotist, and durable medical equipment provider(s).[27,28]

The test and measures recommended for children with DMD are listed in Appendix A: Core Assessment Measures for Neuromuscular Conditions. Different practice settings, their physicians, and rehabilitation specialists, may use or emphasize certain test and measures. The most important factor to consider is that whichever tools may be selected, those tests and measures should be consistently used over time to assess and identify the patients with DMD functional status and disease progression (Appendix B).

There are a variety of types of muscular dystrophies (MDs), but all dystrophy medical diagnoses relate to muscle diseases that over time will weaken the musculoskeletal system. This weakness is caused by the death of muscle cells from defects in the proteins within the muscles themselves. The most common form is DMD, but other varieties include limb-girdle, Becker, facioscapulohumeral, myotonic, congenital, and distal dystrophy.[29] There are a few other types, but they are extremely rare. Males show a higher prevalence of these diseases, although females can also be diagnosed with MD. Although the predominant problem is seen in the peripheral musculoskeletal system, in time all muscle groups can be affected. Thus, the heart and respiratory systems experience critical system failures that ultimately lead to death. With MD, other organ systems, such as the vision, brain, gastrointestinal, and endocrine systems, can also be affected. Because these conditions are inherited and follow different courses, the diagnosis of MD is performed through muscle biopsies, electrocardiogram, electromyography, and DNA analysis. A common thread to these diseases is that the dystrophin gene within the muscles breaks down the muscle tissue itself, which leads to functional motor problems and in time diminishes the individual's ability to participate in normal childhood, adolescent, and adult activities.

The possibility of newborn screening and the anticipated emergence of genetic and molecular disease-modifying treatments for DMD mean that earlier initiation of treatment will become increasingly important in the future. The optimum timing for initiation of new therapies will be a key factor in decisions to implement newborn screening for DMD.[27] Noninvasive prenatal testing for DMD is likely to become clinically available, allowing earlier identification of affected fetuses in women without a family history of DMD.[30]

DMD is the type most frequently seen by physical therapists. A few decades ago, the diagnosis of DMD meant the child would not survive to adulthood. Today, many individuals with DMD survive into adulthood and middle age thanks to the use of corticosteroids and the prevention of other problems such as pneumonia. The introduction of robotic assistive devices has already shown to help maintain the functional mobility in these children and allow them to continue to participate in life.[31,32] Exon-skipping mediated by antisense oligonucleotides (AOS), short single-strand DNAs, has considerable potential for DMD therapy, and clinical trials in DMD patients are currently underway. This exon-skipping therapy changes an out-of-frame mutation into an in-frame mutation, aiming at conversion of a severe DMD phenotypes into a mild phenotype by restoration of truncated dystrophin expression.[33]

Developmental Problems Without Specific Identified Genetic Conditions

Normal development is a lifelong process that is a result of the complex interplay of biological, psychological, cultural, and environmental factors (see Chapter 3). One approach to child development tracks this development within particular domains, such as gross motor, fine motor, social, emotional, language, and cognition skills or behaviors. Within each of these categories are sequences that reflect positive developmental changes and increase the child's ability to become independent in functional activities. These domains within normal development intertwine throughout life. A deficit in one area may cause secondary complications or impairments within another. Developmental delay is a common problem seen in pediatric physical therapy practice.[34] Refer to Table 10-2 for specific developmental milestones within the first 2 years of life.

Many children with abnormal genetic conditions show developmental problems within the first 2 years of life. Similarly, many children have developmental delays without identified genetic correlates. Children born prematurely are at risk of these developmental problems and are usually monitored by developmental specialists, physicians, and physical therapists or occupational therapists. Some of these children will be diagnosed with cerebral palsy (see Chapter 9). For other children without early markers such as MD to identify potential problems, parents are usually the ones to identify that something is wrong with the normal development of their child and ask their pediatricians about these issues. It may be that some of these children have genetic problems and will be diagnosed through genetic tests, whereas others may in time fall into the category of "junk genetics" and have not yet been identified as a genetic problem. Some children may have had some sort of undiagnosed neurological insult in utero that has affected development. But there are many other children who do not reach acceptable developmental milestones who will later be diagnosed with learning disabilities (LDs), IDs, developmental coordination disorders (DCDs), or autism, to mention just a few. Thus, developmental delays are considered delays in milestones that are typically expected of children within a specific age range (Tables 10-3 and 10-4).

Development of a child is so much more than physical size; it refers to the cognitive, social, fine motor, gross motor, and language skills of that individual and how those components interact with activities that are functional as well as societal. The physical therapist or physical therapist assistance may be asked to provide intervention for children with these delays, and it is important for the physical therapist to differentiate whether these delays cross all categories of development or are identified only within specific categories. Children who have consistent delays in all categories usually have generalized retardation, whereas children who have inconsistent delays in developmental categories often fall into a larger group of children with LDs that include motor coordination problems, general academic learning problems, and autism. All of these categories of developmental delays can be the reason why this child and his or her family are referred to physical therapy. Children with general LDs are usually treated within the school system by physical therapists, occupational therapists, and speech pathologists to try to facilitate academic learning.

There are also children with DCDs. These children are usually diagnosed with DCD after the physician has eliminated various LD problems, autism, ID, and genetic abnormalities. DCD is primarily a problem of praxis; the child demonstrates spatial organizational problems that cause the coordination difficulties. The problem affects gross and fine motor development and leads to academic challenges in school because of the demand to write a name, a sentence, or a math problem, as well as the fine motor expressive skills of speech. Prior to attending school, these children are seen as clumsy, and parents are often told they will just grow out of these problems. Whether they are treated by a physical therapist or played with by the parents, the children need repetitive practice in gross and fine motor skill development to help them participate in normal motor activities and thus develop quality in their lives.[35-37] In terms of intervention that can be performed by the physical therapist assistant, the handling techniques presented in Chapter 5 may assist in facilitating mobility in this population of patients. These children do not necessarily have cognitive deficits, but have great difficulty expressing their thoughts when using a hand to write or draw (eg, holding a pencil, crayon, or pen) and when trying to express their thoughts verbally.[38] The specific causation of DCD is not known, but these children have problems with rhythmic coordination, catching and throwing, posture,

Table 10-2
Developmental Milestones in the First 2 Years of Life

Milestone	*Average Age of Attainment (mo)*	*Developmental Implications*
Gross Motor		
Holds head steady in sitting	2	Allows more visual interaction
Can pull to sit, no head lag	3	Muscle tone
Brings hands together in midline	3	Self-discovery
Asymmetric tonic neck reflex disappears	4	Child can inspect hands in midline
Sits without support	6	Increasing exploration
Rolls back to stomach	6.5	Truncal flexion, risk of falls
Walks alone	12	Exploration, control of proximity to parents
Runs	16	Supervision more difficult
Fine Motor		
Grasps rattle	3.5	Object use
Reaches for objects	4	Visuomotor coordination
Palmar grasp disappears	4	Voluntary release
Transfers object hand to hand	5.5	Comparison of objects
Has thumb-finger grasp	8	Able to explore small objects
Turns pages of book	12	Increasing autonomy during book time
Scribbles	13	Visuomotor coordination
Builds tower of 2 cubes	15	Uses objects in combination
Builds tower of 6 cubes	22	Requires visual, gross, and fine motor coordination
Communication and Language		
Smiles in response to face, voice	1.5	Child more active in social participation
Has monosyllabic babble	6	Experimentation with sounds, tactile sense
Inhibits to "no"	7	Response to tone (nonverbal)
Follows one-step command	7	Nonverbal communication with gesture
Follows one-step command without gesture (eg, "Give it to me")	10	Verbal receptive language
Speaks first real word	12	Beginning of labeling
Speaks 4 to 6 words	15	Acquisition of object and personal names
Speaks 10 to 15 words	18	Acquisition of object and personal names
Speaks 2-word sentences (eg, "Mommy shoe")	19	Beginning grammatization, corresponds with more-than-50-word vocabulary
Cognitive		
Stares momentarily at spot where object disappeared (eg, ball dropped)	2	Lack of object permanence (out of sight, out of mind)
Stares at own hand	4	Self-discovery, cause and effect
Bangs 2 cubes	8	Active comparison of objects

(continued)

Table 10-2 (continued)
Developmental Milestones in the First 2 Years of Life

Milestone	*Average Age of Attainment (mo)*	*Developmental Implications*
Uncovers toy (after seeing it hidden)	8	Object permanence
Egocentric pretend play	12	Beginning symbolic thought (eg, pretends to drink from cup)
Uses stick to reach toy	17	Able to link actions and solve problems
Pretend play with doll (eg, gives doll bottle)	17	Symbolic thought

This article was published in *Nelson Textbook of Pediatrics*, 17th ed; Behrman RE, Kliegman RM, Jenson HB, eds; Growth and development; Needlman RD; 44-50; Copyright Elsevier 2004.

Table 10-3
Signs of Possible Delay: First Year of Life

Age of Child	*Problems Encountered*
During Week 2, 3, or 4	• Sucks poorly and feeds slowly • Does not blink when shown a bright light • Does not focus on and follow a nearby object moving side-to-side • Rarely moves arms and legs seem stiff • Seems excessively loose in limbs or floppy • Lower jaw trembles constantly, even when not crying or excited • Does not respond to loud sounds
By the End of 3rd, 4th, and 5th Months	• Does not notice her or his hands by 2 months • Does not follow moving objects with her or his eyes by 2 to 3 months • Does not grasp and hold objects by 3 months • Does not reach for and grasp toys by 3 to 4 months • Still has no motor reflex • Does not seem to respond to loud sounds • Does not babble by 3 to 4 months • Begins babbling but does not try to imitate any sounds by 4 months • Does not bring objects to her or his mouth by 4 months • Does not push down with her or his legs when feet are placed on a firm surface by 4 months • Still has the tonic neck reflex at 4 to 5 months • Has trouble moving one eye or both eyes in all directions • Crosses her or his eyes most of the time • Does not pay attention to new faces, or seems very frightened by new faces or surroundings

(continued)

balance, gait, and sensory perception,[39] and thus are seen by physical therapists.

Task-oriented motor functions have been shown to be the best intervention strategies and fall directly under the scope of practice of physical therapists and occupational therapists. Thus, a physical therapist assistant may very likely see a child with DCD when working in a pediatric setting.[40]

Another population in whom developmental deficits are seen is children with autism. These children may have coordination problems but also have behavioral interaction problems. This pervasive developmental problem needs a multidisciplinary approach. Because of the complexity of these cases, intervention is not often delegated to a physical therapist assistant.

Warning signs of developmental delays, whether caused by genetic factors, DCDs, LDs, or other possible diagnoses, require that the physical therapist assistant identify and recognize these problems when working with children (Table 10-5).

Table 10-3 (continued)
Signs of Possible Delay: First Year of Life

Age of Child	Problems Encountered
By the End of 7th and 8th Months	• Seems very stiff with tight muscles • Seems very floppy like a rag doll • Head still flops back like a rag doll • Reaches with one hand only • Refuses to cuddle • Shows no affection for the person who cares for her or him • Does not seem to enjoy being around people • One eye or both eyes consistently turn in or out • Persistent tearing, eye drainage, or sensitivity to light • Does not respond to sound • Has difficulty getting object to the mouth • Does not turn head to locate sounds by 4 months • Does not roll over in either direction (front to back or vice versa) by 5 months • Seems inconsolable at night after 5 months • Does not smile spontaneously by 5 months • Cannot sit with help by 6 months • Does not laugh or make squealing sounds by 6 months • Does not actively reach for objects by 6 to 7 months • Does not follow objects with both eyes at near ranges (1 to 6 feet) by 7 months • Does not bear some weight on legs by 7 months • Does not try to attract attention through actions by 7 months • Does not babble by 8 months • Shows no interest in games of peek-a-boo by 8 months
By the End of 12 Months	• Does not crawl • Drags one side of body while crawling (for more than 1 month) • Cannot stand when supported • Does not search for objects that are hidden while he or she watches • Says no single word ("Mama" or "Dada") • Does not learn to use gestures, such as waving or shaking head • Does not point to objects or pictures

Adapted from American Academy of Pediatrics, Shelov SP, Hanneman RE, Wray W, Gray A. *Caring for Your Baby and Young Child: Birth to Age Five*. New York, NY: Bantam Books; 1998.

Physical Therapy Management of Children With Genetic and Developmental Conditions: Core Examination Tools

The preceding sections discussed clinical features of the selected genetic conditions and/or developmental delays that may be improved following physical therapy intervention. Problems with fine and gross motor skill development directly affect activities and participation. Impairments such as tone, muscle strength, and balance abnormalities obviously affect skill development and optimal function. Subsystem involvement, such as cognitive deficits, communication disorders, and oral motor delay also confound not only the main problem, but also the potential for habilitation. As the child grows, additional problems, such as loss of range of motion (ROM), weakness, and decreased cardiovascular endurance, further complicate functional progress. Obesity either from dietary habits or immobility can lead to additional problems for these children.

The following section describes in detail some of the more important examination procedures to objectively assess the clinical problems of children with genetic conditions and developmental delays. In the review of the literature, certain assessment tools should be considered to measure the body functions, activity, and participation levels of the children with neuromuscular conditions. The assessment type and assessment tools are listed with a brief description of the tools and which International Classification of Function (ICF) it measures (see Appendix A).

Table 10-4

Signs of Possible Delay: Second to Fifth Years of Life

Age of Child	*Problems Encountered*
By the End of 2 Years	• Cannot walk by 18 months • Fails to develop a mature heel-toe walking pattern after several months of walking or walking on his or her toes • Does not speak at least 15 words by 18 months • Does not use 2-word sentences • By 15 months, does not seem to know the function of common objects (eg, brush, telephone, bell, fork, or spoon) • Does not imitate actions or words • Does not follow instructions • Cannot push a wheeled toy
By the End of 3 Years	• Frequently falls and has difficulty with stairs • Demonstrates persistent drooling or very unclear speech • Cannot build a tower of more than 4 blocks • Has difficulty manipulating small objects • Cannot copy a circle • Cannot communicate in short phrases • No involvement in "pretend" play • Cannot understand simple instructions • Has little interest in other children • Has extreme difficulty separating from mother
By the End of 4 Years	• Cannot throw a ball overhand • Cannot jump in place • Cannot ride a tricycle • Cannot grasp a crayon between thumb and fingers • Has difficulty scribbling • Cannot stack 4 blocks • Still clings or cries whenever the parents leave • Shows no interest in interactive games • Ignores other children • Does not respond to people outside the family • Does not engage in fantasy play • Resists dressing, sleeping, and using the toilet • Lashes out without self-control when angry or upset • Cannot copy a circle • Does not use sentences of more than 3 words • Does not use "Me" and "You" appropriately *(continued)*

Motor Skill Development

Children with motor coordination problems or genetic conditions that affect neurological function will typically manifest with delays in acquisition of motor skills and abnormal movement patterns. Infants and children may have limitations in performing and participating in activities typically performed by age-equivalent individuals. This is true not only of children with genetic problems, but also in a larger community of children with delays in development. Past studies show that the rate of motor development of children with DS is slightly below that of non-DS children. Among children with DS, sitting will be achieved with a 70% probability at 12 months, standing at 24 months, and walking at 30 months. Advanced motor skills are also achieved at around 72 months with a 67% probability for running, 77% for climbing a step, and 84% for jumping forward.[41]

The multisystemic issues present in children with Prader-Willi syndrome contribute to problems in movement and posture. Neurological issues include poor gross motor and fine motor coordination.[42] Their motor skills in

Table 10-4 (continued)
Signs of Possible Delay: Second to Fifth Years of Life

Age of Child	*Problems Encountered*
By the End of 5 Years	• Exhibits extremely fearful or timid behavior • Exhibits extremely aggressive behavior • Cannot separate from parents without major protest • Is easily distracted and unable to concentrate on any single activity for more than 5 minutes • Shows little interest in playing with other children • Refuses to respond to people in general, or responds only superficially • Rarely uses fantasy or imitation in play • Seems unhappy or sad much of the time • Does not engage in a variety of activities • Avoids or seems aloof with other children and adults • Does not express a wide range of emotions • Has trouble eating, sleeping, or using the toilet • Cannot differentiate between fantasy and reality • Seems unusually passive • Cannot understand 2-part commands using prepositions • Cannot correctly give his or her first and last name • Does not use plurals or past tense properly when speaking • Does not talk about his or her daily activities and experiences • Cannot build a tower of 6 to 8 blocks • Seems uncomfortable holding a crayon • Has trouble taking off clothing • Cannot brush his or her teeth efficiently • Cannot wash and dry his or her hands

Adapted from American Academy of Pediatrics, Shelov SP, Hanneman RE, Wray W, Gray A. *Caring for Your Baby and Young Child: Birth to Age Five*. New York, NY: Bantam Books; 1998.

sitting, kneeling, standing, and walking are delayed compared with typically developing children.[43] Hypotonia and severe obesity affects motor development in older children. Later into adult life, these effects are observed in abnormal gait and postural instability. Poor motor coordination can result in delayed acquisition of motor skills.

Specific motor skills and stages of motor development can be measured, monitored, and compared to milestones of other children of comparable age. Several motor skills assessment tests and measures are available and used in physical therapy. These tools are discussed in Chapter 6 and include tests and measures that are appropriate for any child with a delay in development, whether or not that delay is due to a specific genetic deficit. Knowledge of the most frequently used tests can help guide the physical therapist to monitor the effectiveness of the plan of care for specific patients. There are many reliable and valid assessment tools a physical therapist might use to measure progression of a child's functional skills (see Appendix A). No one motor assessment tool is necessarily better than another, and often the determining factor regarding choice is either the physical therapist or the facility within which both the physical therapist and the physical therapist assistant are employed. Two are discussed here.

Gross Motor Function Measure

The Gross Motor Function Measure (GMFM) is a standardized observational criterion-referenced instrument to measure change in gross motor function over time and often used by physical therapists and physical therapist assistants when working with children. The GMFM has undergone revisions from its original form of 88 items to its current form of 66 items.[44] This test was developed to measure gross motor skills of children with cerebral palsy; however, it has been found to be a valid and reliable tool for children with DS and for children with developmental delays.[44-46] This test can describe the child's current level of motor function and help determine treatment goals. Having this information allows clinicians to provide a more concrete way to explain to parents concerns regarding their child's progress and what they might expect as the next step in the progression with their child. The GMFM measures how much of the activity the child can perform instead of how well the child will be able to perform it. The tool measures 5 dimensions of gross motor function: lying

Table 10-5
Warning Signs of a Developmental Delay

Warning Signs
Behavioral
• Does not pay attention or stay focused on an activity for as long a time as other children the same age. • Focuses on unusual objects for long periods of time; enjoys this more than interacting with others. • Avoids or rarely makes eye contact with others. • Gets unusually frustrated when trying to do simple tasks that most children of the same age can do. • Shows aggressive behaviors, acts out, and appears to be very stubborn compared with other children. • Displays violent behaviors on a daily basis. • Stares into space, rocks body, or talks to self more often than other children of the same age. • Does not seek love and approval from a caregiver or parent.
Gross Motor
• Has stiff arms and/or legs. • Has a floppy or limp body posture compared with other children of the same age. • Uses one side of body more than the other. • Has a very clumsy manner compared with other children of the same age.
Vision
• Seems to have difficulty following objects or people with his or her eyes. • Rubs eyes frequently. • Turns, tilts, or holds head in a strained or unusual position when trying to look at an object. • Seems to have difficulty finding or picking up small objects dropped on the floor (after the age of 12 months). • Has difficulty focusing or making eye contact. • Closes one eye when trying to look at distant objects. • Eyes appear to be crossed or turned. • Brings objects too close to eyes to see. • One eye or both eyes appear abnormal in size or coloring.
Hearing
• Talks in a very loud or very soft voice. • Seems to have difficulty responding when called from across the room, even when it is for something interesting. • Has difficulty understanding what has been said or following directions (after the age of 3 years). • Does not startle to loud noises. • Ears appear small or deformed. • Fails to develop sounds or words that would be appropriate at her or his age.
Adapted from Child and Adolescent Services Research Center. How Kids Develop. http://www.howkidsdevelop.com/developDevDelay.html. Accessed May 6, 2005.

and rolling; sitting; crawling and kneeling; standing; and walking, running, and jumping.

Peabody Developmental Motor Scales, Second Edition

Another measure of motor skills used with very young children is the Peabody Developmental Motor Scales, 2nd Edition[47] (PDMS-2). This tool assesses motor skills in children from birth to 5 years of age. There are 6 subtests that can be scored under 2 composites: the gross motor quotient, and the fine motor quotient. The subtests under the gross motor quotient are reflexes, stationary, locomotion, and object manipulation; therapists outside the United States use this tool.[48] The subtests under the fine motor quotient are grasping and visual motor integration. The results of the test can provide the examiner the age equivalents of the infants.[49] This is a frequently asked question of parents, but therapists must always remember to stress what the child can functionally do, and not any specific age norms, because that often leads to misinterpretation of the potential of a small child.

Tone Abnormalities: Hypotonia and Hypertonia

Normal tone refers to that characteristic of muscle in its state of readiness. Tone should be high enough so that muscle activation can be initiated and maintained during a movement or postural contraction, and yet low enough to allow normal range of movement against gravity.[50]

Hypotonia or hypotonicity is a common feature among children with genetic conditions such as DS and Prader-Willi syndrome. Low tone is also often found in children with developmental delays and/or IDs. A systematic review of evidence indicated that there is limited evidence for valid and reliable methods in assessment of hypotonia.[51] Further, this review suggested that a good medical history and proper initial clinical observation are still the best way to determine hypotonicity. Characteristics most frequently observed in children with hypotonia include decreased strength, hypermobile joints, increased flexibility, rounded shoulder posture, delayed motor skills, tendency to lean on supports, poor attention and motivation, and decreased activity tolerance.[52] These characteristics are obtained mainly through observation of the child. At present, the French Angles Factor of the Infant Neurological International Battery is meant to determine hypotonia but fails to discriminate findings from those of hypermobility. The French Angles include the scarf sign, heel-to-ear, popliteal angle, and abductor's angle.[53] The scoring sheet for this battery can be retrieved from https://academic.oup.com/ptj/article-abstract/66/4/548/2728037?redirectedFrom=fulltext. This can guide the therapist on how to perform and score the test. Martin et al[52] proposed that there is a need to develop an operational definition of hypotonia to develop a valid test to determine the presence of this impairment and to assess effectiveness of intervention.

Hypertonicity and *spasticity* are often used interchangeably. However, the difference lies in how they are elicited. Clopton and colleagues[54] pointed out that spasticity is "velocity-dependent resistance of a muscle to stretch," whereas hypertonia is "increased resistance to externally-imposed movement." Both of these types of tone are often seen together. Stiffening of the limbs, tremors and/or clonus, weakness, and difficulty in movement may be present along with spasticity and hypotonia. Children with neurogenetic conditions such as cri du chat exhibit hypertonia. Children with developmental delays, LDs, or IDs do not exhibit hypertonicity or spasticity. Their central nervous system problems are not identified as specific lesions or problems within the motor system that must be correlated with these specific tonal abnormalities. Children with cerebral palsy have specific lesions within the motor system and can simultaneously have delays in development, learning problems, or retardation, but their spasticity or hypertonicity is due to the motor system lesions or deficits.

One way to measure hypertonia is through the Modified Ashworth Scale, which is discussed in detail in Chapter 6 and also found in Table 6-3. The examiner passively moves a joint through its ROM at a standard speed and rates the resistance of the stretched muscles on a 6-point scale. Although prudence is suggested in using this test,[54,55] the grading system can guide therapists to develop realistic expectations when handling patients with hypertonicity. If a grade of 3 or 4 is given, then therapists should be more gentle and patient in moving an extremity. If a grade 1 or 1+ is given, then therapists can expect to move the extremity with ease.

Balance and Coordination Tools

The Pediatric Balance Scale is a revised version of the Berg Balance Scale. The original Berg Balance Scale was modified for use with children by rearranging the order of the test items, reducing time standards for maintenance of static postures, and clarifying directions to suit children.[56] The preliminary test was performed for children from 5 to 15 years with mild to moderate motor impairments, although a more recent study on typically developing children found that the test is more appropriate for children from 2 to 6 years old.[57] The test consists of 14 items arranged in functional sequence, with the most novel tasks placed in the end. Each item requires the tester to score the child from 0 to 4 depending on a set of criteria. The rater will sum up scores for each item; a total score of 56 is expected. To date, interpretation of scores has yet to be performed.

The Four Square Step Test assesses balance in the presence of task and environmental challenge. This test showed excellent interrater reliability when used for children with cerebral palsy and DS.[58] Four canes are used and placed on the floor to come up with 4 squares of 90 cm each. The child is asked to move from one square to the next until the fourth square and then goes back the starting square as fast as possible without touching the canes. The time from start to finish is recorded.

The functionally based Timed Up and Go is shown to be a meaningful outcome measure for children with and without disabilities.[59] The test was modified from its original version when used in adults to accommodate children:

1. The child is asked to sit on a seat with backrest but without armrests. The seat height should allow for a 90-degree knee flexion angle with feet flat on the floor.
2. The child is instructed to stand up, touch a target on a wall 3 meters away from the chair, and then return to the seat to sit down. Time starts as soon as the child's bottom leaves the chair and ends when it touches the chair again.
3. Instructions are repeated during the test.
4. Children are allowed to behave spontaneously (eg, not asked to walk as fast as they can) to get at a more naturalistic performance.

The Timed Up and Go test shows good interrater and test-retest reliability scores when tested for children with disabilities.[59] This test has been used for children with cerebral palsy and spina bifida[60] and for children with

DS.[59,60] The use of this test for children with other medical diagnoses must be done judiciously.

The Timed Floor to Stand-Natural test measures the time to complete the functional task of transition from sitting on the floor, to walking a short distance at a natural place, and returning to sitting on the floor. The test has a good range of intratester reliability and strong intertester as well as test-retest reliability. This test is appropriate for school age children older than 5 years of age.[61,62]

Many of the gross motor measures listed in Appendix A also have the capability to provide insight on the balance and coordination of children with genetic and/or developmental problems.

Physical Therapy Intervention Strategies

Genetic conditions with neuro-developmental concerns often result in motor problems that in turn result in movement dysfunctions. Similarly, children with various types of developmental delays also exhibit movement dysfunction that leads to motor delays. This requires the physical therapist and physical therapist assistant to be essential members of the health care team for these children. The common impairments and activity limitations encountered in these conditions include tone abnormalities (hyper- and hypotonicity), weakness, delay in the development of fine- and gross-motor skills, and problems with balance and coordination. The following are interventions that can usually be delegated to the physical therapist assistant.

Techniques for Managing Tone Problems

Proper positioning in infancy should be implemented at birth. Infants with low muscle tone tend to get into the frog-like posture in which the hips are flexed, abducted, and internally rotated, and the knees are flexed.[63] In a study of low-risk preterm neonates, Vaivre-Douret and associates[64] reiterated the use of proper positioning during infancy to counteract abnormalities in muscle tone. Significant differences in posturing were noted in the treatment group who were reposting every 3 to 4 hours in supine, side-lying, and prone positions during their stay at the neonatal care unit. A support mattress was used to position the infants in side-lying and supine. In side-lying, the infant's head was positioned to be aligned with the trunk. In supine, the shoulders were held back, and the knees were bent forward. In prone, a bolster was placed under the hips to prevent rotation. Figures 10-1 through 10-10 show examples of these positioning techniques.

Handling Techniques to Guide the Child Into Normal Movement Patterns

As children mature and watch others move, they are highly motivated to move themselves. Thus, within the first year, a child will learn to roll, come to sit, sit independently, and come to stand. Some will even cruise independently and walk before their first birthday. These children continue to mature and gain motor control over more complex movement patterns, such as walking, running, climbing stairs, manipulating objects, throwing, independent feeding, and many additional movements that lead to independence and the ability to participate in age-related activities.

Children with developmental delays, no matter the causation, do not experience these same learning opportunities. Thus, they do not develop normal postural control or functional control over moving from one position to another, and they do not gain the independence in motor control over their bodies, thus limiting their ability to participate normally in age-related activities. Handling techniques are designed to move these children through these developmental patterns to allow them the opportunities to gain motor learning experiences and control over their bodies. Handling a child to encourage rolling is usually performed by controlling one of the child's legs, flexing the knee and hip, and guiding the child's pelvis and trunk into a rotation pattern in which the upper body will follow the lower body, followed next by the head. This pattern of rolling elicits a body-on-body-on-head righting reaction. The physical therapist assistant must remember that for the child to learn a motor pattern, that pattern needs to be practiced over and over as the environment is changed by having various textures to roll on, external noises with a slow increase in volume and background sounds, and slight variations in the specific movements of hip and knee flexion with rotation. To get this repetitive practice, the parents or caregivers need to be taught how to move the child consistently and repetitively as part of play. Through handling, a child can be moved from supine to prone, supine to side-lying to sit, through sitting positions, sit to 4-point, 4-point to kneeling, kneeling to half-kneeling, and half-kneeling to standing. The reader is referred to the video on handling techniques that accompanies this text.

One very effective way to learn handling techniques is to play with normal babies and feel their movements as you guide them from one position to another. Excellent resources on observing and development handling techniques can be found in a PowerPoint presentation by Lois Bly in April 2012 and in her books on the treatment of babies.[65,66] Also, spending time watching babies, children, adolescents, young adults, and aging adults is a wonderful way to learn to recognize normal movement and the transitions between one stable position to another as well as the postural control needed to remain over one position such as sitting while reaching with an extremity toward or grasping an object.

Another activity that can be used to help develop the background needed to develop handling techniques is to just move your own body. Start by lying down on the floor and feeling what you experience as you roll over, come to sit, move into various sitting postures, and move from sit to side-sit and then into 4-point. Then, rock back and sit on your knees and come up into hip extension or kneeling, then to half-kneeling and finally standing up. Then go through the same activities but with your eyes closed so you can truly feel using proprioception and vestibular input as to what is normal and what a child should experience when begin handled. Then have a colleague go through those same patterns while you hold onto his or her head, then the arm, and then the leg. By going through these activities, the physical therapist assistant can kinesthetically learn while visually identifying what those movements should look like. Then, as a clinician treating a child with developmental problems, the physical therapist assistant can feel the effort or lack thereof when the child begins to assist with the movement and finally takes control over the patterns. Remember that the goal of treatment is to allow the child to feel normal transitions and experience success with minimal effort as movement is obtained from one position to another. The reader is also referred to Chapter 5 for additional handling ideas under the Neuro-Developmental Treatment section.

Techniques for Facilitating the Development of Muscular Strength

Playing normally is the activity that a child uses to gain the muscular strength necessary to achieve motor control over postural positions and transitions between those postural patterns. A very young child is driven to move through motivation to imitate an older child or to get something it see in space.

A child with developmental delays often lacks control over the necessary power of play, and for that reason has difficulty moving from one position to another, even when the child is motivated to move. Thus, developing the necessary strength needed to independently move may become part of the plan of care for children with these medical diagnoses. Again, strengthening needs to take place through play, and that play needs to be part of the plan of care. Using a ball in play begins with very young children and progresses to all ages. Using a balloon for children who have coordination problems allows them additional time to catch the ball. Medicine balls can have graded weights and can be used to assist in strength training of the upper extremities while giving additional proprioceptive input to their nervous system. If ball play is performed in standing, then having the child pick up the weighted ball can lead to lower limb and trunk strengthening as well. A question that therapists often ask is, "Should strength training be our goal vs using an assistive device?" According to a system review of the Cochrane Database regarding rehabilitation and strength training to prevent foot drop in neuromuscular disease, little long-term effect was found between control and experimental groups. These results may indicate that the use of an orthosis to assist with dorsiflexion of the foot may lead to the best long-term outcome.[67] Thus, identifying evidence that might guide the physical therapist and physical therapist assistant as to whether to begin or continue strength training can help in developing a plan of care for all children.

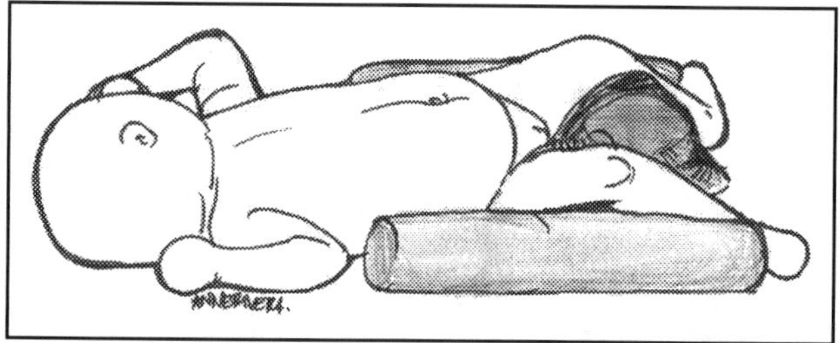

Figure 10-1. In supine, put rolled towels or pillow on lateral sides of the legs to prevent frog-like positioning of the legs. (Illustration by Anne Rivera.)

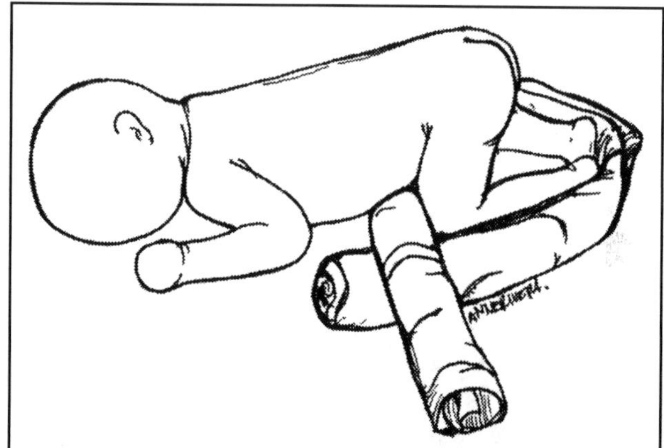

Figure 10-2. In prone, put a rolled towel or blanket to keep legs in midline and hips flexed. (Illustration by Anne Rivera.)

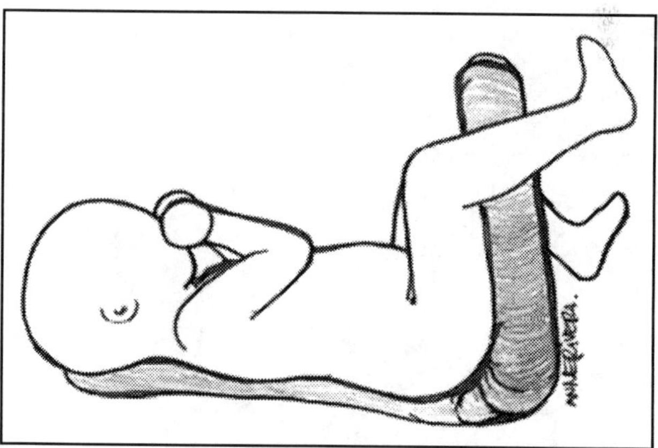

Figure 10-3. In side-lying, put a rolled towel to keep the spine straight and the hips flexed and slightly abducted. (Illustration by Anne Rivera.)

Many children will gain strength and then use that strength to participate and be functionally independent in movement activities valued by the child. But children diagnosed with some of these developmental and genetic delays need to be monitored more closely. Cautions for

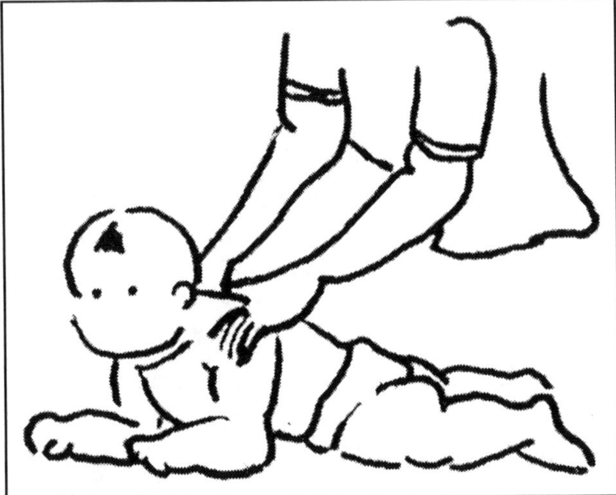

Figure 10-4. Prone on elbows. Support the child in the scapular area. (Illustration by Catherine M. Capio.)

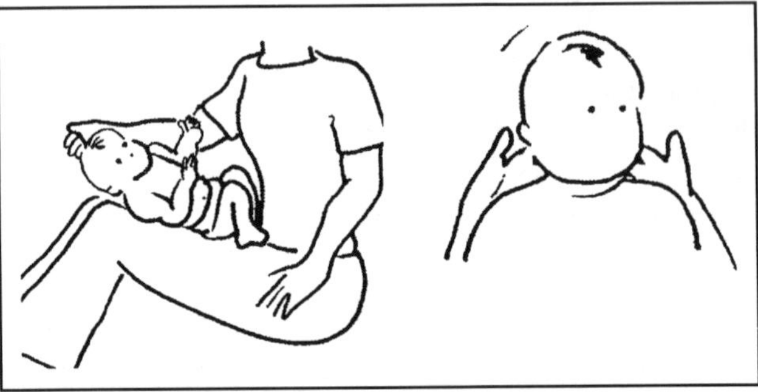

Figure 10-5. Position self in crook-lying facing the child. Give support to scapula and occiput. Lift the child while in this position and allow the child to contract his or her neck muscles. (Illustration by Catherine M. Capio.)

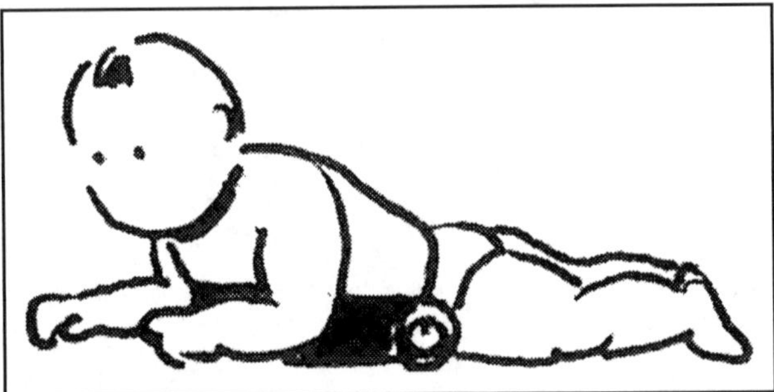

Figure 10-6. Put a rolled towel or blanket or a bolster under the chest to support the trunk in a prone-on-elbows position. (Illustration by Catherine M. Capio.)

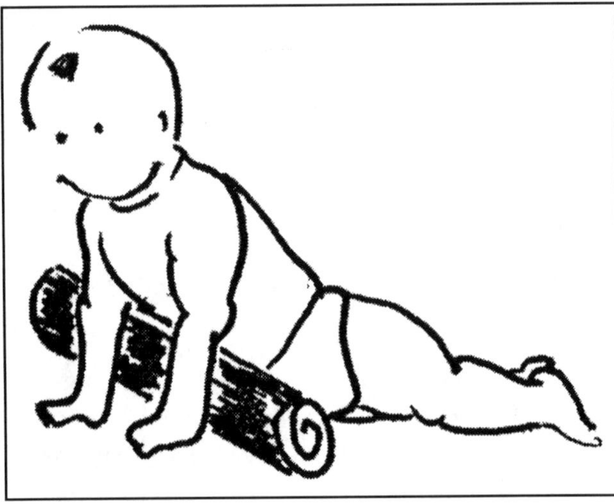

Figure 10-7. Prone-on-hands position with a bolster. (Illustration by Catherine M. Capio.)

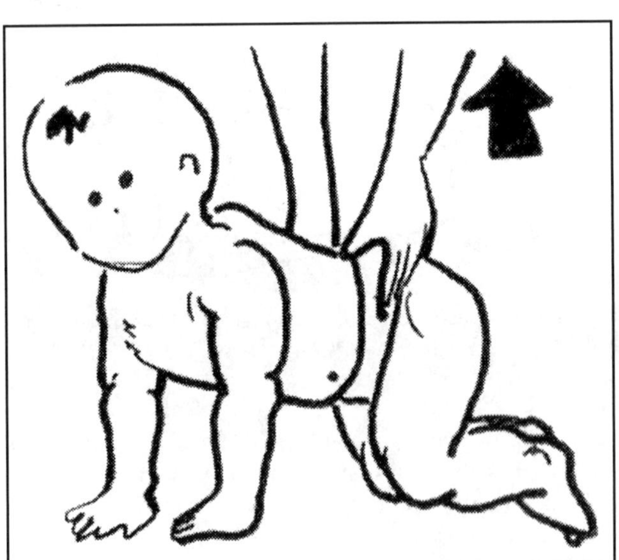

Figure 10-8. From a prone-on-hands position, get the child into a quadruped or all-fours position by lifting the pelvis up and putting weight on the knees. (Illustration by Catherine M. Capio.)

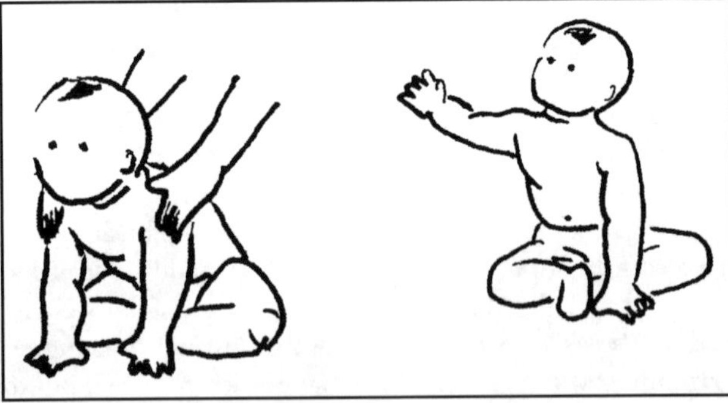

Figure 10-9. Sitting begins with bilateral arm support and progresses with the use of one hand for reaching or manipulating and eventually both hands. (Illustration by Catherine M. Capio.)

specific medical diagnoses are identified in the following few paragraphs.

Progressive resistance training is an effective program to improve strength among adolescents with DS.[68] For 10 weeks, adolescents were placed in a twice-a-week program that was designed according to the recommendations of the American College of Sports Medicine. They performed 6 exercises: latissimus pull-down, seated chest press, seated row, seated leg press, knee extension, and calf raise.

Gupta et al[69] suggested a more specific method for progressive resistance exercise for the lower limbs is to start at 50% of 1 rep maximum. Exercises using sandbags were performed for hip flexors, abductors, extensors, knee flexors and extensors, and ankle plantar flexors. Two sets for 10 reps were performed for each muscle group, and the resistance was increased by half a kilogram when the child was able to complete the sets without difficulty.

Strengthening programs for children with DCD have been reported to be successful when using free weights, body weight, pulley systems, manual resistance, or Pilates-type programs. These studies have[70-72] been shown to improve not only strength in selected muscle groups, but also balance, bilateral coordination, proprioceptive sense, self-esteem, and self-efficacy for exercise. The physical therapist assistant must remember that strength training alone will not necessarily lead to greater functional skills in life activities. Often the therapists need to sequence the strength training into functional activities that motivate the child. Those activities will continue building strength as the child continues to participate in life.

Techniques for Improving Balance and Coordination

Shumway-Cook and Woollacott's research on postural control[10] suggests that treatment should focus on helping children develop and refine their postural responses by way of improving their spatiotemporal coupling between the different muscle groups that act together. These activities should engage children in activating specific muscle groups using appropriate body movements and proper timing. This lack of postural tone is consistent in children with LDs, developmental coordination problems, developmental delays, genetic problems, and IDs. Thus, balance and coordination problems are seen in many children with specific or general diagnoses that have led to delays in motor development.

A study conducted on young children with DS[69] concluded that balance improves when they are given a 6-week exercise training program that includes resistance exercises and balance training. For balance training, children ages 11 to 14 performed horizontal jumps, vertical jumps, one leg stance with eyes open, tandem stance, walking on a line, walking on a balance beam, and jumping on a trampoline. All these activities are within the scope of practice of the physical therapist assistant.

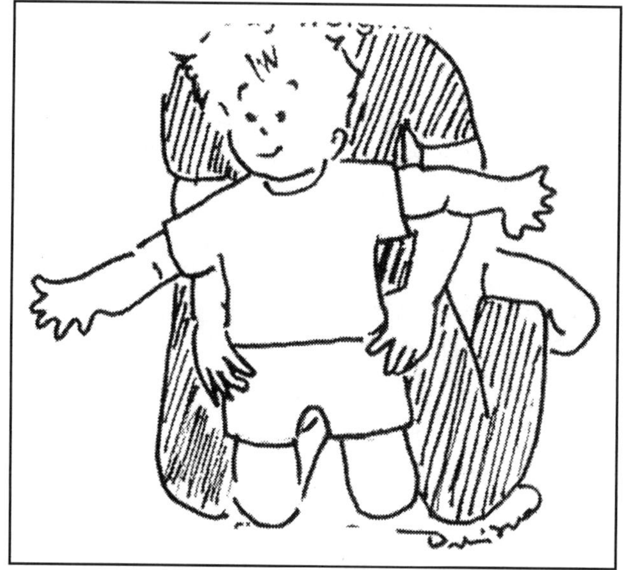

Figure 10-10. Kneeling can initiate standing by allowing the child to feel weight on the hips through the knees. (Illustration by Debbie Qua.)

Physical therapy interventions that facilitate the improvement of postural control are beneficial to this population of patients and clients. For physical therapist assistants, it is important to remember to optimize starting alignment and base of support (BOS) to provide a stable base for the trunk and lower extremity muscles. That allows the musculoskeletal system to be biomechanically optimized and will therefore facilitate more normal and functional movements.[73,74] This can be started with the patient sitting. Before starting an activity, it is important for the physical therapist assistant to make sure that the patient's feet are on the floor to increase the stable BOS. Then the physical therapist assistant can use verbal or tactile cues to improve alignment to ensure a stable proximal segment so that the child can move the distal segments (ie, extremities) more efficiently. In terms of handling and facilitation, the physical therapist assistant could use approximation techniques to facilitate co-contraction or coactivation of the postural muscles to optimize movement. As always, these could be incorporated into play activities. This way the child performs activities that are enjoyable and engaging while training to run motor programs that are not only automatic but also could facilitate cognitive loading or dual tasking.

For example, the physical therapist assistant could start with balloon-tossing activities with the child in sitting with proper support and alignment, with the necessary tactile cues and facilitation to optimize the position. The physical therapist assistant could ask a helper to toss the balloon to the child, first just within a small base, and then progressing so the child moves his or her center of gravity outside the BOS. The same activity could be performed with the patient in kneeling, half-kneeling, standing, or standing on one foot. The physical therapist assistant could provide tactile cues and approximation through the shoulders or pelvis while the child performs the specific activity.

The use of adaptive/orthotic or supportive devices could also be considered, because these items allow for better support and joint protection that could decrease pain and joint stress and facilitate movement.

Exercises that improve balance on compliant and noncompliant surfaces will improve the child's ability to optimize function and increase activity and participation. Going back to the previous example, the sitting and standing activities can be progressed by having the child sit or stand on foam, with appropriate guarding strategies by the physical therapist assistant. A ball may be thrown to the child from different directions. The physical therapist assistant or child could also bounce the ball; this adds another component of complexity because the child will need both anticipatory and reactive control to be able to successfully catch and release the toy. Additionally, there are balls on the market that bounce unpredictably. Those types of balls would offer even more challenge. There is no way to anticipate where the ball will go once it is bounced, and the child would have to respond automatically and quickly.

Another way to increase complexity and link to function is to change the environment to real-world situations. The physical therapist assistant could configure activities outside of the clinic: playing on grass or asphalt or in an open environment where other people are moving, interacting, or playing with the child. This way, the child trains for physical rehabilitation, along with social and emotional interaction.

Higher-level balancing activities disguised as play could also be effective in improving balance and coordination. An obstacle course with a series of starts and stops, perhaps played as part of a game of Simon Says, allows the child to run challenging motor programs while engaging in activities that improve attention and engagement. Playing hopscotch or jump rope allows single- and double-limb support while also moving the upper extremities. As important as these activities are to motor development, the exercises themselves help the cardiovascular and pulmonary systems, improve muscular and pulmonary endurance, increase oxygenation, and improve the child's ability to tolerate more strenuous activities.

Techniques to Improve Soft Tissue Mobility

Soft tissue mobilization (Box 10-3) has been shown to improve muscle tone among toddlers with DS.[75] The tissue mobilization routine used in this study was conducted for 30 minutes twice a week. In supine, the legs and feet, stomach, chest, arms, hands, and, finally, the face were massaged. After this, the child was placed in a prone position and massage was given to the back (Figures 10-11 through 10-15).

Other techniques that involve mobilization of the soft tissues in pediatric populations include myofascial release and craniosacral techniques (see Chapter 18).[76] Both of these techniques require additional training, and the physical therapist assistant is encouraged to seek more information to incorporate these 2 important techniques in the intervention repertoire.

Myofascial release comprises manual techniques that aim to remove fascial restrictions. It is postulated that the fascia is a three-dimensional web of connective tissue that is intricately connected within the entire body. Any trauma, abnormal movements, or decreased mobility could affect the integrity of the fascia, including the formation of scar tissue that limits fascial mobility. Because it is postulated that the fascia is interconnected, it is possible that facial restrictions in one area could affect mobility in remote areas.

Craniosacral techniques also involve a series of specific manual, hands-on techniques that facilitate movements, decrease soft tissue restrictions, improve comfort, and decrease pain. Again, the techniques are highly specialized and require more training for the physical therapist assistant.

Special Focus Topics Specific to Selected Conditions

Care Considerations for Duchenne Muscular Dystrophy

The diagnosis and management of DMD was updated and published in 2018 through a multidisciplinary approach to management across a range of health care specialities.[27,28,77] The rehabilitation management section discuss assessments and interventions pertinent to physical therapy. With prolonged survival, individuals with DMD face unique challenges, and it is important for everyone in the rehabilitation team to be aware of all the medical specialists' and community providers' roles in providing care to their mutual patient. Improvements in function, quality of life, and longevity of patients with DMD have been achieved through a multidisciplinary approach to management across a range of health care specialists.[28]

Fatigue in Children With Duchenne Muscular Dystrophy

Fatigue in children with DMD may indicate the severity of the myopathy.[78] Monitoring the child with DMD during play and watching for development of incoordination or signs of fatigue are critical, and rest periods must be provided when those signs are observed. The muscle loss can be pervasive and progressive, and heavy exercise may lead to further degeneration. Thus, play and strengthening should be of low intensity but regular to maintain the power potential of the child and to allow that child to participate in life.[79-81]

Cardiopulmonary Impairments in Children With Down Syndrome and Other Neuromuscular Diseases

Although not all children with DS have secondary complications, some of them are confronted with cardiopulmonary impairments that, if not identified, can lead to life-threatening problems.[82-84] The physical therapist assistant, when playing with children to create strength training, needs to monitor heart rate and listen to the breathing. If the child begins to breathe heavily or take short but rapid breaths, then the activity may be too taxing for the cardiopulmonary system. If the physical therapist assistant sees these behaviors, documenting and reporting them to the physical therapist is very important. The physical therapist can determine whether the child needs to be referred to the physician or whether the plan of care needs to be changed. Obviously, if the child seems to be in an acute life-threatening situation, the physical therapist assistant needs to call 911 or medical staff immediately.

Trends in Developing Motor Skills

Treadmills

The use of body weight–supported treadmill training has been shown to be an effective way to treat people with cardiovascular anomalies, spinal cord injury, and Parkinson's disease, among others (see Chapters 5, 9, 11, 14, 15, 16 and 19). In recent years, the use of the treadmill for children with neuro-developmental conditions has been reported in the literature, with encouraging results.[37]

For genetic conditions, the treadmill is used for infants and children with DS,[85-89] as well as for children with Rett syndrome.[76] The child can be placed in a body weight–supported harness to take away some of the body weight and need for power or strength. Then the treadmill can be used to trigger gait patterns. As the child improves in balance and strength, the amount of body support given by the harness can be reduced, thus encouraging strength development during movement and as a postural system.[90] The difference in training these children is the slower rate needed for training and the use of a harness that fits the small child. Children with developmental delays without a specific medical diagnosis of a disease or pathology might benefit from this high-tech equipment, but would not qualify through the family's insurance to cover the cost of this type of intervention. When the child exhibits low tone without an abnormality such as spasticity, some parents might be able to adapt their home treadmills with a harness system so their child could get the repetitive practice of gait while having some body weight reduction.

Virtual-Reality Gaming Technology

Another modality being reported in the literature for children with developmental disabilities is the use of virtual reality–based activity, the most common of which is the Wii (Nintendo). Studies have shown that computerized gaming can be used to work on visual-perceptual skills, postural control, and mobility in children with cerebral palsy[91,92]; to reduce hyperactive behavior in children with attention deficit hyperactivity disorder[93]; and to enhance sensory-motor functions in children with DS.[94] Although evidence is still limited as to its effectiveness and outcomes, these studies indicate that gaming can at the very least be an adjunct to regular therapy procedures.[95] These gaming consoles are attractive to children and may help motivate these young individuals to perform physical activities (see Chapter 5 and 19).

Aquatic Physical Therapy

Standard treatment of DMD includes regular physical therapy. Aquatic physical therapy has been prescribed and recommended by more special care physicians following the DMD population since the updated care considerations were published. Although there is little data and evidence available to demonstrate the effectiveness of aquatic physical therapy to land-based exercises, many families are requesting this type of treatment, as physical therapy treatments are provided in a safe aquatic environment and interventions are designed to improve function, aerobic capacity, endurance conditioning, body mechanics and postural stabilization, flexibility, gait and locomotion, relaxation, muscle strength, power, and endurance. Aquatic physical therapies include therapeutic exercises, functional training, manual therapy, breathing strategies, electrotherapeutic modalities, physical agents, and mechanical modalities using the properties of water and techniques unique to the aquatic environment.[96]

A study by Hind et al on aquatic therapy in the United Kingdom highlighted the lack of information on the effectiveness, selection, prioritization, dosage, and practicality of protocols in patients with DMD. Service development should be co-produced with the patient with DMD and their family members, physicians, and rehabilitation team representatives, insurance providers and other community pool providers.[97]

Essential Features in the Management of Neuro-Developmental Conditions

Early Intervention

The strides gained in the field of genetics make it possible for physicians to identify and diagnose various genetic conditions at an early age. Identifying genetic conditions and syndromes as soon as possible allows parents to access medical and other health-related services for their child.

Early intervention is providing necessary and appropriate intervention at the soonest time possible. If patients with genetic conditions can be identified at birth, then referral to early intervention can begin immediately. Similarly, if a child does not progress in what is considered a nor-

Box 10-3

Soft Tissue Mobilization Techniques

1. For the legs and arms, the therapist wraps the fingers around the child's leg/arm and then gives long milking and twisting strokes from the thigh to the ankles or from the upper arm to the wrist (Figure 10-11).
2. For the stomach, slow, circular, rubbing movements are administered to the stomach area using one hand and the palms; slide one palm at a time down the stomach in a hand-over-hand manner in a paddle-wheel fashion (Figures 10-12 and 10-13).
3. For the chest, the therapist places the palms of the hands on the child's sternum and strokes outward across the chest. Start at the sternum and stroke upward and over the top of the shoulders and down the sides of the ribs (Figures 10-14 and 10-15).
4. For the face, make circles to the entire scalp as if shampooing hair; with the flat aspect of the thumbs, while together on midline of forehead, stroke outward toward the temples. Stroke gently on eyes and brows. Progress the stroking from the bridge of the nose, across the cheekbones, to the ears. It is especially important to make circular movements under the chin, around the jaw line, around the ears, to the back of the neck, and to the rest of the scalp (see Figure 10-14).
5. For the back, one described technique starts at the top of the spine, alternating hand strokes across the back working down toward the tailbone but never pressing on the spine. The physical therapist assistant must take care to make sure the hand strokes are not done vertically down along the spine, because that creates an autonomic response and slows down all sympathetic motor responses such as heart rate and breathing. Although this technique can be used to calm or relax an individual, it is not a mobilization technique and thus not used for that purpose.

Source: Hernandez-Reif, Field, Largie, Mora, Bornstein, Waldman, 2006.

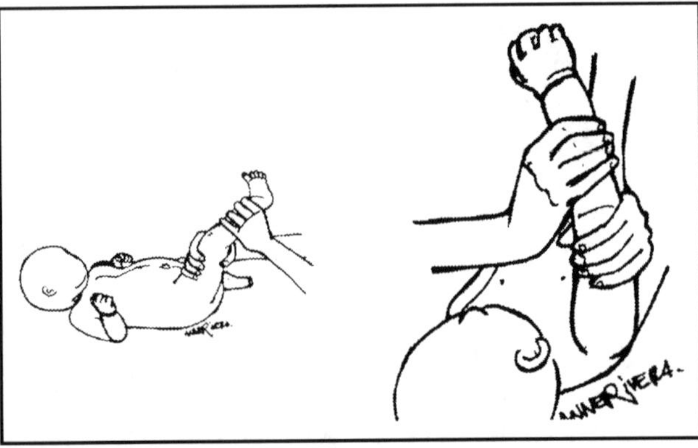

Figure 10-11. The physical therapist assistant wraps the fingers around the child's leg and arm and gives long milking and twisting strokes in a proximal-to-distal direction. (Illustration by Anne Rivera.)

mal developmental progression or rate considered within normal parameters, then that child may qualify for early intervention.

The basic tenet of providing early intervention is to minimize or reduce long-term costs and improve outcomes. For patients with acute or developmental lesions that affect the brain or spinal cord, the basic principles for enhancing neural outcomes include growth of new cells, regrowth of connections, and retraining of existing growths.[88] The chance for each of these neural outcomes to happen depends on factors such as the area that is affected, the extent of damage, and the timing of injury. Regardless, research indicates that activity and specialty training are needed if the physical therapy interventions are to promote neuroplasticity and neuromotor control and to ensure functional outcomes.[88]

In the United States, the Individuals with Disabilities Education Act (IDEA) was amended in 1986 through Public Law (P.L.) 99-457 to include infants and toddlers with disabilities and their families as recipients of appropriate intervention. The amendments recognized the importance of addressing family concerns in the context of having to care for a child with special needs.[98] Bronfenbrenner,[99] in his depiction of the ecology of human development, emphasizes that a developing human being is influenced by and influences his or her immediate institutional structures, such as the family, school, or therapy center. Furthermore, the interactions between these institutions can have an effect on the developing child. These amendments of IDEA, therefore, take this theory into consideration by addressing the family's needs and resources while providing appropriate care for the child with special needs.

Effectiveness of early intervention programs may be attributed to family characteristics, stressors, and resources for support.[100] This review of literature should help physical therapist assistants comprehend the benefits of early intervention. These insights may be applicable to all genetic conditions or developmental delays that affect neuromotor development, such as cognitive disabilities, DCDs, and LDs.

An environment that is generally stimulating through a moderately directive parenting style is found to be favorable in early intervention. To achieve such an environment, therapists must help parents gain confidence and increase their competence in the manner in which they interact

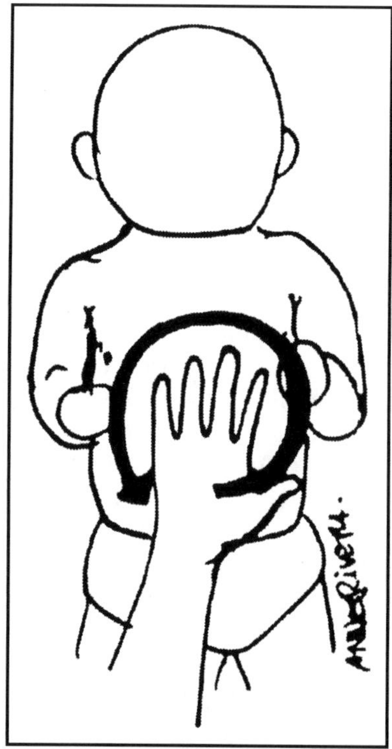

Figure 10-12. Rub the stomach in a slow, circular movement using one hand. (Illustration by Anne Rivera.)

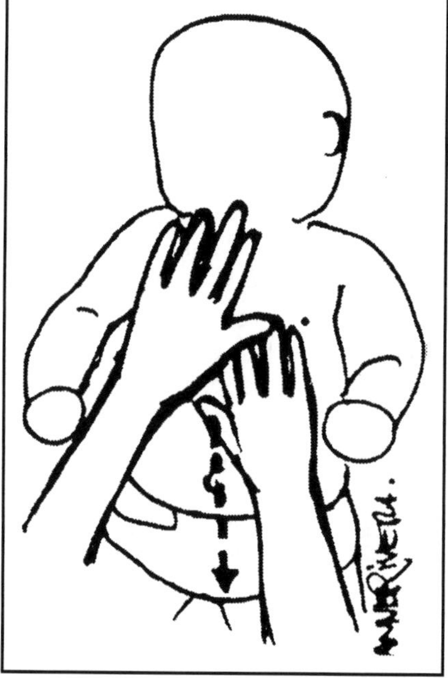

Figure 10-13. Using the palms, slide one palm at a time down the stomach in a hand-over-hand manner in a paddle wheel fashion. (Illustration by Anne Rivera.)

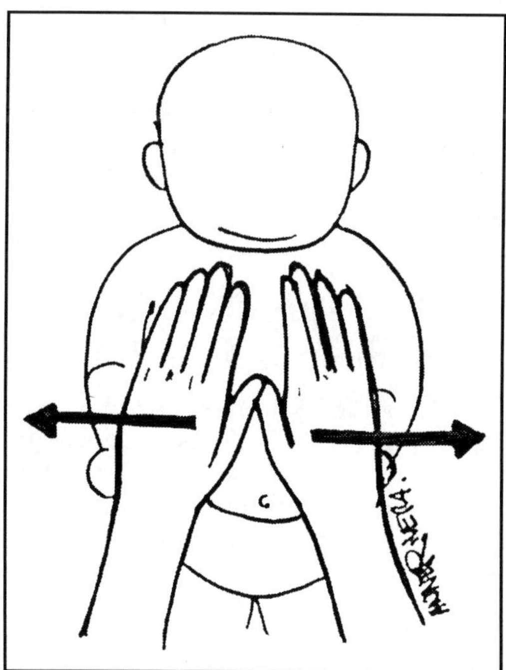

Figure 10-14. Place the palms of your hands on the child's sternum and stroke outward across the chest. (Illustration by Anne Rivera.)

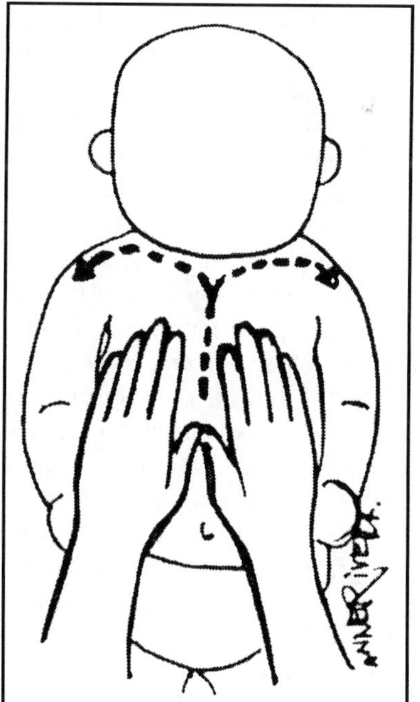

Figure 10-15. For the chest, starting at the sternum, stroke upward and over the top of the shoulders and down the sides of the ribs. (Illustration by Anne Rivera.)

with their infant or toddler with special needs. This indicates that instead of the therapist focusing an entire session working with the child and addressing therapy needs only, adequate time should also be spent in teaching parents how to hold, position, play with, and interact with the child. The parents will be the advocates for the child throughout most of the child's life, and thus should be the ones who gain success from therapeutic intervention. It helps bond the parents to the child while enriching the child's environment. Teaching parents—by instructing, demonstrating, and giving feedback on how they can work with their children at home—can help empower them to care for and properly address their child's special needs. The physical therapist and the physical therapist assistant need to be sensitive to the needs of the parents: their frustrations, their expectations, and their fears. Incorporating the environmental and the personal factors of the parents/family will allow the physical therapist and physical therapist assistant to assess the problems the child will face in addition to those caused by body structure or function when interacting in activities. Refer to Chapter 1 and Figure 1-1 (the International Classification of Functioning, Disability and Health model from the World Health Organization) for additional discussion of impairments in body function, limitations in activities, and restrictions in participation.

Having adequate and timely information regarding the child's condition and possible resources that could help the family can help lessen the stress on the family. Therapists must always be ready to answer parents' questions correctly, provide sufficient and precise information, and lead or guide them to obtain the necessary support and resources that they need. At the time of diagnosis, parents are most interested to know more about whatever the condition might be, what caused the condition, what to expect from the condition, and how the condition will affect their child through life. As a physical therapist or physical therapist assistant, you may not be the first health care professional that the parents have encountered after receiving the medical diagnosis for their child. However, do not assume when you relay crucial data that the parents will immediately absorb all the information. Most parents will need to ask the same question over and over until they understand what either the doctor or the therapist is saying. Always be ready to address the information needs of the parents. It is important that you have accurate information. Apart from knowing about the condition, parents find it helpful if you can direct them to services that they need or for which they are eligible. In areas where a system is in place for early intervention services, knowing the process and reiterating that process to the family is often greatly appreciated.

Social networks can have a positive influence on the family's outlook on the care of the child with a genetic condition or delays in development. It is often valuable to direct families to organizations and groups that support and advocate for that specific condition. It may be a local support group that the family can easily access, or, if those groups are not available in the area, they might find technological advances and support through the internet.

Participation of Children With Disabilities

The ICF promotes an enablement model that focuses on what a person can perform and participate in within important contexts despite physical disabilities.[101] For children, participation is the "active engagement in the typical activities available to and/or expected of peers in the same context."[101] Based on this, children are expected to have interactive relationships in their homes, community, and schools.

In keeping participation and performance of skills congruent, it is important to consider environment and task factors. One way to do this is to use a top-down approach in evaluation and treatment of the child.[101] When using this approach, the therapist first considers the child's or family's chosen participation activities in specific contexts. From here, the therapist explores what factors (ie, tasks, individually or within the environment) need to be addressed to accomplish participation.

For example, a family would want a child with a genetic condition such as DS or DMD to participate in the weekly church activities for children. The therapist can assess the environment in which this activity takes place and see how the child will be able to function. The therapist can recommend supports, assistive devices, and modifications of activities to ensure that the child can perform and participate. Therapy sessions can be directed toward improvement of performance to ensure participation in the activity. Working toward identified participation activities by families, collaboration with parents is important. This is further discussed in subsequent sections of this chapter.

Collaborating With the Rehabilitation Team

A multidisciplinary approach is essential. Recent publications by Birnkrant and colleagues[28] documented that updated care considerations for DMD were driven by multidisciplinary care teams, the survival of patients with DMD, and improvements made with diagnostic and therapeutic approaches. Anticipation of emerging and molecular therapies for DMD and other genetic conditions will necessitate future updates in the care of patients with genetic conditions.

The developmental nature of conditions such as genetic abnormalities or developmental delays requires the involvement of several health care professionals in addressing pertinent problems and concerns. Human development is a complex process that requires attention to the physical, cognitive, and socioemotional aspects of growth and development (see Chapters 3 and 7). The physical therapist assistant must understand the disciplines, and the professionals who may be working with this population.

Parents may often identify their child's delays in motor skills earlier than their child's pediatrician. These parents may obtain their resource information from developmental milestone charts, or from their other children's growth and development if they had children earlier. Some parents may not reach out to their child's pediatrician right away and may wait to see if their child may catch up with their developmental skills. A child with ID may or may not have a genetic condition that is the causation of the limitations in cognitive abilities. One condition of this cognitive disability is that the developmental level across the spectrum of skills (eg, cognitive, fine motor, gross motor, socialization) is constant, whereas a child with LDs, motor coordination deficits, autism, DS, or another problem that causes developmental delays may exhibit areas of strength as well as areas of delay. Children with developmental delays often do not have a medical diagnosis to guide either the therapist or the parents toward available services. Yet, medical institutions have identified mechanisms to help children with developmental delays. Those mechanisms and the team responsible for services may be part of a larger state-run organization. Federal law requires that services be provided once a child's delay reaches certain criteria. Whether those services are part of a state-run children's services agency or are housed within a school-based program, they are often state-specific. As the door to direct access opens more and more to physical therapy, parents may find the resource to share their concerns about their child's motor skills and other areas of development. Parents would have the options to enter into physical therapy services directly, and the physical therapist/physical therapist assistant may engage in interventions that assist the child in learning cognitive and motor skills. Similarly, the physical therapist may need to refer the parents and child to other health care professional to meet the complex nature of the developing child. A brief description of each profession has been included in this section for the physical therapist assistant to become familiar with the entire health care team.

Physical Therapist and Physical Therapist Assistant

Physical therapists and physical therapist assistants are concerned with movement and functional ability.[1] Physical therapists are expected to perform a comprehensive examination of the patient, evaluate findings of the examination, and formulate a diagnosis, prognosis, and plan of care. In addition, physical therapists implement the treatment program, determine outcomes of interventions, and consult with and refer to other experts; physical therapists supervise and direct physical therapist assistants. The physical therapist assistant may implement selected components of the treatment plan, obtain data related to the intervention provided, and make necessary modifications in the intervention at the direction of the physical therapist.[102] Details on pertinent physical therapy management, including the role of the physical therapist assistant, can be found in the next section.

Patients, Parents, and Family Members

To implement client-centered/family-centered care, a change in the development of physical therapy treatment interventions need to change from clinician-driven to client-centered goals. Collaboration and teamwork with the parents and family members can increase the effectiveness of physical therapy services and encourage adherence to home education programs.

The Canadian Occupational Performance Measure (COPM) is an individualized measure to determine, through a semi-structured interview, a client's, parents', and/or family members' perception in the client's self-care, productivities, and leisure time.[103] The client rates the importance, performance, and satisfaction with level of performance of the self-identified occupational performance issues. With this endeavor to improve client-centered services, the therapist can incorporate the findings, and focus on the client's self-identified daily life activities, and develop mutual therapy goals to work on to reach their desired outcome. The physical therapist/physical therapist assistant team can build capacity and share responsibility for the rehabilitation in the child, family in the home, and community.[103]

Clinical Medical Geneticist

The American College of Medical Genetics defines the scope of practice of medical genetics as a broad and unique specialty of medicine that involves all organ systems, periods of life, and disease entities. The American College of Medical Genetics document on the scope of practice[104] identifies members of the genetics health care team to include clinical and laboratory medical geneticists, genetic counselors, nurse geneticists, and metabolic disease dieticians.

Medical or clinical geneticists are physicians who are trained to diagnose and provide therapeutic procedures for patients with genetically linked diseases.[104] They are qualified to diagnose, treat, supervise, coordinate, and case-manage individuals and families with known and suspected genetic disorders.

Genetic Counselor

Genetic counselors are involved in developing, documenting, and assessing family histories and facilitating genetic testing decision-making and patient/family education. They are also able to address the psychosocial needs of patients and families.

Developmental-Behavioral Pediatrician

A developmental-behavioral pediatrician is a medical specialist who has gone through a residency or specialization in pediatrics and further trained for the subspecialty of developmental-behavioral pediatrics.[105] These medical specialists are equipped to evaluate, counsel, and provide treatment for children, adolescents, and families with a wide range of developmental and behavioral difficulties.

Occupational Therapist

Occupational therapy's primary goal is "to help patients and clients to participate in the things that they want and need to do through the therapeutic use of everyday activities."[106] The occupational therapy profession promotes health and well-being through occupation. An occupational therapist can provide a comprehensive and individualized evaluation and treatment plan to improve performance of ADL. For genetic conditions with neurodevelopmental concerns, occupational therapists are helpful in addressing problems that interfere with feeding, attention, and movement. They are also able to provide comprehensive evaluation and recommend modification of the client's home and other significant environmental problems or barriers. Occupational therapists may also recommend and train in the use of assistive devices that will foster occupation.[106,107] A number of occupational therapists work in school systems and focus specifically on the spectrum of problems considered LDs. Children with specific medical diagnoses such as DS, as well as those without medical diagnoses but with delays in motor development, often have LDs or problems that an occupational therapist will treat.

Speech-Language Pathologist

Speech-language pathologists address typical and atypical communication and swallowing in the areas of speech production, resonance, voice, language comprehension and expression, cognition, feeding, and swallowing.[108] Speech-language pathologists are expected to screen, evaluate, diagnose, and provide treatment or intervention to patients with genetic conditions. Their role is more prominent and essential during the preschool and formal school years of children, when communication and socialization play a vital role in children's social and cognitive development. These clinicians often work closely with other professionals addressing problems that stem from language, such as temporal sequencing and how it affects reading or language development.

Audiologists

Audiologists promote healthy hearing and communication competency.[108] These specialists identify, assess, and rehabilitate hearing, auditory function, balance, and other related systems while preventing additional problems within this area. Audiologists are important for children with hearing impairments and auditory problems. They closely work with speech-language pathologists.

The Family as Essential Members of the Team and the Value of Home Programs

The family members are also valued members of the health team. The child's parents and other significant family members collaborate with professionals to determine treatment goals and plans. A family-centered approach promotes the treatment of the child within the context of the family setting to maximize the child's development.[109] Evidence indicates that engaging in a collaborative process improves the child's performance with a moderate effect size, and the family's satisfaction of performance with a large effect size.[110] Furthermore, parents involved in a collaborative process work closely with the therapist and are more confident with their skills in carrying out daily activities. Professionals need to develop and maintain effective communication skills to gain trust and cooperation of family members.

Results of a study that looked into parent and professional perceptions of family-centered programs[109] provide several significant insights into the care and management of children with genetic conditions:

- Communicate information at an appropriate level to encourage parent participation.
- Educate parents on child development and potential problems as the child grows.
- Highlight, or do not overlook, a child's strengths.
- Teach parents how to set goals.
- Provide information regarding community services available to parents and families.
- Consider cultural diversity in assessment and treatment of children.

Exercise programs for children can be prescribed and implemented at home. Providing home exercise programs for children with disabilities proves beneficial for the child and family. Home exercise programs have been shown to help achieve goals, improve motor function,[111] and even cut costs in therapy.[112] A child is expected to participate in home activities. Home exercise programs can be directed so that this can be achieved and everyone has fun. The use of home exercise programs allows parents and family members to have a more concrete and meaningful role in therapy and be part of the positive changes that occur in their child.

In a study that looked at effectiveness of home program for children with autism, parents were asked to observe while a therapist demonstrated and modeled the task with the child. The techniques were explained in detail, and a written program was sent home with the parent. The parent carried out the program at home in the following week. Upon return to the clinic, the parent demonstrated how the program was carried out at home, and the therapist provided suggestions on how to improve and fine-tune the activities. During home visit, the therapist followed-up and checked up with the parents. The results of this study showed improvement in skills of children in the treatment group.[113]

It is important to note, however, that adherence and compliance to home exercise programs is still a challenge for therapists.[111,112] In these studies, factors that affected adherence and compliance negatively were caregiver stress, severity of disability, and perceived family problems. Therefore, therapists must be sensitive to these issues and be able to modify programs as best fits the context of the child and family. It is suggested that incorporating the exercise program within a normal routine and providing activities that are enjoyable may promote adherence.[112]

The Physical Therapist/Physical Therapist Assistant Team: Considerations for Effective Collaboration to Optimize Care

Physical therapist assistants are indispensable members of the rehabilitation team. The physical therapist assistant is tasked to implement activities, conduct exercises, and possibly apply modalities to patients under the physical therapist's direction. A physical therapist assistant may spend a considerable amount of time with the patient and the family, and therefore may have the opportunity to more closely follow the care of the child. When working with this population, the following considerations are important:

- Always remember safety considerations. While many conditions have similarities in presentation, other clinical aspects may be different. The physical therapist assistant must be aware of those differences and must adjust the treatment protocol to accommodate these variations. For example, it may be harder to mobilize extremities of children with hypertonicity such as in Rett syndrome. Forcing an extremity to move through very high tone may result in injury of the child. In contrast, children with DS or Prader-Willi syndrome may be more mobile, but their balance is compromised. The physical therapist assistant must always keep the environment safe to prevent falls and potential injuries to the child.
- Ensure that the child is medically stable. Be sensitive to subtle changes in the child's behavior, participation in therapy, or level of alertness. These may indicate the presence of a medical issue. There may be times that the parents are the ones observing and reporting these changes. Immediately report these issues to the supervising therapist. Seizures are common among children who may have limited mobility. Some children may also experience cardiovascular compromise or other medical system disorders. In both these cases, physical therapy intervention may be altered or stopped completely until the child has been evaluated by an appropriate medical professional.
- Listen to parents' stories and descriptions of their child and family life. Often they will disclose how their personal lives are being affected both positively and negatively by having a child with special needs. It is important that the child is given intervention, but it is just as important to keep the family system working for the child. You may need to report to the physical therapist about these matters that affect therapy to update a plan of care or work out a more feasible and acceptable intervention for the child.

Working with children can be very fulfilling and satisfying. It is also not unusual to find yourself in challenging and frustrating situations. It is best to keep in mind that physical therapy primarily aims to improve mobility and enhance the patient's quality of life.

Care coordination should be a team and family-driven process that improves family and health care practitioner satisfaction, facilitates children's and youth's access to services, improves health care outcomes, and reduces cost associated with health care fragmentation.[114]

Case Studies

Case #1

The patient is a 4-year-old girl whose mother is concerned about her limited mobility skills. The child lives with her mother, a housewife, and father, a driver. She has 2 siblings, aged 21 and 16, who do not live with them anymore. The child was born to a 33-year-old mother and had no remarkable events pre- and perinatally. When the child was 10 months of age, the mother noticed that she was not yet reaching or playing with toys. The child was brought to their local pediatrician, who diagnosed her with global developmental delay and referred her to physical therapy and occupational therapy services. The mother was not able to seek services immediately because of financial issues. The mother noticed that, at the age of 1 year, the child started losing her grip. When the child was 1 year and 3 months old, the mother was finally able to seek physical and occupational therapy services but was unable to go to regular physical therapy once a week and occupational therapy once every 2 weeks. According to the mother's report, at 2 years old, the child was still able to independently W-sit (with hips internally rotated and knees flexed), but eventually lost this skill by age 3.

After consultation with several specialists, the patient was diagnosed as having Rett syndrome. She usually ate finely chopped meat or vegetables and rice. On physical examination, the patient appeared well-nourished. She was non-ambulatory. She appeared lethargic. Tone assessment revealed 1+ spasticity on the Modified Ashworth Scale for both elbows and knees. The child had weak to fair control of her head and neck in sitting; her head lagged when pulled to sit. She rolled from supine to prone and back using the logroll technique. She was able to assume and maintain prone on elbows. She was unable to assume quadruped, cross-sitting, or short-sitting. She was unable to creep or crawl. She was also not able to stand and walk. The child did not reach for any object independently. ROM testing revealed limitations in both hip flexion, both knee extension, and both ankle dorsiflexion and plantar flexion.

The plan of care included the following activities, which were delegated to the physical therapist assistant. Initially mobility or ROM exercises were considered, but current research evidence has shown that ROM or stretching interventions for children with neuromuscular disabilities has minimal benefit to body function and structure so it was not delegated to the physical therapist assistant.[115] Soft tissue mobilization techniques were performed to release any restrictions due to scar tissue. A referral to the orthotist for fitting of posterior ankle splints was also conducted.

The physical therapist assistant was responsible for administering the strengthening exercises for the trunk, postural muscles, and extremities. Examples of these exercises included pull to sit activities, prone extensions on a vestibular ball, and ROM activities in open- and closed-chain positions. Strengthening activities in short-sitting on a bench and cross-sitting on a mat were also performed. Play was incorporated with the child assuming these positions, and the physical therapist assistant providing facilitation and tactile cues to maintain the positions and optimize alignment and BOS. Exercises were performed following a developmental sequence, beginning with the child prone on elbows, prone on hands, and then in the quadruped position. From these positions, the physical therapist assistant trained the child to creep and crawl.

Next, sitting balance activities were performed. The child initially required moderate assistance to maintain the sitting position. The physical therapist assistant optimized the position by correctly positioning the child's feet, keeping the child in proper biomechanical alignment before initiating any activities. In this position, the child performed a bean bag toss, throwing the bean onto a board with targets, with assistance from the physical therapist assistant. The activity was progressed to having the child sitting on foam, then a DynaDisc (Exertools). The patient also performed the activities in standing, first on a flat surface, then on foam. The physical therapist assistant provided facilitation as appropriate to maintain good alignment and optimal engagement of the trunk muscles.

The child then started to perform sit-to-stand activities with the physical therapist assistant. The physical therapist assistant started this activity using a treatment table that could be raised and lowered. The physical therapist assistant started with the table in a high position, and then guided the child to stand up from the sitting position, and then back down to sit. The physical therapist assistant progressively lowered the table and then worked on the same movement, eventually training the child to stand up from sitting in a regular-height chair.

Next, the physical therapist assistant worked on standing balance activities, first working on a hard, noncompliant surface, then progressing to foam. Again, play activities were incorporated, also to work on gross and fine motor movements of the upper extremities.

The child has now started to take a few steps with assistance from the physical therapist assistant. She continues to be engaged in therapy and enjoys the interaction with the therapy staff.

All throughout this episode of care, the rehabilitation team has closely monitored the child's progress. The physical therapist assistant regularly reported to the physical therapist the child's progress and discussed how those changes might affect the plan of care. Once the physical therapist identified the new plan of care, the physical therapist assistant began to work toward those new goals. The physical therapist and the physical therapist assistant also involved the child's family in the rehabilitation process by optimizing adherence to the exercise program and participating in in-clinic activities.

Questions

1. Were any inappropriate interventions delegated to the physical therapist assistant during the intervention periods with this child?
2. If the physical therapist assistant identifies that the child has reached an objective within the plan of care, is it okay to change the plan to progress the child?

Case #2

Jonathan was born at 25 weeks' gestational age with a birth weight of 1 pound, 15 ounces. His mother reported that although Jonathan spent 2 months in the neonatal intensive care unit, he did not have any major medical problems. She stated that Jonathan sat at 9 months, crept on hands and knees at 12 months, cruised at 19 months, and walked at 24 months of age. He was started in an early intervention program upon his discharge from the neonatal intensive care unit and was seen on a twice-a-month basis until his discharge at 3 years old. The physical therapist who saw Jonathan in early intervention was concerned about his motor planning abilities because he had difficulty getting off the sofa, climbing in and out of large boxes, and changing direction when using a small riding toy at the time of discharge. Based on her recommendation, Jonathan was enrolled in a developmental preschool program after being in the early intervention program. At 8 years old, he is enrolled in a regular second-grade class.

At 7 years old, Jonathan was diagnosed as having a DCD by an interdisciplinary evaluation team. He is receiving occupational and physical therapy services through the school system. Jonathan's teacher states he is distractible in the classroom and that he tends to give up if he is stressed by a task. Additionally, he rocks or fidgets frequently while sitting in his desk chair. She also notes that he chews on his pencil or other objects during the day. She further reports that he has difficulty keeping pace with his classmates when walking, and that he bumps into other children frequently when walking in a line. On the playground, he prefers to be by himself and does not like to participate in age-related play.

On examination by the physical therapist, Jonathan was found to exhibit these behaviors:

- Adequate attention span, but distracted by extraneous visual or auditory stimuli
- Good understanding of requests
- Wants feedback often about his performance
- Decreased postural tone, but normal deep-tendon reflexes
- Postural assessment of flat feet, hyperextension of knees in stance, wide BOS during ambulation, increased lumbar lordosis, and protruding abdomen
- Inconsistent use of right and left hands during fine motor tasks; does not have a preferred hand for writing
- Unable to track with either eye, unable to separate eye and head movement, and difficulty with convergence and divergence
- Difficulty with smooth control of movement; during game of Simon Says, he performed movement faster than therapist, and tends to plop when asked to sit down
- *Diadochokinesia* (unable to maintain rhythmical pattern with each arm or with both arms together)
- Unable to perform thumb to finger with either hand/both hands together; difficulty with sequencing
- Good movement of tongue to lower lip, upper lip, and sides
- Co-contraction decreased in arms, shoulders, and neck
- Asymmetric tonic neck reflex quadruped, positive when head turned to the left and right
- Equilibrium reactions include problems with response time when moved quickly in sitting and standing
- Could not assume supine flexion
- Could not assume prone extension
- Slightly uncoordinated when running
- Stands momentarily on either foot; unable to jump with both feet together or on one foot
- Refused to skip

The following lists Jonathan's scores on the Sensory Integration and Praxis Test.

Scores below age expectations:

- Bilateral motor control
- Manual form perception
- Finger identification
- Motor accuracy
- Design copy
- Space visualization
- Standing and walking balance
- Postural praxis
- Sequencing praxis
- Figure ground
- Oral praxis
- Constructional praxis
- Postrotary nystagmus

Scores within age expectations:

- Graphesthesia
- Localization tactile stimuli
- Kinesthesia

The following is a list of physical therapy intervention activities:

1. Increase attention to task using sensory input through use of weighted vest and slanted cushion
2. Increase extensor and flexor tone
3. Improve co-contraction of neck, shoulder, and pelvic musculature
4. Facilitate use of both arms for bilateral motor coordination
5. Improve motor planning using a cognitive approach
6. Facilitate motor learning through the use of repetition and appropriate feedback scheduling

The physical therapist is seeing Jonathan monthly at school, and the physical therapist assistant is scheduled to work with Jonathan on a weekly basis. The physical therapist is giving the physical therapist assistant specific activities to be practiced during the weekly sessions to achieve the stated objectives. When Jonathan has improved his motor function, responds automatically, and may be ready for new activities, the physical therapist assistant should report to the physical therapist and meet to discuss Jonathan's progress. The physical therapist may decide that Jonathan needs more frequent visits, or that he should continue with the same intervention schedule. Once Jonathan's new needs are identified, the physical therapist will delegate treatment to the physical therapist assistant, who will be responsible for continuing practice and monitoring his progress.

Questions

1. What sensory input might be considered to use with Jonathan to increase his postural tone? How could these inputs be incorporated within the classroom setting?
2. Why do you think that Jonathan is rocking and fidgeting in the classroom?
3. What are some activities that might be suggested to encourage Jonathan to use both hands together?
4. Identify 3 activities that could be conducted with Jonathan to improve stability in the pelvic girdle. How would the physical therapist assistant recognize that pelvis stability has been improved and that Jonathan is ready for new activities?
5. What are 2 motor behaviors exhibited by Jonathan that would help the physical therapist assistant know the goals of strength and stability of the UEs are being met?
6. When is it appropriate for the physical therapist assistant to change or advance Jonathan into new movement patterns?

References

1. World Confederation for Physical Therapy. Policy statement: Description of physical therapy. http://www.wcpt.org/policy/ps-descriptionPT. Accessed October 24, 2012.
2. National Human Fenome Research Institute. The Human Genome Project. https://www.genome.gov/human-genome-project. Accessed March 22, 2020.
3. Mburia-Mwalili A and Tyang W. Birth Defects Surveillance in the United States: Challenges and Implications of International Classification of Diseases, Tenth Revision, Clinical Modification Implementation. Hindawi Publishing Corp. International Scholarly Research Notices Volume 2014. Article ID 212874. https://www.ncbi.nlm.nih.gov/pmc/articles/PMC489754/. Accessed March 22, 2020.
4. Long TM, Brady R, Lapham EV. A survey of genetics knowledge of health professionals: implications for physical therapists. *Pediatr Phys Ther.* 2001;13(4):156-163. doi:10.1097/00001577-200113040-00002
5. Sanger WG, Dave B, Stuberg W. Overview of genetics and role of the pediatric physical therapist in the diagnostic process. *Pediatr Phys Ther.* 2001;13(4):164-168. doi:10.1097/00001577-200113040-00003
6. Smith M, Danoff JV, Jain M, Long TM. Genetic disorders: implications for allied health professionals: two case studies. *IJAHSP.* 2007;5(4).
7. Parker SE, Mai CT, Canfield MA, et al; National Birth Defects Prevention Network. Updated National Birth Prevalence estimates for selected birth defects in the United States, 2004-2006. *Birth Defects Res A Clin Mol Teratol.* 2010;88(12):1008-1016. doi:10.1002/bdra.20735
8. Costa ACS. An assessment of optokinetic nystagmus (OKN) in persons with Down syndrome. *Exp Brain Res.* 2011;214(3):381-391. doi:10.1007/s00221-011-2834-5
9. Valentín-Gudiol M, Mattern-Baxter K, Girabent-Farrés M, Bagur-Calafat C, Hadders-Algra M, Angulo-Barroso RM. Treadmill interventions in children under six years of age at risk of neuromotor delay. *Cochrane Database Syst Rev.* 2017;7:CD009242. doi:10.1002/14651858.CD009242.pub3
10. Shumway-Cook A, Woollacott MH. Dynamics of postural control in the child with Down syndrome. *Phys Ther.* 1985;65(9):1315-1322. doi:10.1093/ptj/65.9.1315
11. Centers for Disease Control and Prevention. Data & Statistics on Birth Defects. https://www.cdc.gov/ncbddd/birthdefects/data.html. Accessed March 22, 2020.
12. Head E, Silverman W, Patterson D, Lott IT. Aging and down syndrome. *Curr Gerontol Geriatr Res.* 2012;2012:412536.
13. Cassidy SB, Driscoll DJ. Prader-Willi syndrome. *Eur J Hum Genet.* 2009;17(1):3-13. doi:10.1038/ejhg.2008.165
14. Raspa M, Wheeler AC, Riley C. Public health literature review of Fragile X syndrome. *Pediatrics.* 2017;139(suppl 3):S153-S171. doi:10.1542/peds.2016-1159C
15. Centers for Disease Control and Prevention. Data and Statistics on Fragile X Syndrome. https://www.cdc.gov/ncbddd/fxs/data.html#ref. Published May 30, 2019. Accessed March 9, 2017.
16. Lieb-Lundell CC. Three Faces of Fragile X. *Phys Ther.* 2016;96(11):1782-1790. doi:10.2522/ptj.20140430
17. Cerruti Mainardi P. Cri du Chat syndrome. *Orphanet J Rare Dis.* 2006;1(1):33. doi:10.1186/1750-1172-1-33
18. Smeets EEJ, Pelc K, Dan B. Rett syndrome. *Mol Syndromol.* 2012;2(3-5):113-127. doi:10.1159/000337637
19. U.S. National Library of Medicine. MECP2 gene. http://ghr.nlm.nih.gov/gene/MECP2. Accessed October 24, 2012.
20. Braun S, Kottwitz D, Nuber UA. Pharmacological interference with the glucocorticoid system influences symptoms and lifespan in a mouse model of Rett syndrome. *Hum Mol Genet.* 2012;21(8):1673-1680.
21. Lotan M. Rett syndrome. Guidelines for individual intervention. *ScientificWorldJournal.* 2006;6:1504-1516. doi:10.1100/tsw.2006.252
22. Bharucha BA, Agarwal UM, Savliwala AS, Kolluri R, Kumta NB. Trisomy 18: edward's syndrome (a case report of 3 cases). *J Postgrad Med.* 1983;29(2):129-132.
23. Cereda A, Carey JC. The trisomy 18 syndrome. *Orphanet J Rare Dis.* 2012;7(1):81. doi:10.1186/1750-1172-7-81
24. Merritt TA, Mazela J, Adamczak A, Merritt T. The impact of second-hand tobacco smoke exposure on pregnancy outcomes, infant health, and the threat of third-hand smoke exposure to our environment and to our children. *Przegl Lek.* 2012;69(10):717-720.
25. Janvier A, Farlow B, Wilfond BS. The experience of families with children with trisomy 13 and 18 in social networks. *Pediatrics.* 2012;130(2):293-298. doi:10.1542/peds.2012-0151
26. Bushby K, Finkel R, Birnkrant DJ, et al; DMD Care Considerations Working Group. Diagnosis and management of Duchenne muscular dystrophy, part 1: diagnosis, and pharmacological and psychosocial management. *Lancet Neurol.* 2010;9(1):77-93. doi:10.1016/S1474-4422(09)70271-6
27. Birnkrant DJ, Bushby K, Bann CM, et al. Diagnosis and management of Duchenne muscular dystrophy, part 1: diagnosis, and pharmacological and psychosocial management. *Lancet Neurol.* 2018;17(3):251-267. doi:10.1016/S1474-4422(18)30024-3
28. Birnkrant DJ, Bushby K, Bann CM, et al; DMD Care Considerations Working Group. Diagnosis and management of Duchenne muscular dystrophy, part 3: primary care, emergency management, psychosocial care, and transitions of care across the lifespan. *Lancet Neurol.* 2018;17(5):445-455. doi:10.1016/S1474-4422(18)30026-7
29. Ambardekar N. Muscular Dystrophy Types & Causes of Each Form. WebMD. http://children.webmd.com/understanding-muscular-dystrophy-basics. Published March 31, 2019. Accessed August 24, 2013.
30. Parks M, Court S, Cleary S, et al. Non-invasive prenatal diagnosis of Duchenne and Becker muscular dystrophies by relative haplotype dosage. *Prenat Diagn.* 2016;36(4):312-320. doi:10.1002/pd.4781
31. Esquenazi A, Packel A. Robotic-assisted gait training and restoration. *Am J Phys Med Rehabil.* 2012;91(11)(suppl 3):S217-S227. doi:10.1097/PHM.0b013e31826bce18
32. Huang VS, Krakauer JW. Robotic neurorehabilitation: a computational motor learning perspective. *J Neuroeng Rehabil.* 2009;6(1):5. doi:10.1186/1743-0003-6-5
33. Nakamura A, Takeda S. Exon-skipping therapy for Duchenne muscular dystrophy. *Neuropathology.* 2009;29(4):494-501. doi:10.1111/j.1440-1789.2009.01028.x
34. Needleman H. Lead poisoning. *Annu Rev Med.* 2004;55(1):209-222. doi:10.1146/annurev.med.55.091902.103653

35. Hielkema T, Blauw-Hospers CH, Dirks T, Drijver-Messelink M, Bos AF, Hadders-Algra M. Does physiotherapeutic intervention affect motor outcome in high-risk infants? An approach combining a randomized controlled trial and process evaluation. *Dev Med Child Neurol.* 2011;53(3):e8-e15. doi:10.1111/j.1469-8749.2010.03876.x
36. Magalhães LC, Cardoso AA, Missiuna C. Activities and participation in children with developmental coordination disorder: a systematic review. *Res Dev Disabil.* 2011;32(4):1309-1316. doi:10.1016/j.ridd.2011.01.029
37. Zwicker JG, Mayson TA. Effectiveness of treadmill training in children with motor impairments: an overview of systematic reviews. *Pediatr Phys Ther.* 2010;22(4):361-377. doi:10.1097/PEP.0b013e3181f92e54
38. Flapper BC, Schoemaker MM. Developmental coordination disorder in children with specific language impairment: co-morbidity and impact on quality of life. *Res Dev Disabil.* 2013;34(2):756-763. doi:10.1016/j.ridd.2012.10.014
39. Williams J, Omizzolo C, Galea MP, Vance A. Motor imagery skills of children with attention deficit hyperactivity disorder and developmental coordination disorder. *Hum Mov Sci.* 2013;32(1):121-135. doi:10.1016/j.humov.2012.08.003
40. Wilson PH, Ruddock S, Smits-Engelsman B, Polatajko H, Blank R. Understanding performance deficits in developmental coordination disorder: a meta-analysis of recent research. *Dev Med Child Neurol.* 2013;55(3):217-228. doi:10.1111/j.1469-8749.2012.04436.x
41. Palisano RJ, Walter SD, Russell DJ, et al. Gross motor function of children with down syndrome: creation of motor growth curves. *Arch Phys Med Rehabil.* 2001;82(4):494-500. doi:10.1053/apmr.2001.21956
42. McCandless SE; Committee on Genetics. Clinical report—health supervision for children with Prader-Willi syndrome. *Pediatrics.* 2011;127(1):195-204. doi:10.1542/peds.2010-2820
43. Cimolin V, Galli M, Vismara L, Grugni G, Priano L, Capodaglio P. The effect of vision on postural strategies in Prader-Willi patients. *Res Dev Disabil.* 2011;32(5):1965-1969. doi:10.1016/j.ridd.2011.04.002
44. Russell DJ, Avery LM, Rosenbaum PL, Raina PS, Walter SD, Palisano RJ. Improved scaling of the gross motor function measure for children with cerebral palsy: evidence of reliability and validity. *Phys Ther.* 2000;80(9):873-885. doi:10.1093/ptj/80.9.873
45. Russell D, Palisano R, Walter S, et al. Evaluating motor function in children with Down syndrome: validity of the GMFM. *Dev Med Child Neurol.* 1998;40(10):693-701. doi:10.1111/j.1469-8749.1998.tb12330.x
46. Malak R, Kostiukow A, Krawczyk-Wasielewska A, Mojs E, Samborski W. Delays in motor development in children with Down syndrome. *Med Sci Monit.* 2015;21:1904-1910. doi:10.12659/MSM.893377
47. Folio MR, Fewell RR. *Peabody Developmental Motor Scales.* 2nd ed. Examiner's Manual. Austin, TX: Pro-Ed; 2000.
48. Tavasoli A, Azimi P, Montazari A. Reliability and validity of the Peabody Developmental Motor Scales-second edition for assessing motor development of low birth weight preterm infants. *Pediatr Neurol.* 2014;51(4):522-526. doi:10.1016/j.pediatrneurol.2014.06.010
49. Eldred K, Darrah J. Using cluster analysis to interpret the variability of gross motor scores of children with typical development. *Phys Ther.* 2010;90(10):1510-1518. doi:10.2522/ptj.20090308
50. Boehme R. *Developing Mid-Range Control and Function in Children With Fluctuating Muscle Tone.* Tucson, AZ: Therapy Skill Builders; 1990.
51. Naidoo P. Current practices in the assessment of low muscle tone. *S Afr J Occup Ther.* 2013;43(2):12-17.
52. Martin K, Kaltenmark T, Lewallen A, Smith C, Yoshida A. Clinical characteristics of hypotonia: a survey of pediatric physical and occupational therapists. *Pediatr Phys Ther.* 2007;19(3):217-226. doi:10.1097/PEP.0b013e3180f62bb0
53. Ellison PH, Horn JL, Browning CA. Construction of an Infant Neurological International Battery (Infanib) for the assessment of neurological integrity in infancy. *Phys Ther.* 1985;65(9):1326-1331. doi:10.1093/ptj/65.9.1326
54. Clopton N, Dutton J, Featherston T, Grigsby A, Mobley J, Melvin J. Interrater and intrarater reliability of the Modified Ashworth Scale in children with hypertonia. *Pediatr Phys Ther.* 2005;17(4):268-274. doi:10.1097/01.pep.0000186509.41238.1a
55. Mutlu A, Livanelioglu A, Gunel MK. Reliability of Ashworth and Modified Ashworth scales in children with spastic cerebral palsy. *BMC Musculoskelet Disord.* 2008;9(1):44. doi:10.1186/1471-2474-9-44
56. Franjoine MR, Gunther JS, Taylor MJ. Pediatric balance scale: a modified version of the berg balance scale for the school-age child with mild to moderate motor impairment. *Pediatr Phys Ther.* 2003;15(2):114-128. doi:10.1097/01.PEP.0000068117.48023.18
57. Franjoine MR, Darr N, Held SL, Kott K, Young BL. The performance of children developing typically on the pediatric balance scale. *Pediatr Phys Ther.* 2010;22(4):350-359. doi:10.1097/PEP.0b013e3181f9d5eb
58. Bandong AN, Madriaga GO, Gorgon EJ. Reliability and validity of the Four Square Step Test in children with cerebral palsy and Down syndrome. *Res Dev Disabil.* 2015;47:39-47. doi:10.1016/j.ridd.2015.08.012
59. Williams EN, Carroll SG, Reddihough DS, Phillips BA, Galea MP. Investigation of the timed 'up & go' test in children. *Dev Med Child Neurol.* 2005;47(8):518-524. doi:10.1017/S0012162205001027
60. Nicolini-Panisson RD, Donadio MV. Normative values for the Timed 'Up and Go' test in children and adolescents and validation for individuals with Down syndrome. *Dev Med Child Neurol.* 2014;56(5):490-497. doi:10.1111/dmcn.12290
61. Weingarten G, Kaplan S. Reliability and validity of the Timed Floor to Stand Test—natural in school-aged children. *Pediatr Phys Ther.* 2015;27(2):113-118. doi:10.1097/PEP.0000000000000118
62. Weingarten G, Lieberstein M, Itzkowitz A, Vialu C, Doyle M, Kaplan SL. Timed floor to stand-natural: reference data for school age children. *Pediatr Phys Ther.* 2016;28(1):71-76. doi:10.1097/PEP.0000000000000205
63. Martin K, Kaltenmark T, Lewallen A, Smith C, Yoshida A. Clinical characteristics of hypotonia: a survey of pediatric physical and occupational therapists. *Pediatr Phys Ther.* 2007;19(3):217-226. doi:10.1097/PEP.0b013e3180f62bb0

64. Vaivre-Douret L, Ennouri K, Jrad I, Garrec C, Papiernik E. Effect of positioning on the incidence of abnormalities of muscle tone in low-risk, preterm infants. *Eur J Paediatr Neurol.* 2004;8(1):21-34. doi:10.1016/j.ejpn.2003.10.001
65. Bly L. *Motor Skills Acquisition in the First Year: An Illustrated Guide to Normal Development.* San Antonio, TX: Therapy Skill Builders; 1998.
66. Bly L, Whiteside A, Medvescek R. *Baby Treatment Based on NDT Principles.* San Antonio, TX: Communication Skill Builders; 1999.
67. Sackley CM, van den Berg ME, Lett K, et al. Effects of a physiotherapy and occupational therapy intervention on mobility and activity in care home residents: a cluster randomised controlled trial. *BMJ.* 2009;339:b3123. doi:10.1136/bmj.b3123
68. Shields N, Taylor NF. A student-led progressive resistance training program increases lower limb muscle strength in adolescents with Down syndrome: a randomised controlled trial. *J Physiother.* 2010;56(3):187-193. doi:10.1016/S1836-9553(10)70024-2
69. Gupta S, Rao BK, Kumaran SD. Effect of strength and balance training in children with Down's syndrome: a randomized controlled trial. *Clin Rehabil.* 2011;25(5):425-432. doi:10.1177/0269215510382929
70. Kane K, Bell A. A core stability group program for children with developmental coordination disorder: 3 clinical case reports. *Pediatr Phys Ther.* 2009;21(4):375-382. doi:10.1097/PEP.0b013e3181beff38
71. Kaufman LB, Schilling DL. Implementation of a strength training program for a 5-year-old child with poor body awareness and developmental coordination disorder. *Phys Ther.* 2007;87(4):455-467. doi:10.2522/ptj.20060170
72. Menz SM, Hatten K, Grant-Beuttler M. Strength training for a child with suspected developmental coordination disorder. *Pediatr Phys Ther.* 2013;25(2):214-223. doi:10.1097/PEP.0b013e31828a2042
73. Harris SR. Effects of neurodevelopmental therapy on motor performance of infants with Down's syndrome. *Dev Med Child Neurol.* 1981;23(4):477-483. doi:10.1111/j.1469-8749.1981.tb02021.x
74. Harris SR, Roxborough L. Efficacy and effectiveness of physical therapy in enhancing postural control in children with cerebral palsy. *Neural Plast.* 2005;12(2-3):229-243. doi:10.1155/NP.2005.229
75. Hernandez-Reif M, Field T, Largie S, Mora D, Bornstein J, Waldman R. Children with Down syndrome improved in motor functioning and muscle tone following massage therapy. *Early Child Dev Care.* 2006;176(3-4):395-410. doi:10.1080/03004430500105233
76. Lotan M, Isakov E, Merrick J. Improving functional skills and physical fitness in children with Rett syndrome. *J Intellect Disabil Res.* 2004;48(Pt 8):730-735. doi:10.1111/j.1365-2788.2003.00589.x
77. Birnkrant DJ, Bushby K, Bann CM, et al; DMD Care Considerations Working Group. Diagnosis and management of Duchenne muscular dystrophy, part 2: respiratory, cardiac, bone health, and orthopaedic management. *Lancet Neurol.* 2018;17(4):347-361. doi:10.1016/S1474-4422(18)30025-5
78. Angelini C, Tasca E. Fatigue in muscular dystrophies. *Neuromuscul Disord.* 2012;22(suppl 3):S214-S220. doi:10.1016/j.nmd.2012.10.010
79. Sackley C, Disler PB, Turner-Stokes L, Wade DT, Brittle N, Hoppitt T. Rehabilitation interventions for foot drop in neuromuscular disease. *Cochrane Database Syst Rev.* 2009;(3):CD003908. doi:10.1002/14651858.CD003908.pub3
80. Grange RW, Call JA. Recommendations to define exercise prescription for Duchenne muscular dystrophy. *Exerc Sport Sci Rev.* 2007;35(1):12-17. doi:10.1249/01.jes.0000240020.84630.9d
81. Jansen M, de Groot IJ, van Alfen N, Geurts AC. Physical training in boys with Duchenne Muscular Dystrophy: the protocol of the No Use is Disuse study. *BMC Pediatr.* 2010;10(1):55. doi:10.1186/1471-2431-10-55
82. Chaoui R, Heling KS, Sarioglu N, Schwabe M, Dankof A, Bollmann R. Aberrant right subclavian artery as a new cardiac sign in second- and third-trimester fetuses with Down syndrome. *Am J Obstet Gynecol.* 2005;192(1):257-263. doi:10.1016/j.ajog.2004.06.080
83. Paladini D, Sglavo G, Pastore G, Masucci A, D'Armiento MR, Nappi C. Aberrant right subclavian artery: incidence and correlation with other markers of Down syndrome in second-trimester fetuses. *Ultrasound Obstet Gynecol.* 2012;39(2):191-195. doi:10.1002/uog.10053
84. Zalel Y, Achiron R, Yagel S, Kivilevitch Z. Fetal aberrant right subclavian artery in normal and Down syndrome fetuses. *Ultrasound Obstet Gynecol.* 2008;31(1):25-29. doi:10.1002/uog.5230
85. Angulo-Barroso R, Burghardt AR, Lloyd M, Ulrich DA. Physical activity in infants with Down syndrome receiving a treadmill intervention. *Infant Behav Dev.* 2008;31(2):255-269. doi:10.1016/j.infbeh.2007.10.003
86. Angulo-Barroso RM, Wu J, Ulrich DA. Long-term effect of different treadmill interventions on gait development in new walkers with Down syndrome. *Gait Posture.* 2008;27(2):231-238. doi:10.1016/j.gaitpost.2007.03.014
87. Ulrich DA, Ulrich BD, Angulo-Kinzler RM, Yun J. Treadmill training of infants with Down syndrome: evidence-based developmental outcomes. *Pediatrics.* 2001;108(5):E84. doi:10.1542/peds.108.5.e84
88. Ulrich BD. Opportunities for early intervention based on theory, basic neuroscience, and clinical science. *Phys Ther.* 2010;90(12):1868-1880. doi:10.2522/ptj.20100040
89. Ulrich DA, Lloyd MC, Tiernan CW, Looper JE, Angulo-Barroso RM. Effects of intensity of treadmill training on developmental outcomes and stepping in infants with Down syndrome: a randomized trial. *Phys Ther.* 2008;88(1):114-122. doi:10.2522/ptj.20070139
90. Valentín-Gudiol M, Mattern-Baxter K, Girabent-Farrés M, Bagur-Calafat C, Hadders-Algra M, Angulo-Barroso RM. Treadmill interventions in children under six years of age at risk of neuromotor delay. *Cochrane Database Syst Rev.* 2017;7:CD009242. doi:10.1002/14651858.CD009242.pub3
91. Deutsch JE, Borbely M, Filler J, Huhn K, Guarrera-Bowlby P. Use of a low-cost, commercially available gaming console (Wii) for rehabilitation of an adolescent with cerebral palsy. *Phys Ther.* 2008;88(10):1196-1207. doi:10.2522/ptj.20080062
92. Shih CH, Shih CT, Chu CL. Assisting people with multiple disabilities actively correct abnormal standing posture with a Nintendo Wii balance board through controlling environmental stimulation. *Res Dev Disabil.* 2010;31(4):936-942. doi:10.1016/j.ridd.2010.03.004
93. Shih CH, Yeh JC, Shih CT, Chang ML. Assisting children with Attention Deficit Hyperactivity Disorder actively reduces limb hyperactive behavior with a Nintendo Wii Remote Controller through controlling environmental stimulation. *Res Dev Disabil.* 2011;32(5):1631-1637. doi:10.1016/j.ridd.2011.02.014

94. Wuang YP, Chiang CS, Su CY, Wang CC. Effectiveness of virtual reality using Wii gaming technology in children with Down syndrome. *Res Dev Disabil.* 2011;32(1):312-321. doi:10.1016/j.ridd.2010.10.002
95. Hickman R, Popescu L, Manzanares R, Morris B, Lee SP, Dufek JS. Use of active video gaming in children with neuromotor dysfunction: a systematic review. *Dev Med Child Neurol.* 2017;59(9):903-911. doi:10.1111/dmcn.13464
96. Academy Of Aquatic Physical Therapy. Frequently Asked Questions. https://aquaticpt.org/faq. Accessed June 15, 2018.
97. Hind D, Parkin J, Whitworth V, et al. Aquatic therapy for boys with Duchenne muscular dystrophy (DMD): an external pilot randomised controlled trial. *Pilot Feasibility Stud.* 2017;3(1):16. doi:10.1186/s40814-017-0132-0
98. Bruder MB. Early childhood intervention: a promise to children and families for their future. *Except Child.* 2010;76(3):339-355. doi:10.1177/001440291007600306
99. Bronfenbrenner U. *The Ecology of Human Development: Experiments by Nature and Design.* Boston, MA: Harvard University Press; 1979.
100. Van Hooste A, Maes B. Family factors in the early development of children with Down syndrome. *J Early Interv.* 2003;25(4):296-309. doi:10.1177/105381510302500405
101. Goldstein DN, Cohn E, Coster W. Enhancing participation for children with disabilities: application of the ICF enablement framework to pediatric physical therapist practice. *Pediatr Phys Ther.* 2004;16(2):114-120. doi:10.1097/01.PEP.0000127567.98619.62
102. Gardner K. Role of a Physical Therapist Assistant (PTA). APTA. http://www.apta.org/PTACareers/RoleofaPTA/. Accessed September 9, 2018.
103. Law M, Baptiste S, Carswell A, McColl MA, Polatajko HJ, Pollack N. *Canadian Occupational Performance Measure.* 2nd ed. Ottawa, Canada: CAOT Publications ACE; 1998.
104. American College of Medical Genetics and Genomics. Home. http://www.acmg.net/. Accessed September 9, 2018.
105. American Academy of Pediatrics. Promoting Optimal Development: Identifying Infants and Young Children With Developmental Disorders Through Developmental Surveillance and Screening. https://pediatrics.aappublications.org/content/145/1/e20193449. Accessed March 22, 2020.
106. American Occupational Therapy Association. Practice. https://www.aota.org/practice.aspx. Accessed March 22, 2020.
107. WFOT. About Occupational Therapy. https://www.wfot.org/about/about-occupational-therapy. Accessed March 22, 2018.
108. American Speech-Language-Hearing Association. Scope of Practice in Speech-Language Pathology. https://www.asha.org/policy/SP2016-00343/. Accessed March 22, 2020.
109. Iversen MD, Shimmel JP, Ciacera SL, Prabhakar M. Creating a family-centered approach to early intervention services: perceptions of parents and professionals. *Pediatr Phys Ther.* 2003;15(1):23-31. doi:10.1097/01.PEP.0000051694.10495.79
110. An M, Palisano RJ, Yi C-H, Chiarello LA, Dunst CJ, Gracely EJ. Effects of a collaborative intervention process on parent empowerment and child performance: a randomized controlled trial. *Phys Occup Ther Pediatr.* 2019;39(1):1-15. doi:10.1080/01942638.2017.1365324
111. Rone-Adams SA, Stern DF, Walker V. Stress and compliance with a home exercise program among caregivers of children with disabilities. *Pediatr Phys Ther.* 2004;16(3):140-148. doi:10.1097/01.PEP.0000136006.13449.DC
112. Basaran A, Karadavut KI, Uneri SO, Balbaloglu O, Atasoy N. Adherence to Home Exercise Program among Caregivers of Children with Cerebral Palsy. *Turk J Ph Med Rehab.* 2014;60(2):85-91. doi:10.5152/tftrd.2014.60973
113. Ozonoff S, Cathcart K. Effectiveness of a home program intervention for young children with autism. *J Autism Dev Disord.* 1998;28(1):25-32. doi:10.1023/A:1026006818310
114. Council on Children with Disabilities and Medical Home Implementation Project Advisory Committee. Patient- and family-centered care coordination: a framework for integrating care for children and youth across multiple systems. *Pediatrics.* 2014;133(5):e1451-e1460. doi:10.1542/peds.2014-0318
115. Craig J, Hilderman C, Wilson G, Misovic R. Effectiveness of stretch interventions for children with neuromuscular disabilities: evidence based recommendations. *Pediatr Phys Ther.* 2016;28(3):262-275. doi:10.1097/PEP.0000000000000269

Appendix A: Core Assessment Measures for Neuromuscular Conditions

Legend:
ICF = International Classification of Function
B = Body functions and structures
A = Activity
P = Participation

Types of Assessment	Assessment Tools	Description	ICF Measured
ROM	Goniometry[1]	Measure joint ROM	B
Muscle Strength	Manual Muscle Test[2]	Use 6 basic categories of grading muscle strength (Normal, Good, Fair, Poor, Trace, Zero). Use of plus and minus sign to the basic grade denotes a greater or lesser amount of resistance or ROM.	B
Balance and Coordination	Four Square Step Test[3]	Assess balance in the presence of task and environmental challenge. Test shows excellent interrater reliability when used with children with DS and cerebral palsy.	B
	Functional Reach Test[4]	Assess a patient's stability by measuring the maximum distance he/she can reach forward while standing in a fixed position.	B
	Pediatric Berg Balance Scale[5]	Modification of the Berg Balance Scale (adults) for use with school age children with mild to moderate motor impairments.	B
	Segmental Assessment of Trunk Control[6]	Systematically assess discrete levels of trunk control in children with neuromotor disabilities when sitting balance is delayed.	B
	Timed Up and Go[7]	Assess basic functional ambulatory mobility or dynamic balance.	B
Functional Skills	Brooke Scale[8]	Assess upper extremity function. Grades range from 1 (best function) to 6 (worst).	B
	Vignos Scale[9]	Assess lower extremity function and document progression. Ten-point scale describes activities relating to lower extremities. Ordinal scale 1 (best function) to 10 (worst).	B
	Egen Klassifikation[10]	Specific for wheelchair users. Includes questions on health-based quality of life. Ordinal scale of 0 (highest) to 30 (lowest).	A/P
	Functional Independence Measure[11]	Uniformly measures disability based in ICF; measures the level of a patient's disability and how much assistance is required for the individual to carry out ADL. The 18 measurement items comprise 13 motor tasks, 5 cognitive tasks, and 6 areas of function. Scores range from 18 (lowest) to 126 (highest).	A
	Gross Motor Function Measure[12]	Describes child's current level of motor function in 5 dimensions (ie, lying and rolling; sitting; crawling; standing; and walking, running, and jumping). Uses a 4-point Likert scale.	A
	Hammersmith Motor Ability Score Expanded[13]	Primarily used for patients with Spinal Muscular Atrophy. Scores from 0 (unable) to 2 (fully able). Used in clinical practice and research.	A
	Motor Function Measure Scale[14]	Developed for Neuromuscular Diseases. Comprises 32 items in three dimensions: standing and transfers, axial and proximal motor function, and distal motor function.	B/A

(continued)

Types of Assessment	*Assessment Tools*	*Description*	*ICF Measured*
Functional Skills	Muscular Dystrophy Functional Rating Scale[15]	A disease-specific scale that combines 4 domains to rate mobility, basic ADL, and impairment. Uses a 4-point scale with 1 being unable and completely dependent to 4 means no problem for the activity at normal speed; 132 is the highest total score.	B/A
	North Star Ambulatory Assessment[16]	Specifically designed for children with DMD who are ambulatory; 17 activities are graded as 0 (unable), 1 (with help), and 2 (normal).	B/A
	Pediatric Evaluation of Disability Inventory[17]	Determine functional capabilities and performance, monitor progress in functional skill performance, and evaluate therapeutic or rehabilitative program outcome in children with disabilities. Defined by three categories: self-care, mobility, and social function. There is a caregiver assistance scale.	A/P
	Pediatric Evaluation of Disability Inventory Computer-Adaptive Test[18]	Measure abilities in 3 functional domains of daily activities, mobility, and social/cognitive. Measure the extent to which the caregiver or child takes responsibility for managing complex multi-step life tasks.	A/P
	Wee-FIM (Functional Independence Measure) for Pediatrics[19]	Use an 18-item, 7-level ordinal scale to assess child's typical performance in self-care, sphincter control, transfers, locomotion, communication, and social cognitive; measures need for assistance or severity of disability of children.	A/P
Developmental	Alberta Infant Motor Scale[20]	Identify motor delays and measure motor performance changes over time from birth to 18 months.	B/A
	Bayley-III Scale of Infant Development[21]	Measure rate of infant development and highlight early developmental delays in infants with DMD.	B/A
	Griffiths Mental Development Scales[22]	Measure rate of development in children and highlight early developmental delays in children with DMD.	B/A
	Peabody Developmental Motor Scales-2[23]	Assess child's abilities in early motor development in gross and fine motor skills. Subtest in 6 areas: reflexes, stationary (body control and equilibrium), locomotion, object manipulation, grasping, and visual motor integration. Standardized and norm-referenced tool.	B/A
Endurance	Borg Rating of Perceived Exertion Scale[24]	Measure physical activity intensity level. Scale ranges from 6 ("no feeling of exertion") to 20 ("very, very hard"). Perceived exertion is how hard one feels the body is working during physical activity, including increased heart rate, respiration, or breathing rate, sweating, and muscle fatigue.	B
	6-Minute Walk Test[25]	Through an observational study, evaluate functional capacity in ambulatory boys with DMD; measure ambulatory and cardiopulmonary capacity.	A
	10-Meter Walk Run Test[26]	Assess walking speed in meters/second over a short duration.	A
Pain	Visual Analog Scale (Numeric Pain Scale)[27]	Determine intensity of current state of pain using rating scale of 0 (no pain) to 10 (worst pain).	B
	Wong-Baker FACES[28]	Use 6 levels of facial expressions to determine current state of pain reported by the individual.	B

(continued)

Types of Assessment	Assessment Tools	Description	ICF Measured
Quality of Life/ Participation	Canadian Occupational Performance Measure (COPM)[29]	Detect client's or family member's perception of occupational performance over time. Test self-care, productivity, and leisure.	P
	Children's Assessment of Participation and Enjoyment (CAPE) and Preferences for Activities of Children (PAC)[30]	Examine how children and youths participate in everyday activities outside of their school classes, using a 55-item questionnaire. Provides information about 5 dimensions of participation, including information on intensity and enjoyment of activities.	P
	Pediatric Evaluation of Disability Inventory[17] (see Functional Skills)		
	Pediatric Quality of Life Inventory 3.0-Neuromuscular Module[31]	Assess children in disease areas and health-related quality of life. Multidimensional construct is applicable for young children (5 to 7 years of age) through adolescents (13 to 18 years of age).	P
Upper Extremity Function	ABILHand[32]	Use a questionnaire to measure manual ability in everyday activities.	A/P
	ACTIVLIM[33]	Use a self-reported questionnaire of performing daily activities that require the use of upper extremities, and/or lower extremities activity limitations in children and adults with any neuromuscular disease. Results show a linear progression in difficulty.	A/P
	Assessment of the Functional Abilities of the upper limbs in patients with neuromuscular disease[34]	Evaluate functional state of the upper extremities in patients with neuromuscular diseases. Test 14 items including proximal shoulder and elbow ROM, and distal forearm, wrist, and finger ROM; assess endurance by the number of movement repetition/item.	B

References for Assessment Tools

1. Pandya S, Florence JM, King WM, Robison JD, Oxman M, Province MA. Reliability of goniometric measurements in patients with Duchenne muscular dystrophy. *Phys Ther.* 1985;65(9):1339-1342. doi:10.1093/ptj/65.9.1339
2. Florence JM, Pandya S, King WM, et al. Intrarater reliability of manual muscle test grades in Duchenne muscular dystrophy. *Phys Ther.* 1992;72:115-122. doi:10.1093/ptj/72.2.115
3. Bandong ANJ, Madriaga GO, Gorgon EJ. Reliability and validity of the Four Square Step Test in children with cerebral palsy and Down syndrome. *Res Dev Disabil.* 2015;47:39-47. doi:10.1016/j.ridd.2015.08.012
4. Weiner DK, Duncan PW, Chandler J, Studenski SA. Functional reach: a marker of physical frailty. *J Am Geriatr Soc.* 1992;40(3):203-207. doi:10.1111/j.1532-5415.1992.tb02068.x
5. Franjoine MR, Gunther JS, Taylor MJ. Pediatric balance scale: a modified version of the berg balance scale for the school-age child with mild to moderate motor impairment. *Pediatr Phys Ther.* 2003;15(2):114-128. doi:10.1097/01.PEP.0000068117.48023.18
6. Butler PB, Saavedra S, Sofranac M, Jarvis SE, Woollacott MH. Refinement, reliability, and validity of the segmental assessment of trunk control. *Pediatr Phys Ther.* 2010;22(3):246-257. doi:10.1097/PEP.0b013e3181e69490
7. Podsiadlo D, Richardson S. The timed "Up & Go": a test of basic functional mobility for frail elderly persons. *J Am Geriatr Soc.* 1991;39(2):142-148. doi:10.1111/j.1532-5415.1991.tb01616.x
8. Brooke MH, Griggs RC, Mendell JR, Fenichel GM, Shumate JB, Pellegrino RJ. Clinical trial in Duchenne dystrophy. I. The design of the protocol. *Muscle Nerve.* 1981;4(3):186-197. doi:10.1002/mus.880040304
9. Vignos PJ Jr, Spencer GE Jr, Archibald KC. Management of progressive muscular dystrophy in childhood. *JAMA.* 1963;184(2):89-96. doi:10.1001/jama.1963.03700150043007

10. Steffensen B, Hyde S, Lyager S, Mattsson E. Validity of the EK scale: a functional assessment of non-ambulatory individuals with Duchenne muscular dystrophy or spinal muscular atrophy. *Physiother Res Int.* 2001;6(3):119-134. doi:10.1002/pri.221
11. Stineman MG, Shea JA, Jette A, et al. The Functional Independence Measure: tests of scaling assumptions, structure, and reliability across 20 diverse impairment categories. *Arch Phys Med Rehabil.* 1996;77(11):1101-1108. doi:10.1016/S0003-9993(96)90130-6
12. Harvey A, Robin J, Morris ME, Graham HK, Baker R. A systematic review of measures of activity limitation for children with cerebral palsy. *Dev Med Child Neurol.* 2008;50(3):190-198. doi:10.1111/j.1469-8749.2008.02027.x
13. Main M, Kairon H, Mercuri E, Muntoni F. The Hammersmith functional motor scale for children with spinal muscular atrophy: a scale to test ability and monitor progress in children with limited ambulation. *Eur J Paediatr Neurol.* 2003;7(4):155-159. doi:10.1016/S1090-3798(03)00060-6
14. Bérard C, Payan C, Hodgkinson I, Fermanian J; MFM Collaborative Study Group. A motor function measure for neuromuscular diseases. Construction and validation study. *Neuromuscul Disord.* 2005;15(7):463-470. doi:10.1016/j.nmd.2005.03.004
15. Lue YJ, Su CY, Yang RC, et al. Development and validation of a muscular dystrophy-specific functional rating scale. *Clin Rehabil.* 2006;20(9):804-817. doi:10.1177/0269215506070809
16. Mazzone ES, Messina S, Vasco G, et al. Reliability of the North Star Ambulatory Assessment in a multicentric setting. *Neuromuscul Disord.* 2009;19(7):458-461. doi:10.1016/j.nmd.2009.06.368
17. Haley S, Costner W, Ludlow L, et al. *Pediatric Evaluation of Disability Inventory (PEDI): Development, Standardization, and Administration Manual.* Boston, MA: Trustee of Boston University. 1992.
18. Dumas H, Fragala-Pinkham MA, Haley S, et al. Computer adaptive test performance in children with and without disability inventory computer adapted tests (PEDI-CAT). *Dev Med Child Neurol.* 2012;53:1100-1106.
19. Msail EM, Ottenbachker K, Duffy L, et al. Reliability and validity of the WeeFIM in children with neurodevelopmental disabilities. *Pediatr Res.* 1996;39:378. doi:10.1203/00006450-199604001-02276
20. Piper MC. Darrah J. *Motor Assessment of the Developing Infant.* Philadelphia, PA: WB Saunders; 1993.
21. Connolly AM, Florence JM, Cradock MM, et al; MDA DMD Clinical Research Network. One year outcome of boys with Duchenne muscular dystrophy using the Bayley-III scales of infant and toddler development. *Pediatr Neurol.* 2014;50(6):557-563. doi:10.1016/j.pediatrneurol.2014.02.006
22. Connolly AM, Florence JM, Cradock MM, et al; MDA DMD Clinical Research Network. The MDA DMD Clinical Research Network. Motor and cognitive assessment of infants and young boys with Duchenne muscular dystrophy: results from the Muscular Dystrophy Association DMD Clinical Research Network. *Neuromuscul Disord.* 2013;23(7):529-539. doi:10.1016/j.nmd.2013.04.005
23. van Hartingsveldt MJ, Cup EHC, Oostendorp RAB. Reliability and validity of the fine motor scale of the Peabody Developmental Motor Scales-2. *Occup Ther Int.* 2005;12(1):1-13. doi:10.1002/oti.11
24. Borg G. *Borg's Perceived Exertion and Pain Scales.* Champaign, IL: Human Kinetics; 1998.
25. McDonald CM, Henricson EK, Han JJ, et al. The 6-minute walk test as a new outcome measure in Duchenne muscular dystrophy. *Muscle Nerve.* 2010;41(4):500-510. doi:10.1002/mus.21544
26. McDonald CM, Abresch RT, Carter GT, et al. Profiles of neuromuscular diseases. Duchenne muscular dystrophy. *Am J Phys Med Rehabil.* 1995;74(5)(suppl):S70-S92. doi:10.1097/00002060-199509001-00003
27. Grant S, Aitchison T, Henderson E, et al. A comparison of the reproducibility and sensitivity to change of visual analogue scales, Borg Scales, and Likert Scales in normal subjects during submaximal exercises. *Chest.* 1999;116-1208-1217.
28. Wong DL, Winkelstein ML, Schwartz P, et al. *Wong's essentials of pediatric nursing.* 6th ed. St. Louis, MO: Mosby; 2001.
29. Verkerk GJQ, Wolf MJ, Louwers AM, Meester-Delver A, Nollet F. The reproducibility and validity of the Canadian Occupational Performance Measure in parents of children with disabilities. *Clin Rehabil.* 2006;20(11):980-988. doi:10.1177/0269215506070703
30. King G, Law M. King s, et al. *Children's Assessment of Participation and Enjoyment (CAPE) and Preferences for Activities of Children (PAC).* San Antonio, TX: Harcourt Assessment, Inc; 2004.
31. Uzark K, King E, Cripe L, et al. Health-related quality of life in children and adolescents with Duchenne Muscular Dystrophy. *Pediatrics.* 2012;130(6):130-e1559-1566.
32. Penta M, Tesio L, Arnould C, Zancan A, Thonnard JL. The ABILHAND questionnaire as a measure of manual ability in chronic stroke patients: rasch-based validation and relationship to upper limb impairment. *Stroke.* 2001;32(7):1627-1634. doi:10.1161/01.STR.32.7.1627
33. Vandervelde L, Van den Bergh PY, Goemans N, Thonnard JL. ACTIVLIM: a Rasch-built measure of activity limitations in children and adults with neuromuscular disorders. *Neuromuscul Disord.* 2007;17(6):459-469. doi:10.1016/j.nmd.2007.02.013
34. Mazzone ES, Vasco G, Palermo C, et al. A critical review of functional assessment tools for upper limbs in Duchenne muscular dystrophy. *Dev Med Child Neurol.* 2012;54(10):879-885. doi:10.1111/j.1469-8749.2012.04345.x

Appendix B: Five Stages of Duchenne Muscular Dystrophy and Rehabilitation Management for Each Stage

The physical therapist and physical therapist assistant, as part of the rehabilitation management, should be familiar with the 5 stages of DMD and 11 care consideration guidelines. The 5 stages of DMD are pre-symptomatic, early ambulatory, late ambulatory, early non-ambulatory, and late non-ambulatory. The following chart describes the 5 stages of DMD and the rehabilitation team management areas. The key rehab team member is usually a physical therapist. Other rehab personnel include physicians, occupational therapists, physical therapist assistants, occupational therapy assistants, speech-language pathologists, orthotists, and durable medical equipment providers.

Stage 1: Pre-Symptomatic **Most patients with DMD are not diagnosed during this stage unless there is a family history or blood tests are done for other reasons.**	
Symptoms to Recognize	• Usually noted when child is about 2 to 5 years of age. • Delayed motor milestones, calf muscle hypertrophy, proximal lower limb weakness, learning difficulties, and speech delay.
Tests and Measures	• Tests and measures should be selected based on patient's age and clinical presentation. • During the ambulatory period, the North Star Ambulation Assessment (NSAA) and timed function tests should be done every 6 months. • Other test and measures to consider: Please note those in bold are more specific to use with children with DMD. • ROM, muscle extensibility, posture and alignment, strength, function, ADL, quality of life, and participation, ACTIVLIM, 6-minute walk test, 10-meter walk test, **Brooke Upper Extremity Scale**, **Vignos scale**, and **North Star Ambulatory assessment (NSAA)**.
Therapy Goals	• Reflect on typical development, functional mobility, self-care skills, and participation in the home and community.
Therapy Interventions	• Emphasis is to maintain optimal function and participation. • Keep the children with DMD "functional" for as long as possible.
Preventive Measures to Minimize Contractures	• Home education programs for patient: daily active and passive ROM exercises/stretching of the lower extremities bilaterally. • May consider orthoses or splinting of lower extremities for night use. • NOTE: Ankle-foot orthoses are not typically indicated during ambulation.
Encourage Appropriate Exercises and Activities	• Submaximal aerobic activities such as swimming. • Low resistance exercises. • **Avoid high-resistance strength training and eccentric exercises throughout lifespan due to potential muscle fiber injury.**
Durable Medical Equipment	• For energy conservation: Consider an adapted stroller or manual wheelchair for community outings.
Stage 2: Early Ambulatory **Patients with DMD will start showing a positive Gower's sign, waddling gait, and toe walking. The children with DMD may still climb stairs, but will use a step-to gait pattern.**	
Symptoms to Recognize	• Usually noted when child is about 2 to 5 years of age. • Delayed motor milestones, calf muscle hypertrophy, proximal lower limb weakness, learning difficulties, and speech delay.

(continued)

<table>
<tr><td>Tests and Measures</td><td>• During the ambulatory period, the North Star Ambulation Assessment (NSAA) and timed function tests should be done every 6 months.
• Yearly physical therapy and occupational therapy evaluations are recommended as there will be a significant change in the disease process and increased equipment needs. Need to identify change of status in disease stage.
• Assess pulmonary function at least once a year by using a spirometer to test vital capacity, forced expiratory volume, and peak cough flow.</td></tr>
<tr><td>Therapy Goals</td><td>• Energy conservation.
• Pain management due to back problems, posture, pressure relief, and possible vertebral fractures secondary to glucocorticoid treatment.
• Prevention of ineffective cough, nocturnal hypoventilation, sleep breathing disorder, and daytime respiratory failure.</td></tr>
<tr><td>Therapy Interventions</td><td>• Emphasis to maintain optimal function and participation.
• Keep the children with DMD "functional" for as long as possible.
• Pain management.
• Respiratory management and activities.</td></tr>
<tr><td>Preventive Measures to Minimize Contractures</td><td>• Home education programs for patient, with emphasis on:
  o Energy conservation
  o Daily active and passive lower extremities ROM exercises/stretching bilaterally
• Ankle-foot orthoses are not used during the ambulatory stage, as they limit necessary compensatory strategies the child with DMD may need for ambulation. Ankle-foot orthoses and knee-ankle foot orthoses could be used for night splints.</td></tr>
<tr><td>Encourage Appropriate Exercises and Activities</td><td>• Share information on community resources and parent support groups.
• Encourage submaximal aerobic activities such as swimming.
• Suggest low-resistance exercises.
• Avoid high-resistance strength training and eccentric exercises throughout lifespan due to potential muscle fiber injury.</td></tr>
<tr><td>Durable Medical Equipment</td><td>• Lightweight manual wheelchair for community outings and energy conservation.
• Possible home and adaptive equipment: ramps, stair lifts, bathroom equipment, special beds, mattresses, and vehicle modifications.
• Crutches, canes, and walkers are not used due to increased upper extremity weight-bearing pressures.</td></tr>
<tr><td colspan="2">Stage 3: Late Ambulatory
Patients with DMD will start demonstrating an increasingly labored gait. They will be losing ability to rise from the floor and climb stairs.</td></tr>
<tr><td>Symptoms to Recognize</td><td>• Children most likely will be diagnosed by this stage.</td></tr>
<tr><td>Tests and Measures</td><td>• Monitor patient's status quarterly: Physical therapy and occupational therapy evaluations are recommended as there will be a significant change in the disease process and increased equipment needs. Identify change of status in disease stage. Refer to Stage 1 for the suggested lists of test and measures.
• Assess upper extremities when strength declines.
• Assess for computer and environmental control access, and mobile arm support.
• Ensure pain management due to back problems, posture, pressure relief, and possible vertebral fractures due to glucocorticoid treatment.</td></tr>
<tr><td>Therapy Goals</td><td>• Reflect typical development, functional mobility, self-care skills, and participation.

(continued)</td></tr>
</table>

Therapy Interventions	• Emphasis to maintain optimal function and participation. • Keep the children with DMD "functional" for as long as possible. • Important to maintain good ROM bilaterally and maintain standing and ambulation activities. • Pain management for back pain. • Respiratory management and activities. • Standing programs when weight-bearing—standing or walking becomes more difficult.

Preventive Measures to Minimize Contractures	• Home education programs for patient with emphasis on
	  ◦ Energy conservation
	  ◦ Daily active and passive ROM exercises/stretching bilaterally
	• May consider orthoses or splinting of lower extremities for night use.
	• NOTE: Ankle-foot orthoses are not typically indicated during ambulation.

Encourage Appropriate Exercises and Activities	• Share information on community resources and parent support groups. • Submaximal aerobic activities such as swimming. • Standing programs. • **Avoid high-resistance strength training and eccentric exercises throughout lifespan due to potential muscle fiber injury.**

Durable Medical Equipment	• For long-distance mobility: manual wheelchair with light weight frame, solid seat and back.
	• As upper extremity strength declines, consider evaluation for mobile arm support to be attached to the wheelchair.
	• Power wheelchair may be assessed: Evaluate and consider a power sit-to-stand wheelchair to promote weight-bearing and doing instrumental ADL activities at home and at school.
	• Consider a stander. Depending on financial resources and the child's abilities, height, and weight, there are manual hydraulic standers and power standing devices. (See website information for "**Sit-to-Stand Standers**" below:
	
	• Manual Standers:
	  ◦ https://easystand.com/product/py5500-bantam-medium/
	  ◦ https://easystand.com/product/png50162-evolv-medium/
	  ◦ https://primeengineering.com/symmetry-youth/
	
	• Power Standers:
	  ◦ http://www.permobile.com
	  ◦ http:// www.motionconcepts.com

Stage 4: Early Non-Ambulatory **Patients with DMD will need a wheelchair at this stage. Patients may be able to self-propel a manual wheelchair or may consider a power wheelchair for energy conservation.**	
Symptoms to Recognize	• Children are diagnosed by this stage.
Tests and Measures	• In the older individuals who are non-ambulatory, the Brooke upper extremity scale, Egen Klassifikation scale, and elbow flexion and grip strength should be tested. • Also consider ABILHAND, ACTIVLIM, Brooke Upper Extremity Scale, Vignos scale, and other upper extremity tests.
Therapy Goals	• Energy conservation. • Pain management due to back problems, posture, pressure relief, and possible vertebral fractures secondary to glucocorticoid treatment. • Prevention of ineffective cough, nocturnal hypoventilation, sleep breathing disorder, and daytime respiratory failure. *(continued)*

Therapy Interventions	• Emphasis to maintain optimal function and participation. • Keep the children with DMD "functional" for as long as possible. • Pain management for back pain. • Respiratory management and activities.

Preventive Measures to Minimize Contractures	• Home education programs with emphasis on:
	  ◦ Energy conservation; respiratory exercises
	  ◦ Daily active and passive ROM exercises/stretching bilaterally for all extremities
	• May consider ankle-foot orthoses or knee-ankle foot orthoses or splinting of lower extremities for night use.
	• Thoracic lumbar sacral orthosis may be prescribed by orthopedist.

Encourage Appropriate Exercises and Activities	• Share information on community resources and parent support groups. • Encourage submaximal aerobic activities such as swimming. • **Avoid high-resistance strength training and eccentric exercises throughout lifespan due to potential muscle fiber injury.**
Durable Medical Equipment	• Manual wheelchair: light weight frame, solid seat and back. • Power wheelchair may be assessed: Evaluate and consider a power sit-to-stand wheelchair to promote weight-bearing and doing instrumental ADL at home and at school. • As upper extremity strength declines, consider evaluation for mobile arm support to be attached to the wheelchair. • Consider a stander or a power sit-to-stand wheelchair. Depending on financial resources and the child's abilities, height, and weight, there are manual hydraulic standers and power standing devices. (See website information for standers in Stage 3 in the durable medical equipment row). • Assess assistive technology as upper extremity strength declines. Consider accessible computer, environmental control access such as tongue-touch control system, switch scanning, eye-gaze selection, infrared pointing.
Stage 5: Late Non-Ambulatory **Patients with DMD will find it difficult to use their upper extremities for ADL, and maintaining good posture is increasingly more difficult and complicated as the patient with DMD is in a wheelchair most of their waking hours.**	
Symptoms to Recognize	• Children are diagnosed by this stage.
Tests and Measures	• Assess upper extremities as strength has declined. • ABILHAND, ACTIVLIM, Brooke Upper Extremity Scale, Vignos scale. • Assess for computer and environmental control access, and mobile arm support. • Monitor patient's status more frequently, ie, every quarter of the year.
Therapy Goals	• Monitor patient's status more frequently, ie, every quarter of the year. • Recommend durable medical equipment that best supports independence and participation. • Monitor current equipment for modifications and repairs. • Provide adaptations to assist with eating, drinking, toileting, and transferring to and turning in bed. • Energy conservation. • Pain management due to back problems, posture, pressure relief, and possible vertebral fractures secondary to glucocorticoid treatment. • Prevention of ineffective cough, nocturnal hypoventilation, sleep breathing disorder, and daytime respiratory failure. • ABILHAND, ACTIVLIM, Brooke Timing Protocol, Brooke Upper Extremity Scale, Modified Vignos scale *(continued)*

Therapy Interventions	• Emphasis to maintain optimal function and participation. • Keep the children with DMD "functional" for as long as possible. • Pain management. • Respiratory management and activities.

Preventive Measures to Minimize Contractures	• Home education programs for patient:
	  ◦ Energy conservation; respiratory management
	  ◦ Daily active and passive ROM exercises/stretching bilaterally
	• May consider orthoses or splinting of lower extremities for night use.
	• Thoracic lumbar sacral orthosis may be prescribed by orthopedist.

Encourage Appropriate Exercises and Activities	• Share information on community resources and parent support groups. • Encourage submaximal aerobic activities such as swimming. • Suggest low-resistance exercises. • **Avoid high-resistance strength training and eccentric exercises throughout lifespan due to potential muscle fiber injury.**
Durable Medical Equipment	• Power wheelchair with sit-to-stand component may be assessed: evaluate and consider power sit-to-stand wheelchair to promote weight-bearing and doing instrumental ADL at home and school. • Mobile arm support with wheelchair. • Back-up manual wheelchair: lightweight frame with solid seat and back. • Recommend adaptive equipment to assist with eating, drinking, toileting, and transfers to and turning in bed.

Bibliography for Stages and Duchenne Muscular Dystrophy Management

Birnkrant DJ, Bushby K, Bann CM, et al. Diagnosis and management of DMD, part 1: diagnosis, neuromuscular, rehabilitation, endocrine, and gastrointestinal, and nutritional management. *Lancet Neurol.* 2018;17(3):251-267. doi:10.1016/S1474-4422(18)30024-3

Birnkrant DJ, Bushby K, Bann CM, et al. Diagnosis and management of DMD, part 2: respiratory, cardiac, bone health, and orthopedic management. *Lancet Neurol.* 2018;17(4):347-361. doi:10.1016/S1474-4422(18)30025-5

Birnkrant DJ, Bushby K, Bann CM, et al. Diagnosis and management of DMD, part 3: primary care, emergency management, psychosocial care, and transitions of care across the lifespan. *Lancet Neurol.* 2018;17(5):445-455. doi:10.1016/S1474-4422(18)30026-7

Website Information

Muscular Dystrophy Association. https://www.mda.org/

Parent Project Muscular Dystrophy. https://www.parentprojectmd.org

Duchenne Therapy Network. https://www.cureduchenne.org

Smart phone apps. https://www.google.com/search?q=smartphone+app

Please visit www.routledge.com/9781630915650 to access additional material.

Chapter 11

Clients With Spinal Cord Injury

Brian Hickman, PT, DPT, NCS, GCS, CEEAA; Tony Lema, PT, DPT; Bret Kennedy, PT, DPT, NCS; and Kelly Ryujin, PT, DPT

KEY WORDS Autonomic dysreflexia | Crede | Paraplegia | Sacral sparing | Tetraplegia

Chapter Objectives

- Explain the difference between a complete and incomplete traumatic spinal cord injury (SCI).
- Define sacral sparing.
- Define the motor level and sensory neurological levels of injury.
- Discuss the common characteristics of the clinical picture of a person with an SCI.
- Define autonomic dysreflexia (AD) and discuss why it is a medical emergency and what the physical therapist assistant should do when it occurs.
- Identify complications that may occur with an SCI.
- Discuss why pressure sores occur in people with SCIs and how these sores can be prevented.
- Identify and discuss the purposes of physical therapy for people with an SCI.
- Discuss physical therapy interventions used by physical therapists and physical therapist assistants working with people with an SCI.

SCI is a devastating, life-changing injury that may result in partial or complete loss of sensory function or motor control. Severe SCI affects the systems that regulate bowel and bladder control, breathing, heart rate, and blood pressure (BP). The rate of occurrence in the United States is 54 cases/million.[1] Injuries are classified using the American Spinal Injury Association (ASIA) Impairment Scale to determine the spinal level and grading of the injury for prognostic value. Currently, with advances in technology, more treatment options are available to clinicians to assist their clients in achieving their highest functional capacity.

Treatment for a patient with SCI usually begins in the acute care setting, which may include the intensive care unit. When medically stable, the patient is often transferred to a rehabilitation unit to undergo intensive rehabilitative services. As medical stability improves and necessary functional gains are made, the patient may receive physical therapy services in the home and eventually the outpatient setting. Physical therapist assistants are an integral part of the rehabilitation team. Physical therapist assistants will assist in improving or maintaining joint range of motion (ROM), increasing functional strength and endurance, optimizing safe functional mobility, and educating the patient, family, and caregivers.

Epidemiology of Spinal Cord Injury

Incidence

According to the World Health Organization, 10% of civilian deaths globally are due to traumatic injuries in people aged 5 to 44 years.[2,3] For those suffering spinal trauma, mortality is 17%.[4] As recently as 2017, there were an estimated 54 new cases of SCI/million, or 17,000/year, in the United States. The average age of injury has increased from 29 years during the 1970s to 42 years currently.[1] Males are at most risk in young adulthood (20 to 29) and older age (70 and older). Females are most at risk in adolescence (15 to

Lazaro RT, Umphred DA, eds.
Umphred's Neurorehabilitation for the Physical Therapist Assistant, Third Edition (pp 253-289).

19) and older age (60 and older).[2] It was reported that 81% of new SCI cases are male.[1]

Etiology

Vehicle crashes are the leading cause of injury (38%), followed by falls (30%), acts of violence (14%), and sports/recreation activities (9%). The proportion of injuries due to sports and to violence has decreased over the past 20 years. There has been a rise in SCIs due to falls.[1] Vehicle crashes, sports injuries, and falls were more likely to result in injuries of the cervical region of the spinal cord, whereas SCIs due to violence were more likely to result in injuries to the thoracic or lumbar and sacral regions of the spinal cord.[5]

Costs

Inpatient hospitalization days for SCI patients have greatly decreased recently, but costs associated with SCI remain high, likely due to high rehospitalization rates. The average lengths of stay in the hospital acute care unit after SCI have declined from 24 days in the 1970s to 11 days currently. Average rehabilitation lengths of stay have also declined from 98 days in the 1970s to 35 days currently. About 30% of people with SCI are rehospitalized one or more times during any given year following injury, with urinary tract infections the leading cause of readmission, followed by skin breakdown. Lifetime cost estimates in the United States associated with health care costs and living expenses vary widely from $1.1 million to $4.8 million, depending on age at the time of injury and severity of the injury. Employment rates for persons with SCI remains low: at 1 year after injury, only about 13% are employed, with one-third employed by 20 years post injury.[1]

Life Expectancy

Life expectancy for those with SCIs has not improved significantly since the 1980s and remains less than those without SCIs. Determinants of life expectancy are based on the level and extent of injury; those with a higher level of neurological injuries and/or those individuals who are ventilator-dependent have the lowest life expectancy. Mortality rates are highest within the first year of injury. The leading causes of death in the SCI population are pneumonia and septicemia.[1,6]

Pathophysiology

A traumatic SCI often causes immediate and irreversible damage to the spinal cord. The initial injury involves primary and secondary injuries. The primary injury occurs from an external force or impact and causes immediate vascular hemorrhage and rapid cell death at the site of impact. This may result from compression, transection, distraction, and laceration of the spinal cord. The damage causes spinal shock and resultant flaccid paralysis below the level of the lesion. The initial insult or injury is followed by a cascade of secondary injuries that cause further tissue loss and mechanical damage. Edema around the spinal cord will be present and may spread to higher and lower spinal segments within the first 24 hours,[7] extending the neurological level of injury. The extent of the injury depends on the severity of the primary injury. SCIs are most common in the cervical region, C5 in particular.[8]

Describing the Neurological Injury

Neurological Level and Extent of Lesion

A lesion to the spinal cord can affect the transmission of sensory information to the brain and/or motor information to the periphery, depending on the location of the lesion within the spinal cord. Each spinal nerve root innervates a specific area of the skin called a *dermatome* (sensory) and a group of muscles called a *myotome* (motor). Although dermatomal patterns are similar in all people, the precise area of segmental innervation can vary. By accurately assessing a patient's sensation and muscle strength, a clinician can identify whether an injury is complete or incomplete and establish the neurological level of injury (Figure 11-1). Specific criteria described by the ASIA[9,10] are used to make these determinations. Using these criteria ensures that professionals who work with people with SCIs will speak a common language, that outcomes of research will be comparable, and that functional predictors can be developed.[9,10]

Complete Versus Incomplete Injury

An incomplete SCI as defined by ASIA is the presence of sacral sparing, which is partial or complete preservation of motor function, sensory function, or both in the lowest sacral segments of the spinal cord (S4 and S5). Anal sensation and/or voluntary contraction of the external anal sphincter indicate sensory and motor incomplete injuries, respectively. Based on the sensory and motor evaluation, the ASIA Impairment Scale (AIS) classifies the patient's injury in 1 of 5 categories: A, B, C, D, or E.[9,10] (Table 11-1). With an incomplete injury, motor and sensory function below the injury can vary, depending on the severity of the injury. Remember, a patient may exhibit partial sensory or motor function in segments below the designated neurological level; however, to be considered an incomplete injury, the lowest sacral segments (S4, S5) must have sensory or motor function, known as *sacral sparing*. In patients with a complete injury, a zone of partial preservation may exist.[10] This identifies the most caudal segment with some sensory or motor function.[9,10] For example, if a patient's injury is classified as C5, ASIA A, but has impaired sensation to T1, then T1 is said to be the sensory zone of partial preservation.

Level of Injury

The level of injury describes the neurological level of the spinal cord where normal function remains rather than the vertebral level affected. Specific segments of the cord inner-

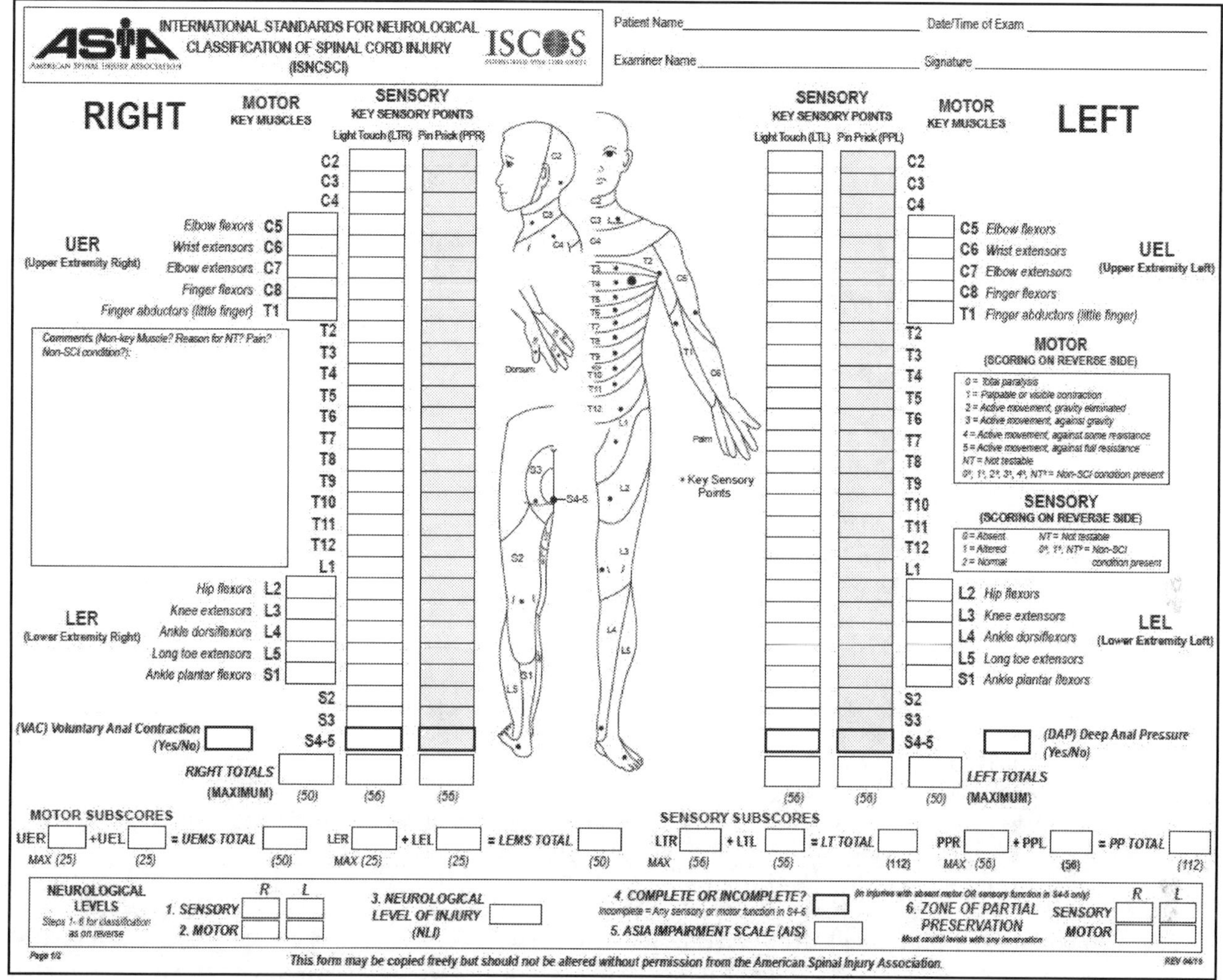

ASIA — AMERICAN SPINAL INJURY ASSOCIATION

INTERNATIONAL STANDARDS FOR NEUROLOGICAL CLASSIFICATION OF SPINAL CORD INJURY (ISNCSCI)

ISCOS

Patient Name ______ Date/Time of Exam ______

Examiner Name ______ Signature ______

RIGHT

MOTOR — KEY MUSCLES

SENSORY — KEY SENSORY POINTS: Light Touch (LTR), Pin Prick (PPR)

C2, C3, C4

UER (Upper Extremity Right): Elbow flexors C5; Wrist extensors C6; Elbow extensors C7; Finger flexors C8; Finger abductors (little finger) T1

Comments (Non-key Muscle? Reason for NT? Pain? Non-SCI condition?):

T2, T3, T4, T5, T6, T7, T8, T9, T10, T11, T12, L1

LER (Lower Extremity Right): Hip flexors L2; Knee extensors L3; Ankle dorsiflexors L4; Long toe extensors L5; Ankle plantar flexors S1

S2, S3, S4-5

(VAC) Voluntary Anal Contraction (Yes/No)

RIGHT TOTALS (MAXIMUM) (50) (56) (56)

LEFT

SENSORY — KEY SENSORY POINTS: Light Touch (LTL), Pin Prick (PPL)

MOTOR — KEY MUSCLES

C2, C3, C4

UEL (Upper Extremity Left): C5 Elbow flexors; C6 Wrist extensors; C7 Elbow extensors; C8 Finger flexors; T1 Finger abductors (little finger)

T2, T3, T4, T5, T6, T7, T8, T9, T10, T11, T12, L1

LEL (Lower Extremity Left): L2 Hip flexors; L3 Knee extensors; L4 Ankle dorsiflexors; L5 Long toe extensors; S1 Ankle plantar flexors

S2, S3, S4-5

(DAP) Deep Anal Pressure (Yes/No)

LEFT TOTALS (MAXIMUM) (56) (56) (50)

MOTOR (SCORING ON REVERSE SIDE)

0 = Total paralysis
1 = Palpable or visible contraction
2 = Active movement, gravity eliminated
3 = Active movement, against gravity
4 = Active movement, against some resistance
5 = Active movement, against full resistance
NT = Not testable
0*, 1*, 2*, 3*, 4*, NT* = Non-SCI condition present

SENSORY (SCORING ON REVERSE SIDE)

0 = Absent
1 = Altered
2 = Normal
NT = Not testable
0*, 1*, NT* = Non-SCI condition present

MOTOR SUBSCORES

UER ___ + UEL ___ = UEMS TOTAL ___ MAX (25) (25) (50)

LER ___ + LEL ___ = LEMS TOTAL ___ MAX (25) (25) (50)

SENSORY SUBSCORES

LTR ___ + LTL ___ = LT TOTAL ___ MAX (56) (56) (112)

PPR ___ + PPL ___ = PP TOTAL ___ MAX (56) (56) (112)

NEUROLOGICAL LEVELS (Steps 1-6 for classification as on reverse) — R, L

1. SENSORY
2. MOTOR

3. NEUROLOGICAL LEVEL OF INJURY (NLI)

4. COMPLETE OR INCOMPLETE? (Incomplete = Any sensory or motor function in S4-5)

5. ASIA IMPAIRMENT SCALE (AIS)

6. ZONE OF PARTIAL PRESERVATION (In injuries with absent motor OR sensory function in S4-5 only) (Most caudal levels with any innervation) — R, L: SENSORY, MOTOR

Page 1/2

REV 04/19

Figure 11-1. Worksheet to consistently document motor and sensory impairments, establish level of injury, and determine ASIA impairment scale in persons with SCI. (Reprinted with permission from the American Spinal Injury Association. *International Standards for Neurological Classification of Spinal Cord Injury, revised 2019*. Atlanta, GA: Reprinted 2019.)

vate specific muscles. ASIA has deliberately chosen specific muscles for determining the motor level. Most of the chosen muscles are innervated by 2 spinal levels; they are easily accessible to test in supine, and they are significant in terms of functional mobility. Motor level of injury is determined by the last spinal segment that innervates key muscles at 3/5 strength, providing that the muscles innervated at the levels above are of 5/5 strength.[9,10] Sensory level of injury is determined by the last spinal segment at which sensation is normal for both light touch and sharp/dull discrimination. People with SCIs may have different motor and sensory levels on the right and left sides of the body.

Tetraplegia Versus Paraplegia

Tetraplegia is the preferred term to describe a person with 4 extremities affected by an SCI, replacing the term quadriplegia. The extent of involvement in a person with tetraplegia can vary from complete loss of sensory and/or motor function of the upper extremities (UEs) and lower body to only partial loss of UE and lower-body function. Tetraplegia refers only to injuries that involve the spinal cord, not to injuries that affect only the peripheral nerves. T2 is the first level of injury at which the person is said to have paraplegia; in paraplegia, the UEs are not affected.

Upper Motor Neuron Lesions (Reflexic) Versus Lower Motor Neuron Lesions (Areflexic)

Most SCIs are considered to be upper motor neuron (UMN) lesions, or *reflexic injuries*, because the spinal cord is a part of the central nervous system. Symptoms of a UMN injury include spasticity, hypertonicity, and pathological reflexes. Lower motor neuron (LMN) lesions, or *areflexic injuries*, are seen when the damage is to peripheral nerves (eg, the cauda equina) or following an infarct to the cord. The clinical picture of an LMN injury includes flaccidity, atrophy, and absence of reflexes. It is possible

Table 11-1

American Spinal Cord Association Impairment Scale

A. Complete. No sensory or motor function is preserved in the sacral segments S4-S5.
B. Sensory Incomplete. Sensory but not motor function is preserved below the neurological level and includes the sacral segments S4-S5 (light touch, pinprick at S4-S5 or deep anal pressure), AND no motor function is preserved more than 3 levels below the motor level on either side of the body.
C. Motor Incomplete. Motor function is preserved at the most caudal sacral segments for voluntary anal contraction (VAC) OR the patient meets the criteria for sensory incomplete status (sensory function preserved at the most caudal sacral segments [S4-S5] by light touch, pinprick, or deep anal pressure), and has some sparing of motor function more than 3 levels below the ipsilateral motor level on either side of the body. (This includes key or non-key muscle functions to determine motor incomplete status.) For AIS C—less than half of key muscle functions below the single neurological level of injury (NLI) have a muscle grade ≥ 3.
D. Motor Incomplete. Motor incomplete status as defined above, with at least half (half or more) of key muscle functions below the single NLI having a muscle grade ≥ 3.
E. Normal. If sensation and motor function as tested with the International Standards for Neurological Classification of Spinal Cord Injury are graded as normal in all segments, and the patient had prior deficits, then the AIS grade is E. Someone without an initial SCI does not receive an AIS grade.
F. Using ND. To document the sensory, motor and NLI levels, the AIS grade, and/or the zone of partial preservation (ZPP) when they are unable to be determined based on the examination results.

For an individual to receive a grade of C or D (eg, motor incomplete status), he or she must have either (1) voluntary anal sphincter contraction or (2) sacral sensory sparing with sparing of motor function more than 3 levels below the motor level for that side of the body. The standards at this time allow even non-key muscle function more than 3 levels below the motor level to be used in determining motor incomplete status (AIS B vs C).

Note: When assessing the extent of motor sparing below the level for distinguishing between AIS B and C, the motor level on each side is used; whereas to differentiate between AIS C and D (based on proportion of key muscle functions with strength grade 3 or greater) the neurological level of injury is used.

Reprinted with permission from the American Spinal Injury Association. *International Standards for Neurological Classification of Spinal Cord Injury, revised 2019.* Atlanta, GA: Reprinted 2019.

for a patient to have both UMN and LMN involvement if there is spinal cord damage and the adjacent spinal root is involved. Areflexia also occurs during the period of spinal shock that follows anatomical or physiological transection or near transection of the cord.[11] During spinal shock, a transient suppression of reflex activity occurs below the injury. Proposed explanations for this phenomenon include decreased excitability of the spinal neurons, decreased descending facilitation, and increased spinal inhibition. The timeframe for spinal shock varies widely, from 4 days to 1 month for early hyperreflexia to begin, and 1 month to 12 months for spasticity and full hyperreflexia to occur.[11,12]

Spinal Cord Injury Syndromes

Damage to specific areas of the spinal cord can result in unique sensory and motor clinical pictures. Based on their clinical presentation, these spinal cord injuries have been categorized into SCI syndromes including Brown-Séquard syndrome (BSS), central cord syndrome, anterior cord syndrome, conus medullaris syndrome, and cauda equina syndrome.[13]

Brown-Séquard Syndrome

BSS results from a hemisection of the spinal cord (Figure 11-2). BSS is defined by a lesion that produces ipsilateral proprioceptive and motor loss and contralateral loss of pain and temperature sensitivity below the level of the lesion. BSS accounts for 1% to 4% of all traumatic SCIs. This type of injury can be caused by a spinal cord tumor, a spinal cord infection (eg, tuberculosis), inflammation of the spinal cord (eg, multiple sclerosis), or penetrating wounds to the spinal cord (eg, knife-stabbing or gunshot wound). Only a limited number of patients have the pure form of BSS—much more common is Brown-Séquard-plus syndrome, which refers to a relative ipsilateral hemiplegia with a relative contralateral hemi-analgesia.[13] BSS has the best prognosis for ambulation of the SCI syndromes. It has been shown that 75% to 90% of patients ambulate independently at discharge from rehabilitation.[14]

Central Cord Syndrome

Central cord syndrome (Figure 11-3) usually occurs in the cervical spine, often in older individuals with cervical spondylosis who have sustained a cervical hyperextension injury from a fall or motor vehicle accident. This type is the most common of the SCI syndromes, accounting for approximately 9% of all traumatic SCIs. The person with central cord syndrome has greater involvement of the UEs than the lower extremities (LEs), usually with urinary retention and varying degrees of sensory loss below the level of injury.[15] The UEs are more affected due to their spinal tracts being more centrally located in the spinal cord (see Figure 11-3). Central cord syndrome has a favorable

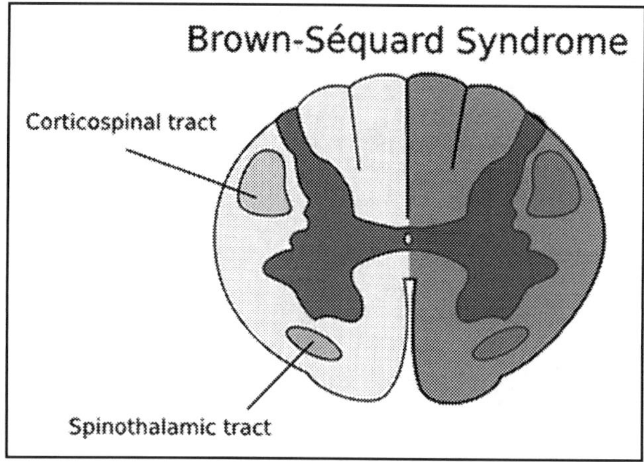

Figure 11-2. BSS. Shading designates areas of injury in this schematic cross-section of the spinal cord. Complete hemisection results in the loss of ipsilateral motor function and proprioception and contralateral light touch and superficial pain sensations below the level of injury. (Reprinted with permission from Olson N. Brown-Séquard syndrome. http://en.wikipedia.org/wiki/File:Cord-en.png.)

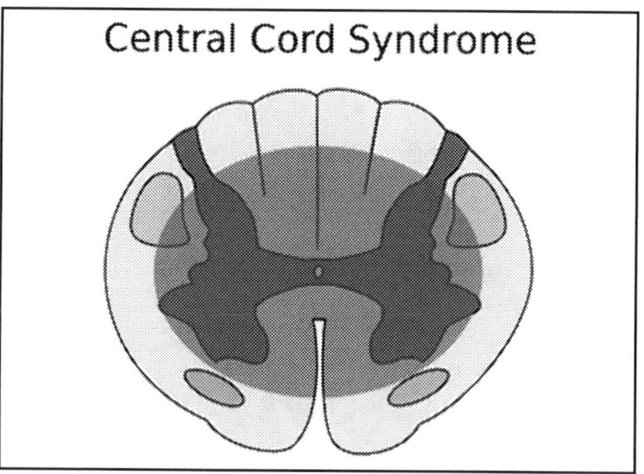

Figure 11-3. Central cord syndrome. Shading designates areas of injury in this schematic cross-section of the spinal cord. There is greater involvement of the UEs than the LEs because neurons within those tracks are organized by cervical, thoracic, and lumbar regions, with the cervical ones more central. (Reprinted with permission from Olson N. Central cord syndrome. http://en.wikipedia.org/wiki/File:Cord-en.png.)

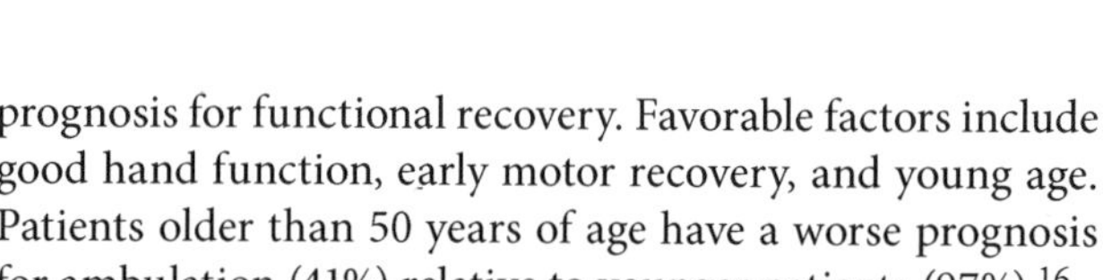

prognosis for functional recovery. Favorable factors include good hand function, early motor recovery, and young age. Patients older than 50 years of age have a worse prognosis for ambulation (41%) relative to younger patients (97%).[16]

Anterior Cord Syndrome

Anterior cord syndrome primarily affects the anterior two-thirds of the spinal cord while sparing the posterior columns. It accounts for 2.7% of all traumatic SCIs.[17] Anterior cord syndrome is usually associated with flexion injuries, direct bone fragments, or injuries causing vascular insufficiency. The primary motor tract (*corticospinal tract*) and a sensory tract (*spinothalamic tract*) are damaged, causing variable motor paralysis with variable loss of pain, temperature, and indiscriminate touch sensation below the level of the lesion. However, because the posterior columns are spared, there is preservation of proprioception, kinesthesia, touch, 2-point discrimination, and vibration sense. Anterior cord syndrome has a poorer prognosis for functional improvement compared with other syndromes.[13]

Conus Medullaris Syndrome

The conus medullaris is the terminal end of the spinal cord, ending at approximately the first or second lumbar vertebrae. Conus medullaris syndrome occurs when there is a lesion in this region, most commonly caused by trauma and tumors. Conus medullaris syndrome presents clinically with a combination of UMN and LMN signs, including saddle anesthesia, areflexic bladder and bowel, and variable degrees of LE weakness.[13]

Cauda Equina Syndrome

Cauda equina syndrome occurs with injury to the lumbosacral nerve roots within the neural canal; therefore, it is not considered to be a true SCI.[13] Cauda equina syndrome is often caused by trauma, tumors, spinal stenosis, disk compression, infection, or post-surgical epidural hematoma. As its etiology suggests, cauda equina syndrome can be caused by an acute process or a slowly progressive condition.[13] Cauda equina syndrome is considered a pure LMN lesion, without UMN signs. Clinically, cauda equina syndrome presents similarly to conus medullaris syndrome with saddle anesthesia, bladder and bowel dysfunction, and variable LE involvement that is often asymmetrical. It is suggested that cauda equina syndrome has a better prognosis than SCIs due to its being a lesion of an LMN, and nerve roots have the potential to regenerate. Early surgical decompression is one of the most important predictors for favorable recovery.[13]

Spinal Cord Injury

Medical Treatment

Emergency personnel, paramedics, and emergency room staff must evaluate the extent of the person's injury while taking measures to save the person's life. This includes using medical treatments to stabilize the person's vital signs. If the spine is unstable because of a fracture or dislocation of the vertebrae or disruption of ligaments, stabilizing the spinal column is required. Stabilization of the bones ensures that loss of nerve function is minimized, and that alignment and integrity of the spinal column are preserved. At the scene of an accident and before vertebral stabilization, care is taken to prevent movement of the neck or back, which could cause further damage to the spinal cord. Late symptoms of cervical instability include pain and tenderness at the site of the fracture or injury, increased radiating neck and arm pain, and increased loss of sensation or strength. When the patient reports symptoms of this nature, treatment must be stopped, and the physical therapist and physician must be notified immediately.

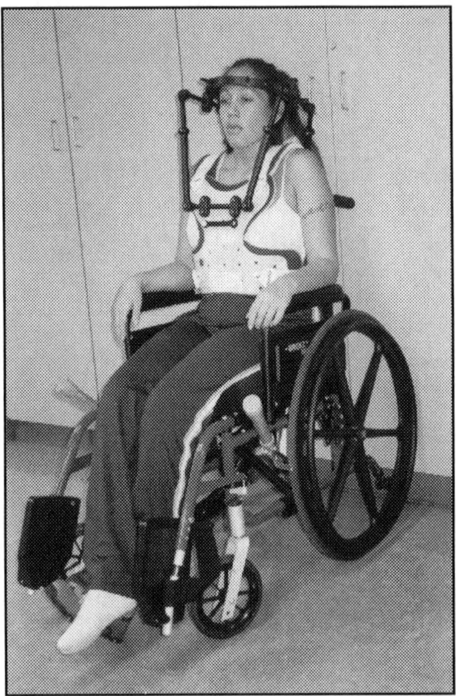

Figure 11-4. Patient with cervical vertebral fracture immobilized in a halo vest.

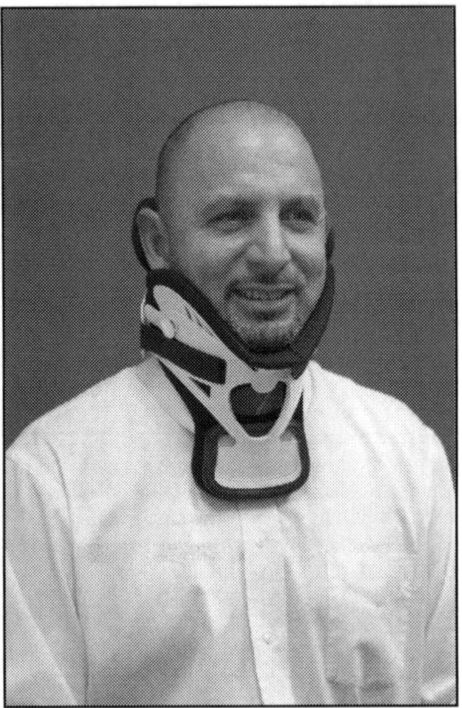

Figure 11-5. Miami collar.

There is strong evidence that early surgical stabilization of patients with unstable spinal columns has favorable outcomes. A systematic review by Dimar et al[18] showed shorter hospital and intensive care unit stays, fewer days on mechanical ventilation, and a lower rate of pulmonary complications. This effect was found in those with more severe injuries.[18]

Nonsurgical stabilization (if not surgically stabilized, and/or in addition to) may allow earlier mobilization. This is achieved by the application of orthotics. Depending on the nature of the injury, the appropriate orthosis (usually custom-made by an orthotist) is applied.

A halo vest (Figure 11-4) or collar (Figure 11-5) for neck injuries or a thoracolumbosacral orthosis (TLSO), also called a body jacket (Figure 11-6), for thoracic and lumbar injuries, may be applied. The length of time the patient wears the device and restrictions on movement and activities during the time of healing depend on the type of fracture and stabilization, how well the fracture heals, and the protocol of the physician and facility. The physical therapist assistant must look for and pay close attention to any restrictions listed in the medical record. It is important to check the patient's skin for redness or breakdown when the brace is being applied or removed and discuss with nursing and the physician if these problems arise.

Clinical Picture

Traumatic SCIs create various clinical pictures. These depend on many factors, including the neurological level of injury, the extent of injury, and medical complications that may accompany the initial injury. However, some common characteristics exist.

Motor Loss

Loss of motor function below the neurological level of injury is present in those with traumatic SCIs. The motor loss may be complete or partial. Based on the segmental innervations of the muscles, ASIA has chosen key muscles to represent each of the neurological levels.[4,9,15,16] A list of the muscles representing each neurological level is provided in the Neurological Classification of Spinal Cord Injury worksheet (see Figure 11-1). These muscles are tested while keeping the patient in a supine position, which is the ASIA standard, and allows safe examination of patients who have an unstable spine. The physical therapist may ask the physical therapist assistant to perform follow-up manual muscle tests of select muscles during the individual's rehabilitation. These procedures should follow the ASIA guidelines.

Respiratory Involvement

Virtually all patients with an SCI will have abnormal pulmonary function and increased risk of chronic respiratory symptoms, additional disability, and higher risk of early death from respiratory complications such as atelectasis and pneumonia.[19,20] Respiratory failure is the highest cause of mortality in the spinal cord–injured population.[21] Those with higher levels of injury may be ventilator-dependent, which in turn is associated with lower functional status and a higher rate of skilled nursing home placement.[20] Those with lower-level injuries will also have compromised pulmonary function due to respiratory muscle involvement.[7] *Forced vital capacity (VC)*, a measure of restrictive

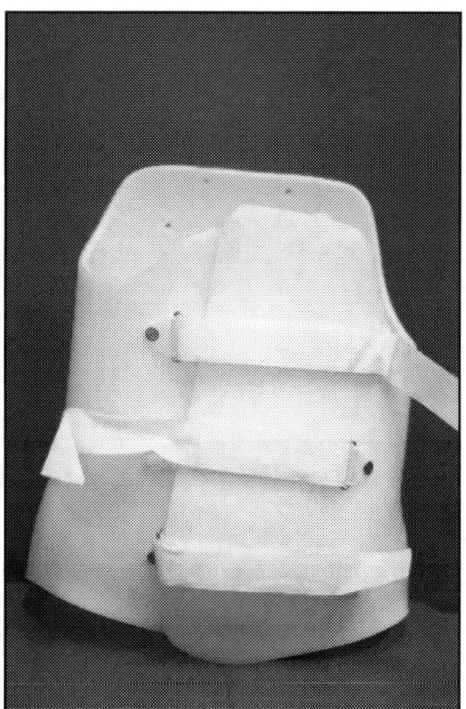

Figure 11-6. TLSO.

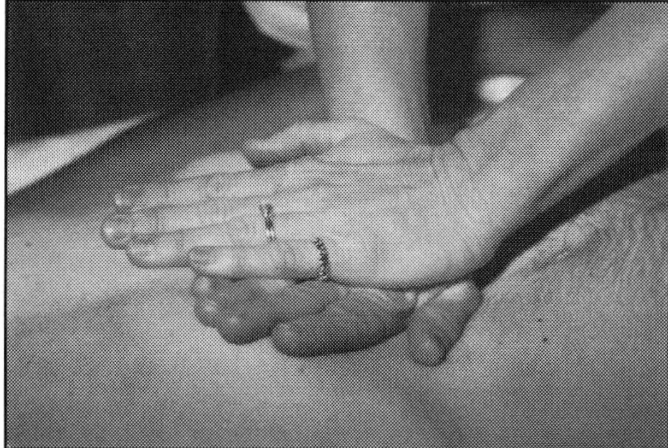

Figure 11-7. Hand position for manual assisted cough. Note how fingers are below the xiphoid process and overlapped to localize force. The patient's head is to the left.

dysfunction; *peak expiratory flow rate*, a measure of cough effectiveness; and *forced expiratory volume in 1 second*, a measure of obstructive dysfunction, increase with ascending SCI level, including pulmonary risk as low as L4.[19]

In people without an SCI, inspiration is carried out by a combination of the diaphragm (innervated by C3 to C5) and intercostal muscles (innervated by T1 to T11). The intercostal muscles are also used in conjunction with the abdominal musculature (innervated by T8 to T12) for expiration, forced breathing, and coughing. The neck musculature (innervated by C2 to C4) is inactive in those without pathology but may show activity in those with cervical lesions.[22]

When adequate diaphragm function is lacking in those with SCI, patients must receive complete or partial mechanical ventilation. Those with injuries above T8 will be profoundly affected by the lack of expiratory effectiveness, limiting clearance of secretions and cough effectiveness, and will be more susceptible to lower respiratory tract infections.[23] Patients may require manual assistance for coughing, a technique taught to patients and caregivers by the physical therapist and physical therapist assistant (Figure 11-7). Abdominal binders have been found to improve respiration by improving diaphragm position.[24] Abdominal or quad coughing can increase stimulation for coughing and increase the cough flow up to 15% to 33%.[20]

Sensory Loss

After a traumatic SCI, a comprehensive physical examination is completed, including sensory testing that will give valuable information regarding injury level and classification and prognosis of neurological recovery.[25] Sensory loss is common in those suffering traumatic SCIs and presents as loss in a dermatomal pattern. Sensory testing according to ASIA standards includes light touch and pinprick in selected dermatomal areas. These areas are identified on an ASIA worksheet (see Figure 11-1). Sensation is graded as normal, impaired, or absent. When the patient is unable to discriminate between sharp and dull input at a given dermatome, sensation for pinprick is considered absent. Proprioception is also tested and graded. The results of proprioception tests help predict functional outcome because patients with impaired or absent proprioception will have difficulty controlling extremity movement, even with favorable motor function.[26] With a complete injury, all sensation is lost below the level of injury. The physical therapist may ask the physical therapist assistant to repeat select sensory testing for individuals with an incomplete SCI to determine whether changes have occurred since the initial physical examination and the physical therapy examination. This may provide valuable prognostic information about recovery.

Spasticity

It has been reported that spasticity is seen in up to 80% of people with SCI, and 41% of individuals report it as a major obstacle in their lives.[27] Spasticity will typically develop after the initial period of spinal shock[28] and can affect skeletal muscles as well as muscles of the bowel, bladder, and sexual organs. The extent of spasticity and the muscles affected varies; it may be minimal, or it may interfere with function and sitting position. Spasticity can have both positive and negative effects. Positives can include assisting with standing or transfers, bone density, and circulation. Negatives include sleep difficulty, pressure ulcers, and pain. Spasticity is measured using the Modified Ashworth Scale. Spasticity is often increased by noxious stimulants such as a full bladder, pressure sores, or urologic infections.

Treatment of spasticity can be difficult. Splinting, bracing, and stretching are common approaches, but patients often need management with medications (eg, baclofen or tizanidine) to reduce spasticity that interferes with their function or quality of life. If spasticity cannot be managed by conventional approaches and is affecting function, some patients may undergo orthopedic surgical interventions such as tendon lengthening to recover ROM and function.[20] More recently, some patients with intractable spasticity are electing to receive an implantable intrathecal programmable pump that delivers spasticity medication (usually baclofen) into a very specific site near the spinal cord. Favorable results have been reported for spasticity and spasm reduction.[28]

Bowel, Bladder, and Sexual Dysfunction

The majority of people with SCI lose total or partial voluntary control of bowel and bladder function. The nature of the bowel and bladder dysfunction will be determined by whether the injury is reflexic or areflexic, and whether it is complete or incomplete. People who lack volitional bladder control will require retraining or implementation of a compensatory voiding program. Methods of voiding urine include using an indwelling, condom, or suprapubic catheter; using intermittent catheterization; or performing a maneuver called *crede*, in which pressing on the bladder forces urine out. This is vital to long-term urinary and renal system integrity. People who lack volitional bowel function may experience incontinence and will require retraining of bowel function and elimination.[29,30] Constipation is very common post-SCI. Prescriptive medications may assist a bowel program. This population is 3 times as likely to have a *cholecystitis* (gallbladder inflammation).[7] Men with reflexive motor function are able to achieve a reflexive erection either spontaneously or by stimulation, but are unable to ejaculate. Most men with areflexic injuries are unable to have erections or ejaculate. Women's menstrual periods stop on average for 4.3 months post-injury and usually not longer than 6 months,[31] but after that time, normal cycles usually return. Women are able to become pregnant following an SCI. Premature infants are a known complication of childbearing in women with an SCI.[7]

Physiological Complications

Blood Pressure

After an SCI, there may be damage to the autonomic nervous system, which can have a variety of effects. Changes in BP are a common result of autonomic dysfunction, and can present in 2 ways: AD and/or orthostatic hypotension (OH).

Autonomic Dysreflexia (Hyperreflexia)

AD is a life-threatening complication that can occur with an SCI at T6 or above, most commonly found in a complete SCI. AD can vary in intensity, from mild discomfort to an emergency situation. It is caused by noxious stimuli leading to an uncontrolled generalized sympathetic response that causes widespread vasoconstriction and can result in a lethal rise in BP.[32] The increase is mostly due to shunting of blood away from the splanchnic vasculature, forcing it to enter the general circulation. The splanchnic nerves, found in the mid-thoracic region, innervate the vessels in the viscera, which is highly vascularized with a large blood supply.

Normally, patients with an SCI at T6 or above have a relatively low systolic BP of 90 to 110 mm Hg in the sitting position. Therefore, a sudden increase of 20 to 40 mm Hg in systolic and diastolic BP over baseline can indicate an AD event is occurring. Paradoxically, bradycardia is often associated with AD due to the parasympathetic nervous system attempting to control the sudden increase in BP. Bladder distention, bowel impaction, pressure sores, catheter irritation, LE hamstring stretching, tight clothing, a restrictive leg bag strap, or medical tests (eg, intravenous pyelogram or barium enema) are common noxious stimuli that can trigger this sympathetic response.[33,34] Signs and symptoms of AD include increased BP; pounding headache; sweating, flushing, or blotchiness of the skin above the level of injury; chills; and blurred vision (Box 11-1).

The following is an example of the normal sequence of events that occurs as the urinary bladder distends for individuals with an intact nervous system. As the bladder fills with urine, the stretch receptors in the bladder walls are activated and transmit impulses to the sacral portion of the spinal cord. As the bladder continues to fill and stretch, the impulses continue to ascend via sensory tracts and synapses in the sympathetic chain ganglia. The impulse continues to ascend to the brain, where the perception of a full bladder is sensed, and the person would likely urinate to inhibit further ascending impulses from the bladder. However, if the bladder is not emptied, there is a sympathetic nervous system response, which includes blood vessel constriction and increased BP. The baroreceptors in the carotid sinus sense this increased BP, and a message is sent to the vasomotor center in the brainstem via the glossopharyngeal nerve. The vasomotor center in turn sends a message down the cord to the sympathetic chain ganglia, triggering a decrease in the sympathetic vasoconstrictive response and ultimately reducing BP.

In individuals with an SCI, as the bladder distends, the sequence of events is similar, as the ascending messages are sent from the bladder up the spinal cord to the sympathetic chain ganglion. However, the individual with an SCI will not experience a normal sensation of a full bladder and cannot react appropriately to relieve the pressure in the bladder. In people with an SCI at T6 or above, the descending impulse sent from the vasomotor center in the brainstem is unable to travel normally down the cord. The message does not reach the sympathetic chain ganglia, and the BP remains high.[33]

During an episode of AD, arterial BP may reach extremely high levels, be prolonged, and cause a cerebrovascular accident and death.[33,35] Because acute elevations of BP represent an immediate threat to the patient's life, AD is considered a medical emergency.[35] The source of the irritation that caused AD must be identified and eliminated.[33-35] Immediate treatment measures by the physical therapist assistant would include monitoring the BP, loosening tight clothing or constrictive devices (eg, binder, stockings, or leg strap), getting the patient into the sitting position, making sure urine flow is unimpeded, and notifying the physical therapist, nurse, and physician. All facilities that treat people with SCIs should establish procedures for addressing this emergency and assign staff who can respond with the appropriate course of action.

The person with SCI must also recognize the importance of treating AD immediately, and must be able to instruct others on how to help. In some facilities, patients receive written instructions for what to do should AD occur at home. AD can sometimes be prevented by careful attention to bowel and bladder training, skin care, clothing, and catheters. If eliminating the precipitating cause is not sufficient to reduce BP, treatment with an antihypertensive drug will be required.[33-35]

Orthostatic Hypotension

OH is a drop in BP that often occurs as patients begin transitioning from the supine position (ie, assuming sitting or standing). The loss of the LE muscle pump and normal muscle tone below the level of the lesion can cause pooling of the blood in the legs and abdomen. Because of a decreased amount of blood and oxygen reaching the brain, a patient may become light-headed or even lose consciousness. An abdominal binder or corset and elastic stockings are used to substitute for lost muscle tone. OH usually resolves over time, although it may persist for 10 to 12 weeks or longer.[36,37] Therapists may often use a tilt table or recliner wheelchair (w/c) to try to acclimate patients to more upright positions, although evidence suggests the effectiveness of these interventions is limited. Medications are often effective in reducing the severity of OH.[36]

Concomitant Injuries Including Dual Diagnosis Spinal Cord Injury With Traumatic Brain Injury

Concomitant injuries may occur at the same time as the SCI. Specific to SCI, they include fractures of the extremities, injuries to the brachial plexus or abdomen, and brain injuries. Studies have found that brain injuries occur in 26% to more than 60% of cases. Increased risk for dual diagnosis of traumatic brain injury and SCI occurs when the mechanism of injury is a motor vehicle accident, higher level of injury, complete injuries, and trauma associated with alcohol.[38] Brain injuries may affect the person's ability to participate in rehabilitation because of deficits in learning abilities or cognitive and emotional deficits.

Heterotopic Ossification

Another complication is heterotopic ossification (HO), an abnormal overgrowth of bone in the joint space and around the joint, which occurs with an incidence of 10% to 20%.[7] Common signs and symptoms are decreased ROM, localized swelling, and pain. It most commonly affects the hips, knees, shoulders, and elbows, in order of prevalence.[7] The physical therapist assistant who works with the patient daily on functional activities and exercise may be the first person to note these changes. In people with an SCI, HO occurs most commonly between the first and fourth month after injury. Risk factors for developing HO include spasticity, age, pressure ulcers, and trauma to the joint.[7] Symptoms may develop, despite having no indication on radiographs, because HO may not be visible until the bone becomes mature. The mechanisms by which HO develops are not well understood, which makes treatment difficult, but treatment will usually include ROM activities, medication, and possibly surgical intervention. Nonsteroidal anti-inflammatory drugs have been shown to help reduce the likelihood of HO developing, and bisphosphonates have the most evidence for helping once HO has developed. Radiation therapy has also shown promise in preventing the development of HO.[39]

Box 11-1

Signs and Symptoms of Autonomic Dysreflexia

- Elevated systolic and diastolic BP
- Pounding headache
- Chills and goose bumps
- Nausea
- Sweating above the level of injury
- Flushing or blotchiness of the face, neck, and arms
- Restlessness or feelings of apprehension
- Bradycardia or tachycardia
- Blurred vision or spots in the visual field
- Nasal congestion
- Minimal or no symptoms other than elevated BP
- Cardiac arrhythmias

Adapted from Acute management of autonomic dysreflexia: adults with spinal cord injury presenting to health-care facilities. Consortium for spinal cord. *J Spinal Cord Med.* 1997;20(3):284-308. doi:10.1080/10790268.1997.11719480

Decreased Bone Mineral Density

Demineralization of bone, or *decreased bone mineral density*, occurs following complete SCI early after onset, and people with paraplegia and tetraplegia exhibit similar changes. Bone mineral density declines significantly during the first 3 months following the SCI and reaches a loss of about 37% by 16 months.[40] Decreases in motor activity and marked decrease in weight-bearing activities are the main contributing factors. Once bone mineral density has decreased 37%, the fracture index has been exceeded, and the person is at risk for fractures.[40] People with an SCI should be aware of this late-occurring risk, and the physical therapist assistant must exert caution when working with these people. Despite caution, fractures may occur during transfers or as the consequence of a fall, unusual movement, or LE-passive ROM, but can go unnoticed.[41]

Deep Vein Thrombosis

Deep vein thrombosis (DVT), a blood clot in a vein (usually of the leg), is associated with being inactive (physically, or lack of muscle contraction) or is due to prolonged bed rest. DVT is of medical concern because the clot could become dislodged, travel to the lungs, and cause a pulmonary embolus, which could be fatal. DVT is treated medically with anticoagulants or, if anticoagulants are contraindicated, with the surgical implantation of an inferior vena cava filter. In the United States it is estimated that 300,000 to 600,000 people will be affected by DVTs every year.[42] Most will occur in the LEs, however 4% to 10% will be in the UEs. Studies have found wide ranges of prevalence of DVTs in the SCI population, ranging from 14% to 100%.[43] Signs and symptoms of DVT include swelling in the extremity, pain or tenderness of the swollen area, increased warmth, and red or discolored skin around in the edematous area. Signs and symptoms of PE include unexplained shortness of breath, pain with deep breathing, and having a bloody cough. Blood tests and ultrasonography are typically used to rule out or confirm the presence of DVT, however there are also clinical models to help guide clinicians in identifying the probability that a DVT is present. The Simplified Clinical Model for Assessment of Deep Vein Thrombosis lists multiple clinical variables, which if present, raise the likelihood of DVT presence. Variables include:

- Active cancer (treatment ongoing or within previous 6 months, or palliative)
- Paralysis/paresis/immobilization of LEs
- Recently bedridden for more than 3 days or more, or a major surgery within previous 12 weeks requiring general or regional anesthesia
- Localized tenderness along distribution of deep venous system
- Entire leg swelling
- Calf swelling at least 3 cm larger than that on the asymptomatic leg (measured 10 cm below the tibial tuberosity)
- Pitting edema confided to the symptomatic leg
- Collateral superficial veins (nonvaricose)[44]

The more variables a patient has, the higher the probability of DVT, unless there is an alternative diagnosis that is as likely or more likely than DVT.[44] Patients with SCI, particularly acutely, will have a higher risk of DVT, the physical therapist assistant will want to consistently monitor the patient and communicate with the rest of the care team if concerns arise. Additionally, if a patient has a DVT and is on anticoagulants for treatment, physical therapist assistants should be aware of the increased risk for bruising and bleeding, and monitor patients accordingly including possibly adjusting treatments to reduce risk of injury.[44]

Another problem that occurs as a result of sympathetic nervous system dysfunction is impaired temperature regulation. The patient may complain about being cold and require warmer clothing. In the heat, however, the patient will be unable to sweat below the level of injury and can be at risk for heat stroke due to difficulty cooling the body. Problems associated with normal aging, such as musculoskeletal[45] and cardiovascular changes,[46] are magnified in people with an SCI; therefore, it is important as a clinician to monitor such situations. Patients with injuries above the T6 level are at greater risk for cardiovascular compromise.[47] Individuals with an SCI will also be at risk for burns given decreased sensation. Patients should be educated about preventing burns in common situations, such as monitoring water temperature while showering, covering exposed sink drainpipes which might contact a patients' legs, and avoiding the use of heated car seats.

Psychological Reaction to Loss

During the initial period following SCI, patients go through a series of adjustment phases of loss and grieving similar to those described by Kübler-Ross for people who are dying.[48] Patient responses to an SCI can vary greatly and may include anger, depression, withdrawal, denial, and having unrealistic expectations about recovery. Those working with the patient can provide better support by understanding this process and helping the patient move through these phases by gaining independence and continuing to modify goals as progress is achieved. Mean prevalence of depression in people after an SCI is 22.2% according to a 2015 review.[49] Depression can contribute to an increased incidence of rehospitalization, fewer functional gains, and a reduced life expectancy.[49] Having fewer positive relationships or less social support is likely to be a predictor of higher depression rates.[50]

Pain

Pain is a very common problem for individuals after an SCI, and can have negative influences on a person's function and ability to participate in life activities (eg, sleep, activities of daily living [ADL], community reintegration, and recreation). In particular, chronic pain is of significant concern and has been reported in up to 96% of cases.[51] Pain can be generated from a variety of sources, and can be described as either *nociceptive* or *neuropathic*. Nociceptive pain is generated by musculoskeletal and visceral sources. Neuropathic pain can occur above, at, or below the level of injury, and from sources including the spinal cord itself, compressive mononeuropathies, complex regional pain syndromes, or nerve root compression.

Research into pain following an SCI has been limited by lack of consistent pain classifications and the inability to identify the mechanisms involved with the development of this pain, particularly with neuropathic pain. The most common site of nociceptive pain in individuals after SCI is in the shoulders. Roughly 50% of adults with SCI will experience shoulder pain, which can last more than a year. Shoulder pain can severely impact performance of ADL and quality of life. Exercise can be beneficial for dealing with shoulder pain, and while it is important to tailor a program to an individual patient, most programs will include strengthening of the rotator cuff and scapular depressors, and maintaining ROM focusing on shoulder external rotation and scapular retraction and depression.[52] Additional treatment options for nociceptive pain include transcutaneous electrical nerve stimulation, which can be effective in reducing musculoskeletal pain.[53]

Neuropathic pain can be much harder to manage, in part because the mechanism of neuropathic pain is not known. There may be maladaptive neuroplasticity that occurs in the brain,[54] and cellular level changes in the neuron that cause and perpetuate neuropathic pain.[55] Given the poor understanding of the underlying mechanisms, treatments of neuropathic pain have not been very effective. A variety of both pharmacological and non-pharmacological treatments have shown promise at times. Pharmacological treatments include pregabalin, gabapentin, tramadol, tricyclic antidepressants, and serotonin-norepinephrine reuptake inhibitors. One review found that tricyclic antidepressants had the best efficacy for treating neuropathic pain.

Non-pharmacological interventions include transcranial direct current stimulation, transcutaneous electrical nerve stimulation, acupuncture, self-hypnosis, and cognitive behavioral training; however a review indicated that there was insufficient evidence to suggest that non-pharmacological treatments are effective in reducing chronic pain in people after an SCI.[56]

Pressure Ulcers

A *pressure ulcer*, also called a bedsore or pressure sore, is damage to the skin and underlying tissues caused by unrelieved pressure, shearing over bony prominences and trauma. Individuals with SCIs are at risk for development of pressure ulcers due to lack of protective sensation and limited mobility. Pressure ulcers are serious and can lead to serious complications such as prolonged hospitalization, bed rest, and amputation. They can become infected and pose a risk of death if not treated. Up to 80% of individuals with an SCI will have a pressure sore during their lifetime, and 30% will have more than one pressure sore. For individuals with an SCI, the prevention of pressure sores is an ongoing, lifelong process. It is estimated that 95% of pressure ulcers are preventable with proper education, equipment, and management.[57]

Common causes of pressure are prolonged sitting without shifting weight, lack of repositioning and padding while in bed, and clothing and shoes that fit too tightly. Shearing and trauma to the skin are commonly caused by poor technique with transfers, improper equipment or seating systems, and spasticity. Associated factors related to SCI that may increase a person's risk for acquiring pressure ulcers include loss of muscle mass, weight gain, decreased circulation, and moisture on the skin. It is important that individuals with SCI maintain a healthy weight, stay active, and manage their bowel and bladder function to limit their risk for skin breakdown.

Pressure ulcers are common over any bony prominence, but some locations are more vulnerable than others depending on the body position the person assumes. For example, the sacrum is at most risk when the person is in supine or sitting in bed with the head of the bed elevated, the ischial tuberosities are vulnerable in sitting, and the heels are most vulnerable in supine.[58] Individuals with an SCI should have a specialized pressure-relieving cushion in their w/c at all times to decrease pressure. The best method of screening for excess pressure in sitting is by palpation of the bony prominences with the physical therapist's or physical therapist assistant's hands. When areas of excess pressure are identified, the cushion or sitting position can be altered to minimize pressures. The physical therapist can perform pressure mapping with computerized pressure-sensing devices to provide additional information about sitting pressures. Pressure can be measured on adaptive equipment, such as mattresses or cushions, and the effectiveness of modified equipment or positions that relieve pressure can be compared. The physical therapist and physical therapist assistant can also use the resulting pressure map as an education tool.

The primary prevention strategy health care providers teach individuals with an SCI is regular performance of pressure relief. When sitting up, pressure relief should be performed every 15 to 20 minutes, and maintained for a duration of at-least 30 to 90 seconds.[57] Pressure relief can be performed in a chair with a "push-up" and lifting of the buttocks from the seat, leaning forward to unweight the sacrum, and leaning from side-to-side to unweight the ischial tuberosities (Figure 11-8). Tilt-in-space systems in power w/cs or specialized manual w/cs change the seat orientation to the ground to decrease pressure over vulnerable areas (Figure 11-9). A tilt angle of 25 to 65 degrees has been shown to provide pressure relief, but 15 degrees or less does not provide any benefit.[57,59] Tilting or reclining only the backrest of the chair does not provide pressure relief, and may actually increase pressure on the vulnerable areas.

Special equipment, such as a mattress, can help relieve pressure over bony prominences or redistribute pressures over larger and less bony areas. Just as in sitting, pressure relief is required in addition to any pressure redistribution provided by the mattress. Pressure relief is provided by turning the person in bed every 2 hours, using an air pressure-changing mattress, or having the person lie prone or semi-prone position. As a general rule, the person should be positioned so that no 2 skin surfaces rest against each other. In the prone or semi-prone position, pillows are

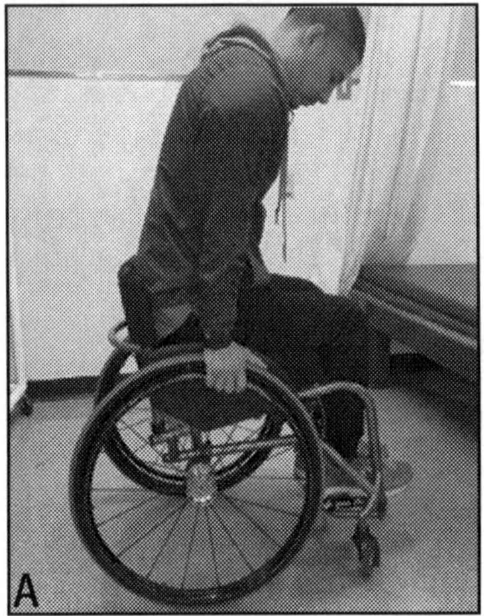

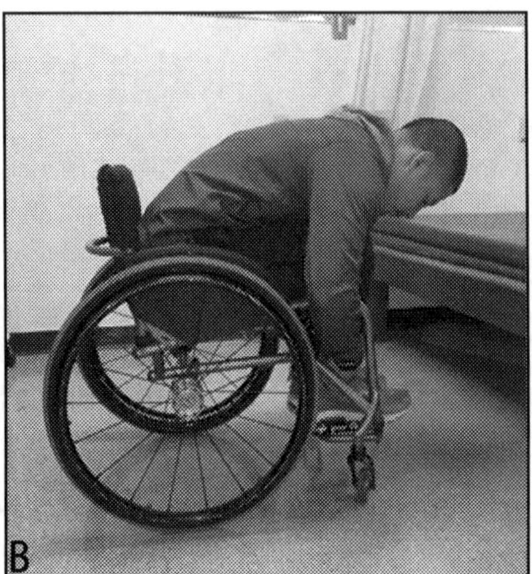

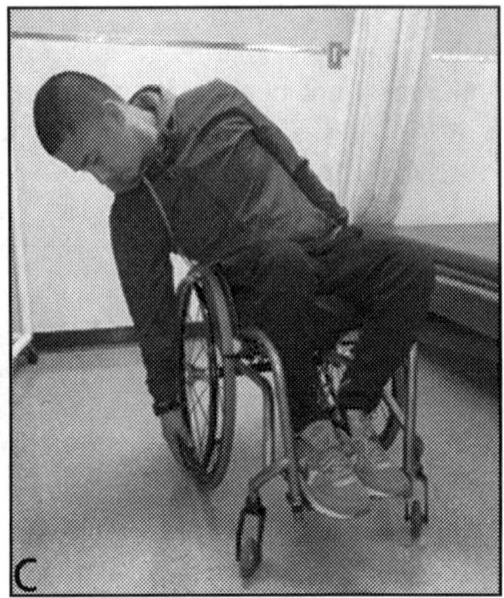

Figure 11-8. Patient with paraplegia performing different types of pressure relief. (A) "Push-up" pressure relief, (B) forward lean, (C) side lean.

used to bridge bony areas, including the pelvis and knees. People who are able to lie in 1 of these positions can sleep for longer periods without turning, because pressure on prominent bony areas is minimized. The person is able to rest better, and the amount of nursing or attendant care required is decreased.

If skin problems do occur, early detection and treatment are essential. Individuals with an SCI should be taught to inspect their skin at least twice/day using a long-handled mirror for hard-to-see areas. Areas to inspect vary depending on type and level of injury, but may include the sacrum and lower back, coccyx, heels of the feet, ischial tuberosities, greater trochanters, elbows, knees, toes, and back of the head. The goal of skin inspection is early detection of changes in skin color, bruises, or cracked, dry skin. The skin should also be felt for hardness, swelling, and warmth that may signal breakdown. If a person wears braces or orthotics, the areas in contact with the braces should be checked every 2 hours.

One of the first signs of a pressure ulcer is red, discolored skin. The skin should be tested with the "blanching test." Press on the discolored area lightly with your finger; the area should go white. Remove the pressure, and the area should return to red or darkened color within 5 seconds. If the skin does not blanch and stays red when you press on it, or the redness persists at least 10 minutes after the pressure is relieved, then this is considered a stage I pressure ulcer. A stage I pressure ulcer may take up to a week to heal. During this time, the person should stay off the area and remove all pressure, keep the skin clean and dry, and inspect the area at least 3 times/day. Often times what is seen on the surface is the smallest part of the pressure ulcer, so all pressure ulcers, regardless of how small, should be regarded as serious.

If the top layer of skin is broken, but the wound does not extend through the second layer of skin, this is considered a stage II pressure ulcer. There may or may not be drainage present with a stage II ulcer. The person should get medical attention right away, as the damage could easily progress deeper into the underlying tissues. There is also a high risk for infection due to the loss of skin integrity, so it is important to keep the area clean and dry. Depending on severity, a stage II pressure sore commonly takes 1 to 3 weeks to heal. During this time, bed rest or severely limited seating time is recommended.[18,57]

If a pressure ulcer progresses to a stage III or stage IV, which involves the tissues or bone below the skin, special wound care and long hospital stays are often required for healing. In these cases, strict bed rest is recommended with a specialized mattress and cushion for a prolonged amount of time. These wounds are very serious and often take at least 3 months to a year for full healing.[57] Many stage III or stage IV pressure ulcers will not heal without surgical intervention (Table 11-2).[60]

Rehabilitation and Recovery After a Spinal Cord Injury

Prognosticating Recovery

The most accurate method used to predict recovery from an SCI is the standardized examination performed by the physician early after injury using the International Standards for Neurological Classification of Spinal Cord Injury. This examination makes it possible for clinicians to classify the degree of impairment and assist in creating a comprehensive plan of care for all disciplines. The Model Spinal Cord Injury Systems database captures the information Model SCI centers gather using the international neurological standards.[61]

Knowledge about the prognosis for neurological recovery following an SCI allows the physician to counsel patients about the time during which recovery occurs and probable functional outcome. Studies have shown that neurological recovery is not related to sex, race, type of fracture, mechanism of injury, or timing or type of surgical procedures.[62] Rather, the most important prognostic variable is completeness of injury. Improved outcomes are seen in younger patients and those with a central cord or BSS; both are incomplete injuries.[36,63] Research completed at the time of this publication has shown that high-dose steroids, usually methylprednisolone, significantly improved neurological outcomes for traumatic SCIs when administered within 8 hours of injury and infused for a period of 23 to 48 hours.[64] Research for the efficacy of using high-dose steroid infusion for older children (8 to 16 years of age) is still under review.[65] Researchers have also shown that methylprednisolone may increase the prevalence of myopathy after high-dose infusion.[66] Motor recovery is the principal determinant of a patient's functional capabilities, and the primary determinant of motor recovery is completeness of injury at 1 month. Most motor recovery occurs within the first 6 months, and only 2% of people experience a late conversion from a complete to an incomplete injury, although many may change ASIA classifications within 30 days of injury and have an improved functional prognosis.[61] Key muscles that are innervated at 1 month following injury usually recover to a grade of 3/5 or greater, while those that are graded at zero are unlikely to recover to a functional level of 3/5.[67,68] Patients with complete injuries are unlikely to walk at a community level,[68] although they may walk with orthoses for exercise. In contrast, 76% of patients with incomplete paraplegia and 46% of those with incomplete tetraplegia are likely to be community ambulators.[68]

Prevent Deformity and Maintain and Protect Joint Range of Motion

Positioning, passive ROM exercises, and the use of orthoses or splints can prevent loss of joint motion. This is especially important when the person is unable to move extremities or when an imbalance between agonist and antagonistic muscles occurs because of the level of injury or hypertonic muscles. For example, an individual with C5 tetraplegia will often rest the elbows in a flexed position because the elbow flexors are innervated but the elbow extensors are not. People with tetraplegia who lack triceps function need full elbow extension and wrist extension, as well as shoulder external rotation, to lock the elbows for functional activities (eg, transfers and sitting balance). Splints can help hold elbows in extension when the person is not using the arms for functional activities, helping avoid elbow flexion contractures. Elbow flexion contractures for individuals with an SCI can be extremely limiting for mobility and ADL, especially for individuals without triceps strength. In people with cervical injuries, the shoulders are particularly vulnerable to developing limited ROM and associated pain. Close attention to maintaining ROM, especially abduction and external rotation of the shoulder, and interventions to reduce pain, such as heat, cold, or

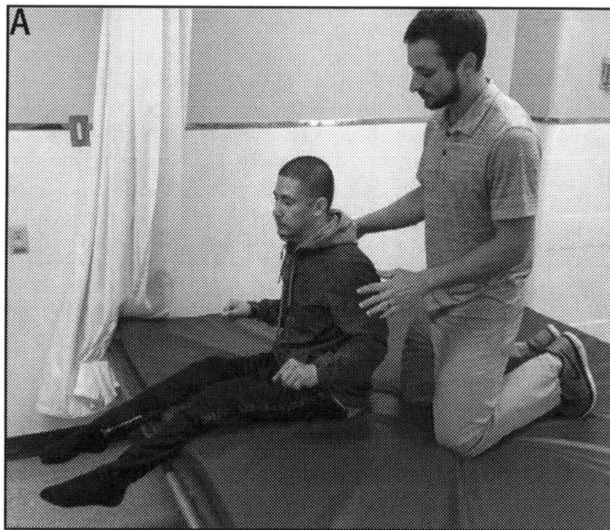

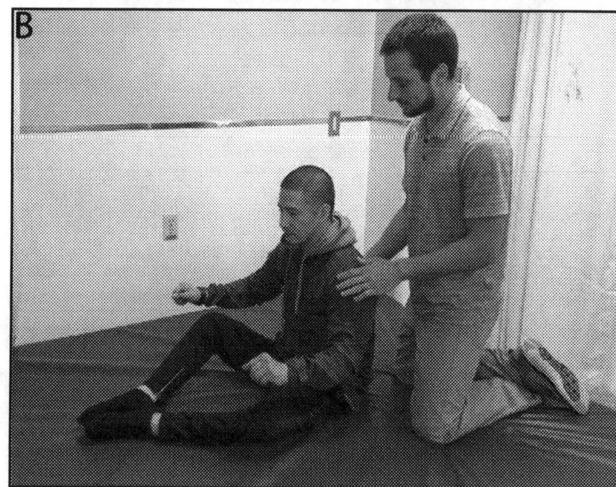

Figure 11-9. If patients have limited hamstring length that makes balancing in long sitting difficult, the physical therapist assistant can modify sitting setup to allow for the patient to maintain balance including (A) placing feet off edge of mat, and (B) using circle (or ring) sitting position.

transcutaneous electrical nerve stimulation, are important to prevent a disabling pain cycle.

All joints should be kept mobile; however, some joints need to be protected from overstretching. Clinicians need to avoid inadvertently overstretching the back extensor muscles; this can occur when the person with tight hamstring muscles leans forward with the knees straight in the long sitting position (Figure 11-10). If the trunk muscles and ligaments are overstretched, the trunk will tend to elongate during transfers, making it more difficult to clear the buttocks. For patients with high cervical injuries, rolling will also be more difficult with an overstretched trunk because the upper trunk will roll without the lower trunk following.

Even individuals with complete tetraplegia, who are not expected to ambulate, must maintain adequate ROM of hips, knees, and ankles. For example, if the hip and knee flexors are tight, there is an increased chance of skin break-

Table 11-2

Classification of Pressure Sores

Stage I	Nonblanchable erythema of intact skin (USPHS). In persons with dark skin, discoloration of the skin, warmth, edema, induration, or hardness may also be indicators.
Stage II	Partial-thickness skin loss involving the dermis, epidermis, or both.
Stage III	Full-thickness skin loss involving damage to or necrosis of subcutaneous tissue that may extend down to, but not through, underlying fascia. The ulcer is a deep crater, with or without undermining adjacent tissue.
Stage IV	Full-thickness skin loss with extensive destruction, tissue necrosis, or damage to muscle, bone, or supporting structures such as tendon or joint capsule.
****Unstageable***	Sore is covered with eschar so that one is unable to determine the condition of the tissue below.

*Used at Rancho Los Amigos National Rehabilitation Center, Downey, CA.

Adapted from Treatment of Pressure Ulcers. *Clinical Practice Guideline #15.* (AHCPR Publication #95-0652) Rockville, MD: US Department of Health and Human Services; 1994.

Note: It is not appropriate to reverse-stage a healing ulcer (eg, stage III will NOT become a stage II). The damaged tissue is not replaced by the same type; it is replaced by granulation tissue. Document the wound improvements by its characteristics (eg, size, depth, amount of necrotic tissue, amount of exudate).

down in the heels and the sacral/coccygeal region when the patient is lying supine. The hip and/or knee flexion contractures will not allow the weight to be distributed through the surface area of the thighs and legs, thereby increasing the pressure on the bony prominences of the pelvis and feet. Patients are encouraged to lie prone to lengthen hip flexors and knee flexors and improve trunk extension. Lying prone for extended periods will also allow improved blood flow to the buttocks and areas that are frequently compromised because of prolonged periods of sitting. Also, ankle plantar flexion contractures can make it difficult for the feet to stay on the w/c footrests and also decrease the stability of the foot/ankle (base of support) during transfers.

People with a complete SCI who will be performing ADL in long sitting (eg, dressing, scooting, recreating, and exercising) need 100 to 110 degrees of hamstring range, as determined by flexing the hip with the knee straight (*straight leg raise* [SLR]). By maintaining approximately 110 degrees of SLR, an individual can rely on the passive insufficiency of the muscles to provide stability in long sitting for ADL. Stretching the hamstrings is most effective when performed for long durations one LE at a time, with the pelvis stabilized as much as possible in the supine position (see Figure 11-10). Initially, physical therapy personnel will need to provide passive LE ROM. People with adequate UE function can learn to perform their own passive LE ROM, typically with the assistance of a strap.

For patients who have wrist extension (C6 innervation) but do not have innervation to the finger flexors (SCI above C8 level), the long finger flexors and the flexor pollicis longus are allowed to become functionally shortened. This allows the patient to flex the fingers and oppose the thumb to the index finger when the wrist is extended. This is called functional wrist tenodesis. Physical therapist assistants play an active role in providing interventions to prevent deformity and increase or maintain ROM, and incorporating tenodesis into functional training, for example, keeping fingers flexed when weight-bearing through the arms during sitting balance training. They may also be involved in teaching the individual and family members how to perform stretching and ROM.

Increasing Strength

Muscles that are innervated below the level of injury will lose function or demonstrate weakness. Bed rest is common after an SCI and is associated with diminished muscle function and endurance. Muscles with remaining function must be strengthened by progressive resistive exercise to provide the maximum strength possible for performing functional activities (Figures 11-11 and 11-12). In people with a complete SCI, the UE muscles must substitute for those lost in the LEs for transfers and w/c propulsion. Specific muscles most vulnerable to fatigue during w/c propulsion are the pectoralis major, supraspinatus, middle and posterior deltoid, subscapularis, and middle trapezius.[69] People with tetraplegia are at greater risk of shoulder pathology because their UE muscles are weaker than those of able-bodied people and people with paraplegia,[70] and activities such as grooming will require different patterns of muscular activity than those used by able-bodied people.[71] People with incomplete injuries also require strengthening of LE muscles. The physical therapist assistant will need to perform periodic manual muscle tests of specific muscles to modify the patient's exercise program and determine when advancing the functional program is warranted.

Develop Endurance

Endurance training is aimed at improving muscular performance and aerobic capacity to improve the efficiency of mobility and improve overall health. Disproportionately high rates of cardiovascular disease and hypertension occur in people with an SCI, compared with able-bodied individuals.[46] Some people have difficulty maintaining an ideal body weight because of their limited ability to exercise, which may cause functional decline. Endurance can be achieved by weight training with low weights and a high number of repetitions, use of a UE ergometer or similar device, and w/c propulsion, all of which are interventions appropriate for the role of the physical therapist assistant.

Promote Respiratory Health

People with thoracic-level injuries initially demonstrate lower respiratory measurements than able-bodied people. Respiratory function returns to able-bodied levels when they undergo UE muscle training.[72] The respiratory program for people with cervical-level injuries focuses on interventions for developing strength and endurance in the respiratory muscles; maintaining rib cage mobility; and learning assisted cough, bronchial hygiene, and postural drainage for home use. People who are ventilator-dependent can learn specialized voluntary breathing techniques, such as neck breathing[73] or glossopharyngeal breathing.[74]

High compliance with a structured inspiratory training program using diaphragm weights (Figure 11-13) or an inspiratory muscle trainer 15 to 30 minutes/day, 5 to 7 days/week for 6 to 8 weeks, has been shown to result in increased VC, inspiratory capacity, and maximal expiratory pressure.[75,76] Lerman and Weiss describe respiratory exercises that can be incorporated into a respiratory program, including breath-holding, taking triple breaths for rib cage expansion, and neck exercises.[76] Exercises can be made more difficult by increasing resistance, increasing the time that the exercise is performed, and changing the patient's position. Weekly VC monitoring is used to assess patients' progress and modify the respiratory program, as needed. VC is greater in people with cervical injuries in supine[14] and in people with lower injuries in sitting. Using a consistent position allows for more accurate assessment of respiratory function. A corset or abdominal binder can assist with respiration when the patient is sitting, as it helps substitute for the abdominal muscles and improve the lung volume. People with C6 injuries require long-term follow-up.[77] Physical therapist assistants working in rehabilitation settings serving patients with SCIs may be actively involved in providing all these interventions, including testing VC.

Functional Training

The person with a complete SCI or residual impairments from an incomplete SCI may need to perform functional activities in a modified manner. The extent of independence achieved and the way in which these activities are performed will depend on the level and completeness of injury. Functional activities include bed mobility and transfers; sitting pressure relief; eating; grooming; dressing; bathing; ensuring good hygiene; ensuring adequate bowel and bladder function; driving, walking, and moving around in the community; preparing meals; and managing the home. See Table 11-3 for a summary of select activities for given levels of SCI, and refer to the Consortium for Spinal Cord Medicine publication, *Outcomes Following Traumatic Spinal Cord Injury: Clinical Practice Guidelines for Health-Care Professionals*, for more detail on expected outcomes.[78] Patients with injuries above C8 can use a tenodesis grip to manipulate objects. Tenodesis is the passive closing of the fingers and opposition of the thumb to the index finger when the wrist is actively extended. When practicing mat activities, like propped sitting, care must be taken to maintain finger flexion for a tenodesis grip; overstretching of the long finger flexors can severely impair hand function for these patients. Patients who have manual muscle grade of 3/5 (fair) in their biceps but lack shoulder strength may be fitted with mobile arm supports (Figure 11-14). This device attaches to the w/c to help support the shoulder while the patient bends his or her elbow for activities such as eating and combing hair.

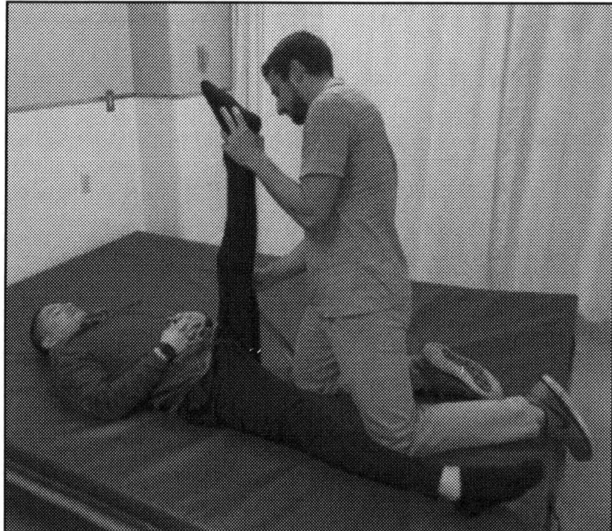

Figure 11-10. Performing straight leg stretch for increasing hamstring muscle length.

Physical therapist assistants play a key role in providing functional training interventions and assessing the current level of assistance required by the patient with an SCI.

Head-Hips Relationship

When teaching new functional mobility skills, it is important to teach the patient the concepts of head-hips relationship, levers, unweighting extremities, and the use of momentum. The concept of head-hips relationship becomes very important in bed mobility and functional transfers. As the patient moves the head in one direction, the hips move in the opposite direction. For example, if the patient is in short-sitting with arms on the mat in elbow extension and moves the head down toward the feet, the hips will lift up; if while lifting the buttocks off the mat with the UEs, the head is turned to the left, the hips will then move to the right.

Mobility Skills

Depending on the level of injury and the amount of neurological injury, a person with an SCI may need to use specific skills to increase independence with mobility. The

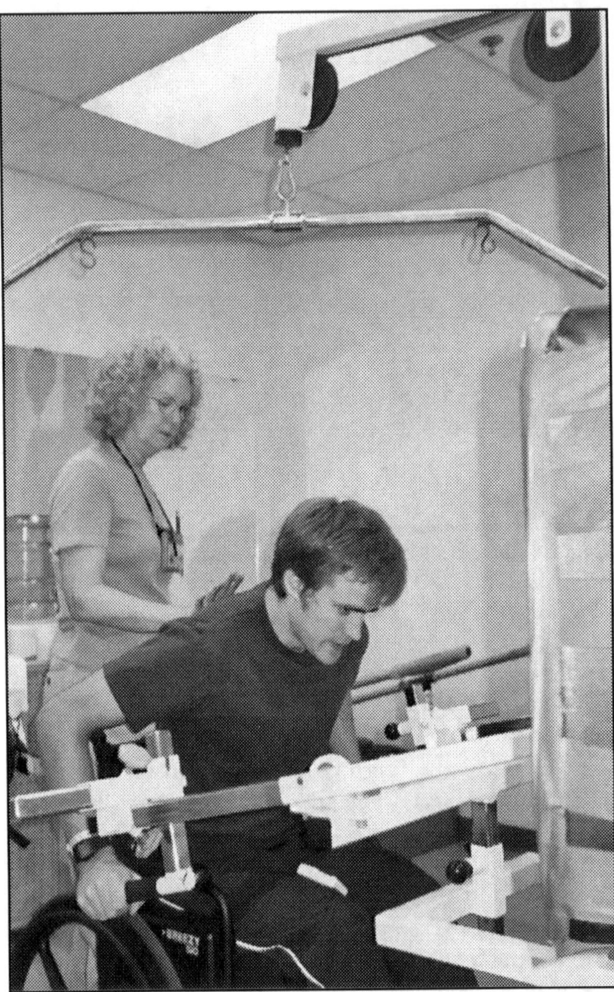

Figure 11-11. The physical therapist assistant helps the patient maintain a forward trunk position while performing UE strengthening exercises. The patient is performing reverse dips to strengthen the elbow extensors and scapular depressors.

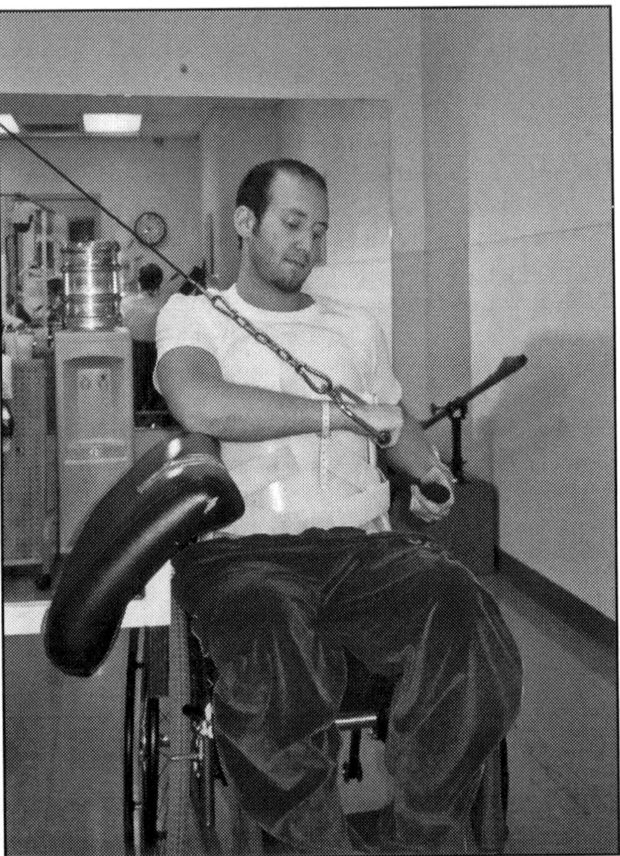

Figure 11-12. Patient performing UE internal rotation exercise with weights. The patient lacks lower trunk musculature and uses his left arm to help stabilize his body while performing the exercise.

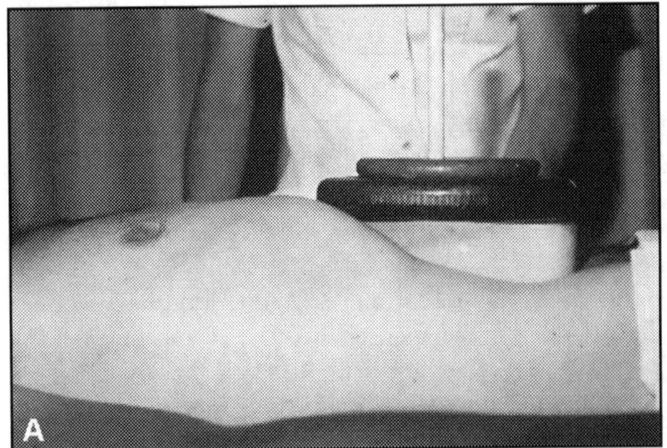

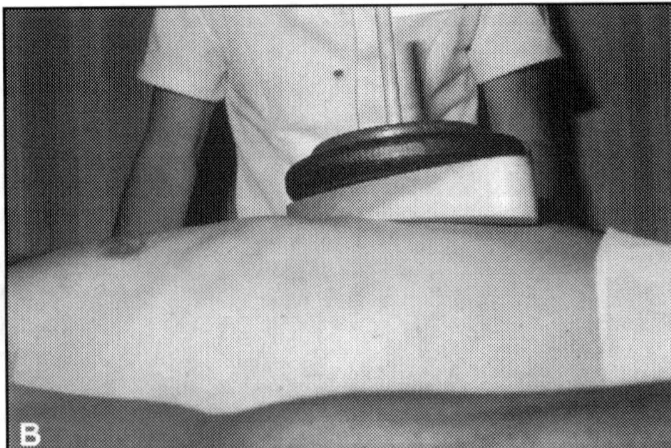

Figure 11-13. Inspiratory training using diaphragm weights. The triangular weight part is designed to fit in the area below the xiphoid process. Note position of the diaphragm (A) before the patient takes a breath, and (B) after. The patient's head is on the left.

main areas of focus during a standard rehab program will include bed mobility, transfers, w/c mobility skills, and possibly gait training.

Bed Mobility

Bed mobility consists of rolling, scooting, moving up and down in bed, doing balance activities, coming to sitting (Figure 11-15), long and short sitting (Figure 11-16) balance, LE management, and self-ROM. Speed of movement and momentum are especially important for patients with tetraplegia.

Bed and Wheelchair Transfers

Transfers allow the person to move from place to place, including to or from a lower or higher surface. For the person with high tetraplegia, a dependent transfer or use of a mechanical lift will be required. A transfer (sliding) board can assist people who have UE weakness or are unstable during movement, whereas people with greater UE strength and better body awareness can often complete level transfers without equipment. The preferred transfer technique for level and uneven transfers is accomplished when the person straightens the elbows, depresses the shoulders, lifts the buttocks off the supporting surface, uses the head-hips relationship, turns, and moves onto a nearby surface (Figures 11-17 and 11-18). Transfers to all surfaces are practiced, including to a mat or the floor, a bed, a toilet, a w/c, a bathtub, a car, the ground, and other sitting surfaces. Teaching patients to transfer can be difficult for clinicians and patients. For both inexperienced and experienced clinicians, collaboration with their colleagues to problem-solve challenging situations will help develop skill and excellence. For patients, transfers are a completely novel movement, and can take substantial practice to master. Initially, most patients fail to lean far enough forward or move their shoulders and head enough to transfer efficiently, possibly due to a fear of falling forward and poor sense of balance. Details on how to perform functional activities for people at varying levels of injury can be found in the book *Spinal Cord Injury: Functional Rehabilitation*, by Somers.[79]

Floor Transfers

There are 3 main approaches to performing floor transfers: side approach, front approach, and back approach. Each of these techniques requires different degrees of strength, ROM, and skill. The side approach is the most common for people with higher levels of injury, as it requires less pectoral and triceps strength, but does require substantial shoulder extension, shoulder abduction, hip flexion, and knee flexion. The side approach uses an exaggerated head-hips movement to lift the hips from the floor onto the higher surface (Figure 11-19). Front-approach transfers need significant pectoralis major, triceps, and serratus anterior strength as the patient pushes up with the hands on the w/c seat (Figure 11-20). During the back approach, patients place the back against the front of the chair and place their hands on the front of the seat before pushing up to the w/c seat. Shoulder extension and internal rotation ROM are key for this technique, which is the least common approach.

Wheelchair Mobility Training

W/C mobility training involves learning to maneuver in tight spaces: over uneven terrain, like gravel or grass; over a threshold; up and down ramps; through doors; and backward, forward, and to the sides. A person using a manual w/c who has sufficient UE motor control may learn more advanced w/c skills, such as how to navigate curbs and go up and down stairs. The position of the wheel axle in relation to the patient's hips, the angle of the seat (anterior to posterior), the amount the wheels flare out (camber), and the patient's position in the w/c are important in maximizing the efficiency of propulsion.

A person in a manual w/c learns to perform a wheelie, balancing on the large wheels while tilted backward. Patients can practice this while attached to an overhead safety cord or being spotted by the clinician, usually using a gait belt attached to a sturdy part of the w/c frame (Figure 11-21). Helping the patient find the balance point while in a wheelie is critical in mastering this skill.

The surface the person pushes on affects velocity, with tile being easier than carpet. In a manual w/c, a person with a higher injury level may push at a slower speed and will likely travel shorter distances than a person with a lower level injury. People with C6 tetraplegia are so limited by UE weakness that they are unable to navigate a 4% grade, and no method of manual propulsion is efficient.[80] Clinicians will need to determine whether a patient is able to be successful with use of a manual w/c vs power or power-assist. Considerations of fatigue, lifestyle, and joint protection, among other factors, will go into determining what type of w/c is most appropriate. Individuals with Assistive Technology Professional (ATP) certification and/or Seating and Mobility Specialist (SMS) certification are experts in w/c assessment and fit, and can be consulted.

Gait Training

Gait training is an important part of functional training for people who have sufficient motor recovery in their LEs, particularly those with incomplete injuries. People with SCIs who ambulate may require LE orthoses to substitute for weak muscles.[67] An ankle-foot orthosis (AFO) can substitute for weak dorsiflexor muscles to prevent foot drop in swing and loading response. An AFO can also substitute for weak plantar flexor muscles by preventing unrestrained dorsiflexion in stance (Figure 11-22). A knee-ankle-foot orthosis (KAFO) is used to substitute for weak quadriceps muscles (Figure 11-23).

An erroneous, yet commonly held, belief of many clinicians is that use of an LE orthosis will prevent a muscle from contracting and, therefore, impede return of strength. This concept has not been supported in research of calf muscle function in people with an SCI,[81] so an AFO should

Table 11-3
Select Functional Outcomes for Persons With Complete Spinal Cord Injury

SCI Level	Muscles Present	Transfer	Functional Capabilities	Equipment
C1 to C3	Scalenes, partial SCM, upper trapezius	Mechanical lift; dependent	• Mouth-stick activities • Electronic aids to daily living • Able to instruct, but dependent with all aspects of self-care • Ventilator full-time for respiratory function	• Power w/c with sip and puff, chin control, or head array with tilt-in-space capability and vent tray (Figure 10-26A-B) • Specialty pressure-reducing mattress
C4	Partial diaphragm, SCM, upper, middle, and lower trapezius	Mechanical lift; dependent	• Mouth-stick activities • Electronic aids to daily living • Able to instruct, but dependent with all aspects of self-care • Ventilator initially, but may be able to wean	• Power w/c with sip and puff, chin control, or head array with tilt-in-space capability and vent tray • Specialty pressure-reducing mattress
C5	Full diaphragm, partial deltoids, biceps, brachialis, brachioradialis, rhomboids, partial serratus, partial pec major	Mechanical lift; possibly slide-board transfers with assist	• UE dressing with assist, LE dressing dependent • Mod/maxA for bathing • Dependent toileting • Mod independent power w/c mobility	• Power w/c with tilt–in-space capability and hand control • Mobile arm support • Wrist supports with U-cuff • Specialty pressure-reducing mattress
C6	Radial wrist extensors, partial pec major, serratus anterior, partial latissimus dorsi	Slide-board transfers from mod independent to maxA	• Mod independent feeding, grooming and UE dressing • Mod/maxA LE dressing • Min/modA bathing • Mod independent to dependent with bowel and bladder program • Mod independent power or manual w/c mobility	• Power w/c with tilt-in-space capability and hand control, or manual ultralight w/c with specialized rims or power-assist • U-cuff • Padded bathroom equipment • Specialty pressure-reducing mattress

(continued)

Table 11-3 (continued)
Select Functional Outcomes for Persons With Complete Spinal Cord Injury

SCI Level	*Muscles Present*	*Transfer*	*Functional Capabilities*	*Equipment*
C7-C8	Full latissimus dorsi, triceps, full wrist extensors, radial wrist flexors, finger flexors/extensors. thumb flexion, extension, abduction	Modified independent transfers with or without slideboard	• Modified independent LE dressing • Min to modified independent for bathing and toileting • Modified independent for writing and electronics • Independent driving with hand controls	• Manual ultralight w/c with pressure-reducing cushion • Padded bathroom equipment with hand-held shower • Hand controls for driving
T1-T9	Intrinsics of the hands, upper interconstals, erector spinae	Modified independent transfers without slideboard	• Modified independent with all ADLs including bathing, toileting, bowel and bladder management, skin care and driving	• Same as C7-C8
T10-L1	Fully intact intercostals, external obliques, rectus abdominus	Modified independent transfers	• Modified independent with all ADLs • Possible short distance ambulation with RGO or KAFOs	• Manual ultralight w/c • Padded bathroom equipment • RGO or KAFO with crutches or walker • Hand controls
L2	Illiopsoas, quadratus lumborum, hip flexors	Modified independent transfers	• Longer distance ambulation with RGO or KAFOs and AD, but primarily for exercise only	• Same as T10-L1
L3	Quadriceps	Possibly stand pivot transfers with AD	• Modified independent ambulation at functional level with AFOs and crutches or walker	• Typically still require ultralight w/c use for longer distances
L4-L5	Tibialis anterior, extensor hallucis longus, knee flexors, hip abductors	Standing or ambulation transfers with or without AD	• Ambulation with AFOs, may or may not require an AD	• Durable medical equipment focused on ambulation, but may require w/c use for longer distances
S1	Gastrocnemius, soleus, hip extensors	Ambulating transfers	• Ambulation with no orthoses or AD	• No w/c required • May require AD for longer distances or community ambulation

Abbreviations: AFO = ankle-foot orthosis; KAFO = knee ankle foot orthosis; maxA = maximum assistance; minA = minimum assistance; modA = moderate assistance; RGO = reciprocating gait orthosis; SCM = sternocleidomastoid muscle.

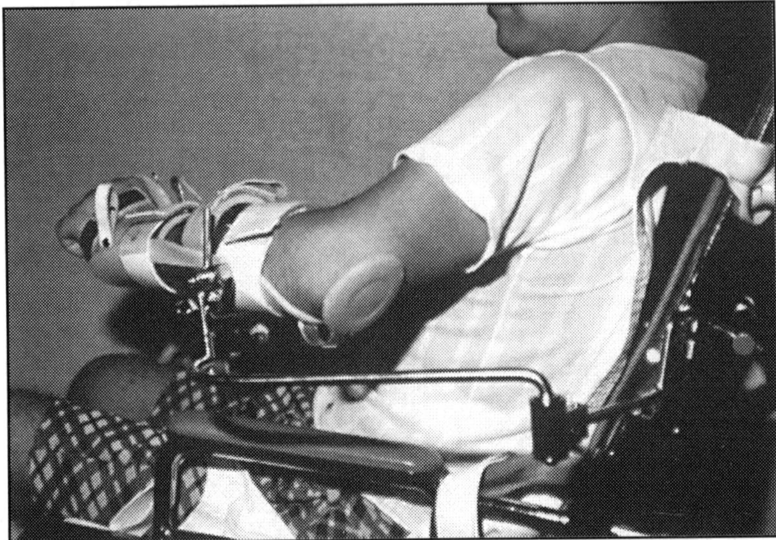

Figure 11-14. Mobile arm support attaches to the back post of the w/c to assist with shoulder flexion and abduction. Functional arm use can be achieved with the patient with weak elbow and shoulder muscles.

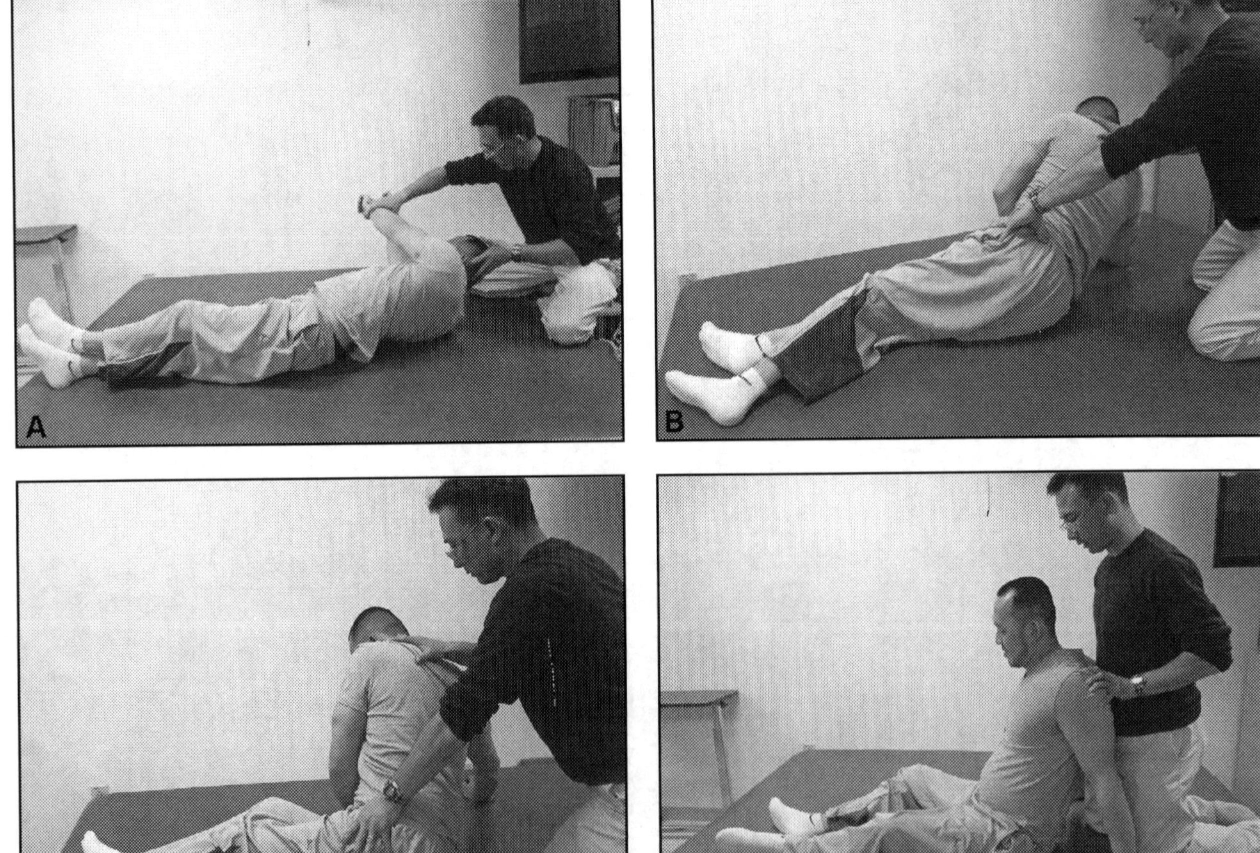

Figure 11-15. Bed-mobility activities with a patient with T7 ASIA A SCI. (A) Coming to sit on the mat. The patient rolls to his side and the physical therapist assistant helps him initiate the sitting movement. (B) The patient moves his arm up on the mat in preparation for pushing to sitting. (C) The patient continues to move his arms around in front of him until he is sitting upright. (D) The patient continues to move his arms around until he is in the long sitting position. With practice, he will be able to do this independently.

be used when it improves patient function during gait or transfers. More extensive orthoses, such as a hip-knee-ankle-foot orthosis, are usually too cumbersome, although a reciprocating gait orthosis (RGO), which controls the hip, may be used to provide assistance in advancing the leg and, therefore, may be used by people with low cervical or thoracic injuries.

Body weight–support devices, provided by an overhead unweighting system, combined with walking on a treadmill or overground, can facilitate ambulation in people with incomplete SCIs (Figure 11-24). Therapists and support staff, or mechanical devices, assist the patient in moving the legs in a normal gait pattern, and speeds approaching those of normal walking are attained. No evidence exists that this intervention has carryover to walking overground in people with complete injuries, but it can also assist in maintaining patient and staff safety from falls.

Although people with complete lesions are usually unable to rely on walking as their primary mode of mobility, they may use it as a form of exercise. The high energy cost of lifting the body with the arms, the slow velocity at which people in KAFOs or RGOs travel, and the demand on the shoulder musculature make this type of walking impractical. Another method of exercise ambulation uses electrical stimulation to activate the LE muscles. The energy cost/meter traveled is similar for walking with KAFOs, RGOs, and electrical stimulation aides.[82]

ROM limitations, such as hip flexion, knee flexion, or ankle plantar flexion contractures, will interfere with the person's ability to walk. Contractures are very difficult to manage. Stretching is a common intervention used to manage contractures; however, a Cochrane review found high-quality evidence to suggest that stretching does not have a clinically important effect, either short- or long-term, on contractures in people with or without neurologic conditions.[83] Additional studies need to be done to determine the effectiveness of splinting and positioning, but those interventions can be used to try to maintain ROM. Standing may be a beneficial position for maintaining ankle dorsiflexion, knee extension, and hip extension ROM. For individuals not strong enough to stand, standing frames or tilt tables may promote weight-bearing while providing additional support. Patients can also be educated on prone positioning to promote hip and knee extension ROM. Serial casting is another intervention used for plantar flexion contractures. Anti-spasticity medications taken orally, delivered via injection, or administered through an implanted pump may assist in managing abnormal muscle tone that can interfere with normal movement patterns.

Robotics, particularly wearable exoskeletons, are becoming more available and used in the clinic. Some are programmable for use with body weight–supported treadmill gait training, and some are programmable, mobile, and battery-operated.[84,85] Promising studies have shown that use of robotics may improve body composition,[86] walking independence, and endurance[87]; however, evidence

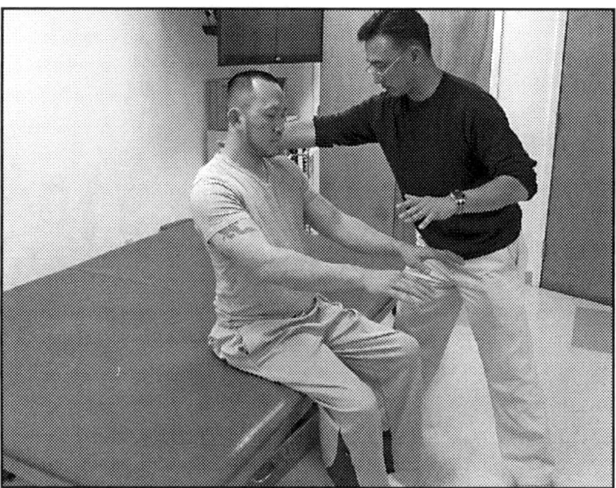

Figure 11-16. Patient with T7 ASIA A SCI in short sitting, practicing balance activities with the physical therapist assistant.

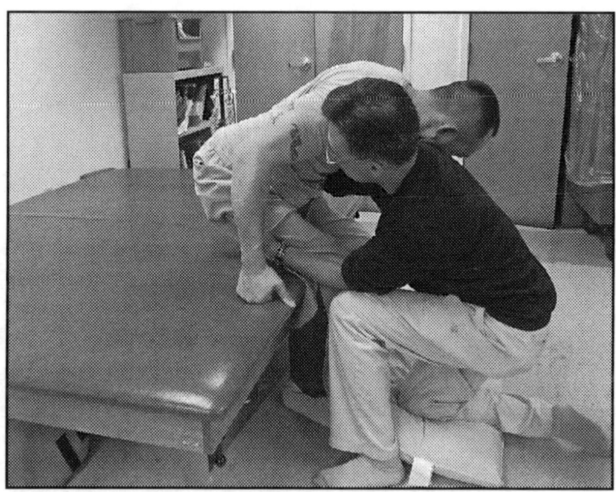

Figure 11-17. The physical therapist assistant assists a patient with T7 ASIA A SCI in practicing a depression lift on the mat. Practicing this skill will make transfers easier to perform.

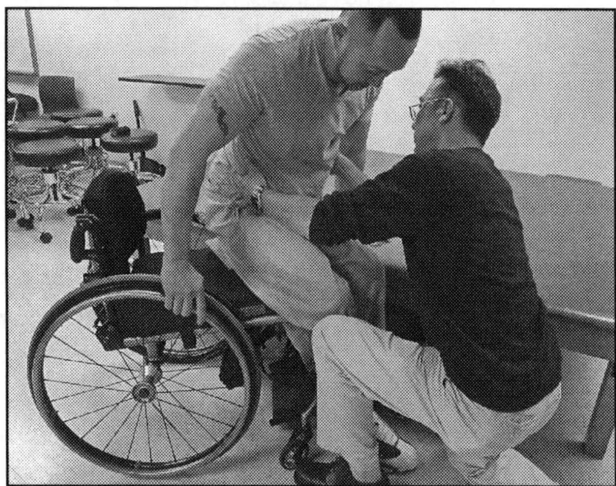

Figure 11-18. The physical therapist assistant assists a patient with T7 ASIA A SCI with depression transfer to the w/c. Note how the patient turns his head to the right as he lifts his body to facilitate movement of his buttocks to the left onto the w/c (head-hips relationship).

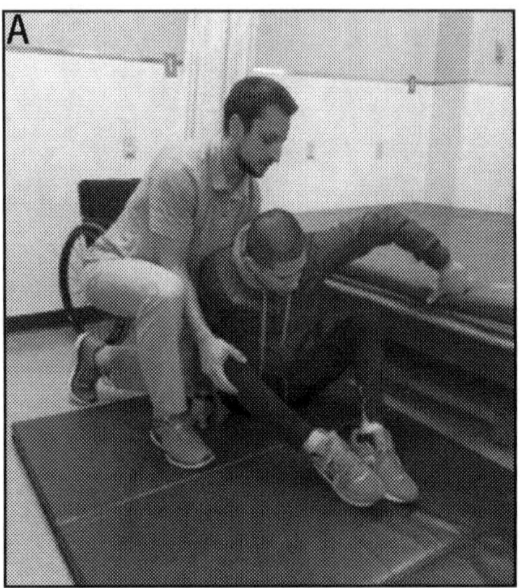

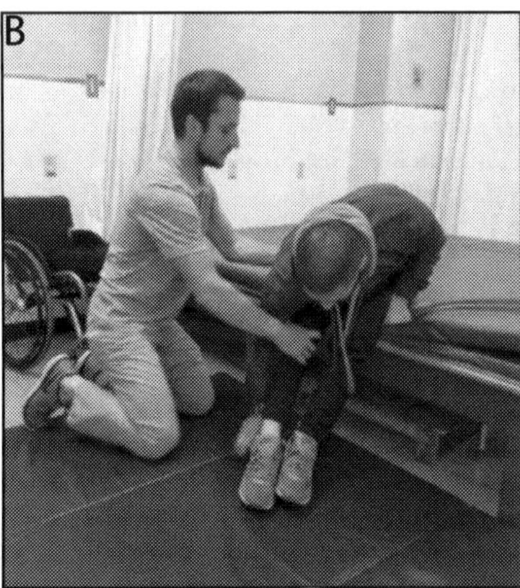

Figure 11-19. A patient using the side approach to complete floor recovery. (A) The physical therapist assistant assists the patient with flexing hips and knees, and balancing, while the patient sets up his hands. (B) The patient needs to use a large head-hips movement to lift the hips into the air onto the higher surface.

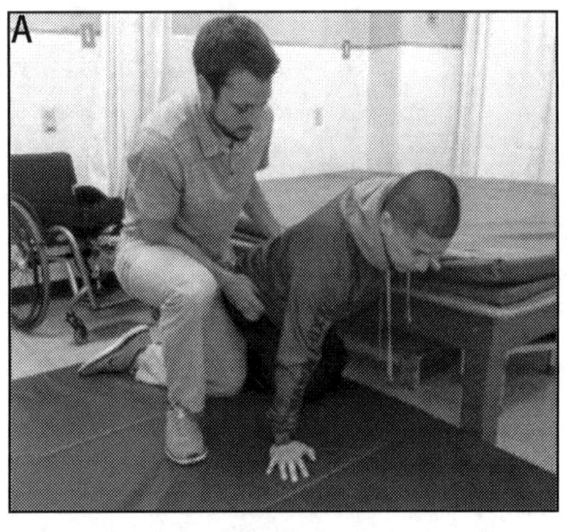

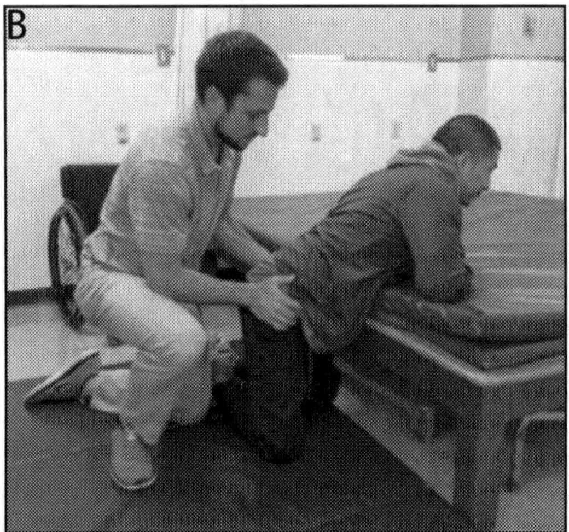

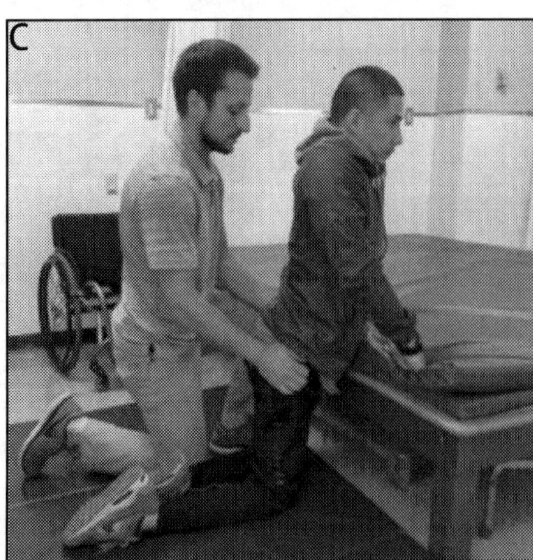

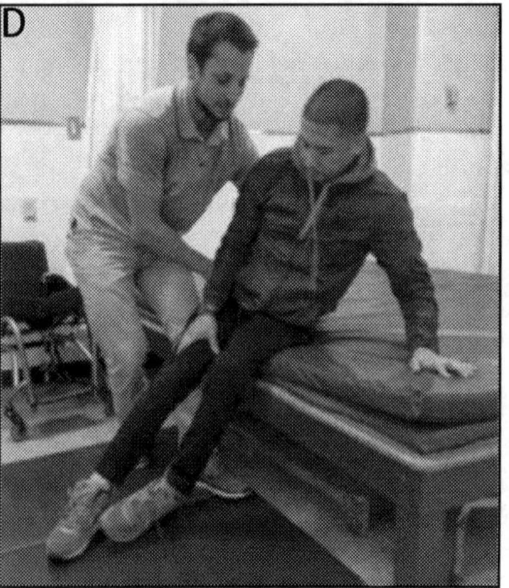

Figure 11-20. A patient completes floor transfers using the front approach. (A) The patient attains a modified quadruped position. (B) Patient transitions into kneeling. (C) Elevating the trunk to begin pressing body up and rotating to move hips onto raised surface. (D) The physical therapist assistant assists at the pelvis to ensure patient lifts and rotates sufficiently.

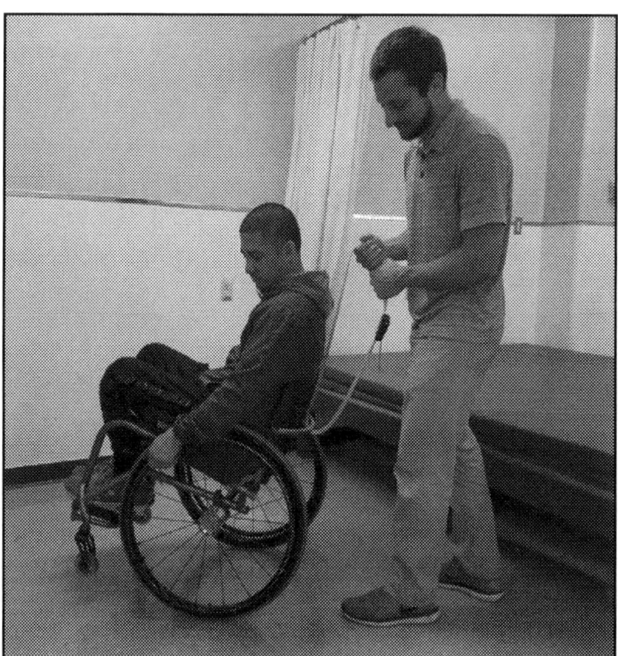

Figure 11-21. The physical therapist assistant is guarding a patient learning to perform wheelies. A gait belt is looped onto the crash bar or axle of the chair to allow the physical therapist assistant to prevent a posterior loss of balance.

remains limited to indicate if, or when, using robotics is better than conventional therapy. Robotic exoskeletons may be used as a gait training tool in the clinic, while others can be purchased by people with an SCI for use on their own as a way to walk in the community when they would otherwise be unable to do so (Figure 11-25).

Patient and Family Education

Family members and hired attendant personnel must learn how to assist the person with an SCI at home. People with SCIs who are unable to care for themselves must learn how to direct others to provide their care. Many rehabilitation programs have classes for patients with SCIs, covering spinal cord regeneration, sexual function, adaptive vehicles, w/c maintenance, w/c vendor relationships, attendant hiring, and other topics for use once the patient has left hospital. Several resources for patients, families, and clinicians are listed at the end of this chapter.

Community Reentry

A multidisciplinary team coordinates visits into the community, with trips to movies, restaurants, or amusement parks; introduction to w/c sports; and similar activities. In some communities, outreach programs provide an opportunity for individuals to participate in competitive sports and outdoor recreation.

Most people with an SCI are discharged home, although people with more severe injuries or fewer resources may require discharge to an assisted living situation, such as a board-and-care, skilled nursing, or subacute facility.

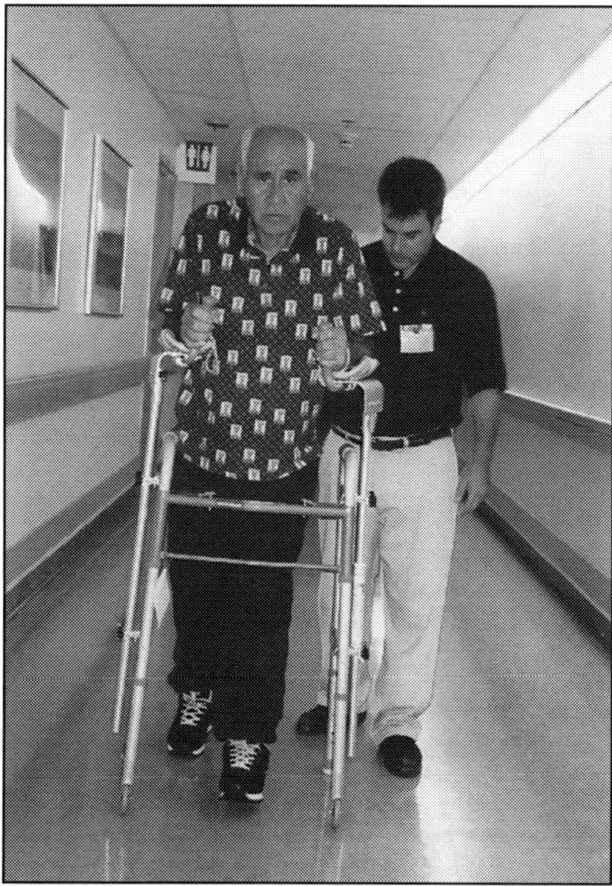

Figure 11-22. The physical therapist assistant walking with a patient with C6 tetraplegia, ASIA D. Bilateral arm troughs on the walker are needed because of weakness in the triceps and finger flexors. Under his trousers, the patient is wearing bilateral polypropylene AFOs with a dorsiflexion assist and dorsiflexion stop. Cosmesis with this type of AFO is excellent.

People with tetraplegia, and some with paraplegia, will require assistance from family members, friends, or a paid caregiver. Some communities have support groups to help people with an SCI and their families continue to cope with the changes in their lives. There are also many online communities where people with an SCI can talk with others who may be having similar experiences. A period of time is required for the person with an SCI to adapt physically and emotionally to the new lifestyle, but successful social and vocational reintegration is an achievable goal. Following discharge from rehabilitation, the person may take advantage of vocational training to determine how the work environment and tasks can be modified for physical limitations, and how adaptive equipment can be used. People who have a valid driver's license may learn to drive with hand controls. Some medical centers have gyms that people with an SCI can access, or they may be able to modify exercise methods to use a commercial gym. Medical follow-up is required to monitor bladder function and overall health and to ensure that late complications are minimized. Each individual with an SCI deserves to have

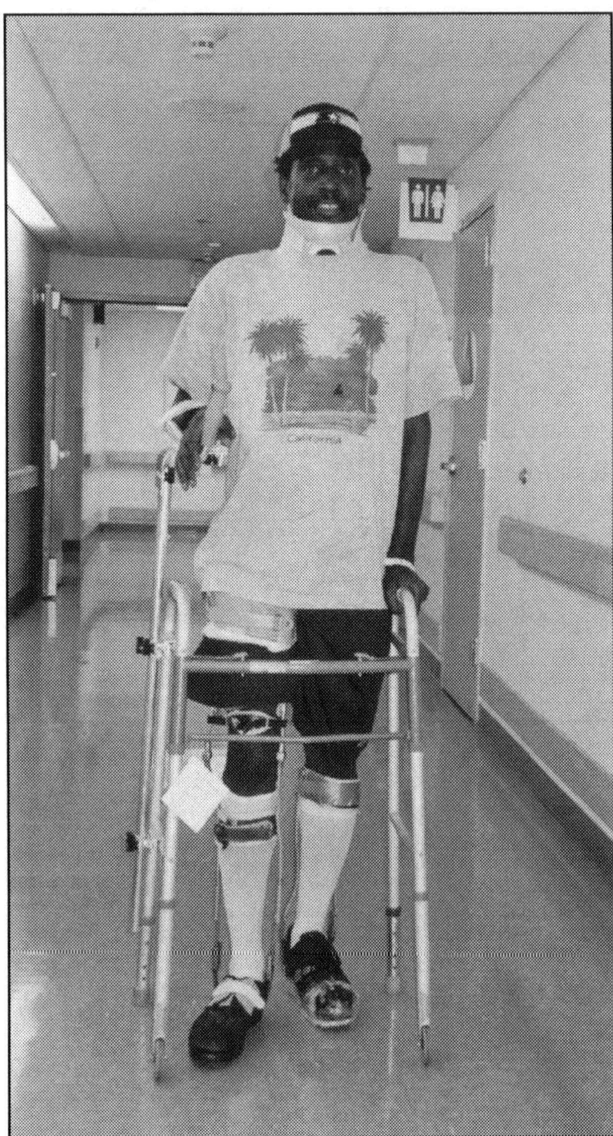

Figure 11-23. Patient with tetraplegia walking with trial orthoses. Using these temporary orthoses—right KAFO and left AFO—allows ambulation before the patient's permanent orthoses are ordered and fabricated. The arm trough helps support the patient's right arm, which has weakness of the triceps muscle.

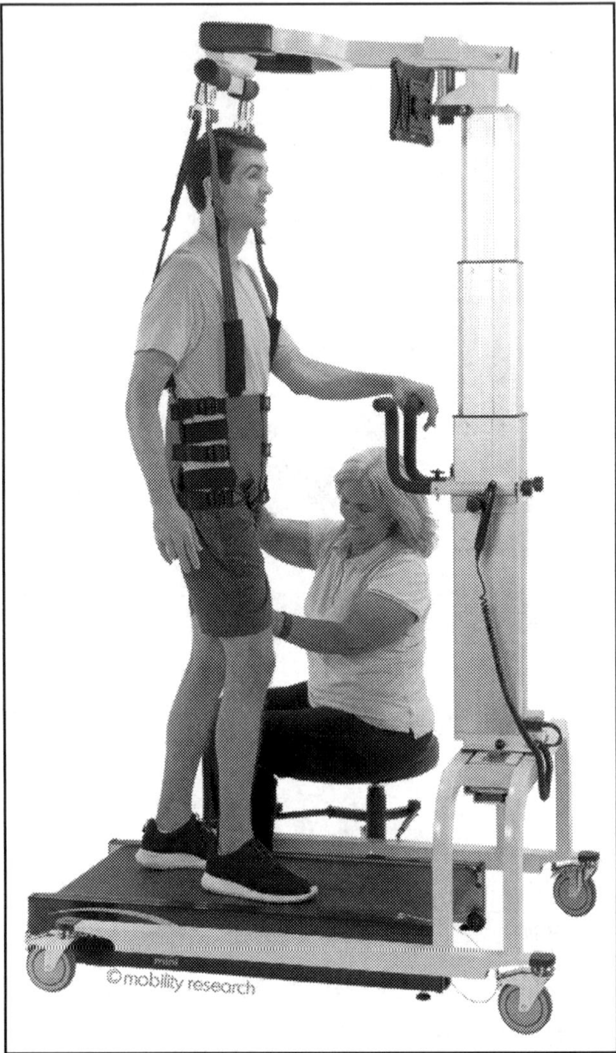

Figure 11-24. Body weight–supported treadmill training. Staff are positioned to assist in moving the legs and to control trunk rotation and weight-shift. (Reprinted with permission from Mobility Research Inc. Tempe, AZ—Makers of LiteGait.)

a fulfilling and meaningful life, and can achieve one with support and assistance.

Wheelchair

Many people with an SCI rely on a w/c for mobility. The most appropriate w/c for depends on factors including the person's level of injury, age, UE strength, vocational or school plans, living situation, resources, and other medical problems. People who are older or weaker or have medical problems may require a power w/c, even with paraplegia or an incomplete injury. Patients with C1 to C4 injuries will require a power w/c with head, chin (Figure 11-26), or sip and puff control to drive the chair. People who lack the ability to perform pressure relief will need a w/c with power recline or tilt. Even people who walk limited distances may require a w/c for community mobility. A rigid-frame ultralight manual w/c (Figure 11-27) is often recommended over a folding w/c for people who are more active or those who require a lighter, more efficient w/c due to UE weakness. The energy cost for pushing a rigid, ultralight w/c is less than for the heavier, collapsible w/cs because the majority of the propulsive energy goes into the wheels rather than into the joints of the collapsible chair.[88] Many w/c components, such as the back height and type, seat-to-floor height, wheel and caster size, tire type, armrests, *dump* (the amount the seat back is lowered compared with the front), wheel *camber* (the amount the wheels flare away from the chair at the floor), and foot plates, can be customized for each patient's needs. Specialized hand rims, such as plastic-covered or with projections, allow better contact with the push surface when hand function is limited, such as in the

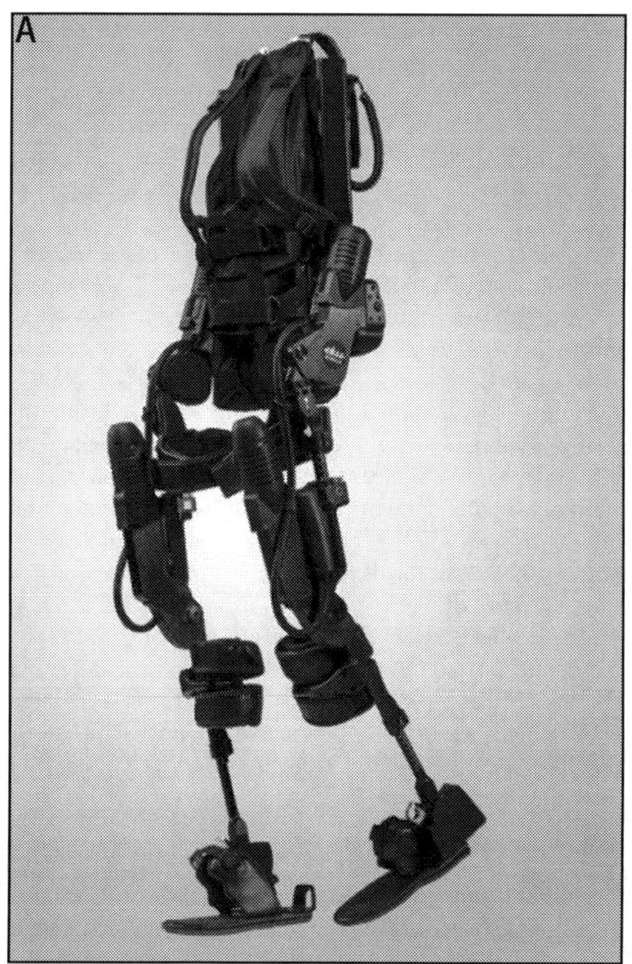

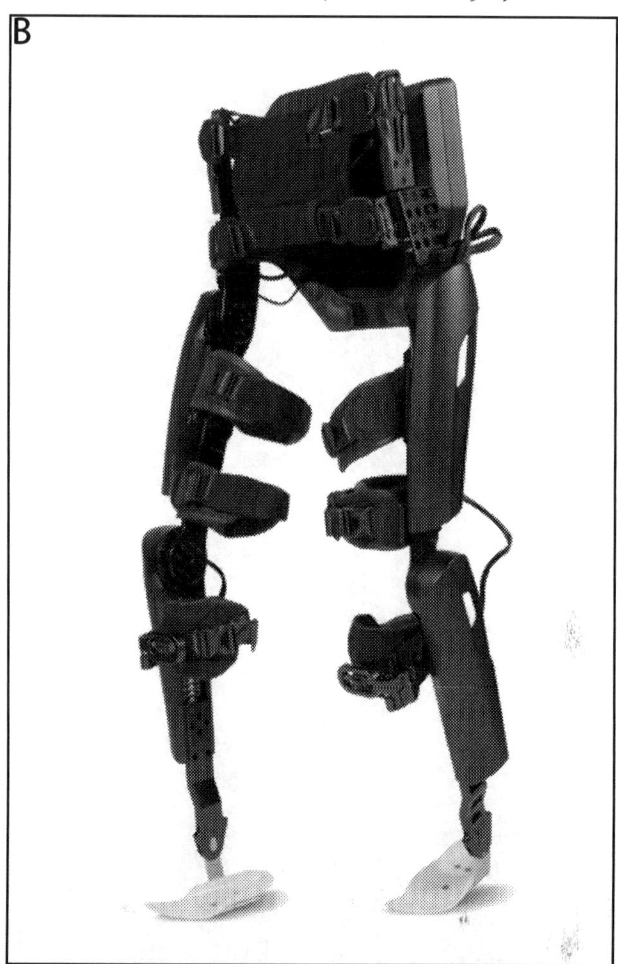

Figure 11-25. Several robotic exoskeletons are available on the market. (A) Ekso GT (Ekso Bionics). (B) ReWalk Personal 6.0 (ReWalk Robotics).

person with C6 to C8 tetraplegia (Figure 11-28). People who will rely on a w/c for mobility must learn enough about w/c maintenance and upkeep to prolong the life of the chair and ensure that it will remain in good working condition.

Obtain Adaptive Equipment

The physical therapist and occupational therapist are responsible for selecting and prescribing most of the appropriate adaptive equipment. The physical therapist may ask the physical therapist assistant for input and suggestions, especially if the physical therapist assistant has been practicing these functional activities with the patient and is more aware of the patient's status. Depending on an individual facility's policies, the physical therapist assistant may be responsible for ordering and obtaining some of the equipment selected by the team.

Adaptive equipment includes a cushion, bathtub bench, raised toilet seat, and equipment that facilitates function, such as a reacher to grab items, a UE orthosis (Figure 11-29), or gloves. A cushion, which helps to better redistribute pressure and provide sitting support, may be foam, gel, air-filled, or a combination (Figure 11-30). Anecdotal reports indicate that standing devices are helpful in reducing bowel and bladder problems, but clinical trials do not exist, and third-party payers may not consider this piece of equipment medically necessary.

Home Assessment

A visit to the individual's home may be recommended to ensure architectural barriers are minimized. The therapist will assess the outside and the interior layouts of the patient's home and make recommendations to maximize functional independence. Possible recommendations may include ramping entryways, moving/removing furniture, changing flooring, lowering commonly used items, altering doorways, removing shower doors, installing a hand-held shower head, arranging placement of medical equipment, and altering the kitchen and bathroom. The physical therapist assistant will assist in contributing to the problem-solving process during and/or after the home visit.

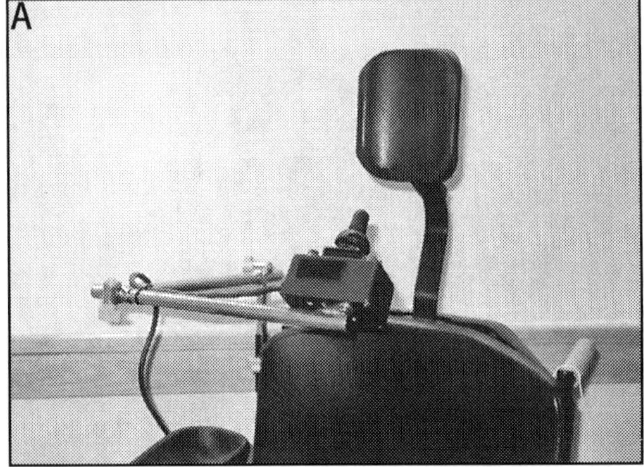

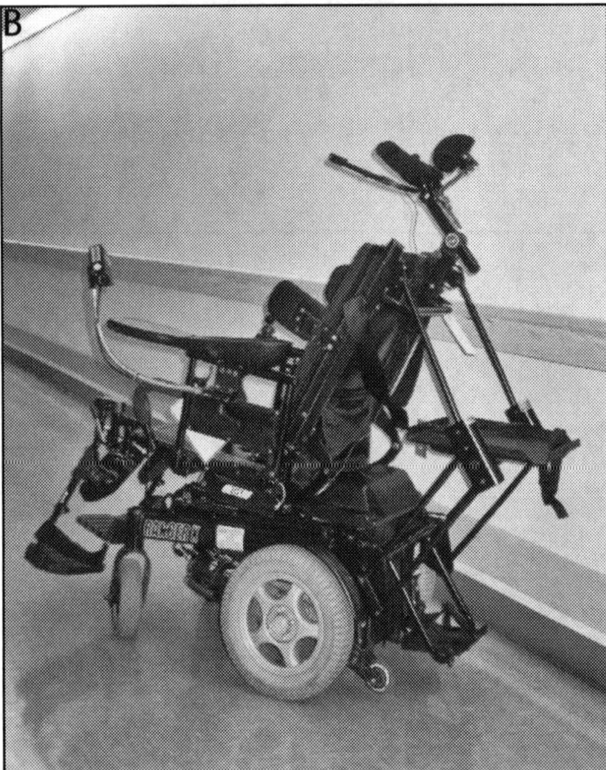

Figure 11-26. (A) Power w/c with head and chin control. (B) Power w/c with ventilator tray. The cheek switch to operate the power recliner is attached to the headrest. Accessories include trunk supports and arm troughs.

Promoting Long-Term Health and Wellness

SCI can be a devastating experience with substantial long-term costs. Rehabilitation immediately post-injury helps patients begin to recover their lives, but people with SCIs will still have to contend with many long-term issues. Physical therapists and physical therapist assistants have an important role in promoting long-term health and wellness through education and treatment. Important areas of emphasis include weight management, metabolic and cardiovascular management, and physical activity.

Systemic changes, both direct and indirect, that happen as a result of an SCI can compromise someone's health. People with an SCI are at a higher risk for developing obesity, which can reduce function and contribute to higher risks of secondary complications. Developing obesity is a function of several factors, but is mostly due to the reduced metabolic rate and reduced physical activity. Muscle mass is an important contributor to metabolic rate, so when muscles atrophy below the level of injury, there will be an associated decline in metabolic activity. If someone is consuming more energy than is being expended, the difference will be stored as fat, and two-thirds of people with SCI are obese.[89] Obesity has physiologic complications, in addition to potentially making mobility more difficult and increasing stress on the shoulders. People with an SCI also have a higher risk for developing diabetes mellitus, which is associated with obesity and reduced physical activity. The most effective way to prevent the onset of obesity is by increasing activity and/or reducing energy intake (eating less). Additionally, staying physically active is associated with reduced rates of hospitalization.[90] Table 11-4 shows exercise recommendations from the American College of Rehabilitative Medicine for people with an SCI.[91]

Shoulder Protection

Shoulder injuries are very common and can be highly debilitating for people after an SCI. One study of people with an SCI found that 46.7% of motorized w/c users, 35.4% of manual w/c users, and 47.6% people using crutches or canes reported having shoulder pain.[92] In some cases, people who rely on their UE to live independently in the community may require hospitalization as a result of shoulder pain. Strengthening should be focused on the rotator cuff, particularly the external rotators, as well as scapular depressors and retractors. It is also important to maintain ROM, especially for shoulder external rotation, and prevent excessive anterior tipping elevation, and protraction of the scapulae, which may lead to abnormal scapulohumeral mechanics that may contribute to developing shoulder pain. If rotator cuff pathology does begin, some patients may find benefit from corticosteroid injections and, in worse cases, surgical repair.[52] Research has also found that people with tetraplegia and limited shoulder ROM at the beginning of their rehabilitation program are more likely to develop shoulder pain over the first 5 years after injury.[93]

Case Study

The following case study illustrates an episode of care in the physical rehabilitation of a person with an SCI.

Background

The patient, Matt, is a 35-year-old man who is married with 2 boys, ages 9 and 12. Prior to his injury, he was

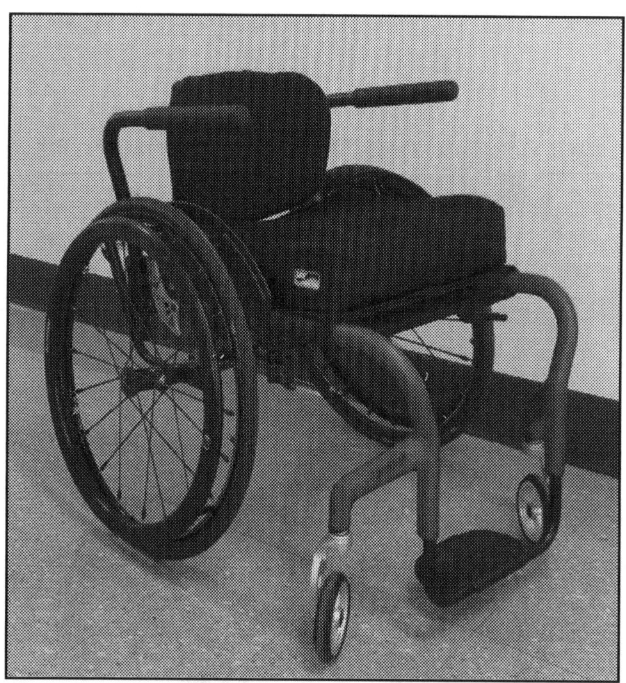

Figure 11-27. Ultralight manual w/c.

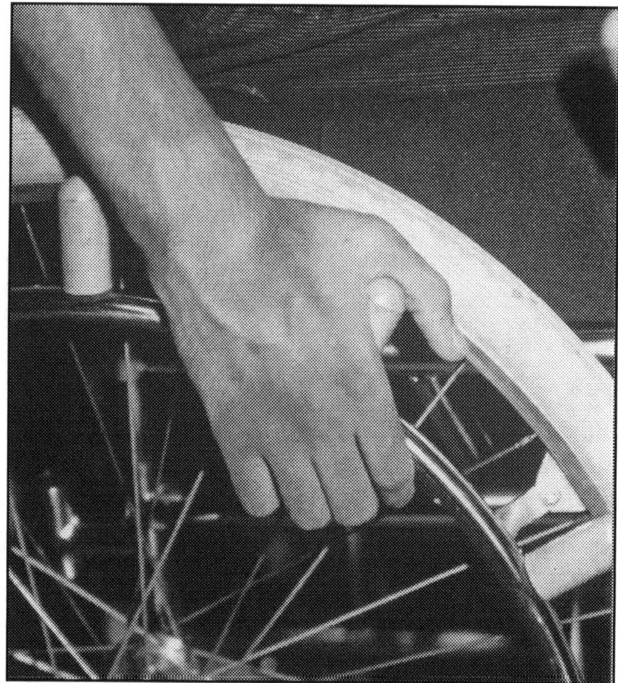

Figure 11-28. Specialized handrims.

employed by an energy company as a senior chemical engineer, managing 16 employees in his department. He enjoys traveling abroad, playing tennis, and watching his children play soccer and baseball. The patient was involved in a motor vehicle accident, sustaining a T4 complete SCI (ASIA A). He lives in a 2-story home, with the bedrooms on the second floor. There are 2 steps to enter the home.

Matt underwent surgery for stabilization with placement of Harrington rods from T2 to T8, and he was given intravenous steroids to reduce inflammation and secondary damage to the spinal cord. He was then admitted to the acute neurological unit for 10 days until he was medically stable. The physician has prescribed a TLSO brace (clamshell type) for the patient to wear for 8 to 10 weeks. Acute therapists worked together to decrease his pain, improve his sitting tolerance, and increase his UE strength and endurance. During treatment, Matt experienced a severe headache; the physical therapist assistant treating him assessed his BP as 180/100, immediately contacted the nurse, and began examining Matt for possible reasons for the rise in BP. The physical therapist assistant found that Matt's urinary catheter was twisted and kinked at the proximal end. After the catheter was straightened, Matt remained sitting up in his w/c; after 20 minutes, his BP came down to his baseline of 92/60. The nurse was prepared to administer nitroglycerin gel if his BP did not return to baseline. This was Matt's first experience of AD. Matt presented with pitting edema in bilateral feet and legs, and prior to Matt's transfer to rehab, his LEs were assessed for DVT using a Doppler ultrasound. He wore compressive thigh-high stockings to help reduce the dependent edema.

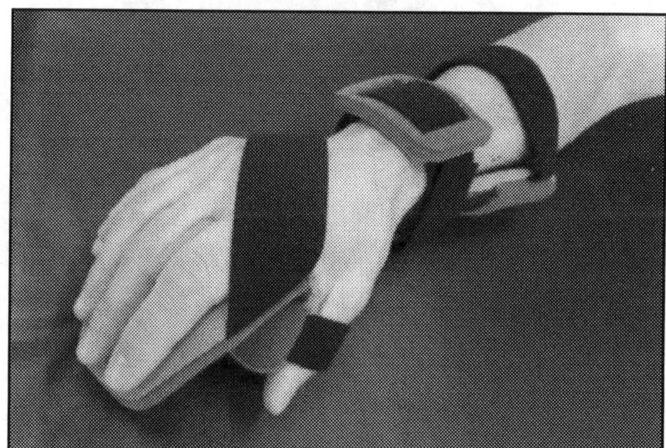

Figure 11-29. A wrist-hand orthosis stabilizes the wrist while the patient performs functional activities. Implements, such as utensils and pens, can be inserted into the palm.

Inpatient Rehabilitation

After he was medically stable and could tolerate an intensive rehabilitation program, Matt was transferred to the inpatient rehab center. The inpatient rehab team evaluating Matt consisted of a physician, registered nurse, physical therapist assistant, occupational therapist, neuropsychologist, dietician, and social worker. During Matt's first week, the clinicians presented their findings to one another at the initial team conference to establish the plan of care. The individualized care plan and his length of stay were based on Matt's medical problems, neurological level and projected functional outcome levels (T4 ASIA A), cognitive and emotional status, physical impairments, functional

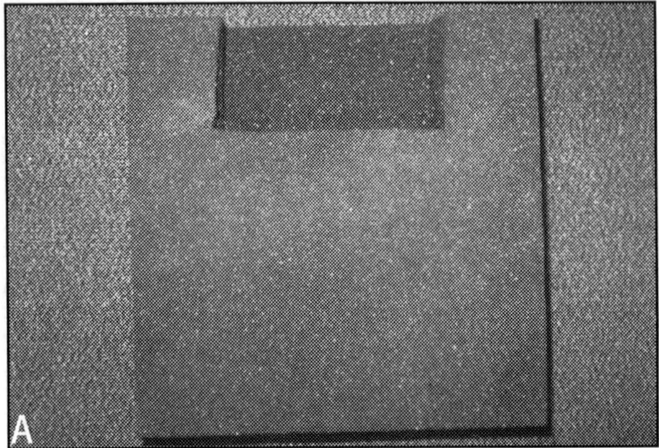

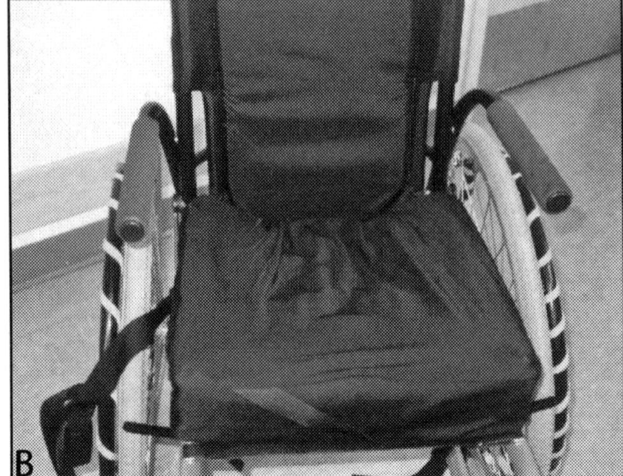

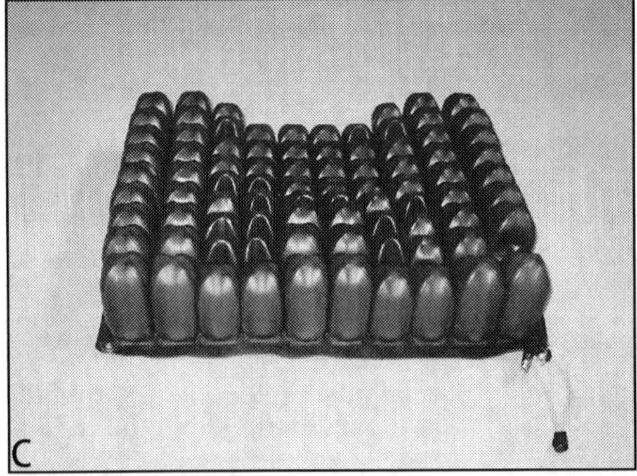

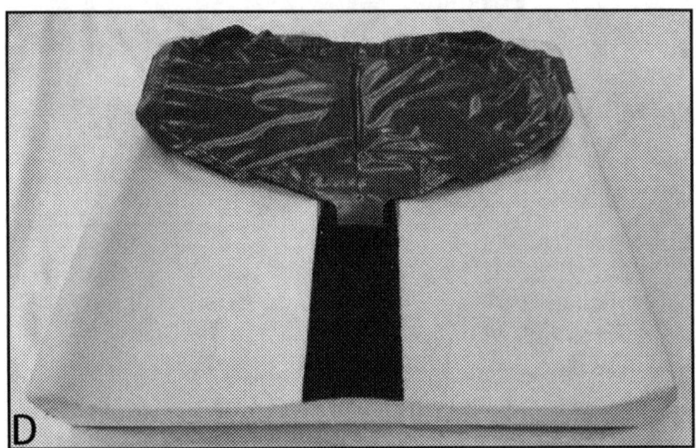

Figure 11-30. Pressure-relieving cushions. (A) Four-inch laminated foam w/c cushion (high density over extra high density) with ischial cutout. The cutout goes three-quarters of the way through the height of the cushion, thereby maintaining integrity of the cushion while eliminating pressure under the ischial tuberosities. (B) Gel cushion over a contoured foam base. Redistribution of sitting pressure is achieved with this cushion. The gel is primarily in the area of the ischial tuberosities. (C) Air w/c cushion. This provides excellent pressure redistribution for persons who have bony deformities of the pelvis. Cushion must be checked daily to ensure that it is inflated adequately to prevent pressure sores. (D) Gel cushion uncovered.

deficits, SCI educational needs, and discharge disposition, as well as his goals and those of his family. Some inpatient rehab centers invite the patient and family members to participate in the team conference. Often, family members offer information that will help the team better understand qualities of the patient and create a more complete treatment plan. In this setting, the patient stated the following goals: take care of himself, return to work, participate in his children's lives, and help care for his family.

The following goals were set during inpatient rehabilitation:

- Be independent with his specific home exercise program for ROM and strengthening areas including UEs and passive ROM.
- Maintain/increase hip, knee, and ankle ROM.
- Independently assume the sitting position from supine with the TLSO on, without using the bedrails (he will continue to require moderate assistance from caregivers to don and doff the TLSO because of spinal precautions).
- Maintain the short sitting position independently at the edge of bed, with UE support.
- Independently transfer from his w/c to a bed, toilet, couch, and tub transfer bench; handle car transfers with transfer board and minimal assistance.
- Demonstrate 3 types of w/c pressure reliefs every 30 minutes.
- Independently propel w/c through doorways and up and down American With Disabilities Act (ADA) compliant ramps.
- Independently propel the w/c over a 2-inch curb, curb cutouts, and uneven terrain. The following goals were set for the family:
    - The family will demonstrate independence with assisting Matt with standard height curbs and stairs.
    - The family will also demonstrate an understanding of how to perform a dependent transfer from floor to w/c for fall recovery.

Table 11-4
Exercise Recommendations for People With Spinal Cord Injury

	Cardiovascular Health	*Muscle Strength and Endurance*	*Flexibility and Range of Motion*
Frequency	Minimum 2 days/week	Minimum 2 days/week	Daily
Intensity	Moderate to vigorous †	8 to 10 reps	30 to 60 seconds/stretch; gentle, slow, pain free
Duration	20 to 30 minutes/session	3 sets; 1 to 2 minutes rest between sets (30 to 60 minutes total)	2 sets; 5 to 15 minutes
Activities	Wheeling, arm cycle, sports, recumbent stepper, aquatics, cycling, circuit training, functional electrical stimulation	Free weights, elastic resistance bands, cable pulleys, weight machines, functional electrical stimulation	Standing in standing frame (if medically cleared); passive and active static stretching

Adapted from SCI Action Canada. www.sciactioncanada.ca/guidelines. Accessed August, 2014.

† Moderate intensity: somewhat hard but can be sustained for long periods without experiencing excessive fatigue; Vigorous intensity: very hard, close to maximum and cannot be sustained for long without experiencing excessive fatigue.

Tests and Measures

Cardiovascular/pulmonary:

- Vitals at rest: BP = 110/70 mm Hg (supine), 96/60 mm Hg (sitting); heart rate = 80 beats/minute; respiratory rate = 20 respirations/minute in sitting; oxygen saturations = 98% in supine, 94% in sitting (using pulse oximeter)

Strength:

- Bilateral UEs = normal (5/5); bilateral LEs = absent (0/5); trunk = intercostal muscles intact to T4 level, abdominal muscles are not innervated

Sensation (sharp/dull discrimination, light touch):

- Bilateral UEs = normal/intact; bilateral LEs = absent; trunk = intact for both sharp/dull and light touch modalities to T4 dermatome, absent below T4

ROM:

- UE active ROM, within normal limits for all UE joints; LE passive ROM, within normal limits, except hip flexion (SLR) = 0 to 60 degrees bilaterally and ankle dorsiflexion to neutral

Deep tendon reflexes (0 to 4):

- Biceps (C5 to C6), 2; brachioradialis (C5 to C6), 2; triceps (C7), 2; quadriceps (L3 to L4), 3; plantar flexors (S1), 4

Functional Abilities

Matt was active and independent for all functional skills prior to his injury. At the time of the evaluation, his functional mobility was as follows:

- **Donning/doffing TLSO**: Matt needed total assistance to don and doff the TLSO brace (clamshell) before getting out of bed. The TLSO brace interfered with all functional mobility skills.
- **Bed mobility**: He needed moderate assistance for rolling, maximal assistance for supine to long sitting position, and maximal assistance from supine to short sitting at the edge of bed. Initially, he needed time to acclimate to the upright position because of OH.
- **Sitting balance**: He needed minimal to moderate assistance to maintain a sitting position at the edge of the bed with bilateral hands either in front or behind his hips (propping). He was not able to change hand position without moderate to maximal assistance to maintain his balance.
- **Transfers**: He needed maximal assistance from one person for all basic transfers, and total assistance for advanced transfers (eg, floor to w/c transfer, car transfers). He was not yet able to apply the head-hips relationship.
- **W/C mobility**: He was independent for propulsion on level terrain for short distances (less than 50 feet). He required total assistance for all high-level w/c skills (eg, steep ramps, wheelies, curbs, and stairs). He was able to demonstrate 3 w/c pressure-relieving techniques with minimal assistance (ie, leaning forward onto thighs to relieve pressure on coccyx and sacrum, leaning laterally to relieve pressure on the ischial tuberosities, and lifting his entire buttocks off the seat using a depression-lift technique).

Physical Therapy Program

- **Team communication**: As Matt continues to improve in his functional mobility, it is important that all members of the team understand his level of assistance needed for activities, as well as movement strategies. A team conference will be held at least weekly, and at some rehab facilities, a team huddle will occur daily or as needed to ensure all team members have current information. An information board is updated daily in Matt's room to keep the staff current and inform Matt and his family about his progress.
- **Teaching problem-solving strategies**: It is important to allow Matt to problem-solve as he is learning new movement strategies. Because of Matt's educational background, he is able to understand the physics and mechanics behind the new skills. However, applying the skills is very challenging without normal sensation or motor control below the level of the lesion. New situations will arise during treatment sessions and throughout his day in rehab; it is important to allow him time to problem-solve on his own to help him become self-sufficient. On a regular basis, the clinicians will ask Matt what his goals are to ensure he is involved in his plan of care.
- **UE-strengthening exercises**: With manual muscle testing, Matt demonstrated having normal strength and ROM throughout his UEs; however, because he will be using his UEs for all functional mobility tasks, the muscle strength of the scapulothoracic and glenohumeral joints is critical to decrease the risk of shoulder pain and injury. Posterior musculature (eg, rhomboids, trapezius, rotator cuff, and posterior deltoids) must be strengthened to avoid a muscle imbalance because the majority of functional movements use primarily the anterior shoulder musculature. The latissimus dorsi, serratus anterior, triceps, deltoids, and pectoralis major muscles are also very important for functional transfers. It is critical for Matt to strengthen his UEs in positions that do not decrease the integrity of the spine surgery or create more kyphosis. The physical therapist and physical therapist assistant will work together to provide an exercise program that he will perform independently using exercise machines, as well as mat exercises using weights or his own body as resistance, or with the physical therapist assistant providing manual resistance through important ROMs specific for functional mobility.
- **Bed mobility skills**: Bed mobility activities require proper technique, speed, momentum, and timing; adequate ROM; and an understanding of how to unweight extremities. Overstretching the back muscles and ligaments will often make rolling more difficult, causing the lower trunk to not move with the upper trunk as it is rotating. The rehab staff will need to help Matt don his TLSO brace prior to teaching bed mobility skills. To roll, Matt needs to use momentum from swinging his UEs while simultaneously rotating and flexing the head/neck. Rolling to the prone position will be useful in reducing pressure on bony prominences on his back, sacrum, coccyx, and heels. Proning is initiated by the therapists for 1 to 2 hours/day, and carried over by nursing; eventually, Matt will be fully responsible for his proning schedule. When Matt is independent, assuming the prone or semi-prone position with pillows protecting bony prominences, he can reduce the amount of turning he must do at night, reducing the amount of assistance required. From the side-lying position, Matt will be able to assume the long sitting position by crawling around toward his feet and then pushing up into long sit. Remember, it is important that his hamstring length is adequate (SLR of 100 degrees to 110 degrees) to prevent excessive posterior pelvic tilt, and overstretching his back when in the long sitting position. Initially, Matt's SLR was inadequate, and he needed to assume the frog-leg position in long sitting (hips abducted and externally rotated, with knees flexed), or the therapist allowed his legs to drape over the edge of the mat. Matt's abdominal musculature is not innervated, but because his ROM and strength in his UEs are within functional limits throughout, he can assume the long sitting position directly from supine using momentum, speed, and power without rolling to the side-lying position. This direct method is more efficient; however, many times the rolling from supine to side-lying to long sit progression will be taught before the supine to long sit progression because it is easier to master. From side-lying or the long sitting position, he will learn how to manage his LEs and trunk to assume short sitting at the edge of the mat/bed.
- **Transfer training and functional activities**: The physical therapist and physical therapist assistant will work together to improve basic transfers and begin advanced transfer training. The natural progression of transfers is usually mastered in the following order: w/c to/from mat, bed, toilet, tub transfer bench, car, and floor. Sitting balance is a critical component in mastering transfers. Although Matt does not have sensation below the nipple level (T4), he will learn to balance himself using his upper trunk, head/neck, and arms. He must learn to maintain balance with his hands in front of his hips and behind his hips, one arm support, and without UE support. As he becomes more dynamic in sitting, counterbalancing is an important mobility skill. For example, positioning his LEs in preparation for a transfer requires balancing on one arm, then counterbalancing to lift and reposition the LE with the other arm. As his long sitting balance and short sitting balance improve, depression lifts are taught, implementing the head-hips relationship. The physical therapist assistant needs to allow Matt to find

his balance point during the lift. It is important to provide Matt with enough space to lean forward, drop his head down, and lift his hips off the mat. While finding his balance point during a depression lift, Matt will often fall quickly backward onto the mat or forward into the clinician; remaining vigilant and in the correct position to catch him is critical. Matt will initially use a transfer board to bridge the distance from surface to surface, until his depression lift-pivot transfer technique is safe to travel over the necessary distance without risk of falling. Because of Matt's need to wear his TLSO brace when out of bed, his ability to master many skills may be difficult. When his TLSO brace is finally discontinued (ie, 8 to 10 weeks), he may have difficulty finding his balance once again and will need to learn how to manage his body during functional activities, and more advanced skills will be taught without the brace interfering (eg, floor transfers). As his mobility and balance improve, he will be taught how to load his w/c independently into a car; he most likely will not be able to master this skill prior to discharge from rehab.

- **W/C mobility exercises**: W/C mobility training involves learning to maneuver in tight spaces, over uneven terrain (eg, gravel or grass), over a threshold, up and down ramps, and through doorways. A person using a manual w/c with sufficient UE motor control may learn more advanced w/c skills, such as how to navigate curbs and go up and down stairs. Matt must be taught how to propel his w/c efficiently on level and uneven surfaces. On a flat, smooth surface, patients will often excessively push their w/c instead of allowing it to coast while resting the UEs. Pushing his w/c on uneven surfaces (eg, grass, steppingstones, or sand) will challenge Matt's balance and his ability to shift weight to maintain traction on the rear wheels. The physical therapist assistant must be sure to secure Matt by using the w/c seat belt, because he may fall forward while practicing high-level skills. Matt has difficulty negotiating doorways, especially those with automatic door closers; he will be taught methods to open and close doors by using the door and the doorframe to get through doorways efficiently. Many ramps are not ADA-compliant in Matt's community. When propelling up ramps, he will be taught to keep his trunk flexed forward to decrease the risk of tipping backward. He will also be taught to descend steep ramps (not ADA-compliant) rolling backward, with his trunk flexed forward on his thighs, and slowly allowing the w/c rims to glide through his hands to manage his speed. Ascending and descending curbs will also be an occasional necessity. In preparation for curbs, wheelies will be taught by using a gait belt around the rear of the w/c frame or rear axle to enable the physical therapist assistant to catch Matt when he falls backward. The clinician will help him find his balance point in the w/c and learn how to keep his hands on the top-most part of the rims, allowing equal movement to push the rims forward and backward when finding his balance. Once Matt has gained some proficiency in performing wheelies, he will practice maintaining a wheelie while propelling the w/c down the hallway (wheelie glide). He will then learn how to ascend and descend a 2-inch curb, popping up the front casters onto the curb, transferring his weight forward, and quickly and forcefully pushing the w/c onto the curb. He will also learn how to descend a curb backward with his trunk flexed forward onto his thighs and also forward in a wheelie glide. Most patients are not proficient or safe with ascending/descending curbs or stairs at discharge from rehab. It is necessary to teach caregivers how to help negotiate curbs and stairs.
- **W/C and cushion prescriptio**n: Because of Matt's neurological level and ASIA classification (T4 ASIA A), it is very unlikely that he will be a functional ambulator; therefore, an ultralight rigid w/c will be prescribed. Factors to consider will be discussed with the patient, such as needing to independently transfer his w/c into a car, have accessibility in his home and work environment, and deal with insurance issues. Matt will try a few w/c models with different specifications and will be educated on their specific features (eg, weight, size, frame dimensions, seat-to-back angle, axle position, camber angle, tires, spokes, and caster size). Matt's body type puts him at high risk for pressure ulcers; therefore, a seating evaluation using a computerized pressure mapping system will be performed to determine the most appropriate w/c cushion. The physical therapist assistant will also work with Matt to teach basic w/c maintenance (eg, fixing a flat tire and adjusting wheel camber, casters, and brakes).
- **Home evaluation**: The physical therapist or physical therapist assistant and an occupational therapist will complete a home evaluation with Matt and his family present. Recommendations for equipment and home modifications will be documented and discussed with the family and the rehab team members. Equipment such as a raised toilet seat, drop-arm commode, bath bench, and grab bars may be recommended. Other home modifications may include installing a ramp in the entrance, removing or installing double-hinged doors to widen entrances, removing sliding bath/shower doors, clearing floors of clutter for w/c accessibility, relocating common items to his level, and removing or securing area rugs. Near the end of his rehab stay, Matt will be scheduled for a day pass with his family to examine some of the potential problems and logistics to returning home.
- **Patient and family education**: Many rehab centers provide educational reading materials and classes

taught by various disciplines on topics specific to SCIs. Matt and his wife will attend classes on bowel and bladder management, pressure ulcer prevention, community resources, and sexuality. SCIs can greatly affect the caregivers physically, mentally, and emotionally. Neuropsychologists and social workers are trained to help caregivers with understanding SCIs, potential issues, and emotional assistance. Matt and his caregivers will be informed regarding area support groups and recreational outreach programs. The internet has become an excellent resource for patients, caregivers, and family members. Many websites and videos provide information on everything from potential movement strategies to the newest technological advancements in mobility.

Final Results

Matt underwent a 5-week rehabilitation program with only a few setbacks, including a small stage II decubitus ulcer on his coccyx and the beginnings of HO in his right hip that was controlled with medication, and passive ROM exercises. During the first week, the physician discussed with him the importance of his rehabilitation program, his current status, and his prognosis. Matt reported that this information was disheartening and at the same time somewhat motivational. During the first 2 weeks, the physical therapist assistant and physical therapist assistant began working with Matt to improve his hamstring ROM, UE strength, bed mobility, sitting balance, performing w/c pressure relief, basic transfer skills, and basic w/c mobility skills. By the end of the third week, Matt was dressing himself with minimal assistance, performing his self-care with supervision/minimal assistance, performing bed mobility skills with supervision assistance and minimal verbal cues for technique, completing tub and toilet transfers with moderate assistance, and performing depression transfers to and from the mat and bed with contact guard/minimal assistance. He was able to pop up into a wheelie and hold it for 3 to 5 seconds. During this week, his physical therapist assistant found his right hip passive ROM was becoming less flexible and reported it to the physical therapist and the physician. He was diagnosed with HO of the right hip and began a course of medication along with continued passive ROM exercises. He was also able to perform self-catheterization independently and check his skin with a flexible mirror independently. Matt was also on a bowel program with nursing. By the end of the fourth week, he was able to perform bed mobility skills with modified independence (after receiving assistance to don/doff the TLSO), transfer from his w/c to the bed with supervision/modified independence, transfer to the toilet and bath bench (managing LEs) with minimal assistance, and transfer to the car with minimal assistance using a sliding board. He was able to perform a wheelie in a w/c and maintain a wheelie while gliding 20 feet with supervision, ascend and descend a 2-inch curb with minimal assistance and verbal cues, propel the w/c up and down a non–ADA-compliant ramp independently, and propel his w/c through grass and gravel with modified independence. The home evaluation was performed during this week by the physical therapist and occupational therapist, who documented and discussed recommendations with the patient and family. A w/c and seating evaluation was performed this week with a vendor; an ultralight w/c with a foam and air combination cushion was ordered because of Matt's history of pressure ulcers and postural concerns. By the end of the fifth week, he was modified-independent with bed mobility skills (except for donning and doffing the TLSO) and w/c transfers to bed, toilet, and tub transfer bench. He required supervision for car transfers with a sliding board. He and his family were educated on how to assist him in the areas of concern, and demonstrated the skills proficiently.

When Matt was discharged from the hospital, the family rented a ramp until a permanent ramp could be built. He then began a course of home health care (including the physical therapist, occupational therapist, registered nurse, and social worker) to adjust to home and to become independent in the home and community. The home health therapists continued making recommendations on home modifications as issues arose. He lived on the first floor of his home for the first 2 months, while a stair glide was installed. The second floor is now accessible to him; however, he needed to purchase another w/c for use on the second floor. After he became independent at home, he was discharged from home health care and then began a course of outpatient therapies to continue working on improving UE strength, maintaining ROM in LEs, advanced w/c skills, advanced transfer techniques, and updating his home exercise program. Matt returned to work at the energy company, continuing his previous level of employment. The company is making efforts to accommodate his disability.

Additional Case Studies

Case #1

John, age 22, a student at a local community college studying computer science, sustained a C6-level SCI, ASIA A, in a motor vehicle accident 2 months ago.

1. What muscles remain innervated?
2. Will he be able to continue using his computer?
3. What kind of adaptive equipment will be required to use the computer?
4. The physical therapist has identified sliding board transfers as a goal for the patient. What activities or interventions might the physical therapist assistant be asked to do prior to initiating or attempting transfers?
5. What kind of w/c will he probably need, given his vocational goals?

Case #2

A patient is on the tilt table having his hamstrings stretched to gain ROM for an SLR. His injury level is T2. He starts sweating and complaining of a headache.

1. What do you suspect has occurred?
2. What should you do first?
3. If his BP is elevated, what should you do?

Case #3

You are working with a patient with an SCI at L1 level, ASIA C, which he sustained 2 months ago. You know that the doctor has talked to the patient about recovery and the level of his injury. The patient now has poor minus (P or 2/5) to poor (P or 2/5) strength in the hip flexor and quadriceps muscles, and trace (Tr or 1/5) in his dorsiflexor, hamstring, and hip abductor muscles.

1. Is it important to continue to strengthen the muscles in his LEs?
2. Can he get stronger?
3. Would he still benefit from exercise if it were 13 months post-injury? Why?

Case #4

A physical therapist assistant was asked to work with a patient who has T6 paraplegia and is sitting on a gel cushion. Yesterday was his first day sitting, and he had no problems with dizziness. The physical therapist asks the physical therapist assistant to implement an education program on pressure relief and prevention of pressure sores.

1. What points would the physical therapist assistant want to cover with this patient?
2. What does the patient need to know about his cushion?

Case #5

The physical therapist has asked the physical therapist assistant to run a class on power w/c mobility for patients with C2 to C5 tetraplegia.

1. What activities would be important for these people to learn to be able to function in the community?
2. What additional activities would be important if it were a class for patients using manual w/cs and at a higher level of function?

Case #6

As part of a plan of care, physical therapist assistant has been asked to work with a patient with T7 paraplegia.

1. What functional activities would the physical therapist assistant work on in preparation for a car transfer?
2. What are some precautions to tell the patient when performing this skill?

Resources

American Spinal Injury Association
An organization for physicians and other health care professionals specializing in care of patients with SCI.
9702 Gayton Road Suite 306
Richmond, VA 23238
www.asia-spinalinjury.org

Christopher & Dana Reeve Foundation
A foundation committed to funding research to develop cures and treatment for paralysis due to SCI. Also provides grants for quality of life for people living with disabilities.
636 Morris Turnpike Suite 3A
Short Hills, NJ 07078
(800) 225-0292
www.christopherreeve.org

United Spinal Association
Provides information on topics related to SCI, and an online newsletter.
120-134 Queens Boulevard Suite 320
Kew Gardens, NY 11415
(718) 803-3782
https://unitedspinal.org/

Paralyzed Veterans of America
Advocate for quality health care, research and education, and civil rights and opportunities for those with SCIs. Provides SCI-related information for patients and families.
801 Eighteenth Street NW
Washington, DC 20006
(800) 424-8200
www.pva.org

The University of Alabama at Birmingham Spinal Cord Injury Model System (UAB-SCIMS)
Provides information about research projects and statistics about SCI, as well as educational materials for patients and families.
Spain Rehab Center
1717 6th Avenue S
Birmingham, Al 35233
www.uab.edu/medicine/sci/

Additional Websites and Social Media

A site of the National Institute of Neurological Disorders and Stroke, National Institutes of Health, which supports biomedical research on disorders of the brain and nervous system.
https://www.ninds.nih.gov/Disorders/All-Disorders/Spinal-Cord-Injury-Information-Page

The Spinal Cord Injury and Disease Resources' site offers general resources, facts, statistics, rehabilitation, email groups and listserves, message boards, newsletters, magazines, articles, and books.

https://www.makoa.org/sci.htm

Facebook

- Life After Spinal Cord Injury
- Spinal Cord Injury Non-Profit Organization
- Spinal Cord Peer Support USA
- United Spinal Association

Twitter

- @faceDisability Peer support for families.
- @spinalinjuries A user-led organization that works to support and promote the well-being of the 40,000 people with an SCI in the United Kingdom.

References

1. National Spinal Cord Injury Center Statistical Center. Spinal cord injury: facts and figures at a glance. Birmingham, AL. https://www.nscisc.uab.edu/PublicDocuments/fact_figures_docs/Facts%202012%20Feb%20Final.pdf. Accessed May 7, 2018.
2. World Health Organization. World Health Statistics 2013. Cause-specific mortality and morbidity, Table 2. http://www.who.int/whosis/whostat/EN_WHS09_Table2.pdf. Accessed May 7, 2018.
3. Hasler RM, Exadaktylos AK, Bouamra O, et al. Epidemiology and predictors of spinal injury in adult major trauma patients: european cohort study. *Eur Spine J.* 2011;20(12):2174-2180. doi:10.1007/s00586-011-1866-7
4. Pirouzmand F. Epidemiological trends of spine and spinal cord injuries in the largest Canadian adult trauma center from 1986 to 2006. *J Neurosurg Spine.* 2010;12(2):131-140. doi:10.3171/2009.9.SPINE0943
5. Jackson AB, Dijkers M, Devivo MJ, Poczatek RB. A demographic profile of new traumatic spinal cord injuries: change and stability over 30 years. *Arch Phys Med Rehabil.* 2004;85(11):1740-1748. doi:10.1016/j.apmr.2004.04.035
6. Krause JS, Saunders LL. Health, secondary conditions, and life expectancy after spinal cord injury. *Arch Phys Med Rehabil.* 2011;92(11):1770-1775. doi:10.1016/j.apmr.2011.05.024
7. LivecchiMA.Spinalcordinjury.*Continuum.*2011;17(3):568-583. doi:10.1212/01.CON.0000399073.00062.9e
8. Oyinbo CA. Secondary injury mechanisms in traumatic spinal cord injury: a nugget of this multiply cascade. *Acta Neurobiol Exp (Wars).* 2011;71(2):281-299.
9. Marino RJ, Barros T, Biering-Sorensen F, et al; ASIA Neurological Standards Committee 2002. International standards for neurological classification of spinal cord injury. *J Spinal Cord Med.* 2003;26(supl)(suppl 1):S50-S56. doi:10.1080/10790268.2003.11754575
10. American Spinal Injury Association. *International Standards for Neurological Classification of Spinal Cord Injury.* Chicago, IL: American Spinal Injury Association; 2002.
11. Atkinson PP, Atkinson JLD. Spinal shock. *Mayo Clin Proc.* 1996;71(4):384-389. doi:10.4065/71.4.384
12. Ditunno JF, Little JW, Tessler A, Burns AS. Spinal shock revisited: a four-phase model. *Spinal Cord.* 2004;42(7):383-395. doi:10.1038/sj.sc.3101603
13. McKinley W, Santos K, Meade M, Brooke K. Incidence and outcomes of spinal cord injury clinical syndromes. *J Spinal CordMed.*2007;30(3):215-224.doi:10.1080/10790268.2007.11753929
14. Roth EJ, Park T, Pang T, Yarkony GM, Lee MY. Traumatic cervical Brown-Sequard and Brown-Sequard-plus syndromes: the spectrum of presentations and outcomes. *Paraplegia.* 1991;29(9):582-589.
15. Schneider RC, Cherry G, Pantek H. The syndrome of acute central cervical spinal cord injury; with special reference to the mechanisms involved in hyperextension injuries of cervical spine. *J Neurosurg.* 1954;11(6):546-577. doi:10.3171/jns.1954.11.6.0546
16. Penrod LE, Hegde SK, Ditunno JF Jr. Age effect on prognosis for functional recovery in acute, traumatic central cord syndrome. *Arch Phys Med Rehabil.* 1990;71(12):963-968.
17. Bosch A, Stauffer ES, Nickel VL. Incomplete traumatic quadriplegia. A ten-year review. *JAMA.* 1971;216(3):473-478. doi:10.1001/jama.1971.03180290049006
18. Dimar JR, Carreon LY, Riina J, Schwartz DG, Harris MB. Early versus late stabilization of the spine in the polytrauma patient. *Spine.* 2010;35(21)(suppl):S187-S192. doi:10.1097/BRS.0b013e3181f32bcd
19. Linn WS, Adkins RH, Gong H Jr, Waters RL. Pulmonary function in chronic spinal cord injury: a cross-sectional survey of 222 southern California adult outpatients. *Arch Phys Med Rehabil.* 2000;81(6):757-763. doi:10.1016/S0003-9993(00)90107-2
20. McKinley WO, Gittler MS, Kirshblum SC, Stiens SA, Groah SL. Spinal cord injury medicine. 2. Medical complications after spinal cord injury: identification and management. *Arch Phys Med Rehabil.* 2002;83(3)(suppl 1):S58-S64, S90-S98. doi:10.1053/apmr.2002.32159
21. van den Berg ME, Castellote JM, de Pedro-Cuesta J, Mahillo-Fernandez I. Survival after spinal cord injury: a systematic review. *J Neurotrauma.* 2010;27(8):1517-1528. doi:10.1089/neu.2009.1138
22. Short DJ, Silver JR, Lehr RP. Electromyographic study of sternocleidomastoid and scalene muscles in tetraplegic subjects during respiration. *Int Disabil Stud.* 1991;13(2):46-49. doi:10.3109/03790799109166683

23. Jain NB, Sullivan M, Kazis LE, Tun CG, Garshick E. Factors associated with health-related quality of life in chronic spinal cord injury. *Am J Phys Med Rehabil.* 2007;86(5):387-396. doi:10.1097/PHM.0b013e31804a7d00
24. Berlowitz DJ, Wadsworth B, Ross J. Respiratory problems and management in people with spinal cord injury. *Breathe (Sheff).* 2016;12(4):328-340. doi:10.1183/20734735.012616
25. Kirshblum S, Millis S, McKinley W, Tulsky D. Late neurologic recovery after traumatic spinal cord injury. *Arch Phys Med Rehabil.* 2004;85(11):1811-1817. doi:10.1016/j.apmr.2004.03.015
26. Chang WK, Jung YS, Oh MK, Kim K. Quantitative assessment of proprioception using dynamometer in incomplete spinal cord injury patients: a preliminary study. *Ann Rehabil Med.* 2017;41(2):218-224. doi:10.5535/arm.2017.41.2.218
27. Strommen JA. Management of spasticity from spinal cord dysfunction. *Neurol Clin.* 2013;31(1):269-286. doi:10.1016/j.ncl.2012.09.013
28. Guillaume D, Van Havenbergh A, Vloeberghs M, Vidal J, Roeste G. A clinical study of intrathecal baclofen using a programmable pump for intractable spasticity. *Arch Phys Med Rehabil.* 2005;86(11):2165-2171. doi:10.1016/j.apmr.2005.05.018
29. Consortium for Spinal Cord Medicine. *Neurogenic Bowel Management in Adults with Spinal Cord Injury.* Washington, DC: Paralyzed Veterans of America; 1998.
30. Benevento BT, Sipski ML. Neurogenic bladder, neurogenic bowel, and sexual dysfunction in people with spinal cord injury. *Phys Ther.* 2002;82(6):601-612. doi:10.1093/ptj/82.6.601
31. Jackson AB, Wadley VA. Multicenter study of women's self-reported reproductive health after spinal cord injury. *Arch Phys Med Rehabil.* 1999;80:1420-1428.
32. Gunduz H, Binak DF. Autonomic dysreflexia: an important cardiovascular complication in spinal cord injury patients. *Cardiol J.* 2012;19(2):215-219. doi:10.5603/CJ.2012.0040
33. Comarr AE. Autonomic dysreflexia (hyperreflexia). *J Am ParaplegiaSoc.* 1984;7(3):53-57. doi:10.1080/01952307.1984.11719608
34. Acute management of autonomic dysreflexia: adults with spinal cord injury presenting to health-care facilities. Consortium for spinal cord. *J Spinal Cord Med.* 1997;20(3):284-308. doi:10.1080/10790268.1997.11719480
35. Naftchi NE, Richardson JS. Autonomic dysreflexia: pharmacological management of hypertensive crises in spinal cord injured patients. *J Spinal Cord Med.* 1997;20(3):355-360.
36. Ditunno JF, Little JW, Tessler A, Burns AS. Spinal shock revisited: a four-phase model. *Spinal Cord.* 2004;42(7):383-395. doi:10.1038/sj.sc.3101603
37. Krassioukov A, Eng JJ, Warburton DER, Teasall R. SCIRE research team. A systematic review of the management of orthostatic hypotension following spinal cord injury. *Arch Phys Med Rehabil.* 2009;90(5):876-885. doi:10.1016/j.apmr.2009.01.009
38. Kushner DS, Alvarez G. Dual diagnosis: traumatic brain injury with spinal cord injury. *Phys Med Rehabil Clin N Am.* 2014;25(3):681-696, ix-x. doi:10.1016/j.pmr.2014.04.005
39. Sakellariou VI, Grigoriou E, Mavrogenis AF, Soucacos PN, Papagelopoulos PJ. Heterotopic ossification following traumatic brain injury and spinal cord injury: insight into the etiology and pathophysiology. *J Musculoskelet Neuronal Interact.* 2012;12(4):230-240.
40. Garland DE. A clinical perspective on common forms of acquired heterotopic ossification. *Clin Orthop Relat Res.* 1991;(263):13-29. doi:10.1097/00003086-199102000-00003
41. Gifre L, Vidal J, Carrasco J, et al. Incidence of skeletal fractures after traumatic spinal cord injury: a 10-year follow-up study. *Clin Rehabil.* 2014;28(4):361-369. doi:10.1177/0269215513501905
42. Beckman MG, Hooper WC, Critchley SE, Ortel TL. Venous thromboembolism: a public health concern. *Am J Prev Med.* 2010;38(4)(suppl):S495-S501. doi:10.1016/j.amepre.2009.12.017
43. Do JG, Kim H, Sung DH. Incidence of deep vein thrombosis after spinal cord injury in Korean patients at acute rehabilitation unit. *J Korean Med Sci.* 2013;28(9):1382-1387. doi:10.3346/jkms.2013.28.9.1382
44. Wells PS, Owen C, Doucette S, Fergusson D, Tran H. Does this patient have deep vein thrombosis? *JAMA.* 2006;295(2):199-207. doi:10.1001/jama.295.2.199
45. Thompson L, Yakura J. Aging related functional changes in people with spinal cord injury. *Top Spinal Cord Rehabil.* 2001;6(3):69-82. doi:10.1310/MEUF-J0A0-FUDK-B49N
46. Bauman WA, Adkins RH, Spungen AM, Kemp BJ, Waters RL. The effect of residual neurological deficit on serum lipoproteins in individuals with chronic spinal cord injury. *Spinal Cord.* 1998;36(1):13-17. doi:10.1038/sj.sc.3100513
47. Sisto SA, Lorenz DJ, Hutchinson K, Wenzel L, Harkema S, Krassioukav A. Cardiovascular status of individuals with incomplete spinal cord injury from 7 NeuroRecovery Network rehabilitation centers. *Arch Phys Med Rehabil.* 2102;93(9):1578-1587.
48. Kübler-Ross E. *On Death and Dying.* New York, NY: Macmillan Publishing; 1969.
49. Williams R, Murray A. Prevalence of depression after spinal cord injury: a meta-analysis. *Arch Phys Med Rehabil.* 2015;96(1):133-140. doi:10.1016/j.apmr.2014.08.016
50. Kraft R, Dorstyn D. Psychosocial correlates of depression following spinal injury: A systematic review. *J Spinal Cord Med.* 2015;38(5):571-583. doi:10.1179/2045772314Y.0000000295
51. Dijkers M, Bryce T, Zanca J. Prevalence of chronic pain after traumatic spinal cord injury: a systematic review. *J Rehabil Res Dev.* 2009;46(1):13-29. doi:10.1682/JRRD.2008.04.0053
52. Van Straaten MG, Cloud BA, Zhao KD, Fortune E, Morrow MMB. Maintaining shoulder health after spinal cord injury: a guide to understanding treatments for shoulder pain. *Arch Phys Med Rehabil.* 2017;98(5):1061-1063. doi:10.1016/j.apmr.2016.10.005
53. Burchiel KJ, Hsu FP. Pain and spasticity after spinal cord injury: mechanisms and treatment. *Spine.* 2001;26(24)(suppl):S146-S160. doi:10.1097/00007632-200112151-00024
54. Jutzeler CR, Curt A, Kramer JLK. Relationship between chronic pain and brain reorganization after deafferentation: A systematic review of functional MRI findings. *Neuroimage Clin.* 2015;9:599-606. doi:10.1016/j.nicl.2015.09.018

55. Kuan YH, Shyu BC. Nociceptive transmission and modulation via P2X receptors in central pain syndrome. *Mol Brain.* 2016;9(1):58. doi:10.1186/s13041-016-0240-4
56. Boldt I, Eriks-Hoogland I, Brinkhof MWG, de Bie R, Joggi D, von Elm E. Non-pharmacological interventions for chronic pain in people with spinal cord injury. [review]. *Cochrane Database Syst Rev.* 2014;11(11):CD009177. doi:10.1002/14651858.CD009177.pub2
57. Skin Care & Pressure Sores. Part 2: Preventing Pressure Sores, 2009. Spinal Cord Injury Model Systems Consumer Information. https://craighospital.org/uploads/Educational-PDFs/Model-Systems/322.Model-System-Preventing-Pressure-Sores.pdf. Accessed May 8, 2018.
58. Treatment of Pressure Ulcers. Clinical Practice Guideline #15 (AHCPR Publication #95-0652). Rockville, MD: US Department of Health and Human Services; 1994.
59. Coggrave MJ, Rose LS. A specialist seating assessment clinic: changing pressure relief practice. *Spinal Cord.* 2003;41(12):692-695. doi:10.1038/sj.sc.3101527
60. Rubayi S, Pompan D, Garland D. Proximal femoral resection and myocutaneous flap for treatment of pressure ulcers in spinal injury patients. *Ann Plast Surg.* 1991;27(2):132-138. doi:10.1097/00000637-199108000-00007
61. Kirshblum S, Millis S, McKinley W, Tulsky D. Late neurologic recovery after traumatic spinal cord injury. *Arch Phys Med Rehabil.* 2004;85(11):1811-1817. doi:10.1016/j.apmr.2004.03.015
62. Pollard ME, Apple DF. Factors associated with improved neurologic outcomes in patients with incomplete tetraplegia. *Spine.* 2003;28(1):33-39. doi:10.1097/00007632-200301010-00009
63. Roth EJ, Lawler MH, Yarkony GM. Traumatic central cord syndrome: clinical features and functional outcomes. *Arch Phys Med Rehabil.* 1990;71(1):18-23.
64. Bracken MB. Steroids for acute spinal cord injury. *Cochrane Database Syst Rev.* 2012;1(1):CD001046.
65. Arora B, Suresh S. Spinal cord injuries in older children: is there a role for high-dose methylprednisolone? *Pediatr Emerg Care.* 2011;27(12):1192-1194. doi:10.1097/PEC.0b013e31823b4d06
66. Qian T, Guo X, Levi AD, Vanni S, Shebert RT, Sipski ML. High-dose methylprednisolone may cause myopathy in acute spinal cord injury patients. *Spinal Cord.* 2005;43(4):199-203. doi:10.1038/sj.sc.3101681
67. Waters RL, Adkins R, Yakura J, Sie I. Donal Munro Lecture: functional and neurologic recovery following acute SCI. *J Spinal Cord Med.* 1998;21(3):195-199. doi:10.1080/10790268.1998.11719526
68. Waters RL, Adkins RH, Yakura JS, Sie I. Motor and sensory recovery following incomplete tetraplegia. *Arch Phys Med Rehabil.* 1994;75(3):306-311. doi:10.1016/0003-9993(94)90034-5
69. Mulroy SJ, Gronley JK, Newsam CJ, Perry J. Electromyographic activity of shoulder muscles during wheelchair propulsion by paraplegic persons. *Arch Phys Med Rehabil.* 1996;77(2):187-193. doi:10.1016/S0003-9993(96)90166-5
70. Powers CM, Newsam CJ, Gronley JK, Fontaine CA, Perry J. Isometric shoulder torque in subjects with spinal cord injury. *Arch Phys Med Rehabil.* 1994;75(7):761-765.
71. Gronley JK, Newsam CJ, Mulroy SJ, Rao SS, Perry J, Helm M. Electromyographic and kinematic analysis of the shoulder during four activities of daily living in men with C6 tetraplegia. *J Rehabil Res Dev.* 2000;37(4):423-432.
72. Silva AC, Neder JA, Chiurciu MV, et al. Effect of aerobic training on ventilatory muscle endurance of spinal cord injured men. *Spinal Cord.* 1998;36(4):240-245. doi:10.1038/sj.sc.3100575
73. Gilgoff IS, Barras DM, Jones MS, Adkins HV. Neck breathing: a form of voluntary respiration for the spine-injured ventilator-dependent quadriplegic child. *Pediatrics.* 1988;82(5):741-745.
74. Warren VC. Glossopharyngeal and neck accessory muscle breathing in a young adult with C2 complete tetraplegia resulting in ventilator dependency. *Phys Ther.* 2002;82(6):590-600. doi:10.1093/ptj/82.6.590
75. Liaw MY, Lin MC, Cheng PT, Wong MK, Tang FT. Resistive inspiratory muscle training: its effectiveness in patients with acute complete cervical cord injury. *Arch Phys Med Rehabil.* 2000;81(6):752-756. doi:10.1016/S0003-9993(00)90106-0
76. Lerman RM, Weiss MS. Progressive resistive exercise in weaning high quadriplegics from the ventilator. *Paraplegia.* 1987;25(2):130-135.
77. Linn WS, Spungen AM, Gong H Jr, Adkins RH, Bauman WA, Waters RL. Forced vital capacity in two large outpatient populations with chronic spinal cord injury. *Spinal Cord.* 2001;39(5):263-268. doi:10.1038/sj.sc.3101155
78. Consortium for Spinal Cord Medicine. Outcomes Following Traumatic Spinal Cord Injury: Clinical Practice Guidelines for Health-Care Professionals. Washington, DC. *Paralyzed Veterans of America.* 1999;9:10-20.
79. Somers MF. *Spinal Cord Injury: Functional Rehabilitation.* Upper Saddle River, NJ: Pearson Education; 2010.
80. Newsam CJ, Mulroy SJ, Gronley JK, Bontrager EL, Perry J. Temporal-spatial characteristics of wheelchair propulsion. Effects of level of spinal cord injury, terrain, and propulsion rate. *Am J Phys Med Rehabil.* 1996;75(4):292-299. doi:10.1097/00002060-199607000-00010
81. Beekman CE, Miller-Porter L, Schoneberger M. Energy cost of propulsion in standard and ultralight wheelchairs in people with spinal cord injuries. *Phys Ther.* 1999;79(2):146-158. doi:10.1093/ptj/79.2.146
82. Waters RL, Mulroy S. The energy expenditure of normal and pathologic gait. *Gait Posture.* 1999;9(3):207-231. doi:10.1016/S0966-6362(99)00009-0
83. Harvey LA, Katalinic OM, Herbert RD, Moseley AM, Lannin NA, Schurr K. Stretch for the treatment and prevention of contractures. *Cochrane Database Syst Rev.* 2017;1(2):CD007455. doi:10.1002/14651858.CD007455.pub3
84. Wu M, Landry JM, Schmit BD, Hornby TG, Yen SC. Robotic resistance treadmill training improves locomotor function in human spinal cord injury: a pilot study. *Arch Phys Med Rehabil.* 2012;93(5):782-789. doi:10.1016/j.apmr.2011.12.018
85. Koopman B, van Asseldonk EH, van der Kooij H, van Dijk W, Ronsse R. Rendering potential wearable robot designs with the LOPES gait trainer. *IEEE Int Conf Rehabil Robot.* 2011;2011:5975448. doi:10.1109/ICORR.2011.5975448
86. Karelis AD, Carvalho LP, Castillo MJ, Gagnon DH, Aubertin-Leheudre M. Effect on body composition and bone mineral density of walking with a robotic exoskeleton in adults with chronic spinal cord injury. *J Rehabil Med.* 2017;49(1):84-87. doi:10.2340/16501977-2173

87. Cheung EYY, Ng TKW, Yu KKK, Kwan RLC, Cheing GLY. Robot-assisted training for people with spinal cord injury: a meta-analysis. *Arch Phys Med Rehabil.* 2017;98(11):2320-2331.e12. doi:10.1016/j.apmr.2017.05.015
88. Beekman C, Perry J, Boyd LA, Newsam CJ, Mulroy SJ. The effects of a dorsiflexion-stopped ankle-foot orthosis on walking in individuals with incomplete spinal cord injury. *Top Spinal Cord Inj Rehabil.* 2000;4(4):54-62. doi:10.1310/Q7AH-NUAL-J7V3-LK85
89. Crane DA, Little JW, Burns SP. Weight gain following spinal cord injury: a pilot study. *J Spinal Cord Med.* 2011;34(2):227-232. doi:10.1179/2045772311Y.0000000001
90. Miller LE, Herbert WG. Health and economic benefits of physical activity for patients with spinal cord injury. *Clinicoecon Outcomes Res.* 2016;8:551-558. doi:10.2147/CEOR.S115103
91. Evans N, Wingo B, Sasso E, Hicks A, Gorgey AS, Harness E. Exercise recommendations and considerations for persons with spinal cord injury. *Arch Phys Med Rehabil.* 2015;96(9):1749-1750. doi:10.1016/j.apmr.2015.02.005
92. Jain NB, Higgins LD, Katz JN, Garshick E. Association of shoulder pain with the use of mobility devices in persons with chronic spinal cord injury. *PM R.* 2010;2(10):896-900. doi:10.1016/j.pmrj.2010.05.004
93. Eriks-Hoogland IE, Hoekstra T, de Groot S, Stucki G, Post MW, van der Woude LH. Trajectories of musculoskeletal shoulder pain after spinal cord injury: identification and predictors. *J Spinal Cord Med.* 2014;37(3):288-298. doi:10.1179/2045772313Y.0000000168

Chapter 12

Clients With Traumatic Brain Injury

Dennis Klima, PT, MS, PhD, DPT, GCS, NCS

KEY WORDS Coma | Coup/contrecoup injury | Diffuse axonal shearing | Glasgow Coma Scale | Persistent vegetative state | Rancho Los Amigos Levels of Cognitive Function | Traumatic brain injury

Chapter Objectives

- Describe major causes of traumatic brain injury (TBI).
- Outline the impact of TBI along the International Classification of Functioning, Disability and Health (ICF) continuum.
- Discuss mechanisms of injury and medical complications associated with TBI.
- Describe the major categories of the Glasgow Coma Scale.
- Outline the major levels and associated cognitive behavior included in the Rancho Los Amigos Levels of Cognitive Function.
- Describe key components of the physical therapist's examination for patients recovering from a TBI.
- Identify common body structure/function, activity, and participation deficits seen in this special patient population.
- List physical therapy management precautions for individuals with TBI.
- Describe major interventions performed for those musculoskeletal and neuromuscular deficits noted in the physical therapist's examination.
- Discuss techniques for integrating both cognitive and functional training strategies to advance the patient toward those established goals.
- Describe key activities associated with patient discharge planning, home programs, equipment procurement, and community integration.
- Describe management interventions for the patient with concussion.
- Describe an exercise progression used to prepare athletes for safe return to play in a designated sport following a concussion injury.
- Describe primary, secondary, and tertiary blast injuries associated with high-order explosion.

Traumatic Brain Injury: Overview

Managing clients with a TBI presents a major challenge for all health care professionals working with this special patient population. More than 2 million people sustain a TBI in the United States annually; furthermore, TBI resulted in 2.8 million emergency department visits, hospitalizations, and deaths in 2013.[1] A *TBI* may be operationally defined as an "alteration in brain function, or other evidence of brain pathology, caused by an external force."[2] While TBI accounts for a large portion of injury-related deaths in the United States, the majority of those treated injuries are classified as mild.[1,3] These include sports concussion injuries.

Major causes of head injury include falls and being struck by an object. Motor vehicle and recreational vehicle accidents are the third leading cause of emergency department visits and hospitalizations.[1,3] Additional causes include intentional self-harm injury. TBI rates are higher for males in all age brackets, and the major cause of TBI-related hospitalization is a fall episode among people 0 to

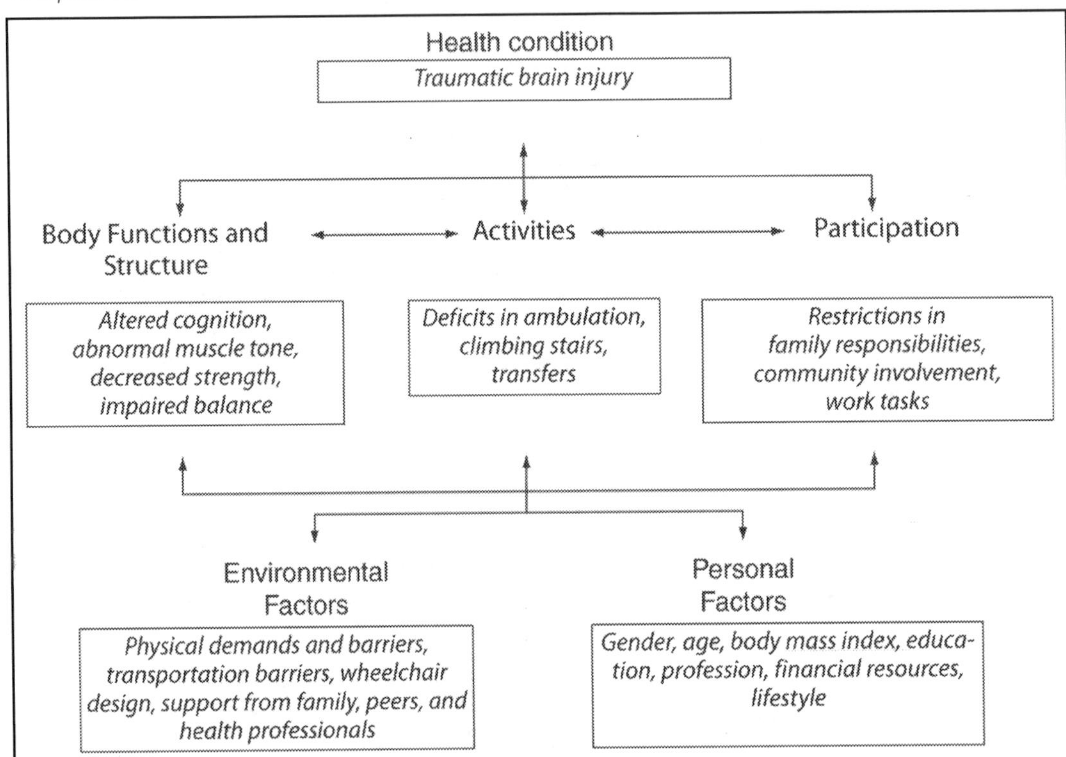

Figure 12-1. Integration of the ICF framework with physical therapy management of clients with traumatic brain injury.

14 years of age and older than 45 years.[1,3] For individuals 65 years or older, the leading cause of TBI mortality is a fall. Hospitalization and death rates are highest among adults 75 years of age and older.[1,3]

Head injury sequelae can be devastating and affect virtually every component of the quality of life: self-care, home management, work responsibilities, and leisure activities.[4] Poor recovery outcomes can eventually lead to long-term institutional placement if caregiving demands exceed available resources in the home environment. Public awareness has increasingly focused on injury prevention through vigilance, with fall prevention strategies for older individuals and increased helmet use during recreational sports and cycling activities. Local and national brain injury associations serve as strong advocacy catalysts for children and adults recovering from a TBI.

Theoretical Framework: The Role of the Physical Therapist Assistant

Physical therapist assistants perform interventions associated with deficits at all levels of the ICF model: body structure/function, activity, and participation components (Figure 12-1).[5] In addition, these domains may be affected by environmental as well as personal factors. Neurological interventions with this special patient population require a level of expertise beyond entry-level practice. Physical therapist assistants working with these clients have gained experience through mentoring, continuing education, and shadowing activities in the clinical arena. Clinical expertise and additional responsibilities may have also developed through a career ladder progression in the rehabilitation setting. Physical therapists and physical therapist assistants with expertise in neurological patient management serve as powerful expert mentors to facilitate clinical expertise among novice clinicians and students.[6] Physical therapist assistants with exceptional clinical expertise in managing patients with TBI and other neurologic diagnoses can elect to be recognized with the formal American Physical Therapy Association's Advanced Proficiency in neuromuscular patient management.

It should be noted that physical therapists and physical therapist assistants may initially elect to approach patient management through a team effort to enhance the physical therapist assistant's intervention skills with patients with TBI. The experienced physical therapist assistant may then be delegated select interventions for more complicated patients for whom patient and situational considerations are less stable and predictable.[7] For example, functional activities with the agitated patient dictate immediate intervention modification given potential outbursts of hostility or inappropriate behavior. Similarly, patients in a minimally conscious state may require ongoing modification of the plan of care from session to session. Effective delegation strategies are enhanced by ongoing communication with the supervising physical therapist to optimize interventions the physical therapist assistant performs in the trajectory of care.

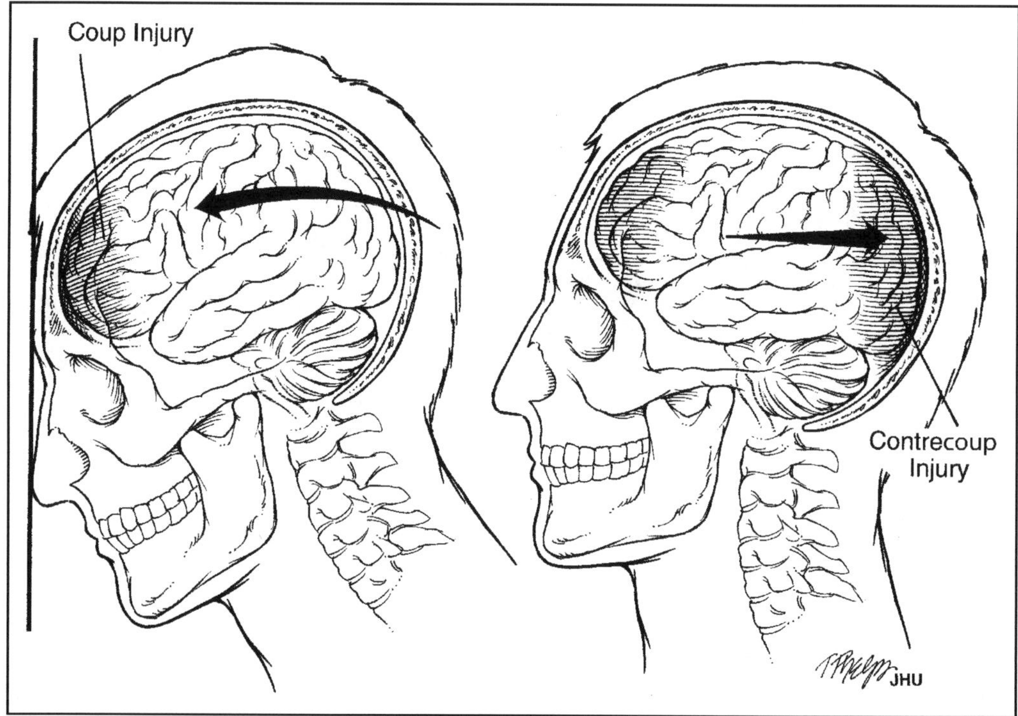

Figure 12-2. Mechanisms of injury: coup and contrecoup injuries. (Illustration by Tim Phelps.)

Medical and Recovery Issues

Mechanisms of Injury

Following a traumatic insult, the initial site of impact to the brain is known as the *coup injury*. Because of the rebound effect that occurs in the cranium following the initial impact, a *contrecoup* injury will often occur (Figure 12-2). The term *diffuse axonal shearing or injury* refers to neuronal damage associated with traumatic rotational acceleration and deceleration of the brain during unrestricted movement.[8] Severe diffuse axonal shearing or injury can result in coma, and extensive brain tissue deformation can occur through shearing forces and inertial loading incurred during the injury. Head injuries generally fall into 2 categories: open and closed. The skull and meninges remain intact following a closed-head injury, whereas open injuries cause fracture and rupture of these protective structures. *Contusions* refer to areas of neuronal death and hemorrhage that occur at the site of injury and are commonly seen in the frontal and temporal regions. Contusions may also occur at a distant site from the initial impact.

Injuries sustained within the cranial vault may also be accompanied by concomitant edema, which adversely increases intracranial pressure (ICP). Normal ICP levels of between 0 and 15 mm Hg can substantially escalate to near-fatal levels. In addition, cerebral perfusion pressure may be impaired following a sustained head injury if neural oxygen supply becomes inadequate.[9] Additional secondary damage results from tissue hypoxemia or infection, with infection more commonly arising when open penetration to the skull occurs during the injury.

Complications

Unfortunately, TBI rarely occurs in isolation without other orthopedic or internal organ trauma. Skull fractures may be present and are classified by the specific type of fracture line or location. Common fractures include linear, depressed, and basilar skull fractures; additionally, each type of fracture is associated with unique characteristics. For example, depressed skull fractures often occur following a blow to the skull, whereas basilar skull fractures are associated with a high incidence of orbital bleeding, cranial nerve damage, and meningitis.[10] In addition to these complications, patients can experience multiple facial fractures and scalp lacerations. Facial fracture severity is outlined in the LeFort classification system. Extremity fractures and internal organ damage further create potential life-threatening complications, which lengthen recovery periods. Common areas of injury include pelvic, femoral, and humeral fractures. The presence of heterotopic ossifications, a condition characterized by abnormal of ectopic bone formation in patients following spinal cord injury and TBI, may cause further joint motion restrictions.[11]

Another complicating factor to recovery is the presence of a hematoma after the head injury (Figure 12-3).[12] Subdural hematomas refer to rupture of the cerebral bridging vein complex with resultant bleeding into the subdural space. Fluctuating periods of lucency characterize this type of complication. An epidural, or extradural, hematoma is

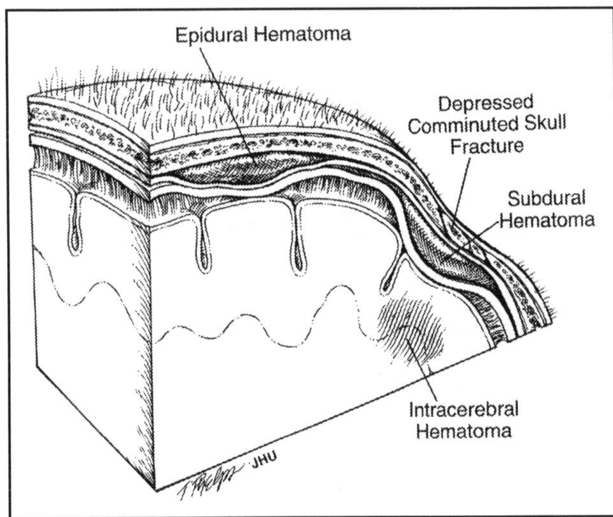

Figure 12-3. Complications from TBI. (Illustration by Tim Phelps.)

usually caused by a tear in the middle meningeal artery. Patients sustaining these types of hematomas can experience varying degrees of altered consciousness, headaches, or other signs and symptoms specific to the areas of the lesion. Intracerebral hematomas are located deeper within the brain and can accompany more severe traumatic injuries. Extensive hematoma formation may require surgical evacuation though a craniotomy procedure. These massive hematomas can potentially cause a hemispheric midline shift because of the size of the space-occupying lesion. People with a midline shift (ie, lateral displacement of the brainstem and medial central nervous system structures, larger than 5 mm) will more likely need ambulation and activities of daily living assistance at rehabilitation discharge.[12] Patients sustaining severe injuries undergo radical craniotomy procedures with and resultant removal of portions of the skull. Subsequent cranioplasty procedures with bone grafting are later performed to ensure neural tissue protection.

Seizures present further medical complications following a TBI and may vary from mild to those of the tonic-clonic variety. Seizures can occur immediately following the injury or can develop later in the course of recovery. Some evidence suggests that the development of late post-traumatic seizures is linked to more extensive brain damage.[13] Patients are placed on prophylactic anticonvulsant medications following a head injury to manage the recurrent seizure activity. Health care professionals who work with patients recovering from TBI should be competent in emergency procedures for those patients having post-traumatic seizure episodes to ensure patient safety during a seizure event. Patients should be protected during the episode, and the type and duration of behavior should be well-documented.

Recurrent, spontaneous seizure activity necessitates medication management. Common medications used for seizure management include Dilantin (phenytoin), Tegretol (carbamazepine), and Luminal or Solfoton (phenobarbital).[14] Pertinent adverse effects of seizure medications should also be recognized in the rehabilitation setting. Specifically targeting the motor cortex, phenytoin inhibits abnormal electrical discharge activity in the brain.[14] Major side effects include ataxia, nervousness, and confusion. Phenobarbital and carbamazepine may both induce drowsiness as a potential side effect, and patients should be monitored for problematic oversedation while in therapy.[14] Zonegran (zonisamide) demonstrates fewer adverse cognitive side effects, although it may induce distal upper extremity dyskinesias.

Intensive Care Unit Management

Following a TBI, appropriate medical intervention must immediately address direct injuries as well as secondary complications. Multitrauma patients are often transported to local or regional trauma centers. Severe injuries necessitate intubation and the need for multiple intravenous lines. An ICP monitor may be placed to record ongoing pressure changes and gradients. Osmotic diuretics are used to decrease adverse ICP.

Damage to the abdominal or thoracic cavities can warrant chest tube placement, and those patients requiring extensive ventricular or fluid monitoring may have a specialized pulmonary artery monitor, the Swan-Ganz catheter, inserted.

In the very acute stage of medical intervention, patients will be evaluated using the Glasgow Coma Scale, and resultant scores will categorize the severity of the injury. The instrument assesses 3 domains of function in individuals following head injury: motor performance, eye opening, and verbal response (Table 12-1).[15,16] The scale is composed of 15 points, and injury severity is depicted through summation of the points from each of the 3 sections. Glasgow Coma Scale scores from 13 to 15 designate mild injury, 9 to 12 moderate injury, and 3 to 8 severe TBI. Patients with mild brain injury generally demonstrate less severe loss of consciousness (less than 20 to 30 minutes) and post-traumatic amnesia (less than 24 hours).[17] Manifestations of moderate and severe brain injury are more pronounced and can be linked to brainstem injury. Factors associated with poorer outcomes include associated secondary injuries, persistent coma, and lingering post-traumatic amnesia.[18] The rehabilitation team members should be aware of the initial Glasgow Coma Scale score and ensuing complications at the time of injury to modify any examination or intervention activities.

Classification of Levels of Recovery

Recovery from TBI depends on factors related to the extent of the injury, associated medical complications, and the patient's premorbid status. The Rancho Los Amigos Levels of Cognitive Function are often used to categorize

Table 12-1

Glasgow Coma Scale

Eyes	Open	Spontaneously	4
		To verbal command	3
		To pain	2
	No response		1
Best Motor Response	To verbal stimulus	Obeys command	6
	To painful stimulus	Localizes pain	5
		Flexion-withdrawal	4
		Flexion-abnormal (decorticate rigidity)	3
		Extension (decerebrate rigidity)	2
		No response	1
Best Verbal Response	Oriented and converses		5
	Disoriented and converses		4
	Inappropriate words		3
	Incomprehensible sounds		2
	No response		1
Total Range			**3 to 15**

Adapted from Teasdale G, Jennett B. Assessment of coma and impaired consciousness. A practical scale. *Lancet.* 1974;2(7872):81-84. doi:10.1016/S0140-6736(74)91639-0.

patients following a TBI and to describe behavioral patterns in the sequence of recovery (Table 12-2).[19] Composed of 8 levels, the original scale illustrates a recovery continuum that begins with the patient's initial unresponsive status and then tracks cognitive improvement to the final behavioral category.[19,20] The initial 3 levels reflect the patient's minimally responsive phase. Level I denotes no response, whereas Level II reflects an observed generalized response to a designated stimulus.[19,20] Such generalized responses often are characterized by gross body movements or an increase in vital signs. Patients in the third level begin demonstrating more specific elicited response patterns, such as a hand squeeze or visual tracking in response to a verbal stimulus. It should be noted that patients with massive injuries and severe brain damage can permanently remain within these initial classification levels. The fourth level of the Rancho scale describes behavior related to the agitated patient. At this level, the patient is unable to integrate the multitude of sensory experiences in the immediate environment. The patient's gross attention to the environment is very limited. Aggression may arise when periods of overstimulation occur, and the patient may become distracted very easily. Young nonverbal pediatric patients may exhibit continual crying at this phase. The physician or physical therapist needs to differentiate agitation from anger. Patients who are angry will often bite, use inappropriate verbal sayings, or strike at the clinician.

Levels V through VIII demonstrate gradual resolution of cognitive deficits toward behavior that is both purposeful and appropriate. In Level V, agitated behavior wanes, although the patient continues to demonstrate substantial deficits in language, memory, and praxis. The patient remains highly distractible and shows difficulty focusing on a specific task and demonstrates inappropriate behavior. Confused appropriate behavior is designated in Level VI, and the patient begins demonstrating increased goal-directed behavior with the ability to follow simple commands.[19,20]

In the remaining 2 Rancho levels (VII-Automatic/Appropriate and VIII-Purposeful/Appropriate), the patient becomes increasingly oriented and demonstrates improved learning capacity. In addition, responses become more automatic. Judgment may continue to remain impaired in the final levels. For example, the patient may have difficulty performing appropriate activities during emergency situations at home.

An updated version of the Rancho scale includes 2 additional stages: Levels IX and X. In Level IX (Purposeful-Appropriate; Standby Assistance), the patient can shift between 2 tasks with accurate completion. However, standby assistance may be required with unfamiliar activities or with escalating task demands. In Level X (Purposeful-Appropriate; Modified Independent), the patient completes multitask activities and can independently modify task

Table 12-2

Rancho Los Amigos Levels of Cognitive Function

I. No Response The patient appears to be in a deep sleep and is completely unresponsive to any stimuli.
II. Generalized Response The patient reacts inconsistently and non-purposefully to stimuli in a nonspecific manner. Responses are limited and often the same regardless of the stimulus presented. Responses may be physiologic changes, gross body movements, and/or vocalization.
III. Localized Response The patient reacts specifically but inconsistently to stimuli. Responses are directly related to the type of stimulus presented. The patient may follow simple commands in an inconsistent, delayed manner, such as with closing of the eyes or squeezing the hand.
IV. Confused/Agitated Behavior is bizarre and non-purposeful, relative to the immediate environment. The patient does not discriminate among people or objects and is unable to cooperate with treatment efforts. Verbalizations are frequently incoherent and/or inappropriate to the environment. Confabulation may be present. Gross attention to the environment is very short and selective attention is often nonexistent. The patient lacks short-term recall.
V. Confused/Inappropriate The patient is able to respond to simple commands fairly consistently. However, with increased complexity of commands or lack of any external structure, responses are non-purposeful, random, or fragmented. The patient has gross attention to the environment, but is highly distractible and lacks ability to focus attention to a specific task. With structure, the patient may be able to converse on a social-automatic level for short periods of time. Verbalization is often inappropriate and confabulatory; moreover, memory is severely impaired. The patient often shows inappropriate use of objects. He or she may perform previously learned tasks with structure but is unable to learn new information.
VI. Confused/Appropriate The patient shows goal-directed behavior but is dependent on external input for direction. He/she follows simple directions consistently and shows carryover for relearned tasks with little or no carryover for new tasks. Responses may be incorrect due to memory problems but appropriate to the situation. Past memories show more depth and detail than recent memory.
VII. Automatic/Appropriate The patient appears appropriate and oriented within the hospital and home settings. He/she goes through daily routines automatically and frequently in a robot-like fashion. The patient has minimal-to-absent confusion but has shallow recall of activities. There is carryover for new learning, but at a decreased rate. With structure, the patient is able to initiate social or recreational activities. Judgment remains impaired.
VIII. Purposeful/Appropriate The patient is able to recall and integrate past and recent events and is aware of and responds to the environment. He/she shows carryover for new learning and needs no supervision once activities are learned. The patient may continue to show deficiencies, relative to premorbid abilities, in quality and rate of processing, abstract reasoning, tolerance for stress, and judgment in emergencies or unusual circumstances.
Reprinted with permission from Hagen C, Malkmus D, Durham P. Levels of cognitive functioning. In: *Rehabilitation of the Head Injured Adult: Comprehensive Physical Management.* Downey, CA: Professional Staff Association of Rancho Los Amigos Hospital; 1979.

demands. Episodic depression can occur in these final stages, with frustration exhibited when activities cannot be performed efficiently or when assistance is required.[21]

Following the acute rehabilitation phase, patients will be discharged to receive further rehabilitation at a subacute facility, rehabilitation center, or nursing home. Patients may even return home provided that sufficient care and monitoring can be provided by the caregiver. Inpatient settings may initially be preferred to offer more intense therapy on a daily basis. Rehabilitation centers, however, often have specific policies that dictate minimum Rancho levels for admission, and placement can be difficult for patients at lower functional levels.[22]

Physical Therapy Management

Examination

The physical therapist will perform an examination prior to the initiation of select interventions by the physical therapist assistant. Given the patient's potential altered mental status, pertinent social history and home environment information may have to be obtained through family members or other caregivers. Families often provide very valuable background information related to the patient's ICF contextual factors such as the home living situation and environmental challenges. In performing a detailed systems review, the physical therapist will ascertain the degree to which the patient's injury has affected the overall baseline cognitive and functional status. Target tests and measures will further assess the extent of deficits along the ICF continuum.

The physical therapist assistant should be clearly aware of those alterations in arousal, mentation, and cognitive status that may be encountered when dealing with patients with TBI. Examination findings may indicate varied levels of arousal impairment consistent with coma or persistent vegetative state. The term *coma* refers to a lack of responsiveness to verbal stimuli, variable responses to other forms of stimuli, and an absent sleep-wake cycle.[23] *Persistent vegetative state* denotes similar patterns of unresponsive behavior and tends to reflect a condition that will be of longer duration. In this condition the patient is unaware of the immediate surroundings despite an intact sleep-wake cycle.

Severe disturbances in cognition, arousal, and communication may impede standard testing procedures. For instance, patients are often able to follow only simple 1-word commands, and examination strategies must be augmented. Key components of the cognitive examination area include orientation, level of consciousness, and memory. Confusion and disorientation may be considerable, and residual lethargy and sluggishness are often associated with delirium following head injury.[24] Furthermore, the patient may exhibit a concomitant period of *post-traumatic amnesia* (the time duration between the injury and subsequent ability to recall people and events) and display persistent memory deficits throughout recovery.

Additional neurological testing will include assessment of select cranial nerve integrity, sensation, and coordination. Patients with cerebellar deficits should be screened for extremity deficits, such as dysmetria and dysdiadochokinesia; moreover, trunk and axial ataxia patterns may be noted in sitting posture or gait activities. Neurological tests may uncover important findings that have implications for interventions by the physical therapist assistant. For example, sensory disturbances may call for therapeutic handling adaptations, and cranial nerve deficits require intervention adjustments because of such conditions as hemianopsia.

A detailed musculoskeletal examination will yield findings related to muscle tone, strength, and joint range of motion (ROM). Abnormalities in tone may be found in any one or all extremities. Patients with more severe injuries may demonstrate postural patterns consistent with decorticate or decerebrate rigidity. Patients with decerebrate rigidity display strong extension posturing in all 4 extremities. Patients with decorticate rigidity demonstrate grossly flexed upper extremities with a similar lower extremity extension positioning. The physical therapist may elect to quantify tonal disturbances through the Modified Ashworth Scale. In this scale, muscle tone is described through varying resistance felt throughout the available ROM.[25] Given the potential for joint contractures and limitations due to abnormal posturing or heterotopic ossification, joint integrity must be thoroughly assessed. Detailed goniometric measurements will underscore pertinent ROM limitations. When cognitive deficits impede formal testing procedures, examination of muscle performance may be completed through motor pattern analysis demonstrated in gravity-eliminated and antigravity planes. Patients at higher functional levels may be candidates for more traditional strength testing techniques.

Examination of the integument involves a systematic skin inspection to detect any possible skin irritation, rashes, or pressure ulcer areas. Patients who have begun posturing extremities are particularly at risk. The therapist must examine those areas that are particularly vulnerable for pressure sore development. These include the ischial tuberosities, greater trochanters, and sacrum. Patients who are bed-confined should be inspected for less common areas of skin compromise, such as the spine of the scapula or olecranon process. Protection devices may be indicated when the patient is unable to volitionally change positions in bed.

For patients at a higher level of function, examination activities will continue with assessment of all areas of functional mobility. Bed mobility activities, including bridging, rolling, and supine-to-sit transitions, will be observed for level of assistance required and qualitative performance strategies. Static and dynamic balance will be assessed to investigate postural control in sitting and standing. Common balance instruments used to identify fall risk in the elderly have been extrapolated to quantify balance performance in individuals with head injury (see Chapter 6) and include the Balance Evaluation Systems Test[26] and the Berg Balance Scale.[27] The physical therapist may elect to use these instruments because of substantial balance deficits, or with geriatric patients who have sustained a head injury because of a fall. Gait examination may be assessed with an emphasis on velocity (4- or 10-meter walk test), or dual task locomotion (Walking and Remembering Test).[28,29]

Careful examination of the patient's gait and locomotion status will identify such important findings as pertinent gait deviations, required level of assistance, and muscle substitution patterns. Lastly, aerobic capacity and functional endurance will be measured through vital sign response to activity, perceived exertion, or other standardized measures of aerobic capacity. These baseline measures are particularly important for patients recovering from severe brain injuries because of reported diminished exercise capacity and fitness levels.[30]

Table 12-3

Practice Patterns Associated With Adult Head Injury

Pattern 5D	Impaired motor function and sensory integrity associated with nonprogressive disorders of the central nervous system acquired in adolescence or adulthood
Pattern 5I	Impaired arousal, ROM, and motor control associated with coma, near coma, or vegetative state

Evaluation, Diagnosis, and Prognosis

Following the examination, the physical therapist will formulate a summation of findings in the evaluation and establish a diagnosis and prognosis. Diagnoses may be related to compromised cognition, motor function, and sensory integrity, and mobility secondary to the TBI. Historically, parameters of management for patients with TBI were delineated in the initial versions of the *Guide to Physical Therapist Practice, Second Edition*. Diagnostic labeling was tied to 2 key practice patterns addressed management of the adult patient with head injury (Table 12-3).[4] More recently, diagnostic clustering has been refined to include target deficits in the body structure/function, activities, and participation domains. Prognostication for patients with TBI is based on characteristics of the injury, comorbidity conditions, and previous level of function. The physical therapist's clinical decision-making process regarding the patient's prognosis will also be based on current evidence to support those short- and long-term goals established. For example, the physical therapist must consider that patients with decreased awareness of their limitations following head injury tend to set less-realistic goals.[31] In addition, brain injury severity, lower-extremity hypertonicity, and concomitant lower-extremity injuries have been shown to predict ambulation potential in children and adolescents following a TBI.[32] Complications such as heterotopic ossification have been associated with poorer functional outcomes following a TBI.[11]

Interventions

Initiating interventions within the physical therapist's plan of care requires careful analysis of those challenges in body structure/functions, activities, and participation. Moreover, the physical therapist assistant must carefully review the results of the physical therapist's tests and measures to effectively target effective interventions aligned with those established goals within the plan of care. Goniometric measurements and muscle test grades will direct types of exercise to be addressed and positional considerations. Furthermore, attention to upper motor neuron deficits will effectively allow the physical therapist assistant to incorporate therapeutic exercise strategies to improve the patient's motor control. Patients recovering from TBI may demonstrate varying levels of hemiplegia in accordance with the severity of the insult. Motor performance may progress from initial flaccidity to isolated movement patterns in the recovery sequence, and active dissociation should be recognized to track and facilitate recovery patterns. For example, the physical therapist assistant must note progress through increased complexity of extremity movement combinations as compared with abnormal synergy patterns. Finally, functional mobility activities will be implemented to address major deficits in bed and wheelchair (w/c) mobility, transfers, balance, and gait performance. Along with the physical therapist examination, the physical therapist assistant should look at the occupational therapy and speech-language pathology documentation for additional information pertinent to the patient's plan of care. These assessments will provide information related to perceptual, communication, and cognitive deficits that impact of essential activities of daily living.

Outcomes

Outcomes collection is an integral part of the Patient/Client Management Model. Outcomes will corroborate to the effectiveness of the plan of care and those interventions that have been rendered. The physical therapist will perform the discharge reexamination to assess the progress achieved since the initial examination. Select tests and measures will be repeated to compare admission and discharge performance. Patients and family members may be surveyed with patient satisfaction questionnaires to obtain data related to quality of services in both the inpatient and outpatient settings.

Specific Body Structure/Function and Activity Interventions

Seating Considerations and Pressure Relief

Careful consideration of all aspects of the patient's condition should be weighed when creating an initial seating system for the patient. The physical therapist assistant may work in conjunction with the supervising physical therapist in making adaptive changes to the w/c to optimize positioning and seating alignment. Patients lacking postural control may benefit from a tilt-in-space w/c with attached head positioning. A recliner w/c may be used for patients with spinal orthopedic devices and associated fractures. For propulsion maneuvers, patients with residual hemiparesis deficits may find a hemi-height w/c effective, given the reduced seat-to-floor height. When adapting any seating system for the patient's needs, it becomes important to recognize the advantages and disadvantages of any change that is proposed. For example, the addition of desk-style armrests to a w/c may be beneficial for approaching any table surface, although it may impede a patient's ability to perform a sit-to-stand maneuver if upper extremity assistance is required.

For a patient first using a w/c, appropriate time should be allotted for instruction in propulsion maneuvers and parts management. Patients should be taught brake-locking maneuvers, leg-rest management, and general propulsion strategies for level surface and turn negotiation. Important points of safety should be reinforced when cognitive deficits exist and judgment is impaired. Frequently, an initial short-term goal for the patient will be to independently propel between the physical therapy department and the rehab gym for scheduled sessions (Figure 12-4). For patients in a minimally conscious state, pressure relief may consist of dependent tilt-positioning in a manual tilt-in-space w/c. As the patient becomes more alert and self-aware, lateral lean and push-up maneuvers are implemented and reinforced.

Therapeutic Exercise

The physical therapist assistant may be delegated selected activities involving the application of therapeutic exercise programs for impaired joint integrity or muscle performance.[4] Given the prevailing weakness that develops from either the injury itself or the adverse effects of bedrest, patients may exhibit considerable deficits in muscle performance. The physical therapist assistant should be cautious in scrutinizing examination findings to discern specific muscle grades of tested muscles or the ratings of muscle tone to effectively position and stabilize affected areas. Appropriate therapeutic exercise programs and mobility activities should be implemented based on these test findings. For example, in an analysis of patients with TBI, Duong et al[33] found that those patients having less than 3/5 lower-extremity strength on admission required greater assistance with transfers and locomotion. Passive ROM and active-assisted strategies may be indicated for flaccid limbs, and the physical therapist assistant may be required to don and doff braces to effectively position an extremity.[34] Splints should be used as an adjunct to treatment.[34] Aggressive-passive ROM regimens are necessary to maintain joint integrity when hypertonicity results in prolonged flexed or extended posturing of extremities. In a study of 105 patients diagnosed with moderate or severe brain injury, it was noted that a major predisposing factor to ankle contracture development included dystonia in the inversion and plantar flexion musculature.[35]

Depending on the resultant hemiparesis from TBI, neurofacilitation techniques may be required to enhance optimum motor performance with upper motor neuron deficits (Figure 12-5). Active dissociation patterns can be used in conjunction with functional activities to promote active use of hemiparetic extremities.[36] In addition, strategies employing techniques such as weight-bearing can facilitate stabilization in flaccid extremities (see Chapters 5 and 13). Physical therapist assistants may elect to have patients perform bilateral extremity patterns for activation of weakened muscle groups.[37]

Interventions involving constraint-induced movement therapy in stroke rehabilitation have also proven to be beneficial in individuals recovering from TBI (see Chapter 5).[38] This procedure involves restraining the patient's unaffected upper extremity in an effort to promote increased functional use of the hemiparetic extremity.

The effective clinician should be innovative in adapting therapeutic regimens around prevailing cognitive deficits. Patients may benefit more from exercise activities within the context of a task rather than conventional cardinal plane performance (Figure 12-6). Patients sustaining additional extremity or spinal fractures may require additional adjustment of therapeutic exercise programs based on the location and severity of the fracture. Caution should be used when handling any extremity with a cast or external fixator apparatus.

Procedural Interventions: Functional Training

Functional training interventions are germane to the patient's rehabilitative success. It is within this domain that physical therapist assistants can effectively and strategically progress the patient toward the short- and long-term mobility goals established by the supervising physical therapist. In accordance with both cognitive and mentation recovery, appropriate mobility maneuvers will guide patients in achieving optimum functional independence. Patients at lower functional or cognitive levels require extensive practical training in transfer techniques and bed mobility sequences.[39] Patients with severely impaired coordination, dense hemiparesis, or orthopedic trauma may initially require a dependent transfer strategy in an effort to maneuver from surface to surface. Patients sustaining a TBI with associated fractures or other complications present a challenge. Extensive fractures and orthopedic complications necessitate modified transfer strategies secondary to weight-bearing restrictions on multiple extremities. Furthermore, fixation devices, such as halo vests, alter balance responses[40] and normal postural transitions, such as supine-to-sit. Sliding boards and upper-extremity fracture platform devices are beneficial to perform transfers and bed mobility tasks.

The physical therapist assistant should guide the patient toward independence in all bed mobility skills, including bridging, rolling, and supine-to-sit. Sit-to-stand transitions may be especially difficult during recovery.[41] Patients having hemiparetic extremities should be taught strategies to use and facilitate use of these limbs. Activities such as bridging merge functional tasks with active dissociation patterns. Adjuncts to treatment, such as physio balls and bolsters, may prove helpful in securing patient positioning.

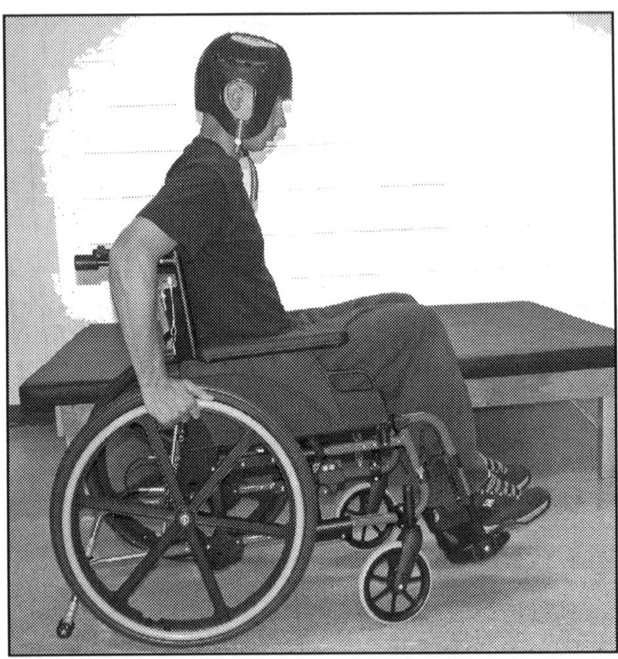

Figure 12-4. Initial short-term goals for the patient include performing w/c parts management independently and propelling to and from therapy sessions.

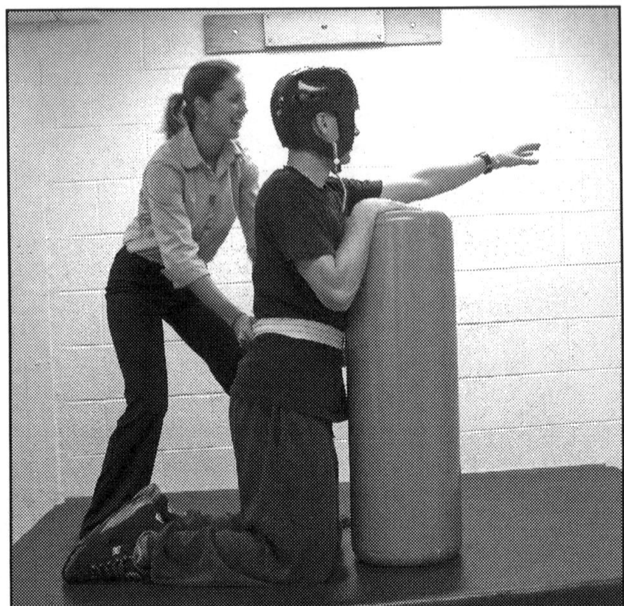

Figure 12-5. Neurofacilitation techniques are performed to enhance optimum motor performance when upper motor neuron deficits are present.

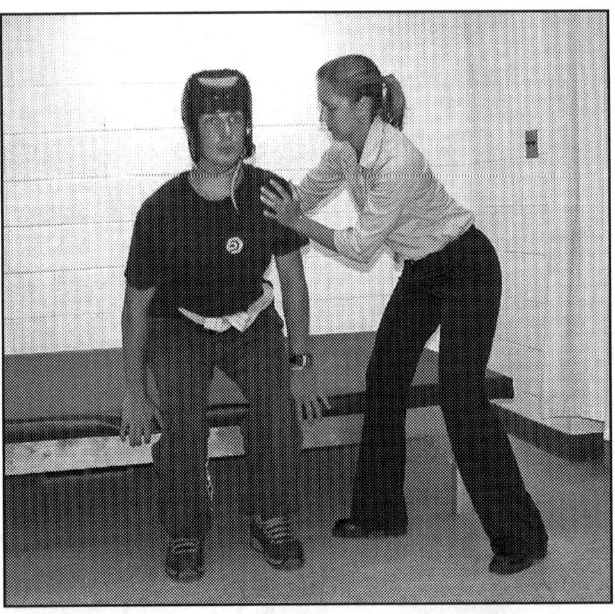

Figure 12-6. Activities such as the sit-to-stand transition allow patients to perform exercise programs within the context of a task.

Interventions for Balance Deficits

Patients recovering from TBI may demonstrate balance impairments related to their injury. Balance interventions are aimed at maintaining the body's center of mass within the limits of stability given environmental factors and the patient's own biomechanics. The regulation of balance reflects contributions by the vestibular, somatosensory, and visual systems to effectively maintain postural control. The physical therapist assistant may elect to challenge or manipulate these sensory systems by having the patient stand on foam or reduce the patient base of support in tandem stance (Figure 12-7). The interaction of these systems illustrates a systems approach to motor control and represents an integrated, multisystem network among structures within the central nervous system to modulate balance responses (see Chapters 5 and 6). This more current model better displays the dynamic nature of the central nervous system compared with previous hierarchical paradigms.

The initial examination by the physical therapist should clarify the extent of the balance impairment and the degree to which functional sitting and standing require attention. The physical therapist assistant should recognize key components, as well as score interpretation, of common balance instruments. The Balance Evaluation Systems Test[26] was developed to assess balance ability through postural adjustments, limits of stability, and reactive stepping tasks. The Berg Balance Scale is a simple battery used to assess an individual's balance control during a series of tasks, which are graded on a 4-point scale. Fifty-six points are possible from performance on the 14 skill categories.[27] Subjects must perform tasks that include a transfer, picking up an object from the floor, and alternately touching a step stool with each foot. For patients at a higher functional level, the therapist may elect to use the functional High-Level Mobility Assessment Tool to assess the ability to perform advanced activities, such as running, hopping, and walking backward.[42] Scores from the physical therapist's initial examination may point to those target interventions that are needed in the rehabilitation program. For example, patients having difficulty with the sit-to-stand maneuver on a standardized balance instrument may require preliminary activities such as strengthening activities or arising from varied surfaces to successfully master the activity.

Patients demonstrating balance improvements from rehabilitation programs may not necessarily have concomitant gait progress.[43] Moreover, medical complications from the patient's acute care hospitalization may affect balance performance. In a multicenter analysis of factors associated with balance deficits among patients recovering from a TBI, it was found that the incidence of medical complications (eg, respiratory complications and urinary tract infections) was strongly related to sitting balance impairment.[44]

Existing muscle weakness can cause or further exacerbate balance deficits. The presence of abductor weakness may result in a compensated abnormal trunk lean in unilateral stance toward the more affected side. This compensation strategy becomes especially treacherous if the patient has a decreased upper-extremity protective response because of hemiplegia or processing latency. Simple light touch contact with a cane or other assistive device may prove beneficial in improving postural control by enhancing hip abductor activation.[45]

Balance training should also reflect activities with attention to designated strategies used to maintain postural control. The sequential ankle, hip, and stepping strategies may be interrupted because of motor control problems or abnormal coactivation. (Refer to Chapter 6, Figures 6-12 and 6-13, for examples.) Also, flexibility limitations at the hip and ankle may further impede strategy activation. Evidence in the application of tai chi techniques suggests that this intervention approach has demonstrated efficacy in improving standing balance with individuals who sustained a severe head injury (see Chapter 18).[46] Patients with severe balance impairments or vestibular dysfunction require more advanced interventions by the physical therapist. Unfortunately, persistent dizziness following a TBI has been shown to be a major barrier to employment return among patients desiring to return to work following their injury.[47]

Gait Training

Gait interventions are an integral component of the patient's functional mobility program. Qualitative and quantitative parameters of gait performance must be addressed. Patients should not be advanced with gait training activities without the appropriate muscle activity or assistive device to support a limb or advance the lower extremities in gait. Patients often achieving independent functional ambulation within 3 months of their TBI include those who are younger, who are less severely injured, and who have a better functional ambulation profile prior to the onset of rehabilitation.[48]

Gait quality for the patient with TBI becomes a major priority in rehabilitation training. Physical therapist assistants should link gait deviation causality to those concomitant impairments. For example, tightness in the gastrocnemius muscle may be linked to a genu recurvatum tendency in stance phase. Likewise, residual weakness in the ankle dorsiflexors may induce a steppage or circumducted swing pattern. Because of the duality in roles of the dorsiflexor muscles in stance and swing phases, an abrupt slap may be observed during the loading response. Persistence of gait deviations should be communicated to the supervising physical therapist to assess the patient for possible orthotic candidacy.

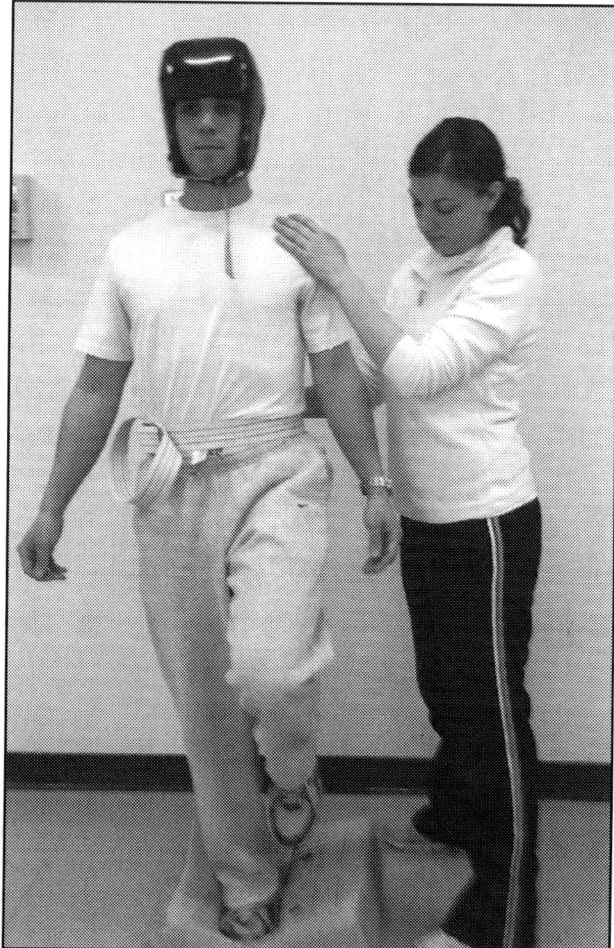

Figure 12-7. The physical therapist assistant can manipulate the sensory systems that modulate balance through the use of foam for higher-level patients.

Patients with resultant spastic hemiplegia in the lower extremities may have additional gait deviations. Particular problematic gait issues include the adductor/scissoring gait, the stiff knee, and the inverted, equinovarus foot.[49] Specific interventions should be employed to address gait quality. Stretching techniques can be performed to elongate spastic muscle groups. Aggressive stretching is indicated following select chemodenervation procedures, such as Botox (onabotulinumtoxinA) injections or phenol nerve blocks, to improve gait quality. In addition, the physical therapist assistant may assist with advanced tone management procedures. The physical therapist frequently elects to perform serial

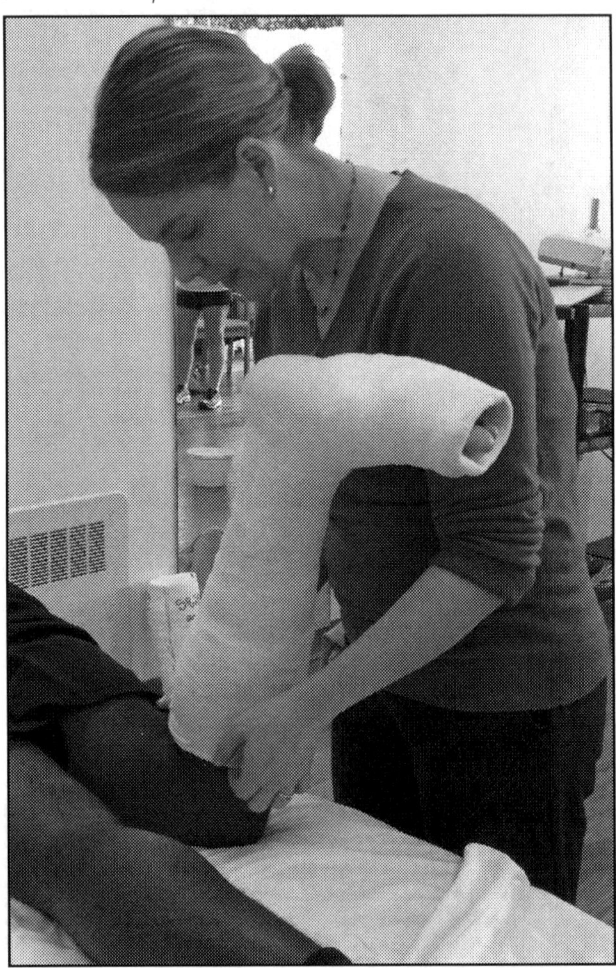

Figure 12-8. The physical therapist may apply a serial cast to gain ankle ROM for patients who have moderate to severe hypertonicity.

casting with a patient who has moderate to severe plantar flexor spasticity to achieve improved ankle ROM for gait or w/c footplate positioning for non-ambulators. The procedure involves the application of a plaster or fiberglass cast for a series of days to achieve the desired ROM gain (Figure 12-8).[50]

Correction strategies during gait and locomotion training are implemented to normalize gait quality and to improve quantitative parameters, such as speed, distance, and base of support. Independence in ambulation for short distances may take 6 months or longer for those individuals recovering from severe injuries and fractures. Selection of the appropriate gait device may be problematic when extensive cognitive deficits persist. Patients exhibit difficulty with sequencing and placement of the cane, crutches, or walker. Patients at higher functional levels should be trained on all surfaces and should perform activities on inclines, curbs, and uneven surfaces. Instruction in floor transfers is also an integral part of the management plan for the patient who is at risk for falls (Figure 12-9). Often slight gait deviations are persistent following a TBI, and patients attempt to maximize safety through a slower walking pattern and increased guardedness.[51] Body weight–support treadmill training interventions have been used to improve gait performance as well as aerobic capacity in the rehabilitation plan of care (Figure 12-10).[52] Robotic training may be implemented for patients that can benefit from sustained mass practice repetition to facilitate step symmetry and increase gait velocity (Figure 12-11).[53]

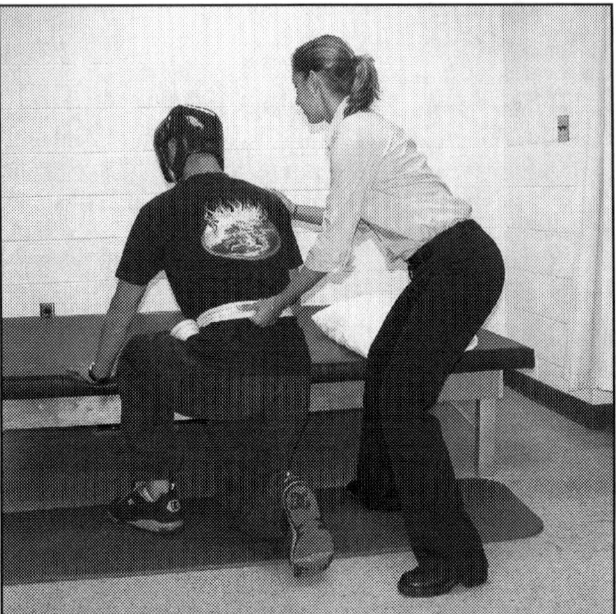

Figure 12-9. Instruction in floor transfers is an integral part of interventions for higher-level patients.

The physical therapist assistant should be aware that walking speed is an integral part of community navigation and the return to participation. A gait speed of 1.2 meters/second is required to effectively navigate the community and cross streets.[54] The physical therapist may initially measure this velocity by timing ambulation across a 4-meter path, with appropriate acceleration and deceleration distances allotted prior to and following the designated path. Gait velocity is determined by dividing 4 meters by this measured time. The physical therapist assistant should incorporate speed drills and dual-task activities to prepare patients functioning at a higher level of motor performance for traffic light changes and changing task demands on the gait cycle. Common gait deviations are noted in Table 12-4, along with key findings from the literature and aligned intervention strategies.

Special Considerations for the Patient With a Brain Injury

Coma Emergence

Patients with a severe TBI may require extensive medical management on the intensive care unit. Following medical stabilization, patients will be discharged to facilities

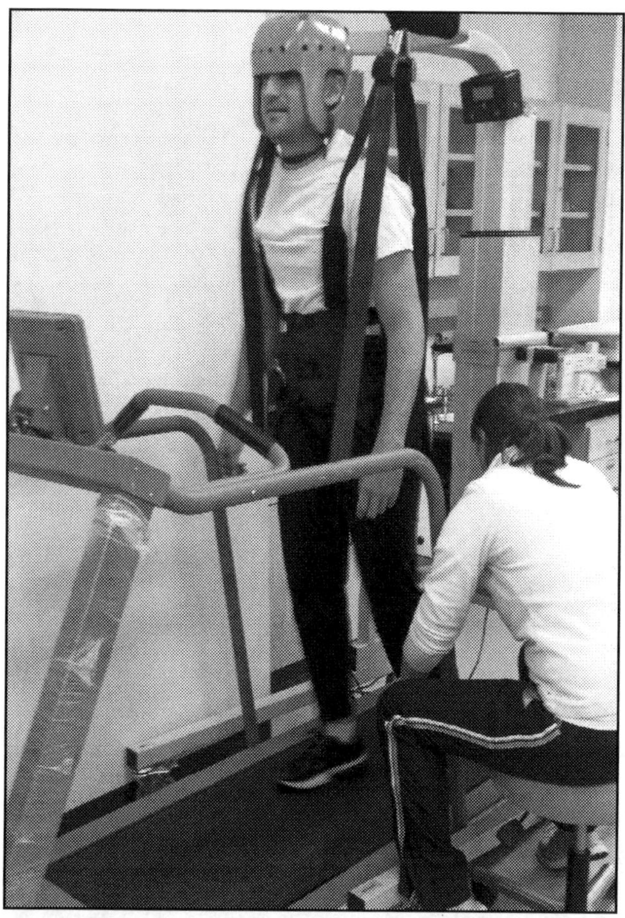

Figure 12-10. The physical therapist may use body weight–support treadmill training to improve gait performance and aerobic capacity.

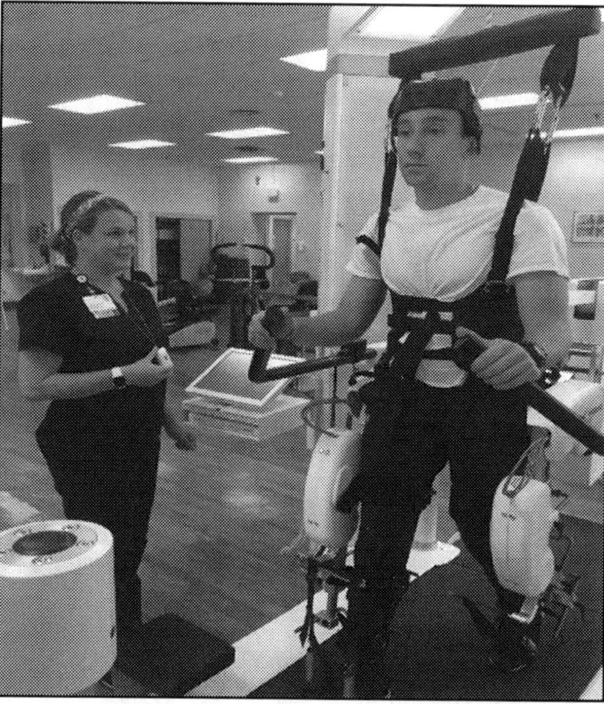

Figure 12-11. Robotic training may be implemented for patients that can benefit from sustained repetition to facilitate step symmetry and increased gait velocity.

where coma-emergence programs may be implemented. The physical therapist may track progress through a standardized coma-emergence rating form. Commonly used instruments include the JFK-Revised instrument.[59] These tools assist in quantifying where designated responses to standardized sensory stimuli are graded. Patients reaching maximum scores on a coma recovery scale may then have more advanced goals and intervention plans established. Patients emerging from minimally responsive states may be progressively mobilized through the use of tilt-table or standing-frame activities (Figure 12-12). Patients are begun on a sitting schedule to gradually increase sitting time. Vital signs should be carefully monitored for orthostatic changes and adverse physiological responses to positional changes. Patients can demonstrate abnormal fluctuations in blood pressure and episodic dizziness. physical therapist assistants often work with supervising therapists in coma emergence programs given the complexity of the multiple medical issues and ongoing need for reexamination. In addition, patients often require 2 people for lifts, positioning, serial casting, and standing activities.

The Agitated Patient

Perhaps one of the most challenging issues for all rehabilitation team members is management of the agitated patient. Significant agitation can contribute to the patient's length of stay, hinder functional independence, and ultimately hinder impending discharge to home.[60] Physical therapists and physical therapist assistants must be attentive to the multitude of sensory experiences that are communicated to the patient during this stage because of potential adverse responses from the patient. Patients often become anxious and aggressive when they cannot process the immediate sensory information within their environment. Moreover, patients may overreact in the presence of relatively minor requests or tasks.

The physical therapist assistant must effectively strategize interventions to deliver appropriate sensory experiences. Sessions should be structured properly to prevent sensory overload. Often, quiet areas are helpful in reducing distractions, and reducing voice volume may be more calming. Treatment sessions may have to be modified to multiple shorter sessions. Time-out periods can be implemented when undesired behavior is unable to be redirected. Caution must be taken with verbal and manual cues during mobility maneuvers, as agitated patients may demonstrate periods of tactile defensive behavior. Before assuming that the agitated or negative behavior presented by the patient is due to the

Table 12-4

Gait Deficits and Intervention Strategies

Gait Deficit	*Key Findings From the Literature*	*Intervention Strategies for the Physical Therapist Assistant*
Slowed obstacle negotiation	People with a TBI demonstrate greater medial lateral sway and dynamic instability with obstacle crossing.[55]	Progressive obstacle negotiation; environmental challenges with surface changes
Slowed velocity	People with a TBI demonstrate slower gait speed, especially when eyes are closed and dual tasks are involved.[56]	Speed drills; task circuit training
Difficulty with running coordination	Self-selected walking speed greater than 1.0 m/sec predicts the ability to run.[57]	Activities that incorporate speed drills and step-to-step bounding
Increased medial-lateral sway in gait	Patients with moderate to severe brain injury present with excessive medial/lateral sway 5 months following injury.[58]	Core stabilization activities; hip abductor strengthening

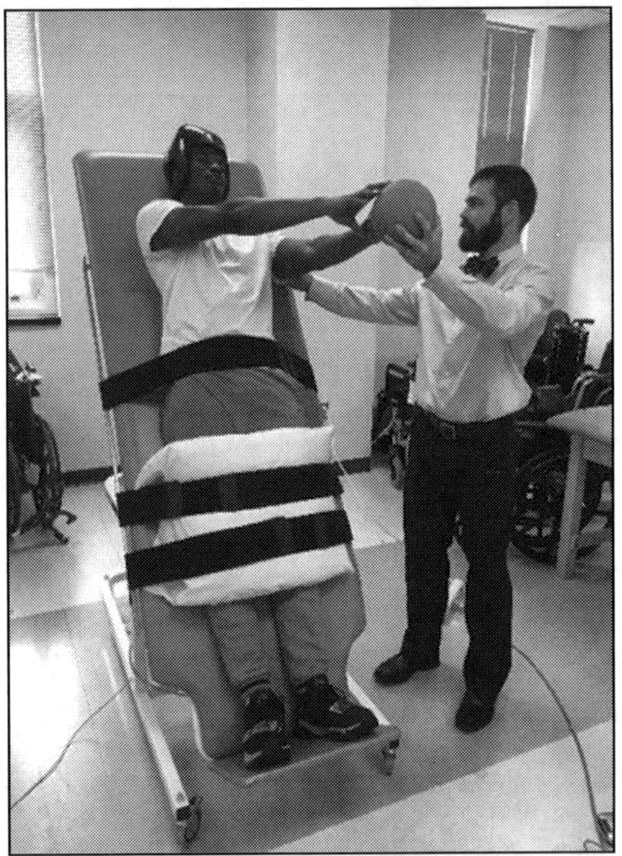

Figure 12-12. Patients emerging from minimally responsive states may be progressively mobilized through the use of a tilt-table.

TBI, the therapist should first assess the environment and behavior of the clinicians to determine if a change in the therapist's techniques or voice or the surrounding environment may eliminate the patient's unwanted behavior.

Integration of Cognitive and Neuromuscular Interventions

The ultimate challenge in head trauma rehabilitation is to integrate cognitive and functional training strategies to effectively guide the patient toward established target goals and to maximize independence. The added cognitive dimension within therapeutic interventions adds a level of complexity that necessitates the skills of the experienced physical therapist assistant. Cognitive impairments following a TBI may be substantial. Sleep disorders arising after the injury can also interfere with treatment sessions.[61] Patients may demonstrate slower processing and require increased time to optimize task performance.[62] Diminished attention span is also apparent, and patients require ongoing redirection to the designated task. Simple strategies, such as reducing background distraction noise can be helpful. The physical therapist assistant must consider that learning often occurs at a considerably diminished rate in the rehabilitation activity. Appropriate time allotment and cue sequence must be constructed within a treatment session to facilitate skill attainment. The effective physical therapist assistant will recognize processing latencies when teaching motor tasks and allow appropriate time for problem solving. Finally, physical therapy clinicians must be reminded that the issue of impaired judgment is still evident, even in the latter stages of the Rancho scale. Cognitive and motor recovery rates do not necessarily occur in synchrony, and while independent in mobility skills, the patient with poor judgment creates a potentially dangerous situation if left unsupervised in the clinic or home environment or out in the community. The rehabilitation team may recommend 24-hour supervision at discharge.

Cognitive and functional interventions are frequently fused. The physical therapist assistant can perform gait interventions while requiring that the patient perform the necessary speed changes needed during an emergency situation, such as exiting a building during a fire drill. Reinforcing safety strategies taught during previous sessions will assist the patient in identifying critical components of a desired task. Physical therapist assistants should employ critical problem-solving strategies to maximize patients' ability to prepare for home or community situations. Such activities might include performing safety maneuvers with rail support in dim lighting during stairs negotiation or practicing dialing 911. A patient's cognitive recovery can be monitored through a cognitive log.[63] This is a simple bedside tool that tracks progress in measures, such as memory, language, attention, and reasoning. Progress achieved and patient outcomes may also be monitored through such assessment measures, such as the Functional Independence Measure tool. This outcomes measure has demonstrated validity with patients recovering from a TBI.[64]

Dual Task Activities and Attention

The ability to perform 2 synchronous activities in the home, work, or community setting is an integral part of daily life.[65] Divided attention refers to a patient's ability to complete 2 concurrent activities. For example, for the patient who must return to restaurant employment, the physical therapist assistant may elect to practice ambulation while carrying a tray with food while responding to customers' orders. In this way, the activity not only meets the objective of being a dual task, but it is also meaningful and, when practiced, simulates a real-world activity necessary for the return to community participation.

Attention-switching requires a shift from one motor task to the next, such as shifting gears when driving and then braking for a sudden emergency stop.[65] When one activity is performed over a longer period of time, sustained attention is being displayed. One example is the patient with balance deficits who performs limits of stability weight-shifting guided by a computer screen avatar for a set time period. When dual-task activities are indicated in the plan of care, the physical therapist assistant should challenge patients' attention deficits with interventions that are in line with functional needs, established goals, and requisite needs for community participation return.

Precautions

Functional mobility programs and interventions for patients with TBI require attention to several key issues. Patients who are agitated should be monitored closely and should never be left alone if 24-hour direct supervision is required. Furthermore, rehabilitation professionals should make sure assistance is immediately available within the treatment area if a sudden occurrence of agitation should occur. Functional activities in enclosed areas, such as stairwells, dictate additional personnel nearby. Policies should be in place for a silent "show of force" pending significant outbursts of aggressive behavior. For example, multiple staff may be required to rush to a patient's room to diffuse a hostile behavioral event. Physical therapist assistants must be cognizant of policies implemented to protect patients who have been victims of family abuse or assault; moreover, alias names are used as part of the facility's procedures to maintain patient protection and confidentiality.

Managing patients at lower levels of function also mandates precautionary measures. Patients who have undergone craniotomy procedures may require helmet use. Patients are regularly required to wear a helmet when out of bed. When patients are mobilized without the helmet, care should be taken not to put excess pressure over the affected area. Rehabilitation team members must also demonstrate competency with management of catheters, oxygen canisters, and tube-feeding lines during treatment sessions.

Discharge Planning and Community Reentry

Equipment Procurement and Family Training

The physical therapist assistant will be involved in all aspects of discharge planning following the designated course of rehabilitation. Appropriate ordering of durable medical equipment will be required at the time of discharge, and the physical therapist assistant will participate in the ordering of required assistive device and ambulation needs. If a w/c is required, appropriate features should be ordered to sufficiently address the patient's needs. For example, appropriate seat width and depth should accommodate the patient's size, and front-rigging features should provide for necessary lower-extremity support and orthopedic considerations. Elevating leg rests may also be required for individuals with lower-extremity fractures or circulatory impairments.

An important component of the discharge disposition will include family training activities for those patients being discharged who require care and assistance at home. The physical therapist assistant will effectively train the caregiver in mobility strategies that are linked to those functional needs of the patient. These activities may include transfer techniques, ambulation guarding, w/c management skills, and supervision of home exercise programs. Family training programs should also address car transfers and both stairs and curb negotiation.

In conjunction with recommendations by the supervising physical therapist, the physical therapist assistant may suggest the need for continued therapy interventions. Patients may require a course of outpatient or home therapy in an effort to continue work toward the long-term goals established for the patient in the plan of care. Patients who are at higher functional levels may benefit from a community reentry program to transition into previous employment and societal roles.

Table 12-5

Key Questions Addressed During the Home Visit

- Will the patient be able to enter and exit the living environment safely?
- What environmental barriers are present?
- Are any grab bars or additional devices needed in the bathroom?
- If a w/c is to be used, will it be able to clear the doorways?
- Where are steps encountered in the home?
- Are rails available in stairways? If so, right or left?
- Are safety devices present, such as smoke alarms or telephone access?
- Will the patient be able to navigate around furniture in all rooms?
- Is lighting sufficient in rooms and stairwells?
- Is there clutter or other potential causes of falls?

Home Assessment

Prior to discharge, the physical therapist assistant or supervising physical therapist may elect to conduct a home visit to assess the patient's home environment and identify potential environment barriers. The setting should be thoroughly inspected for possible safety issues that may arise when the patient returns home. Scrutiny of doorway widths, inclines, and floor surfaces is especially important for the patient who will be returning home in a w/c. In addition, the physical therapist assistant should analyze major entrance and exit passageways to the home. In some rehabilitation settings, patients may be allowed to return home for a scheduled visit prior to discharge for a trial run of mobility skills acquired. Often rehabilitation team members perform a joint home assessment to address multiple areas of potential patient needs (Table 12-5). Occupational therapists will assess the home environment as it relates to activities of daily living performance and make any adaptive recommendations. The physical therapist assistant serves as an important conduit to the supervising physical therapist for identifying issues related to the discharge disposition and recommendations.

Instructional Interventions: Home Programs

Creating an individualized home program following discharge from an inpatient rehabilitation stay requires careful attention to all components of the patient's functional status. Exercise interventions should target weakened muscle groups and incorporate functional activities; moreover, the exercises should be sufficient in quantity to address pertinent needs, yet not overwhelming in number. Home programs should provide for ambulation activity with the caregiver where possible. It is crucial that the program extend beyond a simple instructional sheet. Performance logs will help ensure adherence, especially when caregiver supervision is not optimal. Written instructions should be clearly rendered with large print and should contain key terms familiar to the patient and caregiver. Using medical jargon or unknown terms becomes detrimental to the teaching process. Diagrams are often useful, especially when the physical therapist assistant wants to accentuate important performance strategies or points of emphasis in the program. Effective home programs consider those residual cognitive deficits that may still be pervasive at the time of discharge. Caregivers supervising home programs should receive appropriate instructions regarding strategies to facilitate optimum performance in lieu of any attention or processing deficits. Culturally competent home programs consider key points of emphasis in the patient's native language if English is not spoken.

The Return to Participation: Community Integration

Patients who are recovering from a TBI often begin community reentry activities during the inpatient rehabilitation stay. The rehabilitation team members may accompany patients, for example, on a community outing to the mall or a recreation activity. Patients who display behavior consistent with the final Rancho stages, Levels VII and VIII, are particularly appropriate for such activities, and the physical therapist assistant will be able to observe such phenomena as abstract reasoning processes and social interactions. Gait and locomotion progress within the environmental context can also be analyzed during community outings to gauge the patient's readiness for participation.

Patients may also continue community reentry activities with adult day programs designed for this special patient population. These programs assist patients in transitioning to employment initiatives and also provide important psychosocial support. Important activities aimed at optimizing problem-solving skills are addressed because of those residual cognitive deficits that still exist.[66] Factors associated with a good quality of life following a TBI include inveterate community and social support.[67] Key factors impeding patients' successful return to employment include significant cognitive impairment and low education levels.[68] Day programs can also provide resource assistance for those patients who experience depression, which is one of the most common secondary conditions associated with a TBI.[69]

Special Populations of Patients With Traumatic Brain Injury

Concussion

Recent attention on local and national levels has focused on managing the athlete following a sustained concussion. Operationally, a concussion is a clinically diagnosed brain injury caused by traumatic biomechanical forces with or without a loss of consciousness.[70] It is important to underscore that a concussion, while often mild, is a TBI. From 2001 to 2012, the number of concussions managed doubled, and the American Medical Society for Sports Medicine estimates as many as 3.8 million concussions occur in the United States each year; however, up to 50% may go unreported.[71] Concussions occur through organized and unorganized sports, including bicycling and playground activities. Injuries may also occur with extreme sports. Four major domains have been identified: prevention, identification, evaluation, and management.

Given the current climate for athlete protection and momentum for concussion legislation, athletes are wearing additional headgear, and prohibitive plays have been authorized to prevent dangerous types of hits in contact sports. Following a suspected concussion, athletes undergo a series of neurocognitive batteries to identify the extent of the injury. Tests range from sideline balance and cognitive assessments to ocular testing. The King-Devick Test is a number-identification battery that assesses eye movements and attention through a series of display cards.[72] This test is often used as a sideline diagnostic test to discern sports-related concussion injury. The Immediate Post Concussion Assessment and Cognitive Test is a computerized neuropsychological test battery used to evaluate athletes' neurocognitive function.[73] The instrument comprises 6 individual test modules, including verbal memory, visual memory, reaction time, processing speed, and impulse control. The test also includes a post-concussion symptom scale and a section for demographic and health history information. The neurocognitive battery is computerized, and often school athletes will take the web-based test during pre-season sports training.

Following the primary physical therapist's examination, physical therapist assistants may work with patients following concussion to improve deficits in balance and coordination, and participate in the multidisciplinary effort to safely return an athlete to contact or noncontact play. In their published consensus statement of sports-related concussion (Table 12-6), McCrory and colleagues established guidelines to progress athletes through a continuum of activities and maximize neural preparedness for safe return to play.[70] The physical therapist assistant should recognize that advancement of both ocular and balance exercises should be progressed cautiously secondary to headache development from overstimulation. Vestibular exercises are an integral part of concussion physical therapy management.

Blast Injuries

Soldiers returning from service duty in active military zones have sustained unique injuries associated with warfare: *blast injuries*. These occur when, following detonation, high-order explosives propel expanding gases and create a blast wind. Three types of injuries have commonly been described[74]:

1. Primary injuries occur from the impact of the blast wave. Structures with an air-solid interface, such as the lungs and tympanic membrane, are especially susceptible.
2. Secondary injuries can occur when soldiers are hit by shrapnel (eg, rocks and pellets) from detonated improvised explosive devices.
3. Tertiary injuries occur when soldiers are thrown off their feet and propelled into objects, sustaining traumatic injuries and fractures.

Soldiers returning from active duty with injuries may be managed through the veterans' network continuum of care, including polytrauma rehabilitation centers. Physical therapist assistants working with soldiers in these settings will perform interventions aligned with the severity of injuries, including body weight–supported treadmill training to increase gait endurance and distance.[75] Vestibular and ocular exercises may be performed to alleviate symptoms of dizziness occurring at rest or during activities requiring exertion.[76]

Conclusion

Rehabilitating individuals with a TBI offers the physical therapist assistant the unique opportunity to interlock principles of functional training with key cognitive strategies to improve the overall quality of life for their clients. Carefully planned intervention programs, molded from clinical expertise and best practice evidence, range from bed mobility to locomotion activities to community reentry activities.[77] Interventions by the physical therapist assistant are pivotal components of the ICF and Patient/Client Management Model as they relate to managing patients with TBI.[78] The approach to individuals with complex deficits in body structure/functions and activities should be one of partnership between the physical therapist assistant and the supervising physical therapist to effectively facilitate the patient's return to community participation. The effective physical therapist/physical therapist assistant team will successfully assemble appropriate intervention and reexamination activities, in conjunction with ongoing communication, to optimize functional and neurobehavioral outcomes for the patient.

Table 12-6

Therapeutic Interventions Aligned for Phases of Return to Play in the Management of Athletes With Concussion

Rehabilitation Stage	Functional Intervention Example	Objective
No activity	Complete cognitive and physical rest	Brain recovery
Light aerobic conditioning	Walking, swimming	Add movement
Sport-specific exercise	Running sprint in soccer or lacrosse	Add movement
Noncontact training drills	Passing in football or lacrosse	Multitask Intensity
Full-contact practice	Normal training activities (with medical clearance)	Return to sport-specific intensity

Adapted from McCrory P, Meeuwisse W, Johnston K, et al. Consensus statement on concussion in sport: the 3rd International Conference on Concussion in Sport held in Zurich, November 2008. *Amer Acad Phys Med Rehabil.* 2009;1(5):401-418.

Case Study

The patient, Leszek, is a 19-year-old Polish student who was an unrestrained passenger in a motor vehicle accident. He suffered a right frontal cerebral contusion with diffuse axonal shearing. He also sustained a mild subdural hematoma in the right frontal lobe pole. The initial Glasgow Coma Scale score was 12 in the emergency room. His acute care admission was significant for episodes of post-traumatic seizures, which lengthened his stay considerably. Following medical stabilization, he was transferred to a specialized brain injury unit rehabilitation setting where an initial examination was performed by the physical therapist. The patient's cognitive status was consistent with Rancho Level VI. On admission, the physical therapist performed the following examination.

History

Because of the patient's memory deficits, information was obtained from the patient's family. Leszek's parents are Polish immigrants who moved to this country 16 years ago. He is a student at the university and is majoring in accounting. Leszek works as a waiter at a local restaurant on weekends. His medical history is significant for asthma, and he has had no major surgeries. He enjoys dancing and playing soccer. They characterize Leszek as a "quick learner." He lives with his family in a 2-story home. There are 8 steps between floors. The family has a pet dog, Borek, who is in good health. The patient has one sister, who will be getting married in 1 month. The patient's current medications include Dilantin (phenytoin) and albuterol.

Systems Review

Cardiovascular:

- Blood pressure = 124/76; heart rate = 64 beats/min; lungs = clear to auscultation other than mild congestion heard in upper airways.

Integumentary:

- No areas of skin redness noted over major boney prominences.

Musculoskeletal:

- (+) Proximal weakness in bilateral upper and lower extremities.
- Height:
    - 6 feet 3 inches; 181 pounds.

Neuromuscular:

- Impaired balance and gait activity; required walker assistance in ambulation.

Cognition and communication:

- Oriented to name only; fluent in verbal expression, though confused regarding insight into injury.

Tests and Measures

Mental function:

- Orientation: Oriented to name only. (+) Episodic confusion.
- Arousal: Lethargic; slow in initiating activity.
- Short-term memory: Poor/unable to remember 3 objects.

Cranial nerve integrity:

- Intact: 2, 3 to 6, 7, and 11 to 12

Sensory integrity:

- Intact to light touch and proprioception in all extremities. Patient able to follow simple testing commands.

ROM/joint integrity:

- No upper extremity limitations noted passively. Lower extremity passive ROM is significant for a lack of full hip extension on the right by 5 degrees and a lack of 10 degrees on the left. Knee and ankle joints demonstrate no limitations.

Muscle tone:

- 1+ in right quadriceps/Modified Ashworth Scale.

Muscle performance:

- Upper extremity: 4/5 in major shoulder and elbow muscle groups. 5/5 wrist and hand musculature.
- Lower extremity: Proximal weakness, 3+/5 hip abductors and extensors; 4/5 hip rotators, flexors; 4/5 quadriceps/ hamstrings; 5/5 ankle/foot musculature.

Reflex integrity:

- 2+ biceps, triceps, brachioradialis, 1+ quadriceps, 2+ gastrocnemius.

Coordination:

- Mild right upper extremity dysmetria noted in the finger-to-nose test.

Balance:

- Maintains static unsupported sitting longer than 3 minutes. Patient loses balances when reaching outside base of support.
- Standing: Unable to stand unsupported; demonstrates a (+) Romberg.

Bed mobility:

- Moderate assistance/supine-to-sit; minimal assistance/bridging; minimal assistance/rolling.
- Moderate assistance/sit-to-stand.

Gait:

- Patient ambulates 10 feet with a rolling walker with moderate assistance; he demonstrates decreased step and stride lengths bilaterally and displays strong tendency to shuffle feet in gait. (+) Trendelenburg noted bilaterally.

W/C mobility and locomotion:

- Supervision required for parts management. Propels 20 feet with minimal assistance and extensive cues for turns and direction changes.

Aerobic capacity:

- Resting heart rate of 64 beats/min. Following ambulation: 88 beats/minute. No shortness of breath observed following ambulation.
- Oxygen saturation: Resting, 95%; post-ambulation, 92%.

Goals

Long-term goals (3 weeks):

1. Close supervision with household ambulation with assistive device (distances: 100 feet) with verbalized safety precautions.
2. Modified independent transfers and bed mobility.
3. Close supervision with stairs negotiation with right rail and step-over-step sequencing.
4. Supervision with home exercise program.
5. Hip strength: 4/5 bilaterally and ROM: 15 degrees passive hip extension for step-over-step stairs negotiation with right rail.
6. Durable medical equipment procurement.
7. Completion of family training activities with 100% safe and competent performance by parents.
8. Dancing with supervision with family members in preparation for upcoming wedding participation.

Short-term goals (1 week):

1. Ambulation 40 feet with minimal assistance with rolling walker.
2. Transfers with minimal assistance and minimal cues for safety.
3. Rolling and bridging with supervision and minimal cues; sit-to-stand with minimal assistance.
4. W/C propulsion to and from physical therapy sessions with supervision.
5. Independent w/c parts management.
6. W/C pressure relief with supervision.

Evaluation, Prognosis, and Diagnosis

The physical therapist noted that Leszek demonstrates excellent rehabilitation potential because of his functional profile, age, and minimal restrictions by comorbid conditions. The prognosis for improving his overall functional mobility status is good, although impaired cognition may impede immediate involvement with previous community and work-related activities. The physical therapist's diagnosis conveys impaired motor function and cognition associated with the TBI, along with related balance, transfers, bed mobility, and gait deficits.

Plan of Care

The patient will receive physical therapy for 1 hour daily for gait training, therapeutic exercise, balance activities, and transfers. Appropriate durable medical equipment procurement and family training activities will be included. The patient's estimated length of stay is 3 weeks.

Procedural Interventions

Following the initial examination, the physical therapist assistant began seeing the patient daily. Leszek was also followed by occupational therapy and speech therapy professionals. A w/c and temporary seating system was prepared. Leszek performed a daily regimen of functional training involving those activities included in the plan. Therapeutic exercises included extremity exercise band activities, w/c push-ups, sit-to-stand repetitions, and pelvic lifts. Passive stretching of the hip joint was also included. Gait training focused on increasing distance while decreasing the overall level of assistance required. Consistent with Rancho Level VI, he followed simple directions well, although he displayed difficulty learning new tasks. The physical therapist assistant used repetition and visual cues to enhance the learning process (eg, the w/c brakes were covered with colored tape to serve as a reminder to lock the brakes prior to a transfer). In addition, the physical therapist assistant learned some key Polish terms to emphasize particular skill components. Signs were also placed in the patient's room to indicate times for scheduled activities, and the patient maintained a daily log of activities performed in physical therapy. In each physical therapy session, the patient would verbalize those key safety strategies involved in the performance of the particular skill. Leszek began transporting himself independently to therapy sessions.

The patient steadily progressed through his therapy regimen and incrementally achieved designated goals. Leszek 's cognition also improved, along with his speed of processing in mobility maneuvers. His cognitive behavior displayed many Level VIII attributes. The physical therapist assistant was soon able to introduce a straight cane with contact guarding in ambulation activities. As Leszek's balance progressed, the physical therapist assistant had the family bring in his soccer ball to perform more challenging dynamic activities. Moreover, the ball represented a past activity that he enjoyed and could now revisit in therapy. The physical therapist assistant progressed the patient with more advanced activities, such as floor transfers and uneven surface ambulation. He scored a 48 on the Berg Balance Scale during the physical therapist's reexamination, and he began working on tasks involved with the instrument's most demanding categories. The physical therapist assistant challenged his judgment with emergency maneuvers, such as running to dial 911. In the final week of therapy, he was able to perform a quick polka step in preparation for his sister's upcoming wedding. Discharge planning activities included a family training session and ordering of required equipment. Leszek still required a temporary w/c for longer community ambulation distances. Self-selected gait velocity was 1.0 meters/second. A foam cushion and straight cane were also ordered. His parents demonstrated safe and effective guarding in gait, stairs negotiation, and car transfer techniques. Instructional interventions included a full home exercise program which was reviewed with Leszek and his parents. A course of outpatient therapy was recommended. Two weeks following discharge, the physical therapist assistant received a photo in the mail of Leszek dancing at the wedding.

Physical Therapist/Physical Therapist Assistant Collaboration

Throughout the intervention regimen, the supervising physical therapist and physical therapist assistant discussed the patient's progress toward the established goals. On one occasion, the physical therapist was asked to examine a developing skin rash on the patient's distal upper extremities. In addition, the physical therapist assistant communicated to the therapist that Leszek's gait had been noticeably more unsteady over the past few days. Following the assessment, the physician was notified, and it was determined that the rash was due to an adverse side effect of the patient's Dilantin (phenytoin).

Questions

1. What are some of the red flags seen in the initial evaluation that the physical therapist assistant needs to consider when carrying out the plan of care?
2. Given the long-term goals set by the physical therapist and the plan of care identified, was there anything that was outside the potential scope of practice of the physical therapist assistant?
3. When would it be appropriate for the physical therapist assistant to contact the physical therapist outside of their normal discussion periods regarding this patient?

References

1. Taylor CA, Bell JM, Breiding MJ, Xu L. Traumatic Brain Injury-Related Emergency Department Visits, Hospitalizations, and Deaths - United States, 2007 and 2013. *MMWR Surveill Summ.* 2017;66(9):1-16. doi:10.15585/mmwr.ss6609a1
2. Brain Injury Association of America. Brian Injury Overview. https://www.biausa.org/brain-injury/about-brain-injury/basics/overview. Accessed August 10, 2018.
3. Centers for Disease Control and Prevention. Traumatic brain injury. http://www.cdc.gov/TraumaticBrainInjury/index.html. Accessed August 10, 2018.
4. American Physical Therapy Association. *Guide to Physical Therapist Practice.* 3rd ed. Alexandria, VA: American Physical Therapy Association; 2016.
5. Svestkova O, Angerova Y, Sladkova P, Bickenbach JE, Raggi A. Functioning and disability in traumatic brain injury. *Disabil Rehabil.* 2010;32(1)(suppl 1):S68-S77. doi:10.3109/09638288.2010.511690
6. Jensen GM, Gwyer J, Shepard KF, Hack LM. Expert practice in physical therapy. *Phys Ther.* 2000;80(1):28-43. doi:10.1093/ptj/80.1.28
7. Watts NT. Task analysis and division of responsibility in physical therapy. *Phys Ther.* 1971;51(1):23-35. doi:10.1093/ptj/51.1.23
8. Smith DH, Meaney DF, Shull WH. Diffuse axonal injury in head trauma. *J Head Trauma Rehabil.* 2003;18(4):307-316. doi:10.1097/00001199-200307000-00003
9. Jeremitsky E, Omert L, Dunham CM, Protetch J, Rodriguez A. Harbingers of poor outcome the day after severe brain injury: hypothermia, hypoxia, and hypoperfusion. *J Trauma.* 2003;54(2):312-319. doi:10.1097/01.TA.0000037876.37236.D6
10. Wang H, Zhou Y, Liu J, Ou L, Han J, Xiang L. Traumatic skull fractures in children and adolescents: A retrospective observational study. *Injury.* 2018;49(2):219-225. doi:10.1016/j.injury.2017.11.039
11. Johns JS, Cifu DX, Keyser-Marcus L, Jolles PR, Fratkin MJ. Impact of clinically significant heterotopic ossification on functional outcome after traumatic brain injury. *J Head Trauma Rehabil.* 1999;14(3):269-276. doi:10.1097/00001199-199906000-00007

12. Englander J, Cifu DX, Wright JM, Black K. The association of early computed tomography scan findings and ambulation, self-care, and supervision needs at rehabilitation discharge and at 1 year after traumatic brain injury. *Arch Phys Med Rehabil.* 2003;84(2):214-220. doi:10.1053/apmr.2003.50094
13. Englander J, Bushnik T, Duong TT, et al. Analyzing risk factors for late posttraumatic seizures: a prospective, multicenter investigation. *Arch Phys Med Rehabil.* 2003;84(3):365-373. doi:10.1053/apmr.2003.50022
14. Glenn MB, Hoch DB, Daly L. Anticonvulsants. *J Head Trauma Rehabil.* 2003;18(4):383-386. doi:10.1097/00001199-200307000-00009
15. Teasdale G, Jennett B. Assessment of coma and impaired consciousness. A practical scale. *Lancet.* 1974;2(7872):81-84. doi:10.1016/S0140-6736(74)91639-0
16. Salottolo K, Carrick M, Stewart Levy A, Morgan BC, Slone DS, Bar-Or D. The epidemiology, prognosis, and trends of severe traumatic brain injury with presenting Glasgow Coma Scale of 3. *J Crit Care.* 2017;38:197-201. doi:10.1016/j.jcrc.2016.11.034
17. Kay T, Harrington DE, Adams R, et al. Definition of mild traumatic brain injury. *J Head Trauma Rehabil.* 1993;8(3):86-87. doi:10.1097/00001199-199309000-00009
18. Evans RW. Predicting outcome following traumatic brain injury. *Neurol Rep.* 1998;22(4):144-148. doi:10.1097/01253086-199822040-00007
19. Malkmus D. Integrating cognitive strategies into the physical therapy setting. *Phys Ther.* 1983;63(12):1952-1959. doi:10.1093/ptj/63.12.1952
20. Hagen C, Malkmus D, Durham P. Levels of cognitive functioning. *In: Rehabilitation of the Head Injured Adult: Comprehensive Physical Management.* Downey, CA: Professional Staff Association of Rancho Los Amigos Hospital; 1979.
21. Stenberg M, Godbolt AK, Nygren De Boussard C, Levi R, Stålnacke BM. Cognitive impairment after severe traumatic brain injury, clinical course and impact on outcome: a Swedish-Icelandic study. *Behav Neurol.* 2015;2015:680308. doi:10.1155/2015/680308
22. Gray DS, Burnham RS. Preliminary outcome analysis of a long-term rehabilitation program for severe acquired brain injury. *Arch Phys Med Rehabil.* 2000;81(11):1447-1456. doi:10.1053/apmr.2000.16343
23. Duff D. Review article: altered states of consciousness, theories of recovery, and assessment following a severe traumatic brain injury. *Axone.* 2001;23(1):18-23.
24. Nakase-Thompson R, Sherer M, Yablon SA, Nick TG, Trzepacz PT. Acute confusion following traumatic brain injury. *Brain Inj.* 2004;18(2):131-142. doi:10.1080/0269905031000149542
25. Bohannon RW, Smith MB. Interrater reliability of a modified Ashworth scale of muscle spasticity. *Phys Ther.* 1987;67(2):206-207. doi:10.1093/ptj/67.2.206
26. Horak FB, Wrisley DM, Frank J. The Balance Evaluation Systems Test (BESTest) to differentiate balance deficits. *Phys Ther.* 2009;89(5):484-498. doi:10.2522/ptj.20080071
27. Berg KO, Wood-Dauphinee SL, Williams JI, Maki B. Measuring balance in the elderly: validation of an instrument. *Can J Public Health.* 1992;83(suppl 2):S7-S11.
28. Hirsch MA, Williams K, Norton HJ, Hammond F. Reliability of the timed 10-metre walk test during in-patient rehabilitation in ambulatory adults with traumatic brain injury. *Brain Inj.* 2014;28(8):1115-1120. doi:10.3109/02699052.2014.910701
29. McCulloch KL, Mercer V, Giuliani C, Marshall S. Development of a clinical measure of dual-task performance in walking: reliability and preliminary validity of the Walking and Remembering Test. *J Geriatr Phys Ther.* 2009;32(1):2-9. doi:10.1519/00139143-200932010-00002
30. Bhambhani Y, Rowland G, Farag M. Reliability of peak cardiorespiratory responses in patients with moderate to severe traumatic brain injury. *Arch Phys Med Rehabil.* 2003;84(11):1629-1636. doi:10.1053/S0003-9993(03)00343-5
31. Fischer S, Gauggel S, Trexler LE. Awareness of activity limitations, goal setting and rehabilitation outcome in patients with brain injuries. *Brain Inj.* 2004;18(6):547-562. doi:10.1080/02699050310001645793
32. Dumas HM, Haley SM, Ludlow LH, Carey TM. Recovery of ambulation during inpatient rehabilitation: physical therapist prognosis for children and adolescents with traumatic brain injury. *Phys Ther.* 2004;84(3):232-242. doi:10.1093/ptj/84.3.232
33. Duong TT, Englander J, Wright J, Cifu DX, Greenwald BD, Brown AW. Relationship between strength, balance, and outcome after traumatic brain injury: a multicenter analysis. *Arch Phys Med Rehabil.* 2004;85(8):1291-1297. doi:10.1016/j.apmr.2003.11.032
34. Lannin NA, Horsley SA, Herbert R, McCluskey A, Cusick A. Splinting the hand in the functional position after brain impairment: a randomized, controlled trial. *Arch Phys Med Rehabil.* 2003;84(2):297-302. doi:10.1053/apmr.2003.50031
35. Singer BJ, Jegasothy GM, Singer KP, Allison GT, Dunne JW. Incidence of ankle contracture after moderate to severe acquired brain injury. *Arch Phys Med Rehabil.* 2004;85(9):1465-1469. doi:10.1016/j.apmr.2003.08.103
36. Platz T, Winter T, Müller N, Pinkowski C, Eickhof C, Mauritz KH. Arm ability training for stroke and traumatic brain injury patients with mild arm paresis: a single-blind, randomized, controlled trial. *Arch Phys Med Rehabil.* 2001;82(7):961-968. doi:10.1053/apmr.2001.23982
37. Mudie MH, Matyas TA. Can simultaneous bilateral movement involve the undamaged hemisphere in reconstruction of neural networks damaged by stroke? *Disabil Rehabil.* 2000;22(1-2):23-37. doi:10.1080/096382800297097
38. Karman N, Maryles J, Baker RW, Simpser E, Berger-Gross P. Constraint-induced movement therapy for hemiplegic children with acquired brain injuries. *J Head Trauma Rehabil.* 2003;18(3):259-267. doi:10.1097/00001199-200305000-00004
39. Watson MJ, Hitchcock R. Recovery of walking late after a severe traumatic brain injury. *Physiotherapy.* 2004;90(2):103-107. doi:10.1016/j.physio.2004.02.004
40. Richardson JK, Ross AD, Riley B, Rhodes RL. Halo vest effect on balance. *Arch Phys Med Rehabil.* 2000;81(3):255-257. doi:10.1016/S0003-9993(00)90067-4
41. Zablotny CM, Nawoczenski DA, Yu B. Comparison between successful and failed sit-to-stand trials of a patient after traumatic brain injury. *Arch Phys Med Rehabil.* 2003;84(11):1721-1725. doi:10.1053/S0003-9993(03)00236-3

42. Williams GP, Robertson V, Greenwood KM, Goldie PA, Morris ME. The high-level mobility assessment tool (HiMAT) for traumatic brain injury. Part 2: content validity and discriminability. *Brain Inj.* 2005;19(10):833-843. doi:10.1080/02699050500058711
43. Wade LD, Canning CG, Fowler V, Felmingham L, Baguley IJ. Changes in postural sway and performance of functional tasks after traumatic brain injury. *Arch Phys Med Rehabil.* 1997;78(10):1107-1111. doi:10.1016/S0003-9993(97)90136-2
44. Greenwald BD, Cifu DX, Marwitz JH, et al. Factors associated with balance deficits on admission to rehabilitation after traumatic brain injury: a multicenter analysis. *J Head Trauma Rehabil.* 2001;16(3):238-252. doi:10.1097/00001199-200106000-00003
45. Jeka JJ. Light touch contact as a balance aid. *Phys Ther.* 1997;77(5):476-487. doi:10.1093/ptj/77.5.476
46. Shapira MY, Chelouche M, Yanai R, Kaner C, Szold A. Tai Chi Chuan practice as a tool for rehabilitation of severe head trauma: 3 case reports. *Arch Phys Med Rehabil.* 2001;82(9):1283-1285. doi:10.1053/apmr.2001.25152
47. Chamelian L, Feinstein A. Outcome after mild to moderate traumatic brain injury: the role of dizziness. *Arch Phys Med Rehabil.* 2004;85(10):1662-1666. doi:10.1016/j.apmr.2004.02.012
48. Katz DI, White DK, Alexander MP, Klein RB. Recovery of ambulation after traumatic brain injury. *Arch Phys Med Rehabil.* 2004;85(6):865-869. doi:10.1016/j.apmr.2003.11.020
49. Esquenazi A. Evaluation and management of spastic gait in patients with traumatic brain injury. *J Head Trauma Rehabil.* 2004;19(2):109-118. doi:10.1097/00001199-200403000-00004
50. Singer BJ, Jegasothy GM, Singer KP, Allison GT. Evaluation of serial casting to correct equinovarus deformity of the ankle after acquired brain injury in adults. *Arch Phys Med Rehabil.* 2003;84(4):483-491. doi:10.1053/apmr.2003.50041
51. McFadyen BJ, Swaine B, Dumas D, Durand A. Residual effects of a traumatic brain injury on locomotor capacity: a first study of spatiotemporal patterns during unobstructed and obstructed walking. *J Head Trauma Rehabil.* 2003;18(6):512-525. doi:10.1097/00001199-200311000-00005
52. Mossberg KA, Orlander EE, Norcross JL. Cardiorespiratory capacity after weight-supported treadmill training in patients with traumatic brain injury. *Phys Ther.* 2008;88(1):77-87. doi:10.2522/ptj.20070022
53. Esquenazi A, Lee S, Packel AT, Braitman L. A randomized comparative study of manually assisted versus robotic-assisted body weight supported treadmill training in persons with a traumatic brain injury. *PM R.* 2013;5(4):280-290. doi:10.1016/j.pmrj.2012.10.009
54. Fritz S, Lusardi M. White paper: "walking speed: the sixth vital sign". *J Geriatr Phys Ther.* 2009;32(2):46-49. doi:10.1519/00139143-200932020-00002
55. Vallée M, McFadyen BJ, Swaine B, Doyon J, Cantin JF, Dumas D. Effects of environmental demands on locomotion after traumatic brain injury. *Arch Phys Med Rehabil.* 2006;87(6):806-813. doi:10.1016/j.apmr.2006.02.031
56. Williams G, Galna B, Morris ME, Olver J. Spatiotemporal deficits and kinematic classification of gait following a traumatic brain injury: a systematic review. *J Head Trauma Rehabil.* 2010;25(5):366-374. doi:10.1097/HTR.0b013e3181cd3600
57. Williams G, Schache AG, Morris ME. Self-selected walking speed predicts ability to run following traumatic brain injury. *J Head Trauma Rehabil.* 2013;28(5):379-385. doi:10.1097/HTR.0b013e3182575f80
58. Perez OH, Green RE, Mochizuki G. Characterization of balance control after moderate to severe traumatic brain injury: a longitudinal recovery study. *Phys Ther.* 2018;98(9):786-795. doi:10.1093/ptj/pzy065
59. Kalmar K, Giacino JT. The JFK Coma Recovery Scale—revised. *Neuropsychol Rehabil.* 2005;15(3-4):454-460. doi:10.1080/09602010443000425
60. Bogner JA, Corrigan JD, Fugate L, Mysiw WJ, Clinchot D. Role of agitation in prediction of outcomes after traumatic brain injury. *Am J Phys Med Rehabil.* 2001;80(9):636-644. doi:10.1097/00002060-200109000-00002
61. Castriotta RJ, Lai JM. Sleep disorders associated with traumatic brain injury. *Arch Phys Med Rehabil.* 2001;82(10):1403-1406. doi:10.1053/apmr.2001.26081
62. Ríos M, Periáñez JA, Muñoz-Céspedes JM. Attentional control and slowness of information processing after severe traumatic brain injury. *Brain Inj.* 2004;18(3):257-272. doi:10.1080/02699050310001617442
63. Alderson AL, Novack TA. Reliable serial measurement of cognitive processes in rehabilitation: the Cognitive Log. *Arch Phys Med Rehabil.* 2003;84(5):668-672. doi:10.1016/S0003-9993(03)04842-6
64. Corrigan JD, Smith-Knapp K, Granger CV. Validity of the functional independence measure for persons with traumatic brain injury. *Arch Phys Med Rehabil.* 1997;78(8):828-834. doi:10.1016/S0003-9993(97)90195-7
65. Peterson DS, King LA, Cohen RG, Horak FB, Horak FB. Cognitive contributions to freezing of gait in Parkinson disease: implications for physical rehabilitation. *Phys Ther.* 2016;96(5):659-670. doi:10.2522/ptj.20140603
66. Rath JF, Hennesy JJ, Diller L. Social problem solving and community integration in postacute rehabilitation outpatients with traumatic brain injury. *Rehabil Psychol.* 2004;48(3):137-144. doi:10.1037/0090-5550.48.3.137
67. Kalpakjian CZ, Lam CS, Toussaint LL, Merbitz NK. Describing quality of life and psychosocial outcomes after traumatic brain injury. *Am J Phys Med Rehabil.* 2004;83(4):255-265. doi:10.1097/01.PHM.0000118033.07952.8C
68. Franulic A, Carbonell CG, Pinto P, Sepulveda I. Psychosocial adjustment and employment outcome 2, 5 and 10 years after TBI. *Brain Inj.* 2004;18(2):119-129. doi:10.1080/0269905031000149515
69. Gordon WA. Community integration of people with traumatic brain injury: introduction. *Arch Phys Med Rehabil.* 2004;85(4)(suppl 2):S1-S2. doi:10.1016/j.apmr.2003.08.118
70. McCrory P, Meeuwisse W, Johnston K, et al. Consensus statement on concussion in sport: the 3rd International Conference on Concussion in Sport held in Zurich, November 2008. *Amer Acad Phys Med Rehabil.* 2009;1(5):401-418.
71. Coronado VG, Haileyesus T, Cheng TA, et al. Trends in sports- and recreation-related traumatic brain injuries treated in US emergency departments: The National Electronic Injury Surveillance System-All Injury Program (NEISS-AIP) 2001-2012. *J Head Trauma Rehabil.* 2015;30(3):185-197. doi:10.1097/HTR.0000000000000156

72. Leong DF, Balcer LJ, Galetta SL, Liu Z, Master CL. The King-Devick test as a concussion screening tool administered by sports parents. *J Sports Med Phys Fitness*. 2014;54(1):70-77.
73. Schatz P, Pardini JE, Lovell MR, Collins MW, Podell K. Sensitivity and specificity of the ImPACT Test Battery for concussion in athletes. *Arch Clin Neuropsychol*. 2006;21(1):91-99. doi:10.1016/j.acn.2005.08.001
74. Taber KH, Warden DL, Hurley RA. Blast-related traumatic brain injury: what is known? *J Neuropsychiatry Clin Neurosci*. 2006;18(2):141-145. doi:10.1176/jnp.2006.18.2.141
75. Scherer M. Gait rehabilitation with body weight-supported treadmill training for a blast injury survivor with traumatic brain injury. *Brain Inj*. 2007;21(1):93-100. doi:10.1080/02699050601149104
76. Scherer MR, Shelhamer MJ, Schubert MC. Characterizing high-velocity angular vestibulo-ocular reflex function in service members post-blast exposure. *Exp Brain Res*. 2011;208(3):399-410. doi:10.1007/s00221-010-2490-1
77. Bland DC, Zampieri-Gallagher C, Damiano DL. Effectiveness of physical therapy for improving gait and balance in ambulatory individuals with traumatic brain injury: a systematic review of the literature. *Brain Inj*. 2011;25(7-8):664-679. doi:10.3109/02699052.2011.576306
78. Ptyushkin P, Vidmar G, Burger H, Marincek C. Use of the International Classification of Functioning, Disability and Health (ICF) in patients with traumatic brain injury. *Brain Inj*. 2010;24(13-14):1519-1527. doi:10.3109/02699052.2010.523054

Resources

Academy of Neurologic Physical Therapy
(Outcome measures recommendations for patients with TBI from the TBI EDGE Committee) This website reviews the metric strengths and weaknesses of outcomes measures for patients with TBI in both inpatient and outpatient settings.

http://www.neuropt.org/professional-resources/neurology-section-outcome-measures-recommendations/traumatic-brain-injury

Brain Injury Association of America
This website provides resources information for survivors of TBI and their families. Available links are dedicated to general information about TBI, current research initiatives, and teaching videos and resources.

https://www.biausa.org/

Brainline
This web-based resource offers educational information for people with a TBI, caregivers, professionals, and veterans. Appropriate links are dedicated to TBI basics, caregiver resources, and personal stories and blogs.

https://www.brainline.org/resource-directory

Chapter 13

Adult Clients With Stroke

Becky S. McKnight, PT, MS and James M. Smith, PT, DPT, MA

KEY WORDS Affective disorder | Anosognosia | Aphasia | Apraxia | Body weight–support during gait training | Cerebrovascular accident | Constraint-induced movement therapy | Dysphagia | Dysphasia | Hemiparesis | Hemorrhagic stroke | Homonymous hemianopia | Ischemic stroke | Lacunar infarction | Learned non-use | Pusher syndrome | Shoulder pain after stroke | Stroke | Transient ischemic attack | Unilateral neglect

Chapter Objectives

- Describe the types of cerebrovascular accidents (CVAs).
- Use the physical therapist's initial evaluation appropriately to guide decisions related to the implementation of selected interventions.
- Identify when the directed interventions are beyond the scope of work of the physical therapist assistant.
- Identify when it is necessary to communicate with the physical therapist regarding the patient's status and response to interventions.
- Explain the rationale for selected interventions to achieve patient goals as identified in the physical therapist's plan of care.
- Identify common safety issues and precautions that should be monitored when working with patients who have had a stroke.
- Describe strategies for effective physical therapy interventions, including patient- or client-related communication and instruction and interventions that may be included within a physical therapist's plan of care for a patient who has had a stroke.
- Describe the impairments in body functions and limitations in activities and participation that typically accompany stroke and identify strategies that a physical therapist assistant may use to accommodate for these during the provision of physical therapy interventions.
- Describe strategies and identify tests a physical therapist assistant may use to monitor the patient's response to selected interventions and to determine a patient's progress within the physical therapist's plan of care.
- Describe strategies a physical therapist assistant may use to progress interventions based upon the patient's responses.
- Discuss confounding factors that can affect the patient's ability to participate in physical therapy and describe methods to accommodate the patient's unique needs.

Cerebrovascular disease refers to any disorder involving the blood supply to the brain. When cerebrovascular disease results in the death of brain tissue, a stroke, also called a CVA, occurs. Diverse symptoms can develop depending on the location, the size of the brain injury, and the age of the individual. Stroke is, unfortunately, common; in the United States, about 800,000 strokes occur each year, making it the most common neurological disorder and the leading cause of disability among adults.[1] While often considered a problem experienced by the elderly, it is important to recognize that stroke may occur in younger people, including children and infants (see Chapter 9). Physical therapy interventions are usually indicated for the impairments in body functions and limitations in activities and participa-

Lazaro RT, Umphred DA, eds.
Umphred's Neurorehabilitation for the Physical Therapist Assistant, Third Edition (pp 315-349).

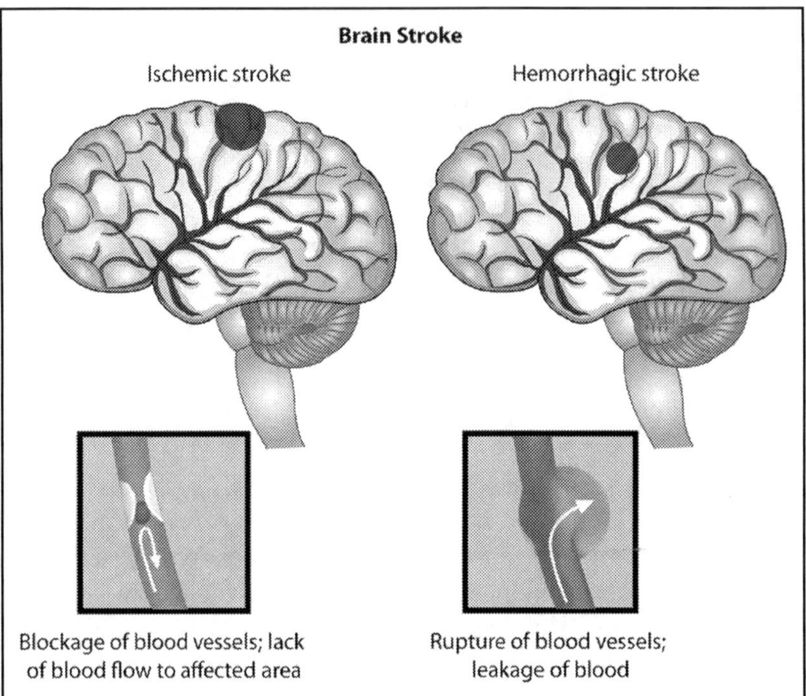

Figure 13-1. Image of ischemic and hemorrhagic stroke.

tion that follow a stroke. Appropriately applied physical therapy interventions can diminish the limitations related to stroke symptoms.[1]

Types of Stroke

There are 2 broad categories of stroke: ischemic and hemorrhagic. *Ischemic stroke*, which is more common, involves loss of the blood supply to part of the brain. This develops because of a blockage of 1 or more arteries that supply blood to the brain. The obstruction can occur from pathological changes that gradually occlude the blood vessel, such as atherosclerosis, or from an embolus that blocks a blood vessel. There are 2 additional categories of ischemic stroke: lacunar infarction and transient ischemic attack (TIA). A *hemorrhagic stroke*, also referred to as an *intracranial hemorrhage*, occurs when a blood vessel in the brain ruptures, resulting in blood flooding into the surrounding tissues (Figure 13-1).

Ischemic Stroke

Ischemia involving the brain is of great concern because of the high-energy demands of brain tissue. There is no mechanism to store metabolic reserves in the brain, so adequate blood supply is required to provide all the glucose, oxygen, and nutrients used by these tissues. When a blood vessel becomes blocked, the blood supply is interrupted distal to the blockage. In the area of complete or near-complete interruption of blood supply, ischemic necrosis, or death of the tissue, occurs within a couple of minutes. This cell damage is irreversible. Surrounding the area of necrosis is an area where the blood supply is diminished but not completely interrupted. The tissues in this area will have diminished functioning during the time of ischemia but can return to normal function if blood supply is restored quickly. If, however, blood supply is not restored within a short period, the necrotic area will expand, resulting in greater tissue death and greater disability. Because of this, immediate medical attention is imperative.[2] The patient's presentation (ie, impairments in body structures and functions and limitations in activities and participation) will depend on the size and location of the lesion as well as the nature and function of the structures involved, the availability of collateral blood flow, and early acute management (Table 13-1).

Lacunar Infarction

Lacunar infarcts are small ischemic strokes deep inside the brain that are named for their crescent-shaped appearance. They are common in the putamen, basal ganglia, thalamus, and internal capsule. As with all strokes, the symptoms associated with lacunar infarctions vary depending on the exact structures that are involved (eg, internal capsule and thalamus). Although these involve a small area, the effects can be quite dramatic because the areas involved can serve a variety of functions and lead to issues including weakness of the face, dysarthria, ataxia, and weakness.[2]

Transient Ischemic Attack

TIAs are caused by a temporary interruption in blood supply to the brain and result in sudden onset of impairments in body functions or limitations in activity, such as extremity weakness, sensory deficits, and difficulties with functional mobility. TIA symptoms vary in duration, but most are resolved within 1 hour. Within 24 hours there is a full recovery from all symptoms. Although the symptoms of TIA do resolve, medical attention is required, as TIAs often precede a stroke.[2]

Hemorrhagic Stroke

The major effects of a hemorrhagic stroke are damage from the lost circulation and damage from the leaked blood itself. The blood that leaks into the brain tissue has volume (ie, it takes up space), but the skull cannot accommodate the increase in volume. This results in compression of brain tissue, which causes direct injury to neurons. It may also compress adjacent blood vessels, resulting in those vessels narrowing or closing. While this effect is greatest in the area of the bleeding, the enclosed nature of the skull may result in an elevated intracranial pressure throughout the brain, requiring special medical management. Another effect of the leaked blood is irritation of the adjacent tissues. The chemical composition of the blood is noxious to brain tissue, causing further damage.[2]

Table 13-1

Body Function Impairments Associated With Cerebrovascular Accident

Primary Impairments
• Impaired muscle strength • Changes in muscle tone • Impairments in motor control • Impaired somatosensation • Impaired perception • Aphasia • Cognitive impairments • Urinary incontinence
Secondary Impairments
• Changes in alignment and mobility • Changes in muscle and soft tissues • Pain • Edema • Diminished cardiovascular endurance • Skin breakdown

Patient Entry Into Physical Therapy Care

A patient who is having a stroke is admitted to an acute hospital for medical intervention. The patient will initially receive medical care to identify the type of stroke and to implement the appropriate medical intervention to minimize the stroke and its sequelae. Of prime importance is to determine whether the stroke is ischemic or hemorrhagic. This is typically accomplished through radiologic imaging (eg, computed tomography). For ischemic strokes, if tissue plasminogen activator can be administered within the first 3 hours of initial stroke, the person is 30% more likely to recover.[2] For this reason it is essential that early signs of a stroke are recognized and that the individual seeks immediate attention. Medical treatment of hemorrhagic stroke depends greatly on the extent of the stroke as well as the underlying cause (eg, arterial malformation). Frequently, medical management consists of administration of antihypertensive medication. Various procedures can also be used to evacuate the hematoma or to repair an arterial malformation or damage.

Physical therapy in the acute care setting is initiated early via a referral from a physician or through a critical pathway established at the institution. In the contemporary health care system, a patient typically has a short stay in the acute care environment. Once the patient has become medically stable, the care team will consider which setting is best suited to provide the rehabilitation necessary to facilitate the patient's recovery. Frequently, patients are moved into an inpatient rehabilitation facility. In this setting patient's recovering from a stroke receive a minimum of 3 hours/day of rehabilitation services from the physical therapy, occupational therapy, and speech therapy departments. Patients who are not able to participate at that level of intensive therapy may qualify to receive therapy services in a skilled nursing facility. Some patients who have mild deficits and an adequate support system at home can be discharged to home to receive therapy through home health services or on an outpatient basis. Patients with limited capacity to improve functioning may be discharged to a nursing home or long-term care setting where physical therapy can be provided. Occasionally patients who have transferred to a skilled nursing facility or nursing home make improvements and demonstrate potential for significant improvements and then are transferred into an inpatient rehabilitation setting for intensive therapy at a later date (Figure 13-2).

Role of the Physical Therapist Assistant

Although symptoms from a stroke can vary widely depending on the size and location of the brain injury, recovery from a stroke often follows a predictable pattern. Once a patient is medically stable and the stroke symptoms appear to be following a predictable prognosis, the physical therapist may choose to direct the physical therapist assistant to provide selected physical therapy interventions. The physical therapist assistant functions as a member of the entire team (Table 13-2), working to assist the patient to meet medical, functional, and social goals. Team members may also include medical personnel, other rehabilita-

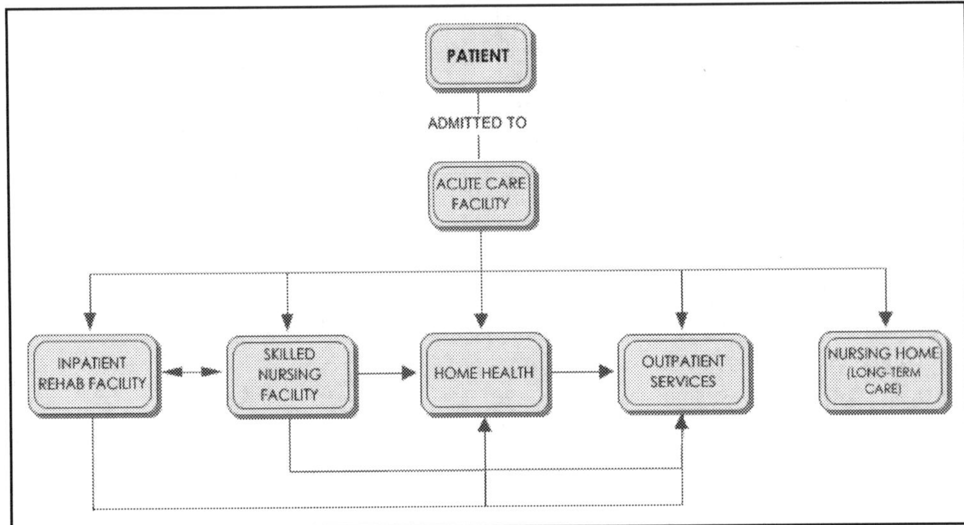

Figure 13-2. Patient pathway through the health care system.

Table 13-2
Team Members Involved in Care of a Patient Who has had a Stroke

- Physician
  - Physiatrist
  - Neurologist
  - Others as appropriate (eg, cardiologist)
- Nursing staff
- Pharmacist
- Neuropsychologist
- Physical therapist and physical therapist assistant
- Occupational therapist and occupational therapy assistant
- Speech therapist
- Recreational therapist
- Orthotist
- Social worker

tion personnel, and other health care professionals (see Table 13-2).

Within this team, the physical therapist assistant provides interventions, as directed by the physical therapist, to address impairments in body functions or limitations in activities and participation. These interventions are designed to help the patient progress from his or her current status to meet therapy goals (set by the physical therapist) focused on helping the patient regain the ability to participate in his or her normal activities. To help structure the intervention session, the physical therapist assistant must take into consideration a variety of factors and pieces of information (Figure 13-3).

Since the physical therapist assistant's primary role is in the implementation of interventions, the physical therapist assistant should order his or her clinical decision-making around interventions directed by the physical therapist. The physical therapist assistant should identify the interventions to be provided, then consider the impairment(s) and activity limitation(s) the physical therapist expects those interventions to address. For example, balance activities can be used to address trunk muscle strength deficits or motor control deficits. It is important for the physical therapist assistant to recognize which impairment is being addressed to choose the specific balance activities and intervention strategies that will be most effective in addressing that problem.

To further refine the intervention choices, the physical therapist assistant also needs to consider the patient's current status as related to the impairment(s) or activity limitation(s) being addressed. These should be addressed in light of the goals the physical therapist has set for these specific deficits. This will allow the physical therapist assistant to plan effective intervention strategies to use. Strategy considerations include assistive or adaptive devices, amount and type of feedback, and specific activities to incorporate in the intervention session. Considering the patient's current status in light of the goals will also help the physical therapist assistant be prepared to progress the patient appropriately. All of these clinical decisions are made within the context of the medical diagnosis and expected prognosis, which is frequently influenced by confounding factors such as comorbidities or other impairments of body factors (eg, communication deficits). Additional factors that can influence patient participation and progress include personal and environmental factors along with preexisting impairment prior to the stroke such as musculoskeletal, cardiac, pulmonary, circulatory, and pain.

To ensure patient safety, the physical therapist assistant must be familiar with common contraindications and pre-

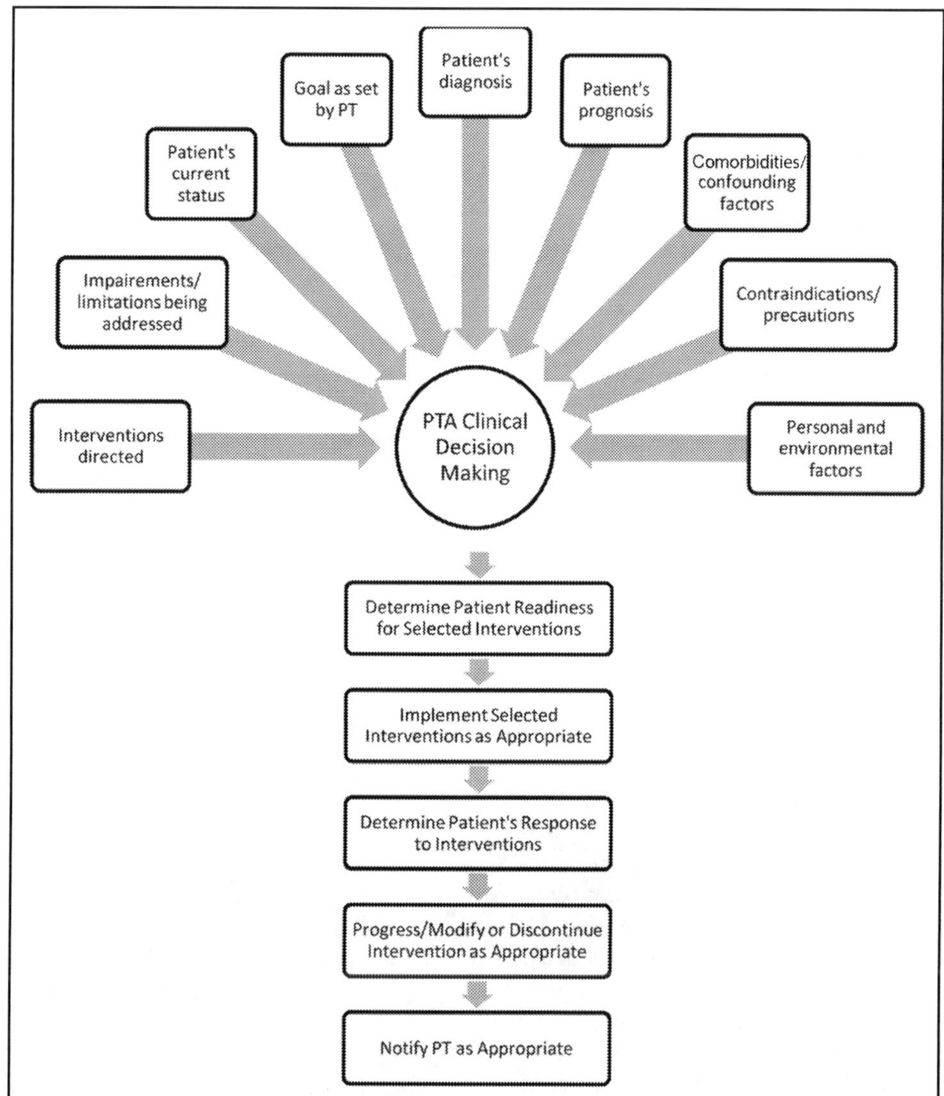

Figure 13-3. Physical therapist assistant clinical decision-making model.

cautions associated with working with patients with CVA as well as those associated with conditions that are frequent comorbidities for these individuals. The physical therapist assistant must take all of these factors into consideration when planning the specific parameters of the interventions prescribed by the physical therapist.

Prior to implementing each session, the physical therapist assistant should determine the patient's readiness for participation. When tests and measures and patient's responses indicate readiness, the physical therapist assistant can then implement the tailor-made intervention activities. The physical therapist assistant uses formal and informal assessment processes during a session, at the end of a session, and at intervals as required by the plan of care to make decisions related to modification, progression, or discontinuation of any or all intervention activities and communicates this to the physical therapist in a timely fashion.

The remainder of this chapter will use this framework to discuss details that the physical therapist assistant should consider when working with patients recovering from stroke. Prior to considering interventions commonly used with patients who have had a stroke, foundational principles of working as a member of the larger team and discussion of the integral nature of patient/client-related instruction will be reviewed.

Coordination, Communication, and Documentation

Because of the diverse symptoms that may be present, coordination of services is very important when working with individuals who have had a stroke. Most patients recovering from a stroke will be receiving care from other health care providers, including a physiatrist, occupational therapist, speech-language pathologist, nurse, neuropsychologist, and others. It is important that all disciplines coordinate the care being provided to ensure the patient will have the time and the energy necessary to participate in all treatment sessions and rehabilitation activities. In some settings (such as an inpatient rehabilitation facility), multidisciplinary meetings will allow for coordination and communication between the different health care providers working with the patient. This will provide the physical therapist and physical therapist assistant with invaluable information regarding the patient's impairments of body structures and functions that are not directly addressed by the physical therapy interventions, the patient's abilities, and strategies to manage these issues. Skilled communication includes verbal interactions between the physical therapist assistant and the physical therapist (and other health care providers) as well as appropriate documentation by the physical therapist assistant that clearly delineates the interventions provided and the patient's response(s) to those interventions. (Refer to Core book series: *Documentation Basics for the Physical Therapist Assistant*, 3rd ed.)[3]

Patient- or Client-Related Instruction

Providing patient- or client-related instruction should be a part of every physical therapy session. This instruction should consist of providing information about the patient's impairments and the implications of those impairments on the patient's functional abilities and daily life including any risk factors which may lead to secondary impairments. In addition, the physical therapist assistant should make sure the patient is actively involved in this process and educated about the specific interventions being used and how these interventions address the goals as outlined in the physical therapist's plan of care.[4]

The physical therapist assistant should document the patient's response to this instruction. Documentation typically includes a description of the individual's ability to follow directions or comprehend instruction as evidenced by the presence or absence of behavioral changes. Patients who learn about their condition, including unique impairments and functional limitations, will be better able to take control over their own care even if independent physical functioning is an unlikely outcome. Additionally, when caring for a patient recovering from a stroke, it is common that the patient's family and caregivers will require education related to providing care and support for the patient. In summary, education should be a priority within the interventions provided to the patient who has had a stroke.

Selected Interventions

The plan of care designed by the physical therapist will be unique to each patient receiving physical therapy following a stroke. Therefore, the physical therapist assistant must be able to interpret that plan of care to address the individual needs of each patient. This can be a daunting challenge, because diverse therapeutic strategies and techniques have been advocated for promoting improvements in body functions and the patient's ability to perform functional activities and participate in a variety of social roles following a stroke. To guide the physical therapist assistant in this process, the authors recommend the conceptual framework for therapeutic interventions for neuromuscular disorders described by Fell.[5] Fell categorized interventions as those related to motor learning and practice, those related to characteristics of a movement or task, and as other parameters for interventions (which will be described shortly). This framework is summarized in Table 13-3 and will be useful for streamlining the clinical decision-making when providing physical therapy interventions to persons who have had a stroke.

The discussion will begin with the area of neuromotor development training that includes motor training and neuromotor reeducation. Principles related to neuromotor reeducation are foundational to working with patients with motor deficits associated with neurological conditions. These basic principles are applied to other types of therapeutic interventions, such as strength training and functional training. This will be followed by discussion of additional interventions commonly used with individuals who have had a stroke.

Therapeutic Exercise for Neuromotor Development

One component of the therapeutic exercise interventions for a patient who has had a stroke is the fostering of a change in abilities through motor learning. The need for learning will vary with each individual and with the types of tasks the individual must perform. Examples include learning how to obtain movement from weakened limbs, learning how to use something new (eg, an assistive device), or learning new strategies for ambulating in crowded areas. To promote learning, the physical therapist assistant must apply strategies that have proven effective for motor learning. Essential strategies include practice, task attention, feedback, and environmental progression.[5] Each of these strategies is discussed in Chapter 4 and will be built on here; in the clinic, the physical therapist assistant should consider these individually and collectively when providing interventions. The physical therapist assistant must remember that sometimes a whole activity is easier than part-learning. For that reason, it may be easier to ask a patient to stand up than to ask him to move the hips forward close to the edge, bend forward, shift weight over the feet, and stand up.

Practice

Practice is a well-recognized technique for improving performance. This applies whether the learner is a canoer learning a paddle stroke, a child learning how to walk, or

Table 13-3

Progressing Therapeutic Intervention in Patients With Neuromuscular Disorders

Parameters Related to Motor Learning and Practice
• Variability in practice (eg, blocked practice → random practice) • Practicing components of movement (eg, part-task training → whole-task training) • Task attention (eg, minimal distractions → cognitive/attentional demands) • Feedback (eg, extrinsic feedback [knowledge of performance, knowledge of results] → intrinsic feedback) • Environmental progression (eg, simple → complex)
Parameters Related to Characteristics of a Movement or Task
• Amplitude or magnitude of movement (eg, small range → large range of movement, mass synergy → isolated movement) • Velocity (eg, slow gait → fast gait) • Amount of work (eg, increase the frequency, intensity or duration of activity/exercise) • Endurance (eg, increase the capacity to persevere at a task) • Regional (eg, isolated movement → multi-joint movement, proximal movements → distal movements)
Other Parameters
• Developmental sequence (eg, low → high center of gravity, large → small base of support) • Supportive device (eg, ankle-foot orthotic or cane) • Assistance given (eg, verbal cues for guidance → minimal cues, moderate assistance → minimal assistance)
Adapted from Fell D. Progressing therapeutic intervention in patients with neuromuscular disorders: a framework to assist clinical decision making. *J Neurol Phys Ther.* 2004;28(1):35-46. doi:10.1097/01.NPT.0000284776.32802.1b.

a person rehabilitating from a stroke who needs to relearn how to move a limb. The physical therapist assistant should recognize that each session of providing physical therapy interventions is the patient's opportunity for practice and that the practice is an essential component of improving the ability to move and to function. Therefore, each session should be designed for motor learning and should include those strategies that will make the act of practicing most successful and efficient for the patient. Skilled applications of motor learning and practice strategies should be applied to all therapeutic exercise interventions so that the patient can gain the optimal benefit from physical therapy.

When designing practice of a new movement or task, a common strategy is to have the patient repeat a single component of the action. For example, the physical therapist assistant may choose to have the patient who has had a stroke repeatedly practice transferring from sitting to standing to sitting, or have the patient practice walking on a flat, smooth surface. This type of practice, which relies on repeating the same component of a task under the same conditions, is called *blocked practice*. Blocked practice assists with the preliminary learning of the movements or components of the task; therefore, it should be used in the early stages of learning. However, "it has been found that recall and transfer of motor skills, as well as learning, retention, and refinement of a skill, are best facilitated by random repetition over blocked repetition."[5] This means that varying the activities being practiced (ie, *random practice*) has the potential to improve the learning. For example, the physical therapist assistant may have the patient practice transferring from sitting to and from standing from chairs of different heights or have the patient practice walking on irregular surfaces or through an obstacle course. An appropriate progression of the intervention would be to advance exercises from the consistency of blocked practice to the variability of random practice of a task.[5] If a patient has difficulty initiating coming to stand, a physical therapist assistant might assist initially and then have the patient begin to sit down and come back up. You might have the patient sit onto a stool initially and back to stand. Then increase the range of motion (ROM) by having the patient move from standing to sitting onto a chair. This can be practiced until the patient can sit from standing and come back to standing. Finally, have the patient in standing come to sitting, relax, and then come back to standing. Once that is easy, then practice initiating from sitting.

Another strategy to advance learning in the early stages of the acquisition of motor learning is part practice (or *part-task training*), in which the movements that constitute a task are practiced. Once these components have been practiced, the intervention should be progressed to whole practice (*whole-task training*) to foster motor learning. For example, a patient who has had a stroke may practice standing weight-shifting, then progress to stepping forward and backward with the non-hemiplegic leg (providing stability in the hemiplegic leg), and then stepping with the other leg for part practice. This may later be progressed to ambulating, which represents the strategy of whole practice.[4]

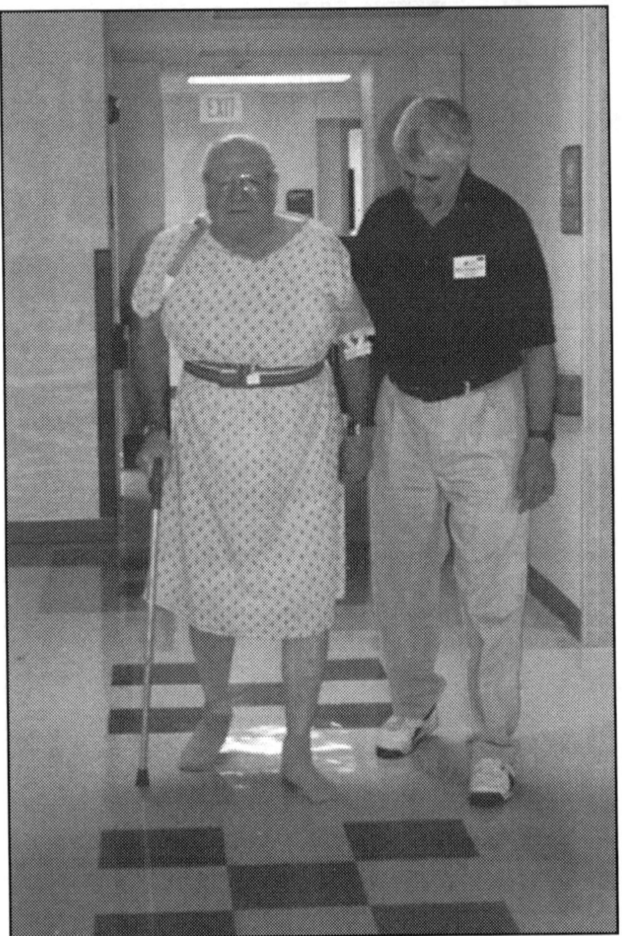

Figure 13-4. Gait training patient in an environment with minimal distractions.

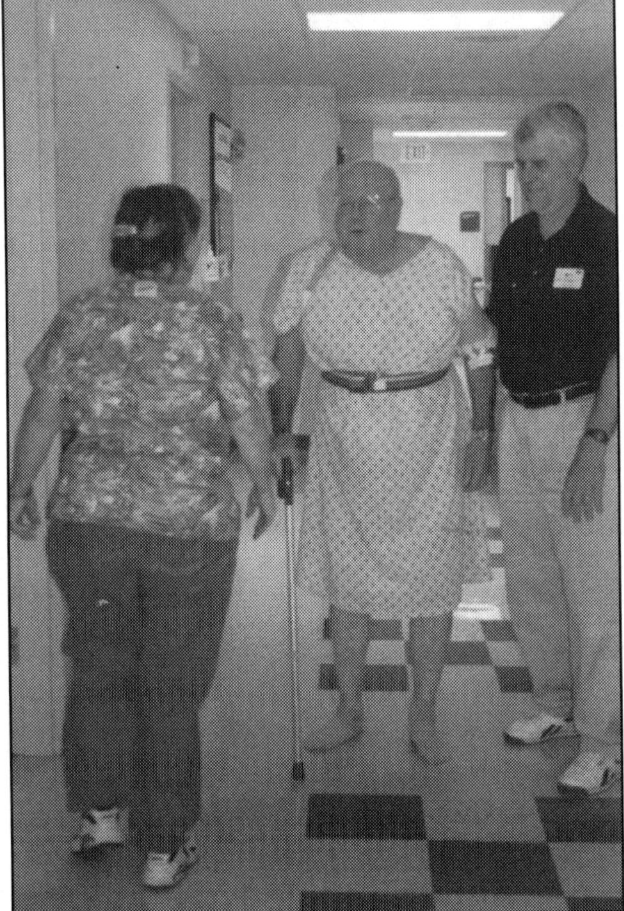

Figure 13-5. As the patient's attention to task improves, the environment should become more complex during the functional activity.

Task Attention

The patient's initial motor learning will be greatest if the patient is able to pay close attention to the task or exercise that is being learned. Since stroke is a type of brain injury, there is a risk for symptoms of altered cognition or attention. Therefore, a physical therapist assistant should choose a setting with minimal distractions. This may mean planning interventions in a quiet room or during quieter periods in the therapy area (Figure 13-4). As learning advances, the physical therapist assistant must also consider the anticipated outcome for the patient. If the patient will need to function in settings with multiple distractions (eg, social gatherings, restaurants, or religious services), the individual will require the ability to manage multiple demands on attention. Therefore, the interventions applied should prepare for those demands by progressing practice sessions toward situations with multiple demands on the patient's attention (eg, walking in a busy hallway [Figure 13-5]) or by increasing cognitive demands (eg, holding a conversation while ambulating).[4]

Feedback strategies used can also impact the patient's attention. Research has shown that post-stroke patients who are provided with explicit information regarding task goals before beginning practice have improved motor learning. Evidence on individuals without neurological impairments suggests that instruction with an external focus (ie, the results of the movement) rather than those with an internal focus (ie, the movement itself) were associated with better outcomes. For that reason, it may be easier to ask a patient to stand up than to ask him to move the hips forward close to the edge, bend forward, shift weight over the feet, and stand up. For example, during gait training to increase step length, the physical therapist assistant can provide instruction for the patient to "put the cane out farther" instead of to "take a larger step."[6]

Feedback

Feedback is any of the sensory information a person uses for learning and improving performance. *Intrinsic feedback* is the sensory information received from an individual's own body, such as the kinesthetic sensations of movement from the limbs. This type of feedback can be augmented by techniques such as using a mirror to allow a patient to observe posture and how the posture changes as a result of movements, although some patients may find the mirror more confusing due to their perceptual problems. A therapist must always be aware of the patient's response when augmenting the environment. *Extrinsic feedback* is when the physical therapy provider gives information to the patient to improve performance. Extrinsic feedback is characterized as knowledge of performance, which is information about the components or quality of movement(s), or knowledge of results, which is information about the outcome achieved from the movement(s). A physical therapist assistant must use feedback as a tool to shape and improve the patient's motor performance and learning. To achieve this, Fell has advised that, as interventions are advanced with a patient, "regardless of the type and source of feedback, there should always be a progressive decrease in extrinsic feedback provided" to promote learning.[5] The physical therapist assistant should also be considerate of the amount of feedback provided, because excessive feedback will distract from the patient's ability to attend to the task at hand. Finally, the timing of feedback should also be considered. In many situations, the optimal time for feedback is delayed for a few seconds following the completion of the task, this allows the patient the opportunity to process the intrinsic feedback, and reflect upon and assess the task performance, prior to receiving external feedback. This helps the patient develop self-regulatory skills and increases the likelihood for motor learning to occur.

Environmental Progression

The environmental context for physical therapy interventions will also influence motor learning. Early learning of tasks may be improved when it occurs in an environment with minimal complexity, so the physical therapist assistant may want to provide interventions in a simple environment with no obstacles and limited items requiring visual processing. In addition to fostering motor learning, by reducing demands for attention, the patient with perceptual or cognitive impairments will be better able to focus on the task and learn from practice.

While this strategy is beneficial early in the learning process, the physical therapist assistant should also consider the desired outcomes and progress the practice sessions to providing relevant experiences. For example, a person returning to community living will need to function in complex environments. To illustrate, consider the demands of walking into a restaurant or place of worship. In these environments, obstacles must be walked around and people will offer greetings. Interpreting and responding to those demands is complex, and it becomes more challenging if the patient also must use an assistive device or deal with visual or other perceptual deficits. Successful function in a complex environment will require practice in similar situations. To accomplish this, the physical therapist assistant should incrementally add environmental complexity in the therapy session. A progression might be adding obstacles the patient must recognize and negotiate, or it might be adding social demands such as talking with the patient during gait training. Progressions such as these should be added singly (rather than making 2 or more progressions at the same time) so the patient can practice and improve in the ability to deal with diverse types of demands.[7]

Another example is drinking from a cup. The progression from performing that task while seated and quiet, to being seated and interacting with others, to standing, to standing and interacting with others is a strategy for advancing the demands placed so the patient achieves motor learning and then advances to increasingly more complex situations.[7] The physical therapist assistant should be able to apply these general concepts for progression of the interventions. This is best achieved by identifying, through the goals established by the physical therapist, the types of environments and demands that the patient is likely to encounter, and advancing according to the patient's response and success of performance. The patient and the family can often provide needed information regarding the environments the patient will interact in once the patient leaves rehabilitation. Once the patient demonstrates success with a task, the physical therapist assistant should consider how to increase the demands (ie, increase the complexity). With this type of practice, the patient will develop the necessary abilities to succeed with the task when performing in the "real world."

Factors Relating to the Movement or Task

The exercises selected by the physical therapist assistant should also be directed at advancing the patient's ability to move a region of the body or complete a task. This will include improving the strength and the quality (skill) of the movement. For example, if a patient who has had a stroke has weakness of the knee extensor muscles requiring assistance to stand up from a chair, the physical therapist assistant could choose from many exercise options that promote strengthening of the knee extensor muscles. However, for the exercise to be therapeutic, the interventions should be designed to both improve strength of the knee extensor muscles and address the function task of rising from a chair. The following are examples of characteristics of a task or movement that should be advanced or progressed as the patient's performance improves:

- The amplitude (or amount) of movement that occurs (eg, progress from moving through a small range to large range of movement or progress from moving large regions of the body to isolated or fine movements).
- The velocity of the movement (eg, progress from training at a slow gait speed to a fast gait).
- The amount of work being performed (eg, increase the frequency, intensity, or duration of the exercise or the task that is being practiced).
- The patient's capacity for work (endurance; eg, increase the repetitions performed or the distance walked during gait training).
- The region(s) of the body being addressed (eg, the challenge may be increased by training for proximal move-

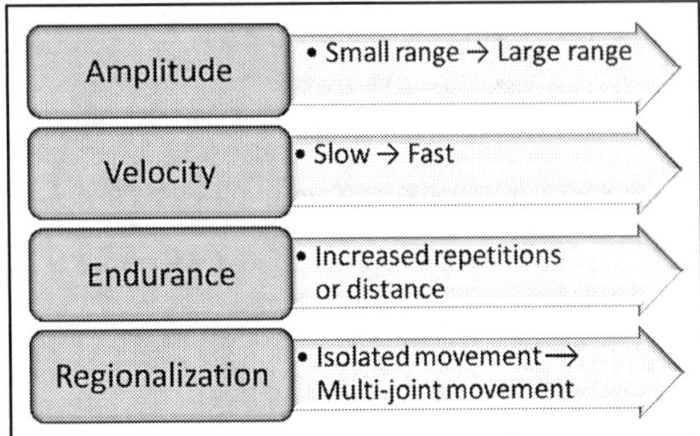

Figure 13-6. Characteristics of a task and how to progress it.

ments before distal movements or for the performance of isolated movement before multi-joint movements; Figure 13-6).[5]

Other Parameters

The ability to perform a task may be improved by using a supportive or adaptive device, allowing for practice and improved capability with that task. For example, a patient may use an ankle-foot orthosis (AFO) to improve the ability to walk, or a grab bar to provide additional support while rolling. Progression may be achieved by reducing the amount of support or the amount of reliance placed on the device, or by adjusting or adapting the device. For example, a patient may initially walk while supporting him- or herself with parallel bars, followed by progression to a quad cane and then a straight cane.[5] Discussion of the use of assistive, adaptive, and supportive devices and orthotics will occur later in this chapter.

Another consideration during the provision of therapeutic exercise interventions is the amount or type of assistance provided by the physical therapist assistant. This progression is commonly recognized for physical assistance, in which the physical therapist assistant gradually and intentionally decreases the amount of support provided, while the patient increases the amount of work performed. Progression can also be achieved by reducing other supports, such as the amount of verbal cues provided for guidance during task performance, with the progression being achieved by intentionally reducing the amount of cues provided to the patient.[5]

Therapeutic Exercise Interventions for Aerobic Capacity/Endurance

An overarching concern when implementing therapeutic exercise interventions is impaired exercise capacity. The American Heart Association has recommended that the major rehabilitation goals following a stroke are preventing inactivity and disuse, decreasing the risk of a recurrent stroke or cardiovascular disorder, and increasing aerobic fitness.[8] To achieve this, each patient should engage in physical exercise as soon as possible to enhance his or her general activity level. The physical therapist assistant providing therapeutic exercise interventions must provide appropriate aerobic challenges, preferably through upright activities (eg, training for gait or stair climbing) while monitoring the patient's response to those exercises.[8] Sample activities are described in Table 13-4. The physical therapist will be a resource for determining precautions and thresholds for aerobic training (eg, target and maximum heart rates and acceptable blood pressure [BP]). However, the physical therapist assistant should also be aware of general guidelines for cardiovascular conditions for patients who demonstrate those comorbidities. Some patients may have inadequate capacity for planned exercise interventions, and in those situations, the physical therapist assistant should modify the intervention appropriately, such as decreasing the exercise intensity or duration while increasing the frequency of exercise sessions (see Chapter 16).

Therapeutic Exercise: Balance and Coordination

Individuals who have had a stroke frequently demonstrate deficits in balance and coordination. These impairments can also be referred to as deficits in postural control and motor control. The deficits are a result of a combination of impairments common for individuals who have had a stroke (see the discussion of impairments later in this chapter). Postural control or balance should be addressed in the sitting and standing positions (as the patient is able). The primary focus of postural control is trunk control. Trunk control is imperative for functional movement, including weight-shifting and reaching. Initially, activities should focus on helping the patient obtain and maintain symmetrical upright control, in which the patient weight-bears equally on both ischial tuberosities in sitting or both feet in standing. Once midline control has been achieved, weight-shifting activities can be initiated. These activities help the patient reestablish the appropriate synergistic relationship between the agonist and antagonist muscle groups. Simple weight-shifting activities are followed by more challenging dynamic activities, such as reaching and manipulating objects or taking steps forward/backward. At each stage, the physical therapist assistant should monitor for appropriate postural control and modify the activity based on the patient's abilities.[6] The importance of initiating sitting activities is emphasized by Carr and Shepherd when they state, "In the acute state post-stroke, major goals are to prevent medical complications associated with the supine position and bedrest and to retrain balance in sitting. Reestablishing sitting balance early is critical since it impacts positively on many functions. It provides greater stimulus for gaseous interchange and facilitates coughing, enables more effective swallowing, encourages eye contact

Table 13-4

Summary of Exercise Programming Recommendations for Stroke Survivors From the American Heart Association

Mode of Exercise	*Major Goals*	*Intensity/Frequency/Duration*
Aerobic		
• Large muscle activities (eg, walking, treadmill, stationary cycle, combined arm-leg ergometry, and seated stepper)	• Increase independence in ADLs • Increase walking speed/efficiency • Improve tolerance for prolonged physical activity • Reduce risk of cardiovascular disease	• 40% to 70% peak oxygen uptake; 40% to 70% heart rate reserve; 50% to 80% maximal heart rate; Borg Rating of Perceived Exertion 11 to 14 (6-20 scale) • 3 to 7 days/week • 20 to 60 minutes/session (or multiple 10-minute sessions)
Strength		
• Circuit training • Weight machines • Free weights • Isometric exercise	• Increase independence in ADLs	• 1 to 3 sets for 10 to 15 reps of 8 to 10 exercises involving the major muscle groups
Flexibility		
• Stretching	• Increase ROM of involved extremities • Prevent contractures	• 2 to 3 days/week (before or after aerobic or strength training) • Hold each stretch for 10 to 30 seconds
Neuromuscular		
• Coordination and balance activities	• Improve level of safety during ADLs	• 2 to 3 days/week (consider performing on the same day as strength activities)

Reprinted with permission from Gordon NF, Gulanick M, Costa F, et al. Physical activity and exercise recommendations for stroke survivors: an American Heart Association scientific statement from the Council on Clinical Cardiology, Subcommittee on Exercise, Cardiac Rehabilitation, and Prevention; Cardiac Rehabilitation, and Prevention; the Council on Cardiovascular Nursing; the Council on Nutrition; Physical Activity, and Metabolism; and the Stroke Council. *Circulation.* 2004;16(109):2031-2041. doi:10.1161/01.CIR.0000126280.65777.A4.

and focusing attention, communication and more positive attitudes, stimulates arousal mechanisms, and discourages learned 'sick role' behavior."[9]

Therapeutic Exercise: Flexibility Exercises

Following a stroke, there is a high risk for losing flexibility in the involved limbs, and traditionally stretching is applied. For example, a patient with involvement of the hand often develops greater activity in the finger flexor muscles over time, with accompanying spasticity and posturing into finger flexion. Stretching is typically provided to prevent or correct for stiffness or contracture involving flexion of the fingers. Evidence has indicated that stretching interventions have no appreciable benefit on joint mobility, spasticity, or pain.[10] Therefore, traditional stretching routines may provide limited benefits for a patient following a stroke. When the physical therapist's plan of care includes specific stretching interventions, based on the unique needs of a patient, strategies the physical therapist assistant should consider include prolonged stretch and relaxation techniques. Prolonged stretch to prevent contracture may include the use of splints for positioning the ankle or the wrist/hand, and positioning the shoulder on the weaker side in external rotation for 30 minutes/day.[1] Relaxation techniques (see Chapter 5) such as constant pressure and gentle oscillations of the limb improve the effectiveness of the stretching by reducing the increased tone usually present following a stroke.

Therapeutic Exercise: Gait and Locomotion Training

Like balance and coordination, much of what is discussed regarding gait and locomotion training falls under motor control and motor learning strategies. In addition, gait training often uses assistive or adaptive equipment. Specifics related to using assistive devices will be discussed in the following paragraphs. Within this section, the

Table 13-5

Common Gait Deviations in Individuals With Hemiparesis

- Heel strike to midstance
  - Excessive forward trunk flexion
  - Limited ankle dorsiflexion
  - Lack of knee flexion
- Midstance
  - Inability to control knee
    - Lack of knee extension
    - Knee hyperextension
  - Limited hip extension
  - Limited ankle dorsiflexion
  - Excessive lateral weight-shift
  - Inability to transfer weight appropriately
- Late stance/preswing
  - Lack of knee flexion
  - Lack of ankle plantar flexion
- Early and mid-swing
  - Limited knee flexion
  - Limited hip flexion
  - Limited ankle dorsiflexion
- Late swing
  - Limited knee extension
- Parameters of gait
  - Decreased walking speed
  - Short and/or uneven step and stride lengths
  - Increased stride width
  - Increased double support phase
  - Dependence on support through UEs

physical therapist assistant will find descriptions of gait deviations that are commonly seen with individuals who have had a stroke, and discussion of general strategies not described in other areas.

Patients who require gait training interventions benefit from repetition to foster motor learning, and specificity of the training (eg, practice in environments similar to their discharge destination and goals) to promote attainment of the abilities needed for activity and participation.[1] During gait training activities, it is important for the physical therapist assistant to monitor and address gait deviations (Table 13-5). Determining the most likely cause of a gait deviation is the responsibility of the physical therapist, as multiple factors can be the cause. Knowledge of common gait deviations displayed by individuals who have had a stroke, however, will allow the physical therapist assistant to be better prepared to provide gait training interventions and make modifications.

There has been interest in using partial body weight–support during gait training. This technique involves gait training on a treadmill or over land while the patient is suspended in a harness that supports the lower trunk and proximal lower extremities (LEs; Figure 13-7). This harness supports a portion of the person's body weight so that the patient may practice the task of walking with a low risk for falling and with a reduction of gait deviation(s). This intervention has achieved restoration of greater walking ability, as demonstrated by significantly less reliance on assistance, greater walking speed, and greater walking endurance.[11,12] Recent studies also support the benefit of mechanically assisted walking (such as robotic devices or an electromechanical gait trainer).[2] Should the physical therapist include one of these devices in the plan of care the physical therapist assistant will require training in the unique application and use of the device.

Locomotor training includes wheelchair (w/c) mobility training. This will be part of the plan of care for patients who will be using a w/c either exclusively or for community integration. W/c mobility includes instructing the patient on how to maneuver the w/c with the stronger extremities. This is frequently accomplished through the patient using the stronger leg to maneuver and propel the w/c with assistance of the stronger arm. Patients should be instructed in maneuvering around obstacles to mimic the environments in which they will be functioning. Instruction should include w/c use up and down ramps, through doors, and on and off elevators.

Therapeutic Exercise: Strength and Endurance Training

Interventions that address strength deficits in individuals who have had a stroke are frequently referred to as *muscle reeducation activities* or *movement reeducation activities*. The strength deficits associated with a stroke, as with other neurological deficits, are due to a unique combination of upper neuron involvement, motor control deficits, and muscular deconditioning (Figure 13-8). As such, several exercise principles come into play when addressing these deficits. Exercise principles that govern all strength programs include the Reversibility Principle, the Overload Principle, and the Specific Adaptation to Imposed Demands Principle[13] (Table 13-6). In addition, aspects of motor control and motor learning discussed earlier in this chapter should guide the physical therapist assistant when making decisions related to strengthening programs for patients who have had a stroke.

Many individuals who have a neurological condition such as a stroke also demonstrate movement patterns that are dominated in a synergistic pattern. To address these abnormal movement patterns, principles of movement reeducation should be implemented. Movement reeducation is designed to increase strength and movement control on 4 levels.

- The first level is the ability to recruit individual muscles. At this level, the physical therapist assistant focuses on helping the patient learn to activate muscles to work selectively with eccentric, isometric, and

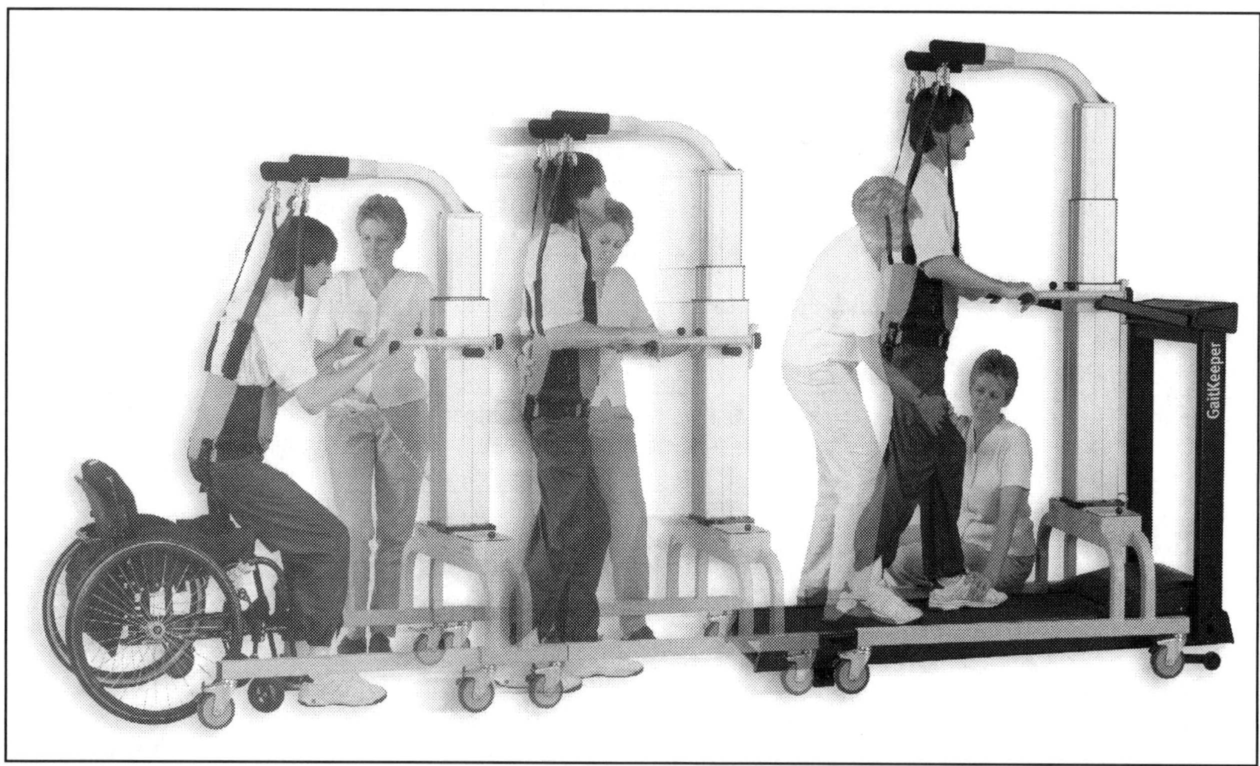

Figure 13-7. Gait training with body weight–support system on treadmill. (Reprinted with permission from Mobility Research, LLC, Tempe, AZ, www.litegait.com.)

concentric contractions without being dominated by synergistic movement patterns. For example, a therapy session may focus on the patient's being able perform elbow flexion without the synergistic movement of shoulder flexion occurring.

- The second level is the movement component level. At this level, groups of muscles in an extremity or the trunk are training to work together synergistically to produce a desired functional movement. For example, the patient will work on bringing a hand to the top of the head.
- The third level is the movement sequence level. At this level, multiple muscles from various body parts are trained to work together. Movement sequences are primarily used for transitional movements, such as rolling.
- The fourth and final level is the functional movement level. At this level, muscles are trained to work together to accomplish complex movements required for function, such as reaching for a glass.[14]

An important consideration of movement reeducation is ensuring appropriate biomechanical alignment during movement. It has been recognized that poor muscle alignment can be a factor in strength deficits and can facilitate inappropriate (even synergistic) muscle activation.

Multiple studies have indicated that strength gains can occur even in patients who are in the chronic stage after traditional therapies are typically discontinued. Therefore, it is important to incorporate strengthening activities at all stages of recovery from a stroke. Strengthening activities can include traditional resistive exercises; however, to facilitate strength gains that are associated with functional activities, task-specific training is preferred.[15-18]

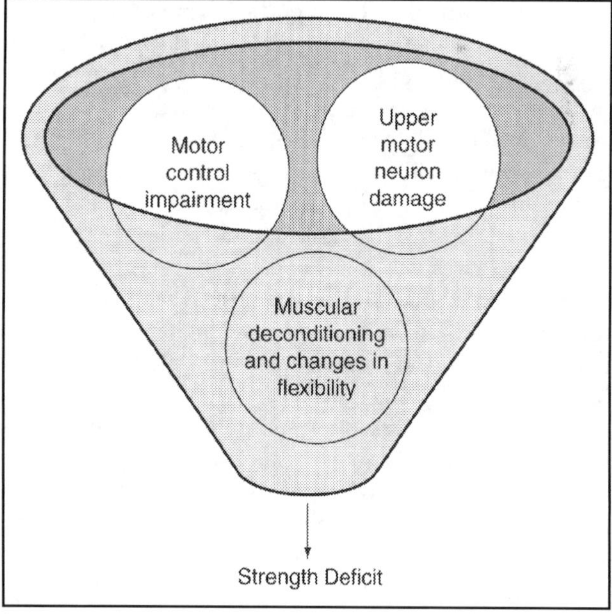

Figure 13-8. Components that lead to strength deficits.

Table 13-6

Principles of Exercise as Applied to Patients With Cerebrovascular Accident

Principle	*Description*	*Application*
Overload	For training adaptation to take place, a greater than normal stress (or load) must be placed on the body system being targeted.	Use interventions that work the patient near the limit of her/his abilities: functionally, aerobically, motorically.
Specific Adaptation to Imposed Demands (SAID)	Certain exercise or type of training produces adaptations specific to the activity performed and only in the body systems stressed by the activity.	Use interventions to train for activities that are relevant to the patient's needs for functioning and participation.
Reversibility	Training-induced changes (such as increased strength) are transient unless regularly used for functional activities.	Engage the patient in behavioral changes that emphasize activity and use of involved body segments (ie, overcome learned non-use).

Functional Training

One challenge when working with patients following a CVA is determining the types of postures or activities that will be used as the foundation for the practice that is necessary to foster the reattainment of functional abilities. A frequently used framework for determining therapeutic exercise interventions is a developmental progression. According to Fell, this is typically biomechanically based and progressed by elevating the center of gravity and/or narrowing the base of support.[5] Examples of activities include exercises in prone or prone on elbows, rolling or crawling activities, exercises in quadruped or during creeping, exercises in kneeling or half-kneeling, and standing and ultimately walking activities (Figure 13-9).[5] For example, a patient who is limited in the ability to transition from supine to a sitting posture should receive exercise interventions addressing that task with activities of a similar nature. Exercises lower on the developmental progression (eg, prone on elbows) will provide insufficient challenge to facilitate improvement, and exercises higher on the developmental progression (eg, standing) will reduce the likelihood of success during practice.

Another framework for determining therapeutic exercise interventions is to choose tasks necessary to the patient, and design exercise interventions to advance ability for that task. This is an important consideration given the wide scope of activities that may be relevant to an individual within the discharge environment (Figure 13-10). These tasks may range from self-care (eg, getting up from the floor or putting on a coat) to recreation (eg, handling a fishing rod or walking on a beach); therefore, potential tasks to be considered are too numerous to list. Instead, the physical therapist assistant must keep the following in mind when choosing postures or activities for exercise interventions: the types of tasks and demands unique to each patient's needs upon discharge from physical therapy, the patient's current functional ability, and those postures or activities that represent a developmental progression that the patient should practice.

The authors recommend that the choice of activities for therapeutic exercise interventions be guided by the following considerations:

- The activity is, or is similar to, a task that is necessary (relevant) to the patient.
- Learning and improved function will be fostered when:
    - The patient is capable of some successful performance of the activity.
    - The activity is sufficiently challenging (difficult) for the patient during the practice sessions.
    - Note that the developmental progression is not a sequential progression or an advancement of activities that should be followed. Also, a patient may be able to skip some activities and should increase practice with those activities that have the greatest relevance to physical therapy goals.[5]

Assistive Technology

Assistive and adaptive devices are used as part of the therapeutic intervention strategy in physical therapy. Some devices are used only during an intervention session to provide additional support or feedback for the patient during task-oriented activities; other devices are used on a temporary basis (eg, days, weeks, or months) to help the patient be more independent and safe while working toward established goals. Some assistive technology, however, is used on a long-term basis as part of a compensatory approach to manage residual deficits. Selecting and using assistive technology should be considered carefully regardless of the time frame for use. Each device should be used in a prescriptive fashion with a clear understanding of the physical therapy goals and intentions for their use. The physical therapist assistant may decide to use some devices, such as an air-sleeve or a knee splint, during an individual treatment session to provide feedback to the patient and to

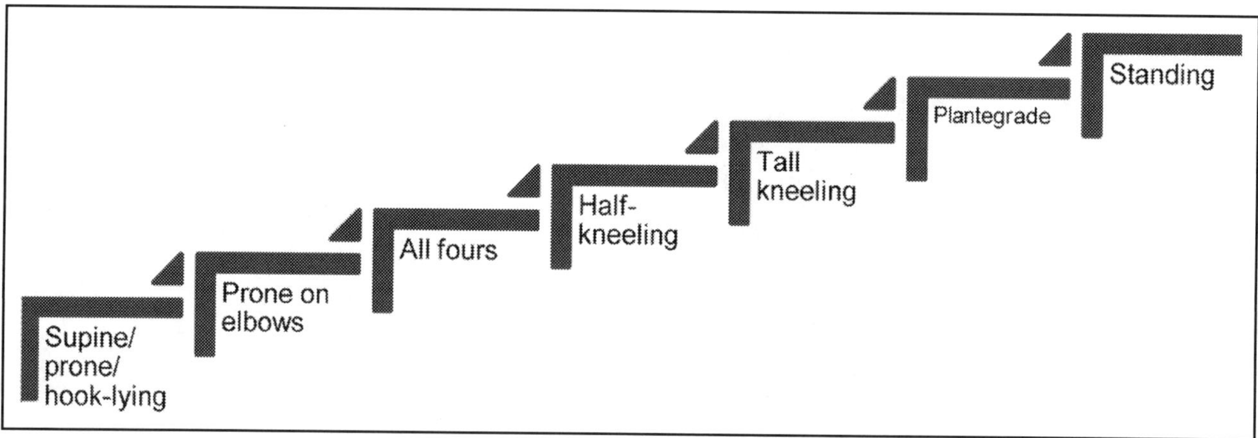

Figure 13-9. Developmental progression framework for functional training.

act as a second pair of hands allowing the physical therapist assistant the opportunity to focus the patient's attention and efforts on other components of the task. For example, a knee splint may be used to stabilize the weaker lower limb during standing balance activities while the physical therapist assistant facilitates appropriate trunk control. Devices used on a temporary (ie, not limited to an individual therapy session) or long-term basis will be the decision of the physical therapist. The physical therapist assistant will be made aware of the physical therapist's expectations through the plan of care. Devices such as a w/c, a hemi cane, or an AFO may be used either on a temporary or a long-term basis. In the event of temporary use, the physical therapist's plan of care will specify the expected time frame when the patient should be advanced to a different device or to independent activity without an assistive device. As with all interventions, the physical therapist assistant will monitor the patient's abilities as related to use of the device. This should include monitoring for appropriate fit and alignment, as well as safe and appropriate use of the device. If the patient's progression is faster or slower than anticipated, the physical therapist assistant should bring this to the physical therapist's attention and make suggestions based on the patient's presentation and response to therapeutic intervention. The following are examples of devices and equipment commonly used with patients who have had a stroke.[19]

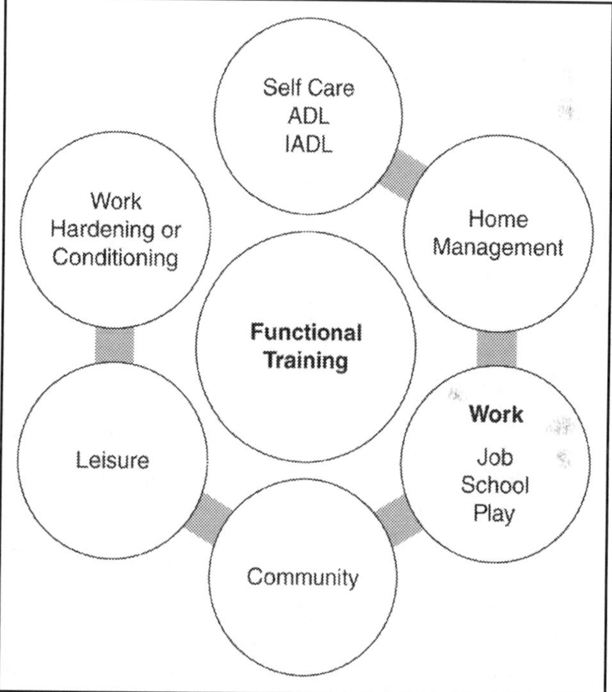

Figure 13-10. Areas of functional training. Abbreviations: ADL; activities of daily living, IADL; instrumental activities of daily living.

Bedside Equipment

Pillows, wedges, towels, and other positioning devices are commonly used, especially in the initial stages of recovery after a stroke. These position the patient in bed or when sitting in a chair to decrease the development of secondary impairments such as ROM deficits or pressure sores. Once the patient can move around in bed, these devices are no longer necessary.

Wheelchairs

When a w/c is used it should have a solid seat instead of a sling seat. A sling seat fosters poor posture and trunk control. In addition, an appropriate seat cushion is required. The type of cushion will depend on the patient's mobility status and prognosis. A lower seat height is preferred to allow the patient to propel the chair with the less affected LE. A supportive device for the affected upper extremity (UE) is also recommended (Figures 13-11 and 13-12).

Canes

Although wheeled walkers (with or without forearm attachments) are on occasion used with patients who demonstrate adequate upper limb strength and movement control, most patients requiring an assistive device for ambulation after a stroke use some type of cane. Cane varieties fall into the basic categories of hemi cane, quad cane,

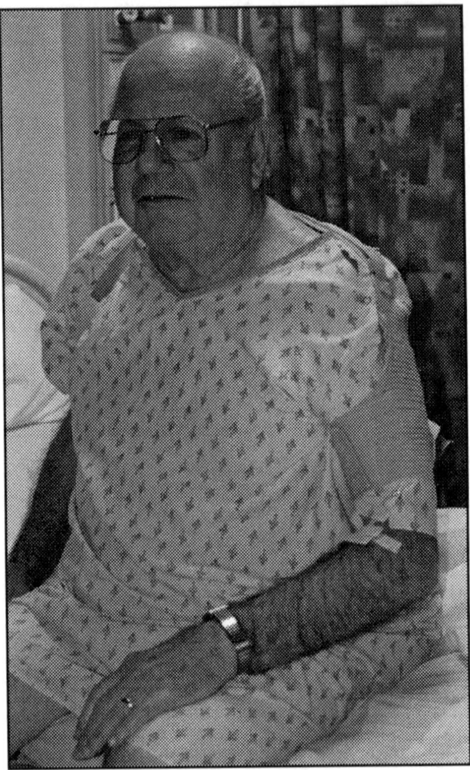

Figure 13-11. Patient with cuff supporting the shoulder of the hemiplegic upper limb.

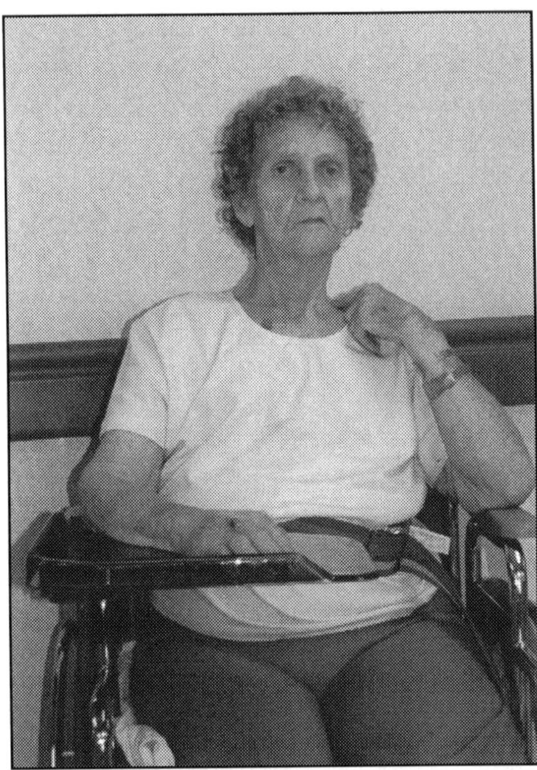

Figure 13-12. Patient using arm support on a w/c to support the weakened UE.

and straight cane. A hemi cane is typically used only early in the recovery process as it provides a very large base of support for initial standing and gait activities and provides a sense of security for the patient. Few patients use a hemi cane on a long-term basis, as its large base of support makes it cumbersome to use. When a patient demonstrates adequate trunk control, frequently a quad cane is used. Quad canes can have larger or smaller bases to accommodate the stability needs of the patient; the larger the base, the more it will slow the patient's walking speed. The least amount of stability is provided by a straight cane. Straight canes can, however, be adapted by adding a large tip. Straight canes are typically used with patients who demonstrate mild balance or LE strength and control deficits.

The physical therapist assistant will instruct the patient on the use of the assistive device during gait on a variety of surfaces congruent with the patient's discharge needs. This may include gait training with an assistive device on stairs, up and down a curb, on uneven terrain (eg, gravel or grass), or on carpet. The physical therapist assistant should monitor for appropriate fit of the assistive device and determine patient safety during use of the device. The patient and/or the patient's caregiver should be instructed on how to clean and adjust the cane, and how to monitor for wear.

Orthotics

The most common orthotic device used with patients who have had a stroke is an AFO. AFOs help ensure foot clearance during the swing phase of gait and help the patient obtain heel strike. AFOs can be set at neutral or into slight dorsiflexion or plantar flexion to produce effects at the knee joint. When a patient demonstrates a tendency toward hyperextension because of poor knee control, the AFO can be set in a mild amount of dorsiflexion to produce a flexion moment at the knee. When a patient uses an orthosis, the physical therapist assistant will need to monitor the patient's skin to ensure proper fit, especially since patients who have had a CVA frequently have altered or absent sensation in their involved limb. The physical therapist assistant should instruct the patient and/or the patient's caregiver how to assess skin integrity and monitor for skin breakdown. In addition, the patient should be taught how to don and doff the device, and how to clean and maintain it.

On occasion, other orthotic devices, such as a knee-ankle-foot orthosis or a hyperextension knee brace, may also be prescribed by the physical therapist for the patient. Basic principles of use and patient training/instruction are the same.

Hand Splints and Slings

Hand splints and slings have traditionally been used to provide support and protection for the more involved UE. Controversy over the use of hand splints has primarily revolved around the evolving understanding of the cause of tonal issues observed in patients with UE involvement from a stroke. A contemporary understanding focuses on providing a neutral functional splint that promotes functional training and hand use. The splint is designed to hold the wrist and hand in a position of orthopedic neutral as opposed to the traditional resting position, which placed the wrist in some extension and the hand in mild flexion. This functional splint is primarily used during the day only.[19]

UE slings are used to support the glenohumeral joint in an effort to prevent subluxation. Various slings are available; however, no research has been conducted that assesses the sling's effect on the trunk or scapular position. No available shoulder sling can provide the scapula with support to maintain the upward rotation required for appropriate scapulohumeral mechanics. As such, use of an UE sling must accompany strengthening and muscle reeducation of the trunk and scapular musculature.

The ideal shoulder sling will help maintain the normal alignment of the glenoid fossa and decrease the tendency for the humerus to internally rotate. Shoulder immobilizer slings should be avoided. Shoulder sling options include shoulder saddle slings, humeral cuff slings, and clavicle supports.[19]

Electrotherapeutic Modalities

Neuromuscular electrical stimulation (NMES) can be effective at increasing movement strength, making it an appropriate physical therapy intervention for some people who have had a stroke. Intervention strategies with NMES vary depending on the impairment or functional limitation being targeted. This intervention should only be a component of, or adjunct to, a therapeutic exercise program. NMES can be applied to the shoulder to reduce glenohumeral joint subluxation and the accompanying pain by stimulating the supraspinatus and posterior deltoid muscles.[20,21]

Another NMES application has been directed at improving UE performance with functional tasks. This strategy requires stimulation to the weakened muscle groups, performed concurrently with a task that requires those muscles. This application may improve patterns of movement that are weak following a stroke, such as impaired strength for wrist and finger extension.[22,23] There have been few reports on the role of NMES interventions to the LEs following stroke. It appears to improve the recruitment of muscles[24] and gait during the stimulation,[25] but the persistence of functional benefits has not been established.

Additional Intervention Strategies in Stroke Rehabilitation

Another strategy for rehabilitation of motor (movement) abilities following stroke is constraint-induced movement therapy. This intervention evolved from a fascinating series of investigations into learned non-use, in which it was discovered in the laboratory of psychologist Edward Taub that a monkey relieved of sensation in a UE will cease to use that limb. The monkey had the potential to use the limb, but doing so was laborious. That level of effort became a negative reinforcement, while use of the limb in which sensation was intact was easy and provided positive reinforcement. The combination reinforced the avoidance of using that limb. Taub has identified this as *learned non-use*. Taub applied this understanding to the development of an intervention in which the limb that is not impaired is constrained by strapping it to the trunk, the monkey is then required to use the impaired limb to feed itself and perform other essential functions. This resulted in constraint-induced movement of the limb and a restoration of the ability to use it functionally.[25]

This technique has proven effective in the rehabilitation of movement ability of either the UE or the LE when the ability to move and use the limb is impaired following stroke, as long as there is some active motion in the limb, although it may be limited. The intervention involves constraint of the less-involved extremity for 14 days. During that period, the patient participates in training activities and tasks using the involved limb for 6 hours each weekday and for additional exercise periods on the weekends. This intervention is effective in increasing the amount and quality of movement in the involved limb and the use of the limb for functional tasks.

The research on this protocol has been impressive in that it confirmed the efficacy of this intervention when massed practice (constraint of the less-involved limb paired with approximately 70 hours of training activities) is provided to the patient.[26-28] The benefits from the intervention are sustained over time.

This intervention is usually used for patients with chronic stroke symptoms (ie, greater than 4 months after the stroke), and the physical therapist will apply criteria to determine which patients are most likely to benefit from constraint-induced movement therapy.[29]

In the past decade, there has been growing interest in using virtual-reality gaming devices to enhance therapeutic exercise interventions. Anecdotal evidence suggests more and more clinical environments are beginning to use gaming devices; many of them are skilled nursing and long-term settings. Recent research has demonstrated that including virtual-reality gaming technology does provide some benefit for motor improvements in individuals who have had a stroke.[1,30,31] Because this is a new strategy, more research is needed to determine parameters to ensure effective use with this patient population.

Typical Impairments and Functional Limitation Being Addressed

Once the physical therapist assistant knows which interventions will be implemented, he or she must confirm which impairments of body function or activity limitation each intervention should address. This is necessary because each intervention can be used to address one or more deficits depending on the patient's problems and the physical therapist's plan to address those problems. For example, using electrotherapeutic modalities can be to address pain issues or to facilitate motor recovery. Parameters will need to be adjusted based on the specific impairment or deficit being addressed (Table 13-7).

It is therefore important that the physical therapist assistant has a basic understanding of common impairments in body functions and limitations in activities seen in patients who have had a stroke. In addition, the physical therapist assistant should be familiar with contemporary intervention strategies that can be used to address them.

Impairments in Motor Planning and Apraxia

Praxis is the performance of intentional action(s) or skills. *Apraxia*, therefore, is an acquired impairment in the performance of purposeful movements. As defined by Shumway-Cook and Woollacott, apraxia "is a disorder of the execution of movement that cannot be attributed to weakness, to incoordination or sensory loss, or to poor language comprehension or inattention to commands."[32] It can develop after a stroke and appears to result from an inability to mentally formulate a plan of action for a motor task. The disruption in the formation or implementation of a plan may result in surprising functional limitations: the inability to comply with a request to lie down on a bed or comb one's hair, consistently putting clothes on inside out, drinking from an empty cup, or attempting to cut one's food with a spoon.[32]

Symptoms among persons with apraxia vary greatly. The following list includes some of the types of apraxia that may be encountered in the clinic[33,34]:

- Ideational apraxia: Failure to conceive or formulate an action, either spontaneously or to command.
- Ideomotor apraxia: The ability to know and remember the planned action, but an inability to execute it with either hand.
- Kinetic limb apraxia: Clumsiness and maladroitness of a limb in the performance of a skilled act that cannot be accounted for by paresis, ataxia, or sensory loss.
- Facial-oral apraxia: Inability to carry out facial movements to command (eg, lick the lips or blow out a match).
- Motor impersistence: An inability to sustain a physical action; usually identified when a patient cannot close the eyes, protrude the tongue, or raise the nonparetic arm on request and persist in the action for 20 seconds.

One-third of patients with a first stroke will have symptoms of apraxia, and it is more common among those who have had a left hemisphere lesion.[35] Apraxia present at the time of hospital admission for a stroke indicates there will be a higher dependency on others to support the patient upon discharge. When providing interventions to a person with apraxia, the physical therapist assistant should recognize the tasks that are impaired by apraxia and focus on the patient's learning of strategies for those tasks.[1] For example, if a patient is impaired in the initiation of an activity, the emphasis should be placed on instruction, and if the problem is one of performance errors, the emphasis should be placed on feedback to enhance error detection.[36]

Diminished Aerobic Capacity

People who have had a stroke have impaired fitness (ie, capacity to perform physical activity and work). The following list includes reasons for this acquired activity intolerance:

- Decreased cardiorespiratory fitness.
- Increased energy demands that accompany hemiparesis, sensory loss, and incoordination.
- Deficient motor planning and deconditioning from bedrest and inactivity.[8,37,38]

In addition, current clinical practices for inpatient rehabilitation appear to contribute to deconditioning because activity levels among individuals receiving rehabilitation services during the 14 days following a stroke are very low. Bernhardt et al found that among patients receiving inpatient rehabilitation, only 13% of an individual's day included participation in therapeutic activities that contribute to the recovery of mobility.[39] The cumulative effect is that the leading cause of mortality among individuals who survive a stroke is vascular disease affecting either the heart (eg, cardiovascular disease) or the brain (eg, stroke).[8]

This has implications for the physical therapy interventions applied following stroke. Gordon et al[8] recommend that exercise programs should be directed at the following goals:

- Regaining the endurance to participate in activities as soon as possible.
- Aerobic training for the benefits of decreasing body fat and improving glucose regulation.
- Improving aerobic fitness to minimize the functional limitations and mortality that accompany stroke.[8]

To achieve these goals, the exercise program, as designed by the physical therapist, may contain elements similar to a cardiac rehabilitation program. That is, the exercise will need to be of sufficient frequency and duration and of a type that the patient can perform to achieve training benefits. To individualize and safely implement the exercises, the physical therapist assistant must collect data about the patient's response during exercise interventions. The data collection should include data on cardiovascular (ie, heart rate, BP, and arrhythmia monitoring) and cardiopulmonary (ie, respiratory rate and oxygen saturation) responses and the patient's perceived exertion.

Impaired Strength or Motor Control

Eighty-nine percent of patients admitted to the hospital following a stroke have weakness.[40] The severity of the weakness or paralysis that develops following stroke varies

Table 13-7
Impairments and Their Corollary Procedural Interventions and Tests and Measures

Impairments	Procedural Interventions: Motor Control	Aerobic Capacity	Balance and Coordination	Flexibility	Gait/Locomotion	Strength and Endurance	Functional Training	Devices and Equipment	Tests and Measures to Objectify Progress
Motor Planning/Apraxia	X		X		X	X	X		• Observation of functional tasks • Nose-finger-nose • Rapid alternating movement • Heel to shin
Decreased Aerobic Capacity/Endurance		X					X		• Observation of patient level of exertion • Heart rate and rhythm • Respiratory rate • BP • O_2 saturation • 6-minute walk test
Decreased Strength	X					X	X	X	• Observation of functional movements • Manual muscle testing • Hand-held dynamometry
Shoulder Pain	X			X		X		X	• Pain scale
Balance Deficits	X		X			X	X	X	• Observation of sitting, standing and functional tasks • Timed Up and Go test • Berg Balance Scale • Timed unipedal standing
Functional Limitations	X	X	X	X	X	X	X	X	• Barthel Index • Fugl-Meyer Assessment of Sensorimotor Recovery After Stroke • Rivermead ADL Scale • National Institutes of Health Stroke Scale

according to the location of the damaged brain tissue. The weakness is more a representation of the locale (ie, structures) damaged than it is the size (ie, volume of brain area) of the stroke.

Hemiparesis describes weakness of either the right or left half of the body, and *hemiplegia* describes a similar unilateral weakness combined with loss of sensation(s). Historically, the weakness that develops following a stroke has been described as hemiparesis or hemiplegia that involves the contralateral side (ie, the extremities and trunk of the half of the body opposite the side of the brain injured from the stroke). However, the loss of strength also involves the extremities and trunk ipsilateral (same side) to the stroke, although to a lesser extent. Therefore, the terms *weaker side* and *stronger side* are recommended for accuracy when describing the pattern of weakness that follows a stroke. This pattern of weakness is important when performing physical therapy interventions, because exercise to improve strength should be directed at both sides of the body and not just to the weaker side.[41]

Fewer than 15% of people who have a stroke will fully recover motor function, and the more severe the weakness, the poorer the prognosis. That is, individuals who have the greatest weakness following a stroke are expected to have a slower recovery and will remain weaker than those with lesser strength deficits. In addition, the severity of post-stroke weakness is related to the severity of functional limitations for transfers, standing, ambulating, and stair climbing.[40]

Shoulder Pain After Stroke

Developing shoulder pain following a stroke can cause psychoemotional distress and limit function. This is a frequent complication, with the literature indicating that it affects 34% to 84% of persons who have had a stroke.[42] Several theories have been proposed to explain the pathology responsible for this disorder, including this summary by Turner-Stokes and Jackson[43]:

- Development of muscle imbalance from the competing symptoms of spasticity and flaccidity, resulting in malalignment of the glenohumeral joint.
- Development of adhesive capsulitis (ie, frozen shoulder) with inflammation of the joint capsule restricting flexibility.
- Joint subluxation with incongruity of the glenohumeral joint developing due to inadequate muscular support to compensate for the tractioning effect of gravity.
- Inflammation of extracapsular structures, such as irritation or tears of the rotator cuff muscles or tendon.
- Nerve damage from traction or entrapment of peripheral nerves.
- Development of complex regional pain syndrome (eg, reflex sympathetic dystrophy).

These theories propose that the pain develops because of irritation or repetitive trauma to the tissues about the shoulder joint, indicating that a proactive approach designed to prevent the development of shoulder pain is the preferred intervention strategy. Unfortunately, strong evidence supporting a single specific method does not exist. Protective strategies have included adhering to a proper (ie, neutral) shoulder positioning program[1] by using a sling or other supportive device for the involved UE. The support devices are used to combat gravity's tractioning pull on the glenohumeral joint. An arm sling will effectively support the limb; unfortunately, it also limits and discourages active use of that UE. Another option is a cuff support that encircles the proximal humerus and is suspended from the upper trunk and opposite shoulder (see Figure 13-11). Placing an axillary roll or pad suspended under the involved limb has fallen out of favor because it does not adequately support the glenohumeral joint. Individuals in a chair can also support the arm in an arm trough attached to a lap tray or directly on the lap tray (Figure 13-12).[43] Patients and their families should be educated about these interventions so they can adhere to the protective positions and behaviors.[1]

Another protective strategy is preserving flexibility about the shoulder joint.[1] This can be achieved through passive ROM. However, care should be taken to inhibit (relax) the shoulder muscles, which may resist the movement because of spasticity or spasm.[43] Overhead pulley systems should not be used to promote flexibility.[1]

NMES is an electrotherapy intervention appropriate for a patient with hemiparesis and can be applied as a component of physical therapy interventions to achieve contraction of the supraspinatus or posterior deltoid muscles. The goal of NMES intervention is to preserve muscle strength in the flaccid or weakened shoulder through peripheral stimulation. By doing so, the subluxation of the glenohumeral joint is reduced or prevented, with benefits of decreased pain or increased mobility.[43]

Balance Deficits

The risk of falling is greater after stroke because of impaired balance. This is expected, because normal balance requires effective performance of the systems for sensation (eg, visual, vestibular, and somatosensation) and motor control (including the strength, coordination, and rate of the person's response), and these abilities are often impaired following stroke. Therefore, a person who has had a stroke may benefit from interventions to remediate impaired balance when sitting, standing, or walking.[1,44]

In addition to these balance disturbances, a subset of about 5% of patients who have had a stroke demonstrate *pusher* behavior. As described by Roller, "*pusher syndrome* in patients post-stroke is characterized by leaning and active pushing toward the hemiplegic side with no compensation for instability"[45] while maintaining the head in a mostly upright position. The person with this disorder will resist correction, and when a caregiver attempts to assist the person toward a neutral (upright) posture, the patient will complain of a feeling of falling, and the pushing behavior will persist.

This pusher behavior develops because the brain injury from the stroke leaves the individual unable to sense and correctly interpret an upright posture (either in sitting or standing). This misinterpretation leads the individual to think the body is upright when, in fact, it is leaning to the side. The individual may also have the sense of falling while being supported in the upright position by the physical therapist or physical therapist assistant. Therefore, the individual's response is to continue to lean, or push, away from the correct upright position.[45] Interventions performed by the physical therapist assistant should include focusing the patient's attention on the available sensations—which may include vision, vestibular sensation, or proprioception—and awareness of the support surface. Interventions should augment this sensory feedback, such as using a mirror or training sitting balance on a firm (rather than soft) surface. Practice is a necessary strategy for improving the patient's ability to detect errors and then to develop corrective strategies.[45,46]

Functional Limitations

The severity of the functional limitations that follow a stroke varies according to the location of the damaged brain tissue and the presence of the previously described impairments. Functional limitations may affect the patient's ability to move alone, change positions, or complete activities of daily living (ADL). The following are functional limitations commonly seen in patients who have had a stroke:

- Difficulty planning movements
- Difficulty with manipulation skills
- Frequent falls
- Loss of balance during ADL
- Difficulty negotiating terrains

Patient's Current Status

The clinical presentation of individuals following a stroke will be diverse and range from individuals requiring total assistance for all ADL to those with no obvious impairments or limitations in functioning. In addition, the stroke may influence any of the brain's functions, so that cognitive skills—such as communication, praxis, or even the ability to stay awake—may be impaired. It is also important to note that the symptoms will vary over time for each patient. To gain a clear picture of the patient's current status to inform intervention-related decisions, the physical therapist assistant will review the physical therapist's evaluation. In addition to indicating deficits that will be addressed by physical therapy interventions, the evaluation will provide information about other impairments in body functions that can influence the patient's ability to participate in therapy and affect the patient's progress. The following section will discuss evaluation tools and measurements used by the physical therapist that can provide useful information to help the physical therapist assistant develop appropriate expectations and make good clinical decisions related to provision of selected interventions. Following this discussion, impairments common to individuals who have had a stroke which are not directly addressed by physical therapy but that may impact therapy will be reviewed.

Examination Tools, Tests, and Measures

The physical therapist's examination will identify baseline measures of the patient's impairments in body functions and limitations in abilities and participation. These data are evaluated by the physical therapist and inform the prognosis and the development of the plan of care. As part of evidence-based practice, physical therapists incorporate standardized tests and measures during the initial examination and evaluation and subsequent evaluations. Some of these standardized tests and measures are referred to as *outcome measurements* or *scales*. Two excellent resources for these types of scales are Lewis and McNerney's *The Functional Toolbox*[47] and *The Functional Toolbox II*.[48] The physical therapist assistant will want to take note of the tests and measures the physical therapist uses in the evaluation to choose the appropriate techniques for data collection to monitor the patient's response to the interventions provided.

Motor Control: Strength and Coordination

As a component of the physical therapist's examination, strength is measured, although the method of collecting these data varies depending on the patient's capabilities (eg, ability to follow instructions, and severity of weakness). Strength measures may be taken through manual muscle testing or hand-held dynamometry, or through a record of functional capabilities (eg, the ability to transfer from sitting to standing). Historically, there has been debate about the role of measuring the strength of patients who have had a stroke or related upper motor neuron lesion (ie, damage to the brain accompanied by symptoms that include spasticity); however, the evidence has indicated that measuring strength following stroke will provide reliable and valid data and that this is valuable information in determining prognosis.[49]

As identified in the section on impaired strength following a stroke, it is common to have weakness that is greater in the extremities opposite from the side of the stroke (eg, following a right middle cerebral artery CVA, the left arm and leg will exhibit more pronounced weakness than the right arm and leg). In a majority of individuals, the strength will improve over time, although impairment of strength will persist.[40]

However, as the strength improves, another impairment that often becomes evident is the inability to isolate extremity movements. That is, when attempting to move a single joint, the other joints in that limb also move in a pattern identified as a *synergy* (see Table 6-4). One of the goals of physical therapy interventions will be to reduce the tendency for movement in these patterns and improve the ability to isolate movements.

Symptoms of coordination impairment that may be affected following stroke include the following:

- *Dysdiadochokinesia*, which is a deficiency in the ability to perform rapidly alternating movements.
- *Dysmetria*, in which the ability to control the distance, power, and speed of movement is impaired.
- *Action tremor*, which indicates that a tremor or shaking occurs during the performance of voluntary (intentional) movements.
- A general slowing of movements, with additional delays in the ability to initiate a movement and to terminate a movement.

Refer to Chapter 6 for testing procedures for coordination.

Flexibility

Passive ROM is usually measured to identify any preexisting impairments that need to be addressed (eg, arthritis). In addition, these baseline data are collected because of the risk for the development of stiffness in the muscles affected by stroke. That is, in addition to the resistance to stretch that accompanies spasticity, the muscles often develop a gradual loss of flexibility because of a reduction of elasticity.

Functional Limitations

Following a stroke, a patient may have limited capabilities with the functions of attaining bed mobility, transferring from sitting to standing or standing to sitting, ambulating, stair climbing, and carrying out many other ADL. Documenting functional abilities may be performed by describing the patient's ability to perform the function, by timing the patient's performance of the function, or by physical therapy outcome measurement scales.

The description of the patient's functional abilities should be based on efficiently and accurately describing the patient's (not the caregiver's) ability or contribution to performing the function. The descriptors from the Functional Independence Measure are effective for this (see Chapter 6).

Timed measurement of a patient's performance of tasks also provides valuable clinical data. Examples include using a stopwatch to time the functions of transferring from sitting to standing and ambulation speed. Transfers can be timed for the time needed to stand up from a chair once, the time needed to stand up 3 consecutive repetitions, or the number of repeated transfers (from sitting to standing to sitting) that can be completed within 10 seconds. Measures such as the 6-minute walk test are designed to measure exercise capacity and may be used for some patients following stroke.[25] However, patients with much lower ambulation or exercise capacity will be better described through measures such as rate of ambulation. One technique is to determine the time it takes an ambulating patient to traverse 10 feet. This should be measured during a period of walking, because starting and stopping will alter the results. Gait speed can then be easily calculated as the distance divided by the duration (eg, feet/seconds). A patient who ambulates across 10 feet in 5 seconds has a gait speed of 2 feet/second, while the speed of a patient who requires 15 seconds is 0.67 feet/second.

Another important distinction in the ability to ambulate is the patient's ability to accommodate to different environments. The surface that is being walked on can alter performance because of the appearance (eg, visual contrast), texture (eg, tile vs carpeting), or presence of obstacles. Environmental complexity will alter performance because the presence of obstacles, local activity (eg, other people walking nearby), or other distractions in the area may impair performance. For example, a patient may be able to walk effectively in a quiet physical therapy department, but his performance may deteriorate when walking in a busy hospital hallway. When this occurs, the difference should be recorded and reported to the physical therapist.

Common standardized examination tools used by the physical therapist during the examination include the Barthel Index, the Fugl-Meyer Assessment of Sensorimotor Recovery After Stroke, the Rivermead ADL Scale, and the National Institutes of Health Stroke Scale. It is helpful for the physical therapist assistant to become familiar with these tools to understand the physical therapist's findings. In addition, some of these tools may be used to determine the patient's response to the intervention(s) provided and objectify the patient's progress. The physical therapist assistant should review the tool with the physical therapist to identify the data collection technique(s) and methods to be used to ensure consistency in the assessment processes.

Balance Measures

Physical therapists use standardized tests to measure balance in the initial evaluation to provide a baseline and to assist the physical therapist in determining the prognosis and plan of care. All of these tools can also be used to demonstrate the patient's progress; therefore, the physical therapist assistant should be able to implement all of them appropriately. The physical therapist assistant should communicate with the physical therapist to ensure the correct performance of the technique. The following are examples of balance measures:

- Timed Up and Go test
- Berg Balance Scale
- Functional Reach Test
- Unipedal standing (timed for duration)

In general, the physical therapist assistant will want to note the patient's balance reactions based on position (sitting vs standing) and in relation to a functional activity. Often, the patient will have increasing difficulty with balance as the demands of the task increase. This information should be noted, documented, and relayed to the physical therapist. Chapter 6 provides more in-depth information on assessing balance.

Cardiovascular Endurance

Exercise capacity is impaired following stroke. Some of this impairment may result from the hemiparesis because the patient must accommodate for weakness. However, cardiorespiratory fitness is also affected. Mackay-Lyons and Makrides reported that within 1 month after the stroke, the capacity to exercise was reduced to 60% of the typical capacity of a healthy, sedentary person, a response that is equivalent to that for a person recovering from a myocardial infarction.[38] The physical therapist's examination will contain measures of the patient's response to exercise to determine the baseline and because the reduced capacity raises the potential for an adverse response during exercise.

The data collected will usually contain information about the amount of exercise and the patient's response to that level of activity. The physical therapist assistant should note the amount of activity, such as whether the patient was able to transfer repeatedly, ambulate a specific distance, or ascend a flight of stairs. This information will aid the physical therapist assistant when determining the exercises and activity expectations for the first intervention session with the patient. The physical therapist's examination should also contain information about the patient's response to exercise. This is usually identified through measuring (at rest and with activity) the patient's heart rate, respiratory rate, BP, and/or oxygen saturation (*pulse oximetry*). The physical therapist assistant should continue to collect these data during exercise interventions to make sure the exercises are within the patient's cardiopulmonary capacity.

Common Impairments Not Directly Addressed by Physical Therapy

Impaired Vestibular Sensation

The vestibular system senses head movement and head position relative to gravity. This information is used to inform the movement system for the extremities and trunk, and to improve visual acuity. When a stroke interrupts the transmission or interpretation of vestibular information, it may cause symptoms of *vertigo* (an illusion of motion), *nystagmus* (involuntary back-and-forth movements of the eye), *disequilibrium* (a sense of imbalance), *ataxia* (incoordination of movement that is not a result of weakness), or a combination of these symptoms. The symptoms of vertigo or disequilibrium may cause nausea, and medications may reduce the nausea sufficiently to allow the patient to participate in physical therapy interventions. The decision to administer medications is outside the physical therapist assistant's scope of practice.

Cognitive Impairments

Cognitive abilities include the mental processes of comprehension, reasoning, and decision-making that guide our behaviors and actions. When a portion of the brain has been injured, there will be a disruption in the way that the brain receives, processes, interprets, or responds to information; the behaviors we observe following a stroke are a result of the disruption of these processes.[32] The cognitive impairments most frequently encountered while working with people who have had a stroke are neglect, apraxia, anosognosia, and communication disorders. These impairments are confusing to recognize and can present barriers to the patients' participation in physical therapy interventions, to their improvement, and to their attainment of goals. Therefore, when providing selected physical therapy interventions, a physical therapist assistant should be able to recognize and respond appropriately to the behavioral expressions of these cognitive impairments.

Another contributor to cognitive performance in some individuals is an alteration in *perception*, which is the process of converting sensations into meaningful and understandable information. Because of the amount and types of sensory disturbances that may occur following a stroke, it is not surprising that these individuals have impaired cognition. When this type of impairment contributes to deterioration in cognitive performance, the physical therapist assistant should work to augment sensory inputs (examples are provided in the following paragraphs) and to educate the patient, family, and other caregivers about strategies to compensate for the sensory or perceptual deficit.

Unilateral Neglect

Unilateral neglect is important to recognize because of its frequency and its influence on the rehabilitation process. The symptoms of unilateral neglect are an inability to report, attend to, or recognize sight, sound, and/or touch opposite to the side of the brain affected by stroke.[50] It is also referred to as *neglect*, *visuospatial neglect*, *hemispatial neglect*, or *left neglect*.

Neglect is a frequently encountered impairment, with a reported incidence following stroke between 10% and 82%.[44] Neglect is classically associated with stroke involving the right half of the brain, causing neglect (ie, inattention or unawareness) of the left environment or body; however, it may also be observed when a left hemisphere lesion causes a right neglect, although that form is more likely to resolve 4 to 8 weeks following the stroke.[51,52]

The physical therapist assistant must be concerned with the functional impact from the symptoms that accompany the inability to attend to the left or right components of the patient's environment. The symptoms will present as deficiencies in the domains of memory (ie, mental representation and recall), action-intention (ie, motor performance), or attention (ie, response to sensations).[51] Neglect involving memory is quite striking because the patients may be impaired in their ability to describe aspects of their home based on the mental perspective from which they are recalling it. For example, a patient with a left unilateral neglect may not be able to recall the railing on his stairs if he is picturing the stairs from the perspective of the bottom of the stairs with the railing on the left, but he will be able to recall the same railing if he changes his perspective to the top of the stairs with the railing on his right. When neglect involves motor intention, the patient will be impaired in his ability to act or plan movements involving the right or left half of the body. This will adversely affect function as seen by behaviors, such as not recognizing that food is on the left side of a plate and, subsequently, not eating that half of a meal; not dressing or applying makeup to half of the body; or not accounting for objects (eg, door frames) to one side and then walking into them, causing injury or falls. When the neglect involves attention, there may not be a response to stimuli that occur within a portion of the individual's environment. For example, a person with a neglect involving the left side of his or her environment may not respond to a sound, sight, and/or touch that originates from the left, regardless of the integrity of those sensations. Another example is when an individual may not be able to identify when a car is approaching from the left side when crossing the street.

Neglect is associated with a poorer outcome following stroke, because people with neglect require longer programs of inpatient rehabilitation, achieve less recovery of functional abilities, and require greater assistance with ADL.[44]

While some symptoms of neglect improve over time, others may respond to interventions. Some of the interventions may be applied during treatment by the physical therapist assistant, such as wearing of special glasses with prisms or with patching to obstruct the intact visual field, cueing for visual scanning into the neglected visual field, or providing stimulation on the neglected side of the body. Other interventions may precede the physical therapy session, such as brain stimulation with transcranial magnetic stimulation.[1]

It is important to appreciate that the evidence on the response to interventions for unilateral neglect is evolving, as the physical therapist may use different strategies for interventions based on the evolving evidence and the patient's symptoms. Given the diverse intervention strategies, it is unlikely for a physical therapist assistant to become trained in applying all of them; therefore, when encountering an unfamiliar technique, the physical therapist assistant must request guidance from the physical therapist.

Anosognosia

Anosognosia is the denial of one's own neurological symptoms, such as weakness, functional limitation, and other deficits. Examples observed following stroke include the denial of hemiparesis, visual loss, aphasia, movement disorder, and apraxia. This is typically observed by the physical therapist assistant through the persistent denial of post-stroke impairments, the minimizing of weakness, and the indifference to the effects of the weakness (eg, blaming it on arthritis, fatigue, or trauma to a limb). Common concurrent stroke symptoms are hemisensory disturbances, unilateral neglect, dressing or constructional apraxia, reduced intellectual functions, motor impersistence, and *prosopagnosia* (impaired recognition of familiar faces), although memory is usually spared. The incidence of anosognosia is greater than is recognized by most clinicians; the literature indicates an occurrence of 28% to 85% among people who have had a right hemisphere stroke, and 0% to 17% among patients who have had a left hemisphere stroke. Although this symptom usually resolves 12 to 22 weeks after the onset of a stroke, the presence of anosognosia is generally considered a poor prognostic indicator for functional recovery.[53,54] The authors are not aware of intervention strategies for those cases in which anosognosia symptoms persist. Fortunately, that occurs among fewer than 10% of people with this symptom.

Communication Disorders

Dysphasia is an acquired impairment of communication, which may include expressive (speaking) ability, receptive (comprehension) ability, or both. *Aphasia* is the term more frequently used in the clinic for this disorder, although that term more accurately refers to the complete loss of these communication abilities.

The brain's cortex contains 2 areas, Broca's and Wernicke's, which are primarily responsible for communication. Communication is a lateralized brain function, meaning that different components of communication are controlled predominantly on each side of the brain. In most people, spoken language is lateralized to the left hemisphere of the brain, and nonverbal communication is lateralized to the right hemisphere (although this rule does not apply to about half of the people who are left-handed). The communication impairments observed after a stroke vary depending on the location(s) affected by the stroke.

Following a stroke that involves Broca's area of the left cerebral cortex, a person will have trouble verbally expressing him- or herself. The impairment is with the process of motor programming for the production or the organization of spoken words. This may present as slow or nonfluent speech, poor articulation, or grammatically incorrect speech.

When a stroke affects Wernicke's area of the left cerebral cortex, an individual will be impaired with the receptive components of communication. The impairment is in the comprehension of language; therefore, these individuals may have difficulty following the physical therapist assistant's spoken instructions. The person with this lesion will retain the ability to speak fluently, but the use of words is impaired, and the patient may demonstrate the use of meaningless words or phrases. In addition to the anticipated frustration that accompanies a disorder of communication, this type of lesion will also contribute to agitation and related emotional reactions.[55]

Nonverbal communication may be impaired following a stroke in the right hemisphere. If Broca's area is involved, the person will be impaired with expression, such as the use of emotional gestures, or with the intonation of speech. If Wernicke's area is involved, the individual will have trouble interpreting nonverbal signals (eg, facial expressions or gestures) from others. A lesion to this area will also cause a deficiency in comprehending spatial relationships (eg, distances).[56]

The following list includes additional communication disorders the physical therapist assistant may encounter[57]:

- *Anomia*: Naming and word-finding impairments.
- *Dysarthria*: Impaired articulation during speech (from incoordination or weakness of the oral-facial muscles).

- *Dyslexia* or *alexia*: Impaired reading (comprehension of written communication).
- *Dysgraphia* or *agraphia*: Impaired ability to communicate through writing.
- *Paraphasia*: The inappropriate substitution of words when speaking.

Communication impairments will adversely affect a patient's response to therapeutic interventions and the ability to function. Because of the complexity of these disorders, the physical therapist assistant should consult with the physical therapist and the speech-language pathologist to identify the optimal communication strategy for each individual.

Affective Disorders

Affect refers to mood or the emotional component of behaviors. It is expected that there will be emotional reactions among patients who have had a stroke, and these may include sadness, denial, passivity, agitation, mood swings, indifference, or the inability to control impulsive or socially inappropriate behaviors.[58] However, the location or type of injury from the stroke may contribute to severe or persistent affective changes that need to be managed within the context of the health care team. Due to the medical management options that may need to be used, the physical therapist assistant should consult with the physical therapist when the following behaviors are encountered: *abulia* (extreme apathy), anxiety, *emotional lability* (rapid swings among emotional states), pathological laughing and crying, and depression (also called *post-stroke depression*).

One challenge for some patients is demonstrating behaviors that are in keeping with the social and cultural expectations for a situation. Stroke may result in a loss of this ability, which is called a *loss of inhibitions* or *disinhibition*. When disinhibition occurs, a patient may act in a manner that would have been unacceptable to the patient before the stroke (eg, telling off-color jokes or physically grabbing at others). The physical therapist assistant should address the inappropriate behavior when it occurs, because the action is not acceptable whether it is the patient's typical behavior or a symptom of stroke, and the physical therapist assistant should clarify the behavioral expectations. A patient with disinhibition may require a comprehensive behavioral shaping program, applied by all members of the health care team, to achieve an appropriate response to typical situations or improvements of behavior.

Dysphagia

Dysphagia is a disorder of swallowing that may result from incoordination or weakness of the oral, pharyngeal, laryngeal, or esophageal muscles. Usually an occupational therapy or speech pathologist work with this impairment. A patient with dysphagia may benefit from treatment to improve control or strength in these muscles. Until this is achieved, the patient may be on a restricted diet to prevent pulmonary aspiration. A common restriction related to dysphagia is the person is only allowed to drink fluids that have had a thickener added, which slows the swallowing process and makes it easier for the individual to swallow correctly. The physical therapist assistant working with a person at this stage of rehabilitation must comply with the dietary restriction because a variation may result in aspiration, which can lead to complications (eg, pneumonia).

Impaired Somatosensation

The somatosensory system conveys information to the brain from the musculoskeletal system and the skin. When a portion of the brain responsible for processing or interpreting this information is affected by a stroke, the person will have an impairment of somatosensation. This will affect safety because the person will be delayed or unable to sense pain and withdraw from harm. It will also impair movement, coordination, and balance, because somatosensation informs us about the position(s) and rate(s) of movement of our limbs and body. Without this information, we cannot move accurately. This is one of the causes of *ataxia* (incoordination of movement that is not a result of weakness).

Another symptom that may develop is *learned non-use*, in which the absence of sensation from a limb contributes to the adaptive behavior of relying on the limb with intact sensation to assist with all functions while the impaired limb is not used to assist with functions. Interventions directed at improving somatosensation may include tactile stimulation through electrical stimulation or stroking of the skin or training for tactile perception through recognition of objects, discrimination of textures, or recognition of positions.[59]

Impaired Vision

A stroke that interrupts the pathways for transmitting or interpreting visual information will cause an impairment of vision. *Homonymous hemianopia* is a commonly encountered visual impairment following stroke and results in defective or lost vision in the right or left half of the visual field. This visual field loss occurs in both eyes and should not be confused with unilateral neglect. Homonymous hemianopia is an impairment of visual sensation, and *unilateral neglect* is an impairment of attention or awareness. These disorders may present concurrently or alone.

Visual acuity may also be impaired following stroke, with symptoms such as blurred vision or *diplopia* (double vision). These develop because of disruption in the ability to stabilize gaze (ie, maintain visual fixation on an object), which is a prerequisite for normal vision. One cause for gaze instability is disruption of the brainstem nuclei responsible for stabilization (which is mediated by the vestibulo-ocular and optokinetic reflexes) or from loss of vestibular or visual sensory input to these nuclei. Another cause is disruption of the movement system for the eyes and control of the muscles that move the eye or the brainstem locations that innervate these muscles, which can result in diplopia or blurred vision.[57]

Goals as Set by the Physical Therapist

Information gathered about the patient's current status should be considered in light of the goals set by the physical therapist. The goals will provide an outline for the physical therapist assistant regarding the expected timing of and activities related to progression of the patient. For example, a patient whose current status includes ambulating with minimal assistance from the therapist along with the use of a small-based quad cane, and whose goal indicates he or she should be ambulating independently with no assistive device within 3 weeks, helps the physical therapist assistant recognize the expected rate of progression and to anticipate the progression (small-based quad cane to straight cane to no assistive device).

Goals common to the acute care setting during the initial stages of therapy include maintaining ROM and protecting the shoulder joint of the more involved UE, educating the patient regarding safety and positioning issues, and facilitating a smooth transition to the subacute setting. Goals in the subacute setting include preventing or minimizing secondary complications, improving movement control with functional tasks, improving postural control and balance, increasing independence with functional tasks such as ADL and gait, and increasing cardiovascular endurance.

The Patient's Diagnosis

A natural part of the physical therapist assistant's clinical decision-making process includes considering the implications of the medical diagnosis of CVA. CVA is an acute focal event that leads to acquired deficits (as opposed to those that are congenital in origin). Although the deficits associated with a stroke may be permanent, the pathology itself is limited. Additionally, because of the normal, neuroplastic capabilities of the brain, the physical therapist assistant should expect a patient who has had a stroke to recover all or some of the body functions and abilities in the absence of confounding factors (discussed later in this chapter).

Although individuals who have had a stroke generally have common deficits (eg, motor control impairments or sensory deficits [see Table 13-1]), specific patterns of deficits depend on the area of vascular compromise. Therefore, it is important for the physical therapist assistant to have a general understanding of the typical pattern of deficits associated with the major cerebral blood vessels (Table 13-8), as well as which deficits are common with each hemisphere (Table 13-9). This will allow the physical therapist assistant to contextualize the information found in the physical therapist's evaluation and to anticipate the patient's presentation. While each person with a stroke will present a unique combination of symptoms, understanding these general patterns of symptoms will improve the physical therapist assistant's ability to identify and respond to the complexities involved with the treatment of patients who have had a stroke.

The Patient's Prognosis

Recovery after an ischemic stroke follows a fairly predictable pattern. Initial recovery of body functions and abilities occurs within the first few days to weeks after the stroke event. This recovery of neurological function is attributed to reduction of edema and improvement in local blood flow to the cerebral tissues. Recovery after this initial time frame is attributed to unmasking of neuropathways and collateral sprouting among surviving neurons. This recovery tends to follow a pattern of improvement over the course of the first 6 months post-stroke. After the 6-month time frame, improvements in function can occur for patients who are motivated and prepared to work diligently to meet their individual goals which can lead to neuroplasticity (see Chapter 4).

Because of this typical course of recovery, the physical therapist assistant's expectation is that the patient will demonstrate improvement in functional abilities in response to physical therapy interventions; this will usually be observed as progress toward, or achievement of, the goals established in the physical therapist's plan of care. The rate of improvement should be communicated to the physical therapist. In some cases, the physical therapist assistant may note a deterioration of functional abilities, and this also should be communicated to the physical therapist. If the physical therapist is not available and the symptoms seem to be deteriorating, quickly call the doctor or 911 if you are in home health. This is particularly important when there is a notable deterioration in functioning or cognitive ability, or when the patient becomes more lethargic, because the patient may be experiencing complications that require acute medical services. Specific expectations related to rate of improvement are highly individualized. The physical therapist assistant should refer to the physical therapy goals to determine what the expected rate of recovery is for each patient. Patient prognosis and rate of recovery are affected by and frequently depend on the presence of comorbidities and confounding problems.

Comorbidities/Confounding Problems

When caring for an individual who has had a CVA, the physical therapist's and physical therapist assistant's major emphasis will be on the impairments of body functions and limitations in abilities that are results of the stroke. These movement disorders are the foundation of the physical therapist's diagnosis. Remember that a medical

Table 13-8

Cerebral Circulation and Common Deficits Associated With Cerebrovascular Accident

Artery	*Cerebral Area Supplied*	*Common Deficits Associated With a Lesion*
Middle cerebral	Lateral cortex of temporal lobe, anterolateral frontal lobe, and parietal lobe	• Contralateral hemiparesis • Contralateral sensory loss • Global aphasia (if dominate side) • UE greater than LE involvement • Perceptual deficits
Anterior cerebral	Medial portions of the frontal lobe, superior medial parietal lobe, basal ganglia and corpus callosum	• Contralateral hemiplegia • Contralateral sensory loss • LE greater than UE Involvement • Mental impairment • Apraxia • Behavioral changes
Posterior cerebral	Occipital lobe, medial and inferior temporal lobe, thalamus, and midbrain	• Abnormal sensation of pain, temperature and proprioception • Hemiplegia • Contralateral ataxia • Drowsiness • Lack of interest in movement • Disturbance in memory
Vertebral and posterior inferior cerebral	Brainstem, medulla and cerebellum	• Vertigo • Ipsilateral ataxia • Ipsilateral sensory deficit • Contralateral hemiparesis • Gait ataxia

diagnosis deals with the pathology or disease, while the physical therapy diagnosis relates directly to the movement dysfunctions. Most individuals who are recovering from a stroke, however, have preexisting medical problems that cannot be ignored. These medical problems can directly affect the patient's ability to participate and progress with physical therapy interventions.

Common cardiovascular diseases found in patients recovering from a stroke include hypertension, coronary artery disease with a history of a heart attack or coronary artery bypass surgery (CABG), and peripheral vascular disease. The physical therapist assistant will need to monitor the cardiovascular status of the individual during therapeutic activities. If the individual has a history of a heart attack or CABG, it is important to know when these occurred so that the appropriate precautions related to exercise intensity can be taken. For example, a patient who recently underwent a CABG and subsequently had a CVA will have precautions related to the amount of pressure that can be put through the UEs during functional activities. This will lead to the need for alternative strategies for sit-to-stand transfers, because the patient cannot push through the hands on the chair.

Common musculoskeletal conditions that may be encountered include arthritis, joint replacement, amputation, osteoporosis, pathologic fractures (eg, hip, wrist, and back), back pain, and rotator cuff injury and repair. Again, impairments and limitations related to these conditions can affect the patient's progress during recovery after a CVA. For example, a patient who has had a transfemoral amputation of the left leg and who now demonstrates hemiparesis of the right side may require a one-arm drive w/c for functional mobility. Precautions related to preexisting conditions must be taken into consideration during provision of interventions (eg, weight-bearing restrictions or total joint precautions).

Other common conditions encountered in this patient population are diabetes and chronic obstructive pulmonary disease. When working with individuals with diabetes, it is important for the physical therapist assistant to be able to recognize symptoms of hypoglycemia so that appropriate action can be taken. A patient with a diagnosis of chronic obstructive pulmonary disease may need oxygen supplementation during therapeutic activities. The physical therapist assistant will need to monitor the patient's response to exercise by noting the respiratory rate and monitoring oxygen saturation using an oximeter.

Table 13-9

Impairments Based Upon Side of Lesion

Right Hemisphere	*Left Hemisphere*
• Left hemiparesis • Left hemisensory loss • Trouble perceiving emotions and non-verbal communication • Trouble sustaining movements • Quick and impulsive • Poor judgment • Difficulty with abstract concepts • Visual-perceptual deficits	• Right hemiparesis • Right hemisensory loss • Speech-language impairments • Trouble planning/sequencing movement • Slow, cautious, anxious • Difficulty processing • Trouble expressing positive emotion

The patient may need verbal cues for appropriate breathing strategies during the physical therapy session. The patient may be limited in endurance for therapy, and the session may need to be divided to allow the patient to rest between activities.

Contraindications/Precautions

The physical therapist assistant must keep in mind any precautions associated with stroke and any accompanying diagnosis that the patient has when interventions are being provided. Although there is no direct contraindication when working with patients who have had a stroke, several conditions are precautions and should be monitored for patient safety. Most of these have been discussed earlier in this chapter but will be mentioned again to highlight their importance.

It is common for the hemiparetic UE to demonstrate joint subluxation due to "inadequate muscular support to compensate for the tractioning effect of gravity."[43] The physical therapist assistant needs to monitor the limb at all times. Positioning strategies and using slings and electrotherapeutic modalities to address this concern have been described. It is also imperative that the patient, the patient's family, and all caregivers be made aware of the concern and be taught to monitor the positioning of the limb at all times. For example, when assisting the patient into standing, that arm should not be used to pull the patient up from a chair. Similarly, the more involved LE can be at risk for injury because of weakness and sensory deficits. It is important to monitor the limb placement and positioning with all activities. This is of special concern during transfers; if the foot is not appropriately positioned and monitored, the ankle may roll as weight is transferred to the limb, resulting in soft tissue injury.

Also discussed earlier was the importance of monitoring the patient's cardiovascular response to activities. Stroke may be the result of underlying cardiovascular disease that could reduce the patient's capacity for exercise, and hemiplegia will create new methods of moving that increase the physical demands imposed on the patient. It is the physical therapist assistant's responsibility to protect the patient through vigilant measuring of vital signs for interpreting the patient's response to interventions.

Although dysphagia is primarily treated by speech therapy rather than physical therapy, it is imperative that physical therapist assistants be aware of the potential for aspiration and seek clarification of any swallowing restrictions. When working with a patient who has had a stroke, it is common for the patient to ask for a drink of water during the physical therapy session. The physical therapist assistant must confirm and comply with the patient's dietary restrictions, which may change from day to day, to protect the patient.

Finally, patients who have had an ischemic stroke are typically on anticoagulation therapy, which can make patients more susceptible to bruising; therefore, extra care should be taken to ensure patients are handled carefully.

Personal/Environmental Factors

When beginning to work with a patient who is recovering from a CVA, the physical therapist assistant must not only consider the limitations due to preexisting medical conditions but also should have an idea of the patient's prior level of functioning as reported in the physical therapist's initial evaluation. Each patient is unique regardless of the diagnostic label(s). Many individuals with multiple medical conditions continue to be active and are reportedly healthy, while other patients have a sedentary lifestyle with obesity and generalized weakness due to inactivity, but may not have any diagnosed medical conditions. Therefore, an understanding of the patient's prior level of function will help to shape the expectations for therapeutic intervention. In addition, knowledge of the patient's prior functional activity will provide insight into the patient's perception of exercise or activity and can guide the physical therapist assistant in determining how to best approach the patient to ensure optimal participation in therapy.

Psychosocial issues that can affect the provision of physical therapy must also be recognized. The patient's cultural background and belief system related to disability and medical intervention must be considered. For example, a social and cultural background that views disability as a personal weakness that must be hidden can result in differing responses. One patient may be motivated to overcome the disability to be able to reenter a previous social role, whereas another individual may become depressed and lose interest in participation with therapy. Regardless, all health care providers must be sensitive to these issues and work within the patient's belief system to ensure optimal recovery. Family and social support can often make the difference in a patient being able to return home or needing alternate discharge arrangements. The physical therapist assistant should review the initial evaluation to gain insight into the social support that is available to the patient and note the prognosis for the discharge environment. Figure 13-13 provides examples of environmental considerations per categories outlined in the International Classification of Functioning, Disability and Health (ICF). A patient with mild limitations in functional mobility may not be able to return to independent living, but if a spouse or other family member is available, this could mean the difference between the individual returning home or needing to move into an assisted living facility. Care must be taken to determine the abilities and the willingness of the family to provide the needed assistance. Patients who have a CVA are often elderly, and many times their spouses are not in good health; it may be dangerous to the patient as well as the spouse if the patient were to return home.

Implementing the Intervention

As Skinner and McVey state in their text *Clinical Decision Making for the Physical Therapist Assistant*, "Effective physical therapist assistants do not simply perform a set of physical therapist prescribed interventions. Instead, they fashion those prescribed interventions into a coherent and logical treatment sequence that best meet the rehabilitation goals. This requires physical therapist assistants to make clinical decisions based on a clear understanding of the conditions and the numerous factors that influence rehabilitation."[60]

Therefore, we have spent the majority of this chapter discussing a model for clinical decision-making and describing factors the physical therapist assistant must consider to be effective. It is only after taking the multiple factors into consideration that the physical therapist assistant will be ready to engage the patient and initiate implementation of selected interventions as directed by the physical therapist. However, during the implementation process, the physical therapist assistant will continue to encounter decisions that need to be made regarding how to proceed with patient care tasks. These decisions include how to determine whether the patient is safe to participate in the planned interventions, how to ensure patient comfort and safety during the intervention, how and when to progress activities, and when to communicate with the physical therapist regarding the patient's response to care. The remainder of this chapter will consider these clinical decisions and discuss factors for the physical therapist assistant to consider when making them.

Determine Patient Readiness to Participate

Prior to initiating any intervention, a physical therapist assistant must always assess the patient to determine if the patient is medically stable and physiologically and psychologically stable enough to engage in the planned activities. In an inpatient environment (eg, acute care, subacute rehab, or skilled nursing facility), this includes reviewing the medical chart to verify that there have not been any changes in the patient's medical status that would affect participation in physical therapy. Direct observation of the patient through measurement of the patient's vital signs (eg, heart rate and BP, at a minimum) and monitoring for changes in the patient's cognitive status are essential to determine whether it is appropriate to initiate physical therapy interventions. These assessments should occur prior to each therapy session.

To make appropriate decisions related to the patient's vital signs, the physical therapist assistant will need to become familiar with the patient's typical vital sign readings found in the medical record. In the days following a stroke, the medical management often includes maintaining a moderately elevated BP to promote blood flow to the brain tissue immediately around the damage from the stroke. These patients may be allowed to have BPs as high as 230/120 mm Hg.[2] Other patients with cardiovascular conditions will have specific parameters that must be maintained. In general, however, the physical therapist assistant can follow basic guidelines for cardiovascular status as listed here to determine whether the patient is responding safely during physical therapy interventions:

- Heart rate less than 130 beats/minute with regular rhythm
- Respiratory rate less than 40 breaths/minute
- Oxygen saturation above 88%
- BP below 140/90 mm Hg, with diastolic pressure remaining above 60

It is not unusual for a patient and family to respond to a stroke with the request to allow the patient time to rest and recover from this devastating medical event. However, physical therapy is the preferred treatment to promote recovery. The physical therapist assistant should clarify that close monitoring of the patient's vital signs will ensure that the patient is safe and responding appropriately to the challenges of therapy.

During this process, it is important to recognize the potential for cognitive and communication deficits.

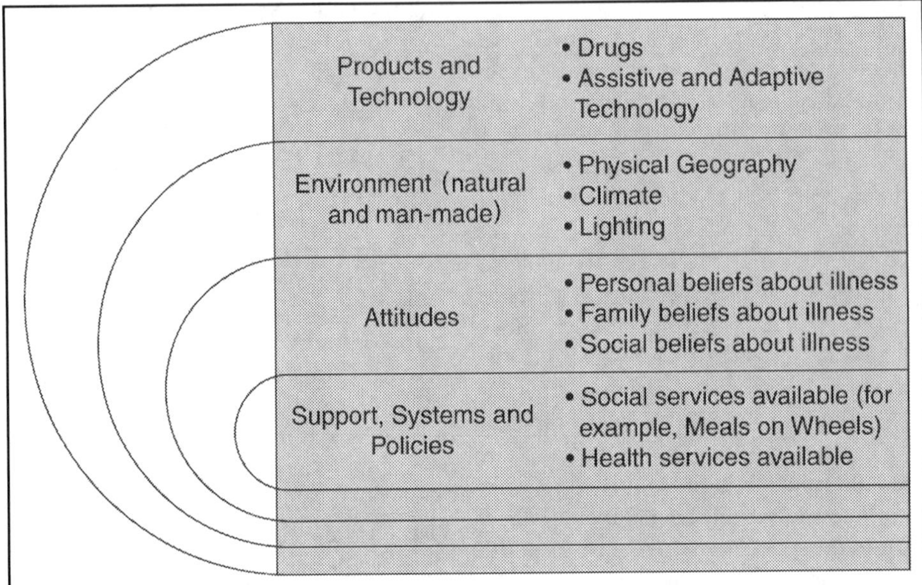

Figure 13-13. Examples of environmental factors based upon the ICF categories.

Excellent strategies for modifying treatment to accommodate a cognitive impairment have been described by Shumway-Cook and Woollacott[32]:

1. Reduce confusion: Make sure the task goal is clear to the patient.
2. Improve motivations: Work on tasks that are relevant and important to the patient.
3. Encourage consistency of performance: Be consistent with goals, and reinforce only those behaviors that are compatible with those goals.
4. Reduce confusion: Use simple, clear, and concise instructions.
5. Seek a moderate level of arousal to optimize learning: Moderate the sensory stimulation in the environment. Agitated patients require decreased intensity of stimulation (eg, soft voice, low lights, slow touch) to reduce arousal levels; stuporous patients require increased intensity of stimulation (eg, brisk, loud commands, and fast movements, working in a vertical position).
6. Provide increased levels of supervision, especially during the early stages of retraining.
7. Recognize that progress may be slower when working with patients who have cognitive impairments.
8. Improve attention: Accentuate perceptual cues that are essential to the task, and minimize the number of irrelevant stimuli in the environment.
9. Improve problem-solving ability: Begin with relatively simple tasks, and gradually increase the complexity of the task demands.
10. Encourage declarative as well as procedural learning: Have a patient verbally and/or mentally rehearse sequences when performing a task.

Implement Selected Interventions

In inpatient settings, patients are frequently seen twice/day for physical therapy. In acute care settings, the time frame is typically limited to the patient's endurance. In the inpatient rehab setting, physical therapy sessions are often 1 hour long. Because several deficits frequently need to be addressed, the physical therapist assistant should consider how to prioritize each session based on factors such as which interventions will target body functions foundational to function (ie, trunk control), which goals are most significant to the patient, how close the patient is to discharge, and what activities previous interventions have addressed. Taking these types of factors into consideration will allow the physical therapist assistant to prioritize and structure each session.

During each session, the physical therapist assistant should begin by clearly communicating the significance of the activity to the patient. As Dutton states, "Explicit knowledge of the task goals before practice for individuals post-stroke appears to improve implicit learning of motor skills."[6] As part of this process, the physical therapist assistant may need to demonstrate the motion or activity desired to provide a visual example. These steps, of course, may be inappropriate for patients with cognitive, visual perceptual, or communication deficits. All patients can, however, be guided through the movement to provide the patients with a kinesthetic input regarding the desired movement. Guided movement should be limited for appropriate motor learning to occur. At this point, the physical therapist assistant will use the motor-learning principles discussed in this section to modify and/or advance the activities appropriately based on the patient's response.

During each individual session, a variety of activities at a variety of levels may be practiced. This variability, when chosen intentionally, can be helpful in the motor learning process. It is important at some point in each session to significantly challenge the patient; however, it is best to finish each session with an activity the patient is able to complete, thus ending on a positive note.

Determine the Patient's Response to Interventions

Another challenge when providing physical therapy interventions to the patient who has had a stroke is the dynamic presentation of the symptoms of the stroke. The physical therapist assistant should expect that changes in symptoms will occur and, therefore, rigorously collect data to inform the process of modifying the intervention(s) to the patient. Changes in response to physical therapy interventions for the symptoms from a stroke may be subtle and observed over several days, or may be sufficient to require intervention progressions to occur repeatedly within a single physical therapy session with the patient.

Much of the assessment will occur through observation of the patient's response rather than through any formal test. The physical therapist assistant will monitor the patient's movements to note muscle substitutions or degradation of movement patterns that indicate fatigue. The physical therapist assistant should also note changes in the patient's attention and cognitive function, which can also indicate fatigue. In addition to general observations, formal assessment processes to monitor patient progress should be used. Choice of test and procedures to use should be based upon the physical therapist's evaluation and plan of care and may include formal measurements of strength or use of a functional test (eg, the Berg Balance Scale).

Formally assessing vital signs during a therapy session is important for patients who have cardiovascular conditions or when the patient is engaged in therapeutic exercise for aerobic/capacity and endurance. Other formal assessment processes such as strength measures and standardized tests will occur based on the plan of care to note progress.

Progress, Modify, or Discontinue

Based on the assessment through observation and data from tests, the physical therapist assistant will decide to progress, modify, or discontinue aspects of procedural interventions. When the patient is demonstrating the expected response, the physical therapist assistant will progress the intervention based on the expectations outlined in the plan of care. Progression may include changing assistive devices (eg, from a hemi cane to a quad cane) or advancing activities (eg, moving from a focus on static sitting balance to dynamic sitting balance). If the patient has met all the established goals, the physical therapist assistant will consult with the physical therapist to determine whether further goals should be established.

Throughout a therapy session, the physical therapist assistant will make multiple modifications to the intervention to challenge the patient as well as to ensure the safety and comfort of the patient. Modification can include the various aspects described related to motor learning. Modification can also be made when the patient is not responding as desired during a therapy session. For example, when attempting to teach a patient how to perform a sit-to-stand transfer, if the patient is unable to perform the task without significant assistance, the physical therapist assistant may choose to raise the surface the patient is sitting on; this allows the patient to work through a shortened range and thus experience more autonomy in movement, and better tap into the appropriate motor program.

Finally, there will be times when a physical therapist assistant will need to decide to discontinue with the current intervention tasks at hand. This should occur any time the patient displays a negative physiological response, a decrease in cognitive functioning, or significant psychological distress as evidenced by inappropriate heart rate and BP response. Exercise should be stopped any time the systolic BP drops 20 mm Hg or more, or is greater than 260 mm Hg, or if the diastolic BP is greater than 115 mm Hg.[61]

Notify the Physical Therapist

To ensure that the most effective and efficient care is being provided, it is imperative that the physical therapist assistant communicate regularly with the physical therapist regarding the patient's response to interventions. The type and frequency of communication will vary based on the patient's needs, the physical therapist's preferences, and the setting where care is being provided. In an inpatient environment where the physical therapist and physical therapist assistant may be working side by side, the physical therapist may be able to observe and monitor the care being provided by the physical therapist assistant and provide guidance when needed, without making specific plans for scheduled communication. The physical therapist assistant's documentation will act as an additional form of communication between the physical therapist assistant and the physical therapist. Some state practice acts regulate the frequency of physical therapist/physical therapist assistant interaction regarding patient care or require the physical therapist to initial all documentation made by the physical therapist assistant. However, regardless of these issues, the physical therapist assistant should ensure the physical therapist is kept up-to-date regarding the patient's status and progress. The physical therapist assistant should inform the physical therapist any time the patient has met a goal or when the patient's progress is not proceeding as expected (eg, whether it is faster or slower than expected). The physical therapist assistant should also make sure the physical therapist is aware of any changes that could affect the patient's goals or plan of care. For example, if the plan was based on the patient being discharged to an assisted-living environment, but the patient's family has decided to take the patient home instead, the physical therapist needs to determine any necessary alterations to the plan of care.

Finally, the physical therapist assistant should immediately inform the physical therapist of any negative responses the patient may display.

Conclusion

Providing interventions for a patient with a CVA is based on the plan of care and considers the individual patient's goals, functional capabilities, and discharge plan. Data collection is critical because the symptoms of the stroke may be changing between, and even within, the physical therapy sessions. While providing skilled interventions, the physical therapist assistant must identify when changes occur, and appropriately modify those interventions provided within the treatment plan established by the physical therapist. Attention must be paid to the progression of interventions, such as therapeutic exercise or gait training techniques, so that the patient is challenged appropriately and advanced toward achieving optimal functional abilities.

The role of the patient, the patient's family, and the other caregivers in this process must also be considered. The selected physical therapy interventions provided will involve only a small portion of the patient's day, but when others are encouraged to be involved in the process, a team effort is available to support the rehabilitation of the patient. This will extend and reinforce the activities and exercises necessary for the patient to achieve an optimal outcome from the process.

Case Studies

Case #1

A 64-year-old man was admitted to an acute rehabilitation facility 6 days after having a CVA, which was diagnosed as a left internal capsule infarction. The patient displayed mild right extremity and trunk weakness. The patient also displayed diminished sensation throughout the right extremities. He demonstrated impaired balance and motor control and required minimal assistance for gait activities due to apraxia. The patient required constant verbal cues when ambulating and became easily distracted in cluttered environments or when other individuals walked past him. He had poor insight into his deficits and demonstrated impulsivity that placed him as a safety risk. The patient previously lived alone in a home with 5 steps to enter, and his goal was to return to that environment. The physical therapist's plan of care called for therapeutic exercise to improve strength and motor control, gait training on level and uneven surfaces, and patient education.

Questions

1. What impairments of body functions, limitations in activities, and restrictions in participation does this patient demonstrate?
2. Within the plan of care, what activities could be used to address the right LE strength deficits? What parameters would be used (eg, frequency or intensity)?
3. This patient demonstrates safety issues during gait due to motor apraxia and anosognosia. How do you want to progress the environmental context in which this patient is practicing gait activities?
4. What feedback strategies could you use related to the patient's functional mobility deficits?
5. Using the concepts of movement sequencing, what other postures and activities might you choose to use with this patient to address the deficits of motor apraxia noted during gait?
6. What are you going to observe in this patient's movements to determine if the intervention strategies being used are effective?

Case #2

A 72-year-old woman was on vacation with her sister when she had a left middle cerebral artery CVA. She was transported from her hotel room to the hospital via an ambulance. The patient displayed strength of 0/5 throughout the right UE. The patient had sufficient strength to initiate the movements of hip extension and adduction, but demonstrated severe weakness and decreased tone throughout the right LE musculature. The patient required maximal assistance with all mobility, including the tasks of rolling, supine-to-and-from-sit, and sit-to-and-from-stand transitions; as well as the tasks of transferring from the bed to the w/c and from the w/c back to the bed. When standing, she needed maximal assistance and a hemi cane and was unable to support weight through her right leg. The patient's sitting balance was diminished, requiring minimal to moderate assistance to maintain an upright posture. The patient demonstrated mild pusher behavior and required frequent verbal cues to shift her weight to the left. The patient also demonstrated global aphasia. She did not attempt to speak and communicated only with head nods and shakes. The speech therapist's notes indicated the patient had only 50% accuracy with head nods and shakes. The patient was able to follow simple commands with physical and visual cues with 90% accuracy. Discharge plans are for the patient's son to assist with transporting the patient back to her hometown, where she will enter an inpatient rehabilitation unit. She will travel by commercial air. The son will need to be taught how to transfer the patient from a w/c into and out of a car, and needs to practice a simulated transfer from a w/c into and out of an airplane seat.

Questions

1. What impairments of body functions, limitations in activities, and restrictions in participation does this patient demonstrate?
2. How will this patient need to be positioned when sitting in a w/c?

3. How you will approach this patient in relation to her aphasia?
4. What activities can you describe that can be used to help facilitate the patient's use of her right leg?
5. What parameters would be appropriate when addressing transitional movements (eg, variability, and components of movement)?
6. What approach will you use when teaching the patient's son how to assist the patient in transfers?

References

1. Winstein CJ, Stein J, Arena R, et al; American Heart Association Stroke Council, Council on Cardiovascular and Stroke Nursing, Council on Clinical Cardiology, and Council on Quality of Care and Outcomes Research. Guidelines for adult stroke rehabilitation and recovery: a guideline for healthcare professionals from the American Heart Association/American Stroke Association. *Stroke.* 2016;47(6):e98-e169. doi:10.1161/STR.0000000000000098
2. Fuller KS. Stroke. In: Gooman CV, Fuller KS, eds. *Pathology: Implications for the PT.* 3rd ed. St. Louis, MO: Saunders-Elsevier; 2009.
3. Erickson ML, McKnight R. *Documentation Basics for the Physical Therapist Assistant.* 3rd ed. Thorofare, NJ: SLACK Incorporated; 2018.
4. American Physical Therapy Association. Guide to Physical Therapist Practice 3.0. http://guidetoptpractice.apta.org/. Accessed April 18, 2018.
5. Fell D. Progressing therapeutic intervention in patients with neuromuscular disorders: a framework to assist clinical decision making. *J Neurol Phys Ther.* 2004;28(1):35-46. doi:10.1097/01.NPT.0000284776.32802.1b
6. Dutton LL. Adult nonprogressive central nervous system disorders. In: Cameron MH, Monroe LG, eds. *Physical Rehabilitation: Evidence-Based Examination, Evaluation and Intervention.* St. Louis, MO: Saunders; 2007:405-435. doi:10.1016/B978-072160361-2.50019-3
7. Gentile AM. Skill acquisition: action, movement and neuromotor processes. In: Carr J, Shepherd R, Gordon J, et al, eds. *Movement Science: Foundations for Physical Therapy in Rehabilitation.* Rockville, MD: Aspen Publisher; 1987:93-154.
8. Gordon NF, Gulanick M, Costa F, et al. Physical activity and exercise recommendations for stroke survivors: an American Heart Association scientific statement from the Council on Clinical Cardiology, Subcommittee on Exercise, Cardiac Rehabilitation, and Prevention; Cardiac Rehabilitation, and Prevention; the Council on Cardiovascular Nursing; the Council on Nutrition; Physical Activity, and Metabolism; and the Stroke Council. *Circulation.* 2004;16(109):2031-2041. doi:10.1161/01.CIR.0000126280.65777.A4
9. Carr J, Shepherd R. *Stroke Rehabilitation: Guidelines for Exercise Training to Optimize Motor Skill.* Edinburgh, Scotland: Butterworth-Heinemann; 2010.
10. Katalinic OM, Harvey LA, Herbert RD. Effectiveness of stretch for the treatment and prevention of contractures in people with neurological conditions: a systematic review. *Phys Ther.* 2011;91(1):11-24. doi:10.2522/ptj.20100265
11. Hesse S. Rehabilitation of gait after stroke: evaluation, principles of therapy, novel treatment approaches, and assistive devices. *Top Geriatr Rehabil.* 2003;19(2):109-126. doi:10.1097/00013614-200304000-00005
12. Visintin M, Barbeau H, Korner-Bitensky N, Mayo NE. A new approach to retrain gait in stroke patients through body weight support and treadmill stimulation. *Stroke.* 1998;29(6):1122-1128. doi:10.1161/01.STR.29.6.1122
13. Kisner C, Colby LA. *Therapeutic Exercise: Foundation and Techniques.* 5th ed. Philadelphia, PA: FA Davis; 2007.
14. Ryerson S, Levit K. *Functional Movement Reeducation.* Philadelphia, PA: Churchill Livingstone; 1997.
15. Ouellette MM, LeBrasseur NK, Bean JF, et al. High-intensity resistance training improves muscle strength, self-reported function, and disability in long-term stroke survivors. *Stroke.* 2004;35(6):1404-1409. doi:10.1161/01.STR.0000127785.73065.34
16. Ferrarello F, Baccini M, Rinaldi LA, et al. Efficacy of physiotherapy interventions late after stroke: a meta-analysis. *J Neurol Neurosurg Psychiatry.* 2011;82(2):136-143. doi:10.1136/jnnp.2009.196428
17. Jørgensen JR, Bech-Pedersen DT, Zeeman P, Sørensen J, Andersen LL, Schönberger M. Effect of intensive outpatient physical training on gait performance and cardiovascular health in people with hemiparesis after stroke. *Phys Ther.* 2010;90(4):527-537. doi:10.2522/ptj.20080404
18. Bean JF, Kiely DK, LaRose S, O'Neill E, Goldstein R, Frontera WR. Increased velocity exercise specific to task training versus the National Institute on Aging's strength training program: changes in limb power and mobility. *J Gerontol A Biol Sci Med Sci.* 2009;64(9):983-991. doi:10.1093/gerona/glp056
19. Ryerson S. Hemiplegia. In: Umphred DA, Lazaro RT, Burton GU, eds. *Umphred's Neurological Rehabilitation.* 5th ed. St. Louis, MO: Mosby; 2007.
20. Faghri PD, Rodgers MM, Glaser RM, Bors JG, Ho C, Akuthota P. The effects of functional electrical stimulation on shoulder subluxation, arm function recovery, and shoulder pain in hemiplegic stroke patients. *Arch Phys Med Rehabil.* 1994;75(1):73-79.
21. Price CI, Pandyan AD. Electrical stimulation for preventing and treating post-stroke shoulder pain: a systematic Cochrane review. *Clin Rehabil.* 2001;15(1):5-19. doi:10.1191/026921501670667822
22. Gritsenko V, Prochazka A. A functional electric stimulationassisted exercise therapy system for hemiplegic hand function. *Arch Phys Med Rehabil.* 2004;85(6):881-885. doi:10.1016/j.apmr.2003.08.094
23. Sullivan JE, Hedman LD. A home program of sensory and neuromuscular electrical stimulation with upper-limb task practice in a patient 5 years after a stroke. *Phys Ther.* 2004;84(11):1045-1054. doi:10.1093/ptj/84.11.1045

24. Newsam CJ, Baker LL. Effect of an electric stimulation facilitation program on quadriceps motor unit recruitment after stroke. *Arch Phys Med Rehabil.* 2004;85(12):2040-2045. doi:10.1016/j.apmr.2004.02.029
25. Burridge JH, Taylor PN, Hagan SA, Wood DE, Swain ID. The effects of common peroneal stimulation on the effort and speed of walking: a randomized controlled trial with chronic hemiplegic patients. *Clin Rehabil.* 1997;11(3):201-210. doi:10.1177/026921559701100303
26. Taub E, Uswatte G, Pidikiti R. Constraint-Induced Movement Therapy: a new family of techniques with broad application to physical rehabilitation—a clinical review. *J Rehabil Res Dev.* 1999;36(3):237-251.
27. Blanton S, Wolf SL. An application of upper-extremity constraint-induced movement therapy in a patient with subacute stroke. *Phys Ther.* 1999;79(9):847-853. doi:10.1093/ptj/79.9.847
28. Kunkel A, Kopp B, Müller G, et al. Constraint-induced movement therapy for motor recovery in chronic stroke patients. *Arch Phys Med Rehabil.* 1999;80(6):624-628. doi:10.1016/S0003-9993(99)90163-6
29. Zablotny C, Hershberg J, Parlman K. Stroke: PTNow Clinical Summaries [educational series online]. https://www.ptnow.org/ClinicalSummaries/quick-detail/stroke-2 Accessed March 30, 2020.
30. Saposnik G, Levin M; Outcome Research Canada (SORCan) Working Group. Virtual reality in stroke rehabilitation: a meta-analysis and implications for clinicians. *Stroke.* 2011;42(5):1380-1386. doi:10.1161/STROKEAHA.110.605451
31. Saposnik G, Teasell R, Mamdani M, et al; Stroke Outcome Research Canada (SORCan) Working Group. Effectiveness of virtual reality using Wii gaming technology in stroke rehabilitation: a pilot randomized clinical trial and proof of principle. *Stroke.* 2010;41(7):1477-1484. doi:10.1161/STROKEAHA.110.584979
32. Shumway-Cook A, Woollacott M. *Motor Control Theory and Practical Applications.* 2nd ed. Philadelphia, PA: Lippincott Williams & Wilkins; 2001.
33. Adams RD, Victor M, Ropper AH. *Principles of Neurology.* 6th ed. New York, NY: McGraw-Hill; 1997.
34. Kertesz A, Nicholson I, Cancelliere A, Kassa K, Black SE. Motor impersistence: a right-hemisphere syndrome. *Neurology.* 1985;35(5):662-666. doi:10.1212/WNL.35.5.662
35. Donkervoort M, Dekker J, van den Ende E, Stehmann-Saris JC, Deelman BG. Prevalence of apraxia among patients with a first left hemisphere stroke in rehabilitation centres and nursing homes. *Clin Rehabil.* 2000;14(2):130-136. doi:10.1191/026921500668935800
36. van Heugten CM, Dekker J, Deelman BG, Stehmann-Saris JC, Kinebanian A. Rehabilitation of stroke patients with apraxia: the role of additional cognitive and motor impairments. *Disabil Rehabil.* 2000;22(12):547-554. doi:10.1080/096382800416797
37. Kelly JO, Kilbreath SL, Davis GM, Zeman B, Raymond J. Cardiorespiratory fitness and walking ability in subacute stroke patients. *Arch Phys Med Rehabil.* 2003;84(12):1780-1785. doi:10.1016/S0003-9993(03)00376-9
38. Mackay-Lyons MJ, Makrides L. Exercise capacity early after stroke. *Arch Phys Med Rehabil.* 2002;83(12):1697-1702. doi:10.1053/apmr.2002.36395
39. Bernhardt J, Dewey H, Thrift A, Donnan G. Inactive and alone: physical activity within the first 14 days of acute stroke unit care. *Stroke.* 2004;35(4):1005-1009. doi:10.1161/01.STR.0000120727.40792.40
40. Hendricks HT, van Limbeek J, Geurts AC, Zwarts MJ. Motor recovery after stroke: a systematic review of the literature. *Arch Phys Med Rehabil.* 2002;83(11):1629-1637. doi:10.1053/apmr.2002.35473
41. Andrews AW, Bohannon RW. Distribution of muscle strength impairments following stroke. *Clin Rehabil.* 2000;14(1):79-87. doi:10.1191/026921500673950113
42. Vuagnat H, Chantraine A. Shoulder pain in hemiplegia revisited: contribution of functional electrical stimulation and other therapies. *J Rehabil Med.* 2003;35(2):49-54. doi:10.1080/16501970306111
43. Turner-Stokes L, Jackson D. Shoulder pain after stroke: a review of the evidence base to inform the development of an integrated care pathway. *Clin Rehabil.* 2002;16(3):276-298. doi:10.1191/0269215502cr491oa
44. Murphy MA, Roberts-Warrior D. A review of motor performance measures and treatment interventions for patients with stroke. *Top Geriatr Rehabil.* 2003;19(1):3-42. doi:10.1097/00013614-200301000-00003
45. Roller ML. The "pusher syndrome". *J Neurol Phys Ther.* 2004;28(1):29-34. doi:10.1097/01.NPT.0000284775.32802.c0
46. Pérennou DA, Amblard B, Laassel M, Benaim C, Hérisson C, Pélissier J. Understanding the pusher behavior of some stroke patients with spatial deficits: a pilot study. *Arch Phys Med Rehabil.* 2002;83(4):570-575. doi:10.1053/apmr.2002.31198
47. Lewis CB, McNerney T. *The Functional Toolbox: Clinical Measures of Functional Outcomes.* Washington, DC: Learn Publications; 1994.
48. Lewis CB, McNerney T. *The Functional Toolbox II: Clinical Measures of Functional Outcomes.* Washington, DC: Learn Publications; 1997.
49. Bohannon RW. Measurement, nature, and implications of skeletal muscle strength in patients with neurological disorders. *Clin Biomech (Bristol, Avon).* 1995;10(6):283-292. doi:10.1016/0268-0033(94)00002-O
50. Pierce SR, Buxbaum LJ. Treatments of unilateral neglect: a review. *Arch Phys Med Rehabil.* 2002;83(2):256-268. doi:10.1053/apmr.2002.27333
51. Swan L. Unilateral spatial neglect. *Phys Ther.* 2001;81(9):1572-1580. doi:10.1093/ptj/81.9.1572
52. Stone SP, Wilson B, Wroot A, et al. The assessment of visuospatial neglect after acute stroke. *J Neurol Neurosurg Psychiatry.* 1991;54(4):345-350. doi:10.1136/jnnp.54.4.345
53. Maeshima S, Dohi N, Funahashi K, Nakai K, Itakura T, Komai N. Rehabilitation of patients with anosognosia for hemiplegia due to intracerebral haemorrhage. *Brain Inj.* 1997;11(9):691-697. doi:10.1080/026990597123232
54. Pedersen P, Jorgensen HS, Nakayama H, Raaschou HO, Olsen TS. Frequency, determinants, and consequences of anosognosia in acute stroke. *Neurorehabil Neural Repair.* 1996;10(4):243-250. doi:10.1177/154596839601000404

55. Ross E. Acute agitation and other behaviors associated with Wernicke aphasia and their possible neurological basis. *Neuropsychiatry Neuropsychol Behav Neurol.* 1993;6(1):9-18.
56. Lundy-Ekman L. Neuroscience: *Fundamentals for Rehabilitation*. Philadelphia, PA: WB Saunders; 2002.
57. Waxman SA. *Correlative Neuroanatomy.* 23rd ed. Stamford, CT: Appleton and Lange; 1996.
58. Ghika-Schmid F, Bogousslavsky J. Affective disorders following stroke. *Eur Neurol.* 1997;38(2):75-81. doi:10.1159/000113164
59. Bohannon RW. Evaluation and treatment of sensory and perceptual impairments following stroke. *Top Geriatr Rehabil.* 2003;19(2):87-97. doi:10.1097/00013614-200304000-00003
60. Skinner SB, McVey C. *Clinical Decision Making for the Physical Therapist Assistant.* Sudbury, MA: Jones and Barlett; 2011.
61. Elokda AS, Helgeson K. Deconditioning. In: Cameron MH, Monroe LG, eds. *Physical Rehabilitation: Evidence-Based Examination, Evaluation and Intervention.* St. Louis, MO: Saunders/Elsevier; 2007. doi:10.1016/B978-072160361-2.50026-0

Chapter 14

Clients With Degenerative Diseases

Parkinson's Disease and Amyotrophic Lateral Sclerosis

Amanda A. Forster, PT, DPT, NCS and Rolando T. Lazaro, PT, PhD, DPT

KEY WORDS Amyotrophic lateral sclerosis | Degenerative disease of the central nervous system | Parkinson's disease | Rigidity | Therapeutic exercises

Chapter Objectives

- Discuss the signs and symptoms of Parkinson's disease and amyotrophic lateral sclerosis (ALS), and explain their implications to physical therapy examination and intervention.
- Discuss common intervention strategies for patients and clients with degenerative diseases of the central nervous system (CNS).
- Identify some clinical pearls that can assist a physical therapist assistant in treating patients and clients with degenerative conditions of the CNS.

Many patients and clients referred for physical therapy intervention have conditions caused by the degeneration of specific portions of the CNS, specifically those that involve or influence movement. The degeneration may be caused by the normal aging process, mediated by genetic abnormalities, exacerbated or hastened by harmful environmental agents, or be a combination of 2 or more of these factors. As movement specialists, physical therapists and physical therapist assistants have an important and unique role in helping patients and clients with degenerative neuromuscular diseases achieve and/or maintain their highest functional capacity and optimum health and well-being. A thorough understanding of the specific functions of the structures of the CNS will allow the clinician to make inferences on potential movement disorders based on the structures involved in the disease process. This knowledge will facilitate appropriate clinical decision-making and allow the physical therapist assistant to determine what to expect (assuming a typical presentation of the condition) and will empower the physical therapist assistant to communicate to the physical therapist possible changes in the patient's condition that do not follow the specific presentation for the disease. For example, if the physical therapist assistant who is treating a patient with Parkinson's disease (PD) notices that this patient has developed paralysis on one side of the body, the physical therapist assistant should communicate this finding to the physical therapist, because this is not consistent with a medical diagnosis of PD.

Impairment in motor performance is a common problem seen in patients with degenerative conditions. The physical therapist assistant can use several intervention approaches to improve this problem. It is important for the physical therapist assistant to monitor the patient's response to these interventions, because this will indicate whether the overall plan of care is meeting the anticipated goals and expected outcomes. In people with degenerative conditions, it is important to be aware of undesired responses, especially in

Lazaro RT, Umphred DA, eds.
Umphred's Neurorehabilitation for the Physical Therapist Assistant, Third Edition (pp 351-361).

relation to fatigue and further loss of strength. This will be discussed in more detail later in the chapter.

This chapter will focus on 2 common degenerative diseases in adults: PD and ALS.

Parkinson's Disease

PD is a medical condition that results in a variety of movement disorders that impair an individual's ability to perform normal everyday tasks. In the United States, it is reported that one million individuals have this condition, with 1% of those being older than 60 years of age.[1] Sources indicate that approximately 50,000 people are diagnosed with PD annually in the United States.[2]

A person with PD may exhibit one or more of the following motor impairments: *bradykinesia* (ie, extreme slowness of movement), rigidity, resting (unintentional) tremors, postural instability, and festinating gait.[3] Bradykinesia in PD is also associated with "on-off phenomenon," characterized by freezing episodes in which the person appears to be fixed or "stuck " in space, usually seen during a gross motor activity.[4] Other physical traits associated with PD include increased thoracic kyphosis and decreased lumbar lordosis, producing a stooped and flexed posture.[3] This posture can also be a compensatory mechanism to account for loss of stability when weight is shifted posteriorly, as is often indicated on the pull test.[5] People with PD may feel as though they are losing balance posteriorly and thus exaggerate the anteriorly shifted posture. Each of these manifestations of PD impairs the gross motor function of all extremities, thus negatively affecting balance. Poor balance leads to falls that, when combined with other comorbidities associated with aging, can create life-threatening results. One study, which used a questionnaire that reported on the frequency of falls in patients with PD, stated that more than one-third of these patients had fallen, and more than 10% fall at least once a week. Causes of these falls were attributed to postural instability, movement dysfunction, gait abnormalities, and difficulty with transfers.[6] Falls may occur because of the delayed motor responses when standing, walking, turning, and sitting without back support.[7] As normal individuals age, falls become an increasing problem. With age and a preexisting diagnosis of a disease such as PD, an individual may not only be at risk of falling, but the resulting problems following a fall may also have greater consequences.

Because PD is due to a progressive degeneration of the basal ganglia, people with PD present with increasingly altered posture, rigidity, and bradykinesia, which become more significant over time and lead to a decreased ability to balance. Eventually, movement requires so much energy that the individual may become bedridden, with a fixed trunk and flexion contractures. In the advanced stages, inspiration is decreased, coughing is difficult, and bronchopneumonia may be one of the reasons for morbidity.[3]

Traditionally, drug therapy has been the primary intervention to delay the progression of impairments, activity limitations, and participation restrictions related to PD. The general effect of these PD medications is to replenish the brain's supply of dopamine, a neurotransmitter that is important in basal ganglia function. Common medications for PD include Sinemet (carbidopa levodopa). The "next-generation" medications that have been approved include Permax (pergolide mesylate) and Mirapex (pramipexole), which are dopamine agonists that bind to and stimulate cerebral dopamine receptors to improve motor performance.[8] While on these medications, patients may experience motor fluctuations causing unpredictable on-off episodes, which interfere with performance of activities of daily living (ADL) and ambulation. Recent research indicates that physical exercise can also alter the disease process and allow medications to work more effectively.[9,10] Many studies are being conducted to further evaluate the effect of physical exercise on the underlying health condition of PD, as well as the changes in outward physical presentation of persons with PD.[11-15] This information is exciting and pertinent to rehabilitation professionals working with persons with PD, and an indication for specific physical therapy intervention with these patients and clients.

The progression of PD has been classified by the Hoehn and Yahr stages.[16] This scale was modified in 2004 to include intermediate stages in the progression of the disease.[16] These stages are medically diagnosed by a physician or other health care provider licensed to determine medical diagnoses. Physical therapy interventions and goals will vary depending on the stage of PD. The following describes the stages, patient presentation, and appropriate physical therapy approaches.[17]

Early Stages (Hoehn and Yahr, Stages 1 to 2.5)

Early stages involve axial, unilateral to bilateral extremity involvement. In these stages, physical therapy interventions are aimed at encouraging movement to prevent the deleterious effects of inactivity. The patient is encouraged to join exercise groups to improve mobility and strength and to promote an active lifestyle.

Middle Stages (Hoehn and Yahr, Stages 2 to 4)

In the middle stages, the patient presents with increasing impairments causing limitations in activity and participation. In these stages, the patient may require more assistance in ADL. The patient will present with postural instability, leading to problems with ambulation and falls. Physical therapy interventions typically start at this stage with the goal of improving mobility, balance, and gait, and reducing risks for falls. Task-specific interventions with cueing and cognitive movement strategies are incorporated into the treatment plan.

Late Stage (Stage 5)

In the late stage, the patient is significantly debilitated and typically wheelchair (w/c) ambulatory. In this stage, physical therapy is aimed at preventing skin breakdown and contractures. Interventions include family/caregiver training on proper bed/w/c positioning and ROM exercises.

Amyotrophic Lateral Sclerosis

ALS, also known as *Lou Gehrig's disease*, is the most common progressive neurodegenerative disease affecting adults. This disease involves the progressive degeneration of the motor neurons in the brain and spinal cord. Progression of the disease is rapid, and death due to compromise of the respiratory system is typically noted within 2 to 5 years.[18]

Clinical symptoms include *fasciculations* (involuntary twitching of muscle fibers), muscle cramps, fatigue, weakness, and atrophy. There is a highly varied pattern of onset in ALS, with the most common pattern being lower extremity (LE) onset, followed by upper extremity (UE) onset and bulbar onset; the least common pattern demonstrates symptoms in the distal musculature of the UEs and LEs. With each pattern of onset, the eventual progression of ALS is similar for most patients, with a spread of weakness to other muscle groups ultimately leading to complete paralysis. The cause of death is usually related to respiratory failure.[18]

Several phases and stages characterize the progression of ALS (Box 14-1).[18] Depending on the stage of the disease, physical therapy interventions and goals will vary.[19]

Box 14-1

Summary of the Stages of Amyotrophic Lateral Sclerosis

- Phase I: Independent
  - Stage 1: Patient exhibits only mild weakness with no limitation in function.
  - Stage 2: Patient exhibits definite weakness in some muscle groups.
  - Stage 3: Patient's muscle weakness affects ADL, especially in the extremities, although independence is still demonstrated and compensation observed. Respiratory function is beginning to be compromised.
- Phase II: Partially Independent
  - Stage 4: Patient able to perform most ADL with adaptations, but fatigues quickly. Mobility is primarily through the use of a w/c.
  - Stage 5: Both UE and LE demonstrate severe weakness, limiting the individual's ability to function independently.
- Phase III: Dependent (Final Phase)
  - Stage 6: Patient is bed-dependent and requires maximal assistance for all activities.

Phase I

Phase I is termed *independent* phase and is characterized by the patient's ability to perform most everyday activities without any limitation. There are 3 stages under phase I. In stage 1, the patient exhibits mild weakness and complaints of clumsiness. Stage 2 is characterized by more evident weakness affecting certain muscle groups, often in the extremities. It is also in this stage that a noticeable decrease in the ability to perform ADL appears. Stage 3 shows more severe selective weakness in the distal portions of the extremities. Respiration is also starting to be affected in this stage, as shown by increased fatigue and slight increase in breathing effort.

Phase II

Phase II is termed *partially independent*. As the name implies, the patient requires assistance in several ADL in this phase. Phase II has 2 stages: stages 4 and 5. In stage 4, the patient is still able to perform most ADL but tires easily. In terms of locomotion, the patient is mostly using a w/c at this point. Muscular weakness is present, and tone abnormalities (*spasticity*) may be evident. More affectation in functional performance due to progression of the disease is evident in stage 5, which is characterized by significant weakness of the LEs and moderate to severe weakness of the UEs. Because of decreased mobility, the risk of skin breakdown is also evident in this stage.[18,19]

Phase III

Phase III is termed the *dependent* phase of the disease. There is 1 stage under this phase: stage 6. In this stage, the patient is bed-bound and requires maximal assistance in ADL. Respiratory function is severely compromised.[20,21]

Examination and Evaluation: The Role of the Physical Therapist Assistant

Several factors must guide the physical therapy examination of a patient with degenerative disease. First, it is important to identify from the patient's perspective the impact of the presenting signs and symptoms on the ability to function. It is important to determine, in terms of activity, what the patient can and cannot do, and then hypothesize the impairments that may be causing the identified activity limitations. The *Guide to Physical Therapist Practice*[22] (the *Guide*) is a helpful tool to guide the clinician in identifying the pertinent tests and measures that will provide the best representation of the patient's functional level. The physical therapist assistant may be delegated portions of a reexamination (see Chapter 6), and it is of the utmost importance for the physical therapist assistant to clearly communicate the results of the tests and measures to the physical therapist.

The physical therapist assistant must identify the specific signs and symptoms associated with the condition, monitor these signs and symptoms, and communicate to the supervising physical therapist any significant changes in the patient's presentation, which may indicate the progression of symptoms, ineffectiveness of the prescribed physical therapy intervention, medication issues, or the possibility of other comorbidities. The rehabilitation team must be cognizant of other signs and symptoms that may necessitate referral to other medical practitioners. For example, symptoms of chest congestion, difficulty breathing, increased coughing, and mucus may be indicative of aspiration pneumonia and must be resolved expediently. This congestion may have been precipitated by decreased respiratory function (eg, chest expansion, decreased inability to clear secretions, or ineffective cough) and is a fairly common complication in patients with degenerative neuromuscular disorders.

In looking at examination, it is important to identify the patient and family goals in determining exercises and activities that will be implemented. Standardized functional tests often provide the clinician useful information regarding the impact of the disease progression on the patient's function. Serial testing of function allows the clinician to generate objective function documentation; however, it should always follow a thoughtful interpretation of the results afforded by the physical therapist. Examples of general functional tests that could be administered to patients with PD, multiple sclerosis (MS), or ALS include the Performance-Oriented Mobility Assessment,[20] Berg Balance Scale,[21] Functional Reach Test (FRT),[23] or Timed Up and Go.[24] These tests give the clinician insight regarding the patient's level of function and risk of falls. Disease-specific tests include the United Parkinson's Disease Rating Scale.[25]

It is also important to include measures of participation, self-efficacy, and quality of life. Examples of these measures include the Parkinson's Disease Quality of Life Questionnaire[26] and ALS-specific quality of life instrument.[27]

All the examination areas mentioned in Chapter 6 must be assessed in patients with degenerative diseases to provide the clinician with a clear picture of the patient's impairments, activity limitations, and participation restrictions.

Intervention

Physical therapy intervention for patients with degenerative disorders should be based on the correction of, remediation of, or compensation for the identified activity limitations and impairments. The procedural interventions physical therapists commonly use when treating patients with PD and ALS could be delegated to a physical therapist assistant as long as the patient is stable and does not need ongoing (formal) assessment during the intervention period.

Aerobic and Endurance Conditioning and Reconditioning

The ability of the patient to have the cardiopulmonary capacity to be able to perform functional activities is central to optimal health and well-being. Graded exercise must allow the patient to perform activities within the safe levels of cardiopulmonary functioning to allow the patient to tolerate increased activities. ADL training, gait, and locomotion activities can be incorporated into therapeutic intervention, as appropriate. Aquatic exercise programs also allow the patient to perform these activities with less impact on the joints; however, increased workload due to increased hydrostatic pressure must be monitored accordingly. Examples of aerobic and endurance conditioning and reconditioning include the use of an upper body ergometer, LE pedal exerciser or exercise bike, treadmill training, or walking using an appropriate assistive device, increasing distance as tolerated while ensuring that vital signs are within safe limits. In terms of ADL training, the therapist can start with facilitation of simple ADL tasks (eg, maintaining sitting balance while the patient puts on socks and shoes) and then progress to those activities that require higher demands on the system in terms of postural control, coordination, endurance, and safety. The use of progressive resistance exercise has been shown to improve mobility and muscular strength in people with PD, so this is a consideration when performing physical therapy interventions and prescribing a home exercise program for these patients and clients.[28] Similar types of resistive exercises need to be carefully monitored with individuals diagnosed with ALS, while individuals with MS may benefit as long as prolonged fatigue does not set in.

Balance, Coordination, and Agility Training

There must be an emphasis on decreasing the risk of falls to avoid the deleterious effects of decreased activity and the medical complications following such an incident. Task-specific performance training could be used to improve performance of everyday tasks, increase confidence in mobility activities, and improve quality of life. Vestibular training might be indicated to heighten the role of the vestibular system in balance tasks and compensate for loss in somatosensory and visual systems. Examples include standing weight-shifting activities with eyes open and eyes closed, standing or balancing on foam, tandem walking, braiding, practicing tai chi, and maintaining balance while performing functional tasks such as brushing teeth, getting something from the refrigerator or kitchen cabinets, or putting on socks and shoes. Some of these activities can be performed in groups, which helps increase the socialization of these individuals and make them feel included as a whole. Thus, when working on balance, multiple individuals can be throwing and catching balls, which causes weight-shifting as well as perturbations as the individual catches the ball. Increasing and decreasing the weight of the ball can change the activity. In a group setting, multiple balls can be used and switched to increase the challenge and enjoyment of these interactions.

Balance exercises may be incorporated with ADL, gait training, or endurance training. The therapist could start by having the patient sit upright, providing adequate support as necessary, instructing the patient to "sense" the upright position, improving stability in this position via compression (approximation through the shoulder will allow co-contraction and, therefore, stability) or proprioceptive neuromuscular facilitation rhythmic stabilization. Then the therapist could work on strengthening the postural muscles using proprioceptive neuromuscular facilitation or progressive resistance using manual and machine-generated resistance.

Once the patient achieves relative stability in the static sitting position, the therapist can progress to working on dynamic sitting. To achieve this, the therapist could incorporate ADL training. For example, the therapist could ask the patient to reach for an object that is outside the patient's base of support, and then guide the patient to make sure that the patient maintains balance. Performing isometric holds when the patient is in varying degrees of leaning will allow the patient to be stable in those increments of motion and achieve improved proprioceptive input in that position. The patient can then use the newly learned balance strategies in more ADL (eg, putting on shoes and socks while sitting) or in recreational activities (eg, tossing a balloon, playing beanbag basketball, or throwing darts). These same principles can be performed while facilitating static and dynamic standing balance. Regardless of the degenerative disease, the physical therapist assistant must monitor the patient's response to the activity to determine its value to the patient's therapeutic environment. Oftentimes, maintaining function is the goal of therapeutic intervention, rather than regaining function. Physical therapy cannot prevent the progressive nature of a degenerative disease, but often function can be maintained for a period of time in spite of the progressive nature of the disease process by maintaining the highest level of motor performance possible.

Flexibility Exercises

It is important for patients with degenerative diseases to maintain or improve their range of motion (ROM) and flexibility to allow for normal excursions of the body during functional tasks, thereby decreasing the risk of falls. Flexibility exercises also allow for easier transfers from one surface to another or easier performance of ADL, such as lower-body hygiene and grooming. These exercises can also potentially improve or normalize tone, which is commonly a major issue for patients with PD, MS, or ALS. Because daily ROM is important, the patient must be taught how to perform self-assisted ROM activities, and the family must also be instructed on performing these activities. If the patient has cognitive deficits that prevent the performance of a self-ROM program, family members and caregivers should perform these activities. They must understand the importance of adequate joint mobility and muscle length on the patient's functional abilities. Examples include passive to active-assisted to active ROM of shoulder (eg, flexion, abduction, and internal-external rotation), elbow (eg, flexion and extension), forearm (eg, pronation and supination), wrist and hand (eg, flexion, extension, abduction, and adduction), hip (eg, flexion, extension, abduction, and internal-external rotation), knee (eg, flexion and extension), and ankle and foot (eg, dorsiflexion, plantar flexion, inversion, and eversion) movements.

Muscle Performance

The physical therapist assistant must incorporate interventions that increase muscle performance, including activities that improve muscular strength, power, and endurance. Often, activity limitations result from lack of strength, power, or endurance to perform an activity. Weakness in the LEs has also been associated with increased fall risk, decreased gait velocity, and decreased functional performance.

The physical therapist assistant must appropriately apply the principles of therapeutic exercise in terms of accurately identifying the patient's threshold, dosing, and response to ensure that the exercise prescription achieves the goal of improving muscular performance while preventing excessive overheating and fatigue (especially for persons with MS) or extreme muscle soreness. All modes of strengthening exercise can be applied to these patients. In patients with MS, the recommended protocol for strengthening includes 2 to 3 training sessions every week, with 1 to 3 sets for 8 to 15 reps for major muscle groups, with the patient in the seated position if necessary. The resistance is increased by 2% to 4% when 15 reps are easily performed.[29] More research is being conducted regarding the potential for exercise to positively affect persons with MS and potentially slow disease progression.[30-33] There are no specific recommendations for people with PD; however, several studies have confirmed the importance of strengthening exercises to facilitate muscle hypertrophy, improve mobility, and decrease fall risk. The exercise modes vary from low- to high-intensity activities, performed with supervision in the clinic or home as part of a home program.[34-36] There are also no suggested protocols regarding exercise in people with ALS, but evidence also supports the benefits of exercise in this population.[37] However, caution must be exercised to not overfatigue the patient; therefore, submaximal exercise dosage has been suggested when working with this population.[38] There is evidence that indicates that submaximal exercise is beneficial in delaying the decline in motor performance in people with ALS.[39]

Relaxation

An often-forgotten, but nevertheless important, component of a successful rehabilitation program for patients with degenerative disorders is relaxation training. Relaxation in the form of breathing exercises allows for increased oxygenation of the muscles and vital organs, thereby leading to increased performance and endurance, which may lead to improved swallowing and speech while allowing chest expansion and improved posture in the process. Examples of activities include rhythmic breathing, progressive relaxation by contracting and relaxing muscle groups, and using imagery or music. Since diminished respiratory capacity can be a factor in PD, MS, and ALS, the importance of diaphragmatic breathing should be emphasized with these patient populations. There are many ways to teach patients to breathe using their diaphragm. For example, the patient lies supine on a firm but comfortable bed or mat with a pillow to support the head, and another pillow under the knees. The therapist instructs the patient to put one hand on the diaphragm and another on the sternum. The patient is then asked to breathe in through the nose and breathe out using pursed lips. The patient is instructed to feel the rise of the hand placed on the diaphragm, to indicate correct technique. The therapist further instructs the patient to make sure that the upper chest does not rise with inspiration; if it does, the patient is using accessory muscles, and the technique must be corrected. Once the patient has gained the correct techniques, the therapist then instructs the patient to feel the shoulders, and then the back and the neck, relax while breathing deeply.

Neuromuscular Education or Reeducation

It is important to maintain the patient's ability to run normal functional motor programs to optimize functional performance. If this is impaired because of PD, MS, or ALS, the physical therapist assistant could facilitate the performance of these functions using neurological approaches that aim to allow for a window by which more normal tone is achieved. These approaches facilitate the performance of normal movement while that window is open, and consciously and consistently open that window so the patient might eventually run an entire program sequence in the most efficient, effective, and functional manner possible. Examples of these neurological approaches include the use of proprioceptive neuromuscular facilitation or neuro-developmental treatment to strengthen muscle and facilitate functional mobility, transfers, or gait. If the physical therapist has specific methods or strategies that employ these approaches, open communication with the physical therapist assistant will help improve continuity of care and improve intervention outcomes. An example of how to narrow and then open a window to a functional activity might be analyzing the activity of sit-to-stand-to-sit. If an individual cannot sit down in a controlled and safe manner (as often seen in people with PD), the physical therapist assistant can start the activity in standing. If a high/low mat table is available, the physical therapist assistant could start by having the patient sit on the mat, elevating the mat to a height where the patient is almost standing, then asking the patient to perform several sit-to-stands from this table height. This way, the physical therapist assistant narrows the available range to allow the patient to perform this activity safely and correctly. Once the patient is able to perform this activity correctly, the physical therapist assistant may decide to lower the mat so the patient is now performing the activity with a wider range and a greater challenge to improve strength, range, balance, and skill. The mat is lowered further until the patient reaches a mat height that is similar to a regular chair. To facilitate task-specific training, the same principle can then be used, but this time using bar stools of varying heights, from tallest to shortest, and then transitioning to performing sit-to-stands using a regular armless chair. Once the entire fluid movement is within the capability of the patient, then the patient should sit back in the chair, relax, and then come back to stand. Many functional activities can be narrowed into programs that patients can control, and then reintroduced with a wider ROM or need for additional power or other variables that aim to improve motor performance.

Gait and Locomotion Training

Gait or locomotion training is also important to the patient's functional independence. Being able to ambulate functional distances will allow the patient more freedom in movement (eg, the ability to walk from the bedroom to the dining room or bathroom), as well as allowing the patient to be a more social and productive member of the community. A physical therapist assistant might be asked to perform gait training with any of these individuals with degenerative CNS problems. Certainly maintaining functional gait will empower the patient. How best to regain or maintain ambulation skill varies based on the balance, strength, endurance, speed of ambulation, ability to run feedforward programs for walking, ROM, desire to ambulate, and dysfunction caused by the disease itself. All these variables can lead to variance in the specific treatment protocol. Whether the individual needs assistive devices, such as a quad-cane, a walker, or a single upright cane,[40] or whether the physical therapist thinks using a body weight–support system while ambulating on a treadmill or overground[41] is the best selection for intervention, the physical therapist assistant must be able to sequence the intervention toward the established goals. If gait is not realistic, the ability of the patient to safely and independently use an appropriate mobility device (eg, a w/c) will improve endurance while allowing the patient to be as functional as possible.[42] Examples include w/c mobility training and gait training using the appropriate assistive device on level or uneven surfaces while progressively decreasing assistance, as appropriate. Selection of noncompliant surfaces as the training site (eg, hardwood, tile, or linoleum) vs compliant surfaces (eg, rugs, grass, or dirt) can vary the training environment and demands placed on the patient's CNS.[43]

Activities of Daily Living Training

All activities must have the ultimate goal of facilitating improvements in the performance of ADL to allow the patient the highest level of independence possible. Examples include training for activities such as dressing, grooming, bathing, transfers, and bed mobility.

Monitoring Response to Exercise Interventions and Level of Fatigue

The physical therapist assistant must always monitor the patient's response to the plan of care. In people with degenerative conditions, it is especially important to look for abnormal responses to interventions that should improve motor performance. Degenerative conditions that result in damage to the lower motor neuron could present with muscle weakness because of the decrease in the amount of functioning motor units. Strenuous strengthening exercise in this case may lead to further deterioration of the remaining intact motor units, thereby causing a further decline in strength. It is suggested that moderate exercise could still be an effective way of maintaining or improving strength. However, with damage to motor units resulting in grades below a fair (3/5) grade, improvement is unlikely; therefore, the physical therapist assistant is advised to focus on stronger muscles.[43]

Other degenerative conditions show a similar abnormal response to strengthening exercises. It is hard to differentiate whether loss of muscle function is due to a progressive disease process or due to overwork. For that reason, the physical therapist assistant must be aware that exercises at a level to cause a positive effect in a normal muscle may damage diseased muscle. Thus, keeping exercise at a functional level and not too strenuous is important. Exercise will not prevent the progression of the disease, but it will often maintain the functional skills for a longer period as well as keep the individual interacting with the physical world. Mild or gentle exercises often increase ROM and maintain muscle function, which often can decrease pain and muscle stiffness.[44-46]

In individuals with degenerative diseases, there are additional recommendations with regard to exercise interventions.[43] First, a combination of individual and group exercises may improve adherence to the therapeutic programs. Group exercises are of particular importance in creating opportunities for social interaction and a feeling of accomplishment or success. It has also been suggested that strengthening should focus on concentric more than eccentric contractions, with adequate rest periods to avoid fatigue. Finally, muscle strength should be closely monitored in those individuals who participate in unsupervised movement activities (eg, home treadmill exercises, elliptical machines, or other available gyms) because these individuals may be exercising too strenuously and causing further decline in their muscular strength.

Clinical Pearls

The following are suggestions from the field for approaches that might help patients with degenerative diseases.

Focus 1: Parkinson's Disease

- Rotation is important. Trunk rotation should be part of any physical therapy intervention for PD unless contraindicated because of spinal conditions or surgery or other conditions that contraindicate trunk rotation. Rotation decreases the tone of the axial musculature, thereby decreasing trunk rigidity, and opens a window that will allow the patient to perform movements that are more normal and functional.[47] Rotation can be performed supine in bed in the morning (lower trunk rotations) before the patient gets up, in sitting throughout the day, and in standing (as long as the patient is safe in this position). Rocking also decreases tone.
- Encourage the patient to participate in group exercises. Group exercises allow the patient to engage in social activities, talk to other individuals who may have a similar condition or situation, and improve flexibility, strength, and endurance. Using a ball while throwing and catching with others in the group will encourage rotation, total body activities, and eye-hand coordination while interacting with other people.[47] Tai chi is becoming a more recognized form of group exercise and can also be incorporated into a person's individual home exercise program.[48,49]
- Imagery may help. Incorporating visual imagery may assist in motor performance, whether contraction or relaxation. Teaching the patient to visualize being "strong and stable like a tree" may assist in improving standing balance; also, visualization may assist in relaxation (eg, "Imagine that you are relaxing in your favorite place. . .").[50]
- Music and rhythm may help. Music often gives the individual a rhythmical beat that overrides the freezing episodes and can be used very effectively with walking or gait interventions.[51] Incorporate large amplitude movements in interventions and recommend safe performance of these movements as part of a home exercise program. Recent research has indicated that amplified movements during specific exercises can have a positive and prolonged effect on tasks such as walking, arm swinging, and having the ability to turn around.[10]

Focus 2: Amyotrophic Lateral Sclerosis

- Optimize cardiopulmonary function.[19] Maintaining good cardiopulmonary health is very important in patients with ALS to avoid the rapid decline in functional level due to secondary complications arising from decreased oxygenation. (Chapter 16 offers additional recommendations.) Examples of interventions include diaphragmatic breathing exercises, assisted cough (as necessary), and postural exercises to maintain optimal trunk alignment, which is important in efficient breathing. More complex equipment and intervention may be necessary with some patients or with patients in the more advanced stages of the disease, and a referral to a physician and a respiratory therapist may be appropriate.
- Maximize functional performance.[19] While maximizing functional performance may be important when discussing the rehabilitation of all patients, maintaining the highest functional performance is of utmost importance with patients and clients with ALS. Emphasis must be on achieving and maintaining the ability to perform vital activities, such as having mobility in bed, transferring, ensuring locomotion, having sitting and standing balance, and mastering toileting and hygiene activities. Patients will benefit from a ROM and muscle-strengthening program to prevent contractures and to maintain and improve strength. A home program consisting of these exercises, performed independently by the patient initially or assisted by the caregiver, is appropriate. The use of adaptive equipment may allow for performance of activities without assistance and should be considered. This equipment ranges from orthotic appliances to assist in ambulation or improve ROM to reacher sticks and dressing aids. Adaptive equipment also includes personal care aids, which will assist in optimizing function when used.
- Discuss with the physical therapist the options available to improve communication. Because patients with ALS eventually lose the ability to communicate verbally because of paralysis of the muscles of speech, alternative communication strategies may be considered.[52] These communication aids may be in the form of a basic communication board or more complex computer equipment.
- Optimum psychological health is important.[53] Maintaining a positive mental outlook decreases stress, which is detrimental to the body's immune response. Examples of approaches to achieving good psychological health include daily exercise, participating in support groups, psychological consultation, and good nutrition, among others. It is important to remember that a potential reason for an observed decline in functional performance is depression. The physical therapist assistant should communicate this finding to the physical therapist.

Conclusion

Patients and clients with degenerative diseases of the CNS often access and can benefit from physical therapy services. Appropriate intervention is based on the identified activity's limitations and impairments. The physical therapist assistant can effectively carry out an individualized treatment program developed by the physical therapist. Many treatment approaches have been presented in this chapter. Communication between the physical therapist and the physical therapist assistant is important to ensure that the patient receives care that is appropriate and evidence-based, to optimize the patient's level of health and wellness.

Case Studies

Case #1

MG is a 72-year-old man who was diagnosed with PD 12 years ago. Current medical diagnosis indicates that MG is at Hoehn and Yahr stage 3 when his medications are at their optimum. The client resides in an independent living facility with his wife. The environment provides the client with a wide spectrum of social interaction and cognitive challenges as well as good access to health care. MG is cognitively aware of his surroundings and the effects of his illness. He cites unsteadiness when walking and dressing, poor night vision, and occasional drooling as symptoms that he experiences.

The client currently takes Sinemet and Mirapex. He reports that he experiences freezing episodes when his medications wear off. As a result, he and his wife carefully plan outings around peak medication times. The client reports increasing difficulty with ambulation and ADL, such as transfers, dressing, and bathing. The client also reports increased falls in the past several weeks. He is afraid that he might sustain severe injuries following a serious fall. He owns a single-point cane and a front-wheeled walker, both of which he intermittently uses.

The client presents with a stooped posture, rounded shoulders, and thoracic kyphosis. He ambulates to the department carrying (not using) a single-point cane in the left hand, with a festinating gait pattern. He also presents with pill-rolling tremor in the right greater than the left UE at rest. He transfers from the bed to the mat with minimal assistance. Functional mobility testing shows that the client is independent with bed mobility but requires minimal assistance to sit from the supine position. He requires minimal assist to perform sit-to-stand. Sitting balance is good, while standing balance is fair. ROM is within functional limits to all 4 extremities. He demonstrates weakness in his bilateral LEs, as well as truncal rigidity. The client scored a 17/28 in the Tinetti balance and gait tests, indicating risk for falls. He scored 6 inches in the FRT, and this also indicates a risk for falls. The Berg Balance Scale test was also administered, and the client scored a 38/56, further indicating a risk for falls.

Questions

1. What presented impairments and activity limitations can you identify?
2. What potential interventions can be performed by the physical therapist assistant to assist in improving the patient's functional performance?

Case #2

RW is a 58-year-old man with a medical diagnosis of ALS. He reports that he was diagnosed with the condition 2 years ago. He is a retired truck driver and lives in a double-wide trailer with his girlfriend, who is his primary caregiver. He receives home health supportive services: a nurse visits every month, and a home health aide visits every other day to assist him with self-care activities.

The client is still capable of speech communication, but his caregiver reports that his speech is getting worse. The client also reports difficulty in breathing at night and gets supplemental oxygen via nasal cannula. During the time of the examination, the client's vital signs are as follows: blood pressure is 120/90, pulse is 88, and respiration is 20. The client is incontinent of bladder and has a Foley catheter in place. Inspection of the skin reveals a slightly reddened sacral area.

He is able to move in bed with minimal assistance and use of the overhead trapeze bar. He requires minimal assistance to get up from supine-to-sit and to transfer from the bed to the w/c using a slideboard. The client demonstrates poor sitting and standing balance. He is able to stand with minimal assistance and a front-wheeled walker, and take a few steps with moderate assistance, but he is unable to functionally ambulate. The client uses a manual w/c as his primary mode of locomotion, with his girlfriend or caregiver pushing the w/c. He is unable to afford a power w/c.

The client demonstrates bilateral plantar flexion contractures and some tightness of both hamstrings. He has spasticity of both LEs (grade 2 on the Modified Ashworth Scale). Strength of both LEs and UEs is generally 3/5 to 3+/5. The client demonstrates absent proprioception for both LEs and impaired light touch sensation bilaterally.

Questions

1. What presented impairments and activity limitations can you identify?
2. What potential interventions can be performed by the physical therapist assistant to assist in improving the patient's functional performance?

References

1. DeMaagd G, Philip A. Parkinson's disease and its management: part 1: disease entity, risk factors, pathophysiology, clinical presentation, and diagnosis. *P T.* 2015;40(8):504-532.
2. National Institute on Aging. Parkinson's disease. https://www.nia.nih.gov/health/parkinsons-disease. Accessed April 8, 2020.
3. Melnick ME, Allen DD. Basal ganglia disorders. In: Umphred DA, ed. *Umphred's Neurological Rehabilitation.* 6th ed. St. Louis, MO: Elsevier; 2013. doi:10.1016/B978-0-323-07586-2.00029-7
4. Marsden CD. On-off phenomena in Parkinson's disease. In: Rinne UK, Klinger M, Stamm G, eds. *Parkinson's Disease: Current Progress, Problems, and Management.* Amsterdam, The Netherlands: Biomedical Press; 1990.
5. Mille ML, Creath RA, Prettyman MG, et al. Posture and locomotion coupling: a target for rehabilitation interventions in persons with Parkinson's disease. *Parkinsons Dis.* 2012;2012:754186. doi:10.1155/2012/754186
6. Koller WC, Glatt S, Vetere-Overfield B, Hassanein R. Falls and Parkinson's disease. *Clin Neuropharmacol.* 1989;12(2):98-105. doi:10.1097/00002826-198904000-00003
7. Aita JF. Why patients with Parkinson's disease fall. *JAMA.* 1982;247(4):515-516. doi:10.1001/jama.1982.03320290053035
8. Mirapex. https://www.centerwatch.com/drug-information/fda-approved-drugs/drug/290/mirapex. Accessed April 8, 2020.
9. Ahlskog JE. Does vigorous exercise have a neuroprotective effect in Parkinson disease? *Neurology.* 2011;77(3):288-294. doi:10.1212/WNL.0b013e318225ab66
10. Fox C, Ebersbach G, Ramig L, Sapir S. LSVT LOUD and LSVT BIG: behavioral treatment programs for speech and body movement in Parkinson's disease. *Parkinsons Dis.* 2012;2012:391946. doi:10.1155/2012/391946
11. Li F, Harmer P, Fitzgerald K, et al. Tai chi and postural stability in patients with Parkinson's disease. *N Engl J Med.* 2012;366(6):511-519. doi:10.1056/NEJMoa1107911
12. Rafferty MR, Schmidt PN, Luo ST, et al; all NPF-QII Investigators. Regular exercise, quality of life, and mobility in Parkinson's disease: a longitudinal analysis of national Parkinson foundation quality improvement initiative data. *J Parkinsons Dis.* 2017;7(1):193-202. doi:10.3233/JPD-160912
13. Cugusi L, Solla P, Zedda F, et al. Effects of an adapted physical activity program on motor and non-motor functions and quality of life in patients with Parkinson's disease. *NeuroRehabilitation.* 2014;35(4):789-794. doi:10.3233/NRE-141162
14. Lauzé M, Daneault JF, Duval C. The effects of physical activity in Parkinson's disease: a review. *J Parkinsons Dis.* 2016;6(4):685-698. doi:10.3233/JPD-160790
15. Rosenthal LS, Dorsey ER. The benefits of exercise in Parkinson disease. *JAMA Neurol.* 2013;70(2):156-157. doi:10.1001/jamaneurol.2013.772
16. Goetz CG, Poewe W, Rascol O, et al; Movement Disorder Society Task Force on Rating Scales for Parkinson's Disease. Movement Disorder Society Task Force report on the Hoehn and Yahr staging scale: status and recommendations. *Mov Disord.* 2004;19(9):1020-1028. doi:10.1002/mds.20213
17. Keus SHJ, Hendriks HJM, Bloem BR, et al. Clinical practice guideline for physical therapy in patients with Parkinson's disease [KNGF-richtlijn Ziekte van Parkinson]. *Ned Tijdschr Fysiother.* 2004;114(suppl):3.
18. Hallum A. Neuromuscular diseases. In: Umphred DA, ed. *Umphred's Neurological Rehabilitation.* 6th ed. St. Louis, MO: Elsevier; 2013. doi:10.1016/B978-0-323-07586-2.00026-1
19. Dal Bello-Haas V, Kloos AD, Mitsumoto H. Physical therapy for a patient through six stages of amyotrophic lateral sclerosis. *Phys Ther.* 1998;78(12):1312-1324. doi:10.1093/ptj/78.12.1312

20. Tinetti ME. Performance-oriented assessment of mobility problems in elderly patients. *J Am Geriatr Soc.* 1986;34(2):119-126. doi:10.1111/j.1532-5415.1986.tb05480.x
21. Berg K. Measuring balance in the elderly: validation of an instrument. *Physiother Can.* 1989;41:304. doi:10.3138/ptc.41.6.304
22. American Physical Therapy Association. Guide to Physical Therapist Practice 3.0. http://guidetoptpractice.apta.org/. Accessed August 1, 2018.
23. Duncan PW, Weiner DK, Chandler J, Studenski S. Functional reach: a new clinical measure of balance. *J Gerontol.* 1990;45(6):M192-M197. doi:10.1093/geronj/45.6.M192
24. Podsiadlo D, Richardson S. The timed "Up & Go": a test of basic functional mobility for frail elderly persons. *J Am Geriatr Soc.* 1991;39(2):142-148. doi:10.1111/j.1532-5415.1991.tb01616.x
25. Stebbins GT, Goetz CG. Factor structure of the Unified Parkinson's Disease Rating Scale: motor examination section. *Mov Disord.* 1998;13(4):633-636. doi:10.1002/mds.870130404
26. de Boer AG, Wijker W, Speelman JD, de Haes JC. Quality of life in patients with Parkinson's disease: development of a questionnaire. *J Neurol Neurosurg Psychiatry.* 1996;61(1):70-74. doi:10.1136/jnnp.61.1.70
27. Simmons Z, Felgoise SH, Bremer BA, et al. The ALSSQOL: balancing physical and nonphysical factors in assessing quality of life in ALS. *Neurology.* 2006;67(9):1659-1664. doi:10.1212/01.wnl.0000242887.79115.19
28. David FJ, Rafferty MR, Robichaud JA, et al. Progressive resistance exercise and Parkinson's disease: a review of potential mechanisms. *Parkinsons Dis.* 2012;2012:124527. doi:10.1155/2012/124527
29. White LJ, Dressendorfer RH. Exercise and multiple sclerosis. *Sports Med.* 2004;34(15):1077-1100. doi:10.2165/00007256-200434150-00005
30. Döring A, Pfueller CF, Paul F, Dörr J. Exercise in multiple sclerosis—an integral component of disease management. *EPMA J.* 2011;3(1):2. doi:10.1007/s13167-011-0136-4
31. Hebert JR, Corboy JR, Vollmer T, Forster JE, Schenkman M. Efficacy of balance and eye-movement exercises for persons with multiple sclerosis. *Neurology.* 2018;90(9):e797-e807. doi:10.1212/WNL.0000000000005013
32. Farup J, Dalgas U, Keytsman C, Eijnde BO, Wens I. High intensity training may reverse the fiber type specifc decline in myogenic stem cells in multiple sclerosis patients. *Front Physiol.* 2016;7:193. doi:10.3389/fphys.2016.00193
33. Dalgas U, Stenager E. Exercise and disease progression in multiple sclerosis: can exercise slow down the progression of multiple sclerosis? *Ther Adv Neurol Disorder.* 2012;5(2):81-95. doi:10.1177/1756285611430719
34. Hirsch MA, Toole T, Maitland CG, Rider RA. The effects of balance training and high-intensity resistance training on persons with idiopathic Parkinson's disease. *Arch Phys Med Rehabil.* 2003;84(8):1109-1117. doi:10.1016/S0003-9993(03)00046-7
35. Ashburn A, Fazakarley L, Ballinger C, Pickering R, McLellan LD, Fitton C. A randomised controlled trial of a home based exercise programme to reduce the risk of falling among people with Parkinson's disease. *J Neurol Neurosurg Psychiatry.* 2007;78(7):678-684. doi:10.1136/jnnp.2006.099333
36. Dibble LE, Hale TF, Marcus RL, Droge J, Gerber JP, LaStayo PC. High-intensity resistance training amplifies muscle hypertrophy and functional gains in persons with Parkinson's disease. *Mov Disord.* 2006;21(9):1444-1452. doi:10.1002/mds.20997
37. de Almeida JP, Silvestre R, Pinto AC, de Carvalho M. Exercise and amyotrophic lateral sclerosis. *Neurol Sci.* 2012;33(1):9-15. doi:10.1007/s10072-011-0921-9
38. Kent-Braun JA, Miller RG. Central fatigue during isometric exercise in amyotrophic lateral sclerosis. *Muscle Nerve.* 2000;23(6):909-914. doi:10.1002/(SICI)1097-4598(200006)23:6<909::AID-MUS10>3.0.CO;2-V
39. Carreras I, Yuruker S, Aytan N, et al. Moderate exercise delays the motor performance decline in a transgenic model of ALS. *Brain Res.* 2010;1313:192-201. doi:10.1016/j.brainres.2009.11.051
40. Constantinescu R, Leonard C, Deeley C, Kurlan R. Assistive devices for gait in Parkinson's disease. *Parkinsonism Relat Disord.* 2007;13(3):133-138. doi:10.1016/j.parkreldis.2006.05.034
41. Frenkel-Toledo S, Giladi N, Peretz C, Herman T, Gruendlinger L, Hausdorff JM. Treadmill walking as an external pacemaker to improve gait rhythm and stability in Parkinson's disease. *Mov Disord.* 2005;20(9):1109-1114. doi:10.1002/mds.20507
42. Karmarkar AM, Dicianno BE, Graham JE, Cooper R, Kelleher A, Cooper RA. Factors associated with provision of wheelchairs in older adults. *Assist Technol.* 2012;24(3):155-167. doi:10.1080/10400435.2012.659795
43. Kilmer DD, Aitken S. Neuromuscular disease. In: Frontera WR, Dawson DM, Slovik DM, eds. *Exercises in Rehabilitation Medicine.* Champaign, IL: Human Kinetics; 1999:253-266.
44. de Almeida JP, Silvestre R, Pinto AC, de Carvalho M. Exercise and amyotrophic lateral sclerosis. *Neurol Sci.* 2012;33(1):9-15. doi:10.1007/s10072-011-0921-9
45. Dal Bello-Haas V, Florence JM. Therapeutic exercise for people with amyotrophic lateral sclerosis or motor neuron disease. *Cochrane Database Syst Rev.* 2013;(5):CD005229. doi:10.1002/14651858.CD005229.pub3
46. Aksu S, Citak-Karakaya I. Effects of exercise therapy on pain complaints in patients with amyotrophic lateral sclerosis. *Pain Clin.* 2002;14(4):353-359. doi:10.1163/15685690260494924
47. Schenkman M, Donovan J, Tsubota J, Kluss M, Stebbins P, Butler RB. Management of individuals with Parkinson's disease: rationale and case studies. *Phys Ther.* 1989;69(11):944-955. doi:10.1093/ptj/69.11.944
48. Corcos DM, Comella CL, Goetz CG. Tai chi for patients with Parkinson's disease. *N Engl J Med.* 2012;366(18):1737-1738. doi:10.1056/NEJMc1202921
49. Liu T, Lao L. Tai chi for patients with Parkinson's disease. *N Engl J Med.* 2012;366(18):1737-1738. doi:10.1056/NEJMc1202921

50. Tamir R, Dickstein R, Huberman M. Integration of motor imagery and physical practice in group treatment applied to subjects with Parkinson's disease. *Neurorehabil Neural Repair.* 2007;21(1):68-75. doi:10.1177/1545968306292608
51. McIntosh GC, Brown SH, Rice RR, Thaut MH. Rhythmic auditory-motor facilitation of gait patterns in patients with Parkinson's disease. *J Neurol Neurosurg Psychiatry.* 1997;62(1):22-26. doi:10.1136/jnnp.62.1.22
52. Adams MR. Communication aids for patients with amyotrophic lateral sclerosis. *J Speech Hear Disord.* 1966;31(3):274-275. doi:10.1044/jshd.3103.274
53. Rowland LP, Shneider NA. Amyotrophic lateral sclerosis. *N Engl J Med.* 2001;344(22):1688-1700. doi:10.1056/NEJM200105313442207

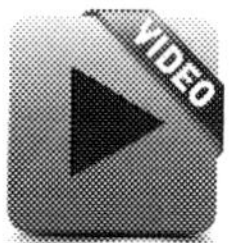

Chapter 15

Clients With Multiple Sclerosis and Guillain-Barré Syndrome

Germaine Ferreira, PT, DPT, MSPT, BHMS; Kristen Barta, PT, PhD, DPT, NCS; and Rolando T. Lazaro, PT, PhD, DPT

KEY WORDS Acute inflammatory demyelinating polyneuropathy | Guillain-Barré syndrome | Movement dysfunction | Multiple sclerosis | Rehabilitation

Chapter Objectives

- Discuss the pathophysiology and medical management of individuals with multiple sclerosis (MS) and Guillain-Barré syndrome (GBS).
- Discuss the movement problems associated with the medical diagnosis of MS and GBS.
- Understand the role of the physical therapist assistant in the rehabilitation management of a person with MS or GBS.

Multiple Sclerosis

MS is the most common neurological condition affecting young adults. It is characterized by degeneration and subsequent loss of myelin scattered throughout the central nervous system (CNS), primarily in the white matter. In this condition, plaques of demyelination are accompanied by destruction and inflammation of oligodendroglia, which form part of the supporting structure of the CNS. Because of the degeneration of the myelin, neurotransmission is disrupted and will manifest as delayed or absent transmission of nerve impulses.[1] It is a chronic demyelinating disease affecting the CNS. Since demyelination can occur anywhere in the CNS, the resulting signs, symptoms, and clinical manifestations can vary based on the areas affected. The degenerative nature of the condition causes progressive and irreversible disability.[2]

Etiology and Pathology

The cause of MS is unknown, but the condition is believed to be triggered by immunologic, environmental, infectious, and other factors.[3] An abnormal immune-related response triggers the inflammatory process and damages the myelin coating of the axons. Environmental factors thought to contribute to the risk of developing MS include geography (MS "clusters"), low levels of vitamin D, smoking, and obesity. Certain bacteria and viruses comprise the infectious factors causing MS. While MS is not an inherited disease, there may be a genetic risk that can be inherited.[3]

Clinical Manifestations

Signs and symptoms associated with MS can develop slowly over days and weeks, or rapidly within hours. Common symptoms include fatigue, motor weakness, paresthesias, unsteady gait, double vision, tremor, and bladder and/or bowel dysfunction. Fatigue is the most common symptom of MS and is frequently misunderstood by family, friends, and employers because it is not a visible symptom. Some researchers and clinicians have noted that the fatigue experienced by patients with MS increases as the day pro-

Lazaro RT, Umphred DA, eds.
Umphred's Neurorehabilitation for the Physical Therapist Assistant, Third Edition (pp 363-372).

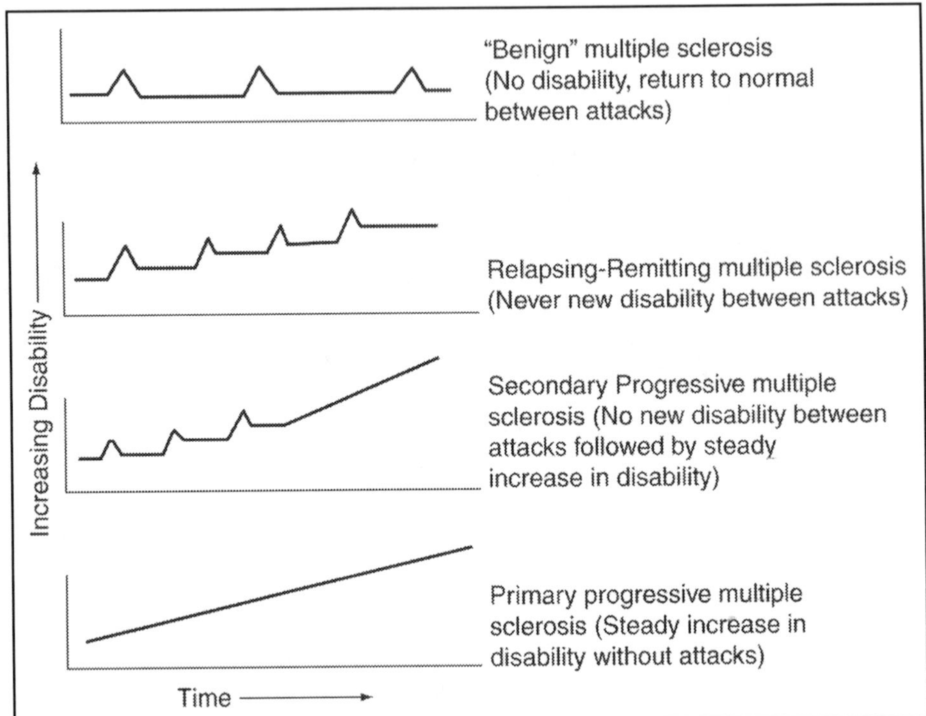

Figure 15-1. Types of MS. (Reprinted with permission from Wikimedia. https://commons.wikimedia.org/wiki/File:Ms_progression_types.svg.)

gresses and can also vary depending on the climate and environmental temperature.[1]

In terms of the pattern of the disease, the classic presentation is characterized by periods of *exacerbations* (relapses) and *remissions* (partial or total disappearance of symptoms). As the disease progresses, the periods of exacerbations become more frequent and longer, while the periods of remissions become more limited. Most individuals afflicted with this disease then demonstrate progressive deterioration of function. Factors that have been associated with exacerbations include excessive fatigue, hot weather, and rise in body temperature due to fever, trauma, and hot baths or showers.[1] Figure 15-1 illustrates the types of MS.

Over the past 2 decades, treatment with disease-modifying agents has been developed. These agents have been found to reduce the frequency and severity of relapses, reduce the numbers of brain lesions as shown on magnetic resonance imaging, and possibly reduce future impairments, activity limitations, and participation restrictions.

Fatigue and heat intolerance are 2 important symptoms that are common in people with MS. Fatigue is reported by 65% to 97% of people with MS, with almost half of them stating that this symptom most significantly affects their functional performance.[1] Primary fatigue, otherwise known as *lassitude*, is a direct result of the demyelination process, causing abnormalities in nerve conduction. Secondary fatigue often results from deconditioning and other associated conditions from the disease (eg, infections, disturbances in sleep, and inadequate nutrition).[1] Fatigue can lead to inactivity causing disuse and deconditioning, which further perpetuates the deterioration to affect mobility, balance, and ambulation. A significant proportion of people with MS also report worsening of symptoms following an increase in core body temperature due to physical exercise or a hot climate.[1]

Other clinical manifestations worth noting from a physical therapy standpoint include spasticity, pain, mobility limitations, balance impairments leading to increased risk of falls, ataxia, incoordination, and vestibular dysfunction. Spasticity can interfere with functional movement and cause limitations in joint range of motion (ROM) and problems with self-care. Patients with MS often report both nociceptive and neuropathic pain, which again affects their ability to move and function. Mobility limitations, balance dysfunctions, and increased risk of falls are caused by a combination of the disuse and deconditioning process as well as the impairments of CNS structures due to the demyelination and disease progression. Ataxia and vestibular dysfunctions are often a result of the disease process affecting the cerebellum and the vestibular system.

Additionally, other medical complications related to MS progression include bowel and bladder dysfunctions, dysphagia and dysarthria, cognitive impairments, and depression.

Examination and Evaluation of Clients With Multiple Sclerosis: The Role of the Physical Therapist Assistant

The physical therapy examination of a patient with MS must be guided by several factors. First, it is important to identify from the patient's perspective the impact of the presenting signs and symptoms on the ability to function. It is important to determine, in terms of activity, what the patient can and cannot do, and then hypothesize the impairments that may be causing the identified activity limitations. The *Guide to Physical Therapist Practice* (the *Guide*)[4] is a helpful tool to guide the clinician in identifying the pertinent tests and measures that will provide the best representation of the patient's functional level. The Multiple Sclerosis EDGE contains a listing of outcome measures that are recommended for use corresponding to the International Classification of Functioning, Disability and Health (ICF) level, and also in different practice environments.

The physical therapist assistant may be delegated portions of a reexamination (see Chapter 6). Whenever possible, it is important to use the same examination tools that were used by the physical therapist upon initial examination to document that change has occurred.

It is very important for the physical therapist assistant to clearly communicate the results of the tests and measures to the physical therapist to determine if the plan of care needs to be revised. The physical therapist assistant must identify the specific signs and symptoms associated with the medical condition and associated movement dysfunctions, monitor these signs and symptoms, and communicate to the supervising physical therapist any significant changes in the patient's presentation, which may indicate the progression of symptoms, ineffectiveness of the prescribed physical therapy intervention, medication issues, or the possibility of other comorbidities. The rehabilitation team must be cognizant of other signs and symptoms that may necessitate referral to other medical and health care practitioners.

In looking at examination, the physical therapist must identify the patient and family goals in making the determination regarding exercises and activities that will be implemented, and communicate that to physical therapist assistant. Standardized functional tests often delegated to the physical therapist assistant provide the clinician useful information regarding the impact of the disease progression on the patient's function and thus reassessment is an important aspect of ongoing treatment. Serial testing of function allows the clinician to generate objective documentation of function; however, it should always follow a thoughtful interpretation of the results afforded by the physical therapist. Examples of highly recommended tests and measures to administer in people with MS for inpatient and outpatient settings include the following: 6-minute walk test, Timed Up and Go with Cognitive and Manual, Berg Balance Scale, 9-hole peg test, and MS Quality of Life Scale.[5]

All the examination areas mentioned in Chapter 6 must be assessed in patients with neuromuscular degenerative diseases to provide the clinician with a clear picture of the patient's impairments, activity limitations, and participation restrictions.

Therapeutic Interventions

Therapeutic interventions for people with MS must be geared toward optimizing function and preventing or reducing complications to allow for optimal participation and quality of life. Clinicians must focus on addressing impairments, activity limitations, and participation restrictions that have been identified as important to the patient. People with MS present significant variability in their presentations and rate of progression of the condition. Clinicians need to consistently assess and adjust their treatment plans and closely partner with the patient to achieve the mutually negotiated goal and plan of care.

Literature over the past 2 decades has shown that physical therapy management has been one of the best ways to improve movement function leading to activity and participation. Exercise-based physical activity has been shown to significantly reduce fatigue as reported by patients. However, there is still a need to identify specific treatment designs, dosage, and modalities that would lead to best practice for this patient population.[6] There is growing evidence on the importance of exercise as a major intervention in MS. Exercise helps manage many of the symptoms associated with MS such as fatigue, muscle weakness, impaired joint ROM, and decreased cardiovascular endurance. At the same time, it is beneficial to the person's general health and physical and psychological well-being. Increased activity following exercise has been proven to be neuroprotective in people with neurological conditions. In people with MS, exercise has been proven to decrease the amount of inflammation markers in the blood, which may suggest that exercise may have a role in altering the disease process itself. It can therefore be argued that regular exercise must be started early in the disease process. The growing number of studies supports the critical role of exercise in inducing neuroplasticity that assists recovery in people with neurological conditions.[7] However, optimal exercise parameters (eg, type, frequency, and intensity) are still unknown. Underdosed exercise programs will not likely result in improvements in outcome measures, while too much may result in fatigue, overexertion, and possible relapse. Closely monitoring the symptoms from MS and using that information to provide the appropriate exercise dosage could be an effective way of progressing a person's exercise program. Box 15-1 shows recommendations for exercise programs for a person with mild to moderate disability following MS.

Box 15-1

Endurance Exercise Program Recommendations for Persons With Mild to Moderate Disability Secondary to Multiple Sclerosis

- Regular exercise 2 to 3 sessions/week
- 65% to 75% of maximum heart rate
- 20 to 30 minutes/session
- 1 to 3 sets with 15 to 18 reps/session, with a goal of increasing to 3 to 4 sets
- 12-week program[1]

Management of MS-related fatigue should be a major rehabilitation consideration because it is not only a frequent complaint, but it is also the most disabling in this population. There are very few options to treat primary fatigue, and only suggestions to manage secondary fatigue, such as energy conservation, use of a cooling suit, progressive exercise training, and patient education.[8] Graded exercise that is dosed appropriately has the potential of improving muscle strength that has been impaired due to deconditioning or disuse which could in effect decrease fatigue.

It is important for the physical therapist assistant to always monitor the patient's response to the plan of care. Proper exercise dosing is important and optimally achieved by keeping exercise at a level that is functional but not too strenuous and does not cause prolonged fatigue. Exercise will not prevent the progression of the disease, but it will often maintain the functional skills for a longer period, while keeping the individual interacting with the physical world. Mild or gentle exercises often increase ROM and maintain muscle function, which often can decrease pain and muscle stiffness.[9]

A combination of individual and group exercises may improve adherence to the therapeutic programs. Group exercises are of particular importance in creating opportunities for positive social interaction and a feeling of accomplishment or success. Finally, muscle strength should be closely monitored in those individuals who participate in unsupervised movement activities (eg, home treadmill exercises, elliptical machines, or other available gyms) because these individuals may be exercising too strenuously, causing a level of fatigue that may be harmful.

Spasticity is often a common problem with individuals diagnosed with MS and certainly causes pain and limitations in the ability to function in daily life. Appropriate management of spasticity will facilitate a window of normal movement that can potentially be expanded with targeted task-specific physical therapy interventions. Pharmacological agents can be integrated in the patient's plan of care to manage spasticity. Physical therapy approaches include stretching, application of cold, application of electrotherapeutic agents, and use of orthotic and supportive devices. These interventions are commonly seen in physical therapy practices, and further studies are needed to establish efficacy.

Physical therapy interventions are used to improve balance and postural control problems of people with MS. While the choice of intervention depends on the underlying cause of the balance or postural control problem, a multidisciplinary approach to this issue allows the patient to improve mobility, decrease the risk of falling, and improve quality of life. Numerous studies have confirmed the importance of balance training in improving balance related outcomes in patients with MS.[10-14] Training protocols include resistive strength training, aerobic exercise, balance training and task-specific training are some of the options. The patient must be invested in these interventions, as they will likely carryover into life activity once the individual is no longer in treatment.

Guillain-Barré Syndrome

GBS is an acute, inflammatory, demyelinating condition that results in motor and sensory deficits. There is a rapid progression of ascending symmetrical muscle weakness, areflexia, and mild sensory motor weakness.[15] GBS affects males more than females.[15,16] The degree of loss varies and may result in long-term disability.[17] Many patients present with cognitive psychosocial issues, further complicating the disability.[18] In the United States, the incidence annually is 1 to 2 cases/100,000; worldwide, the annual incidence varies from 1.1 to 1.8 in every 100,000 adults including pregnant women, and 0.6 in every 1,000,000 children.[15,19-23] GBS has the potential to occur in all ages.[19] It is not uncommon for GBS to develop in pregnant women during the third trimester or during the first 2 weeks of the post-partum period.[22,24] Young adults and those in their fifth through eight decade of life are the most-frequently diagnosed.[15,21]

Etiology and Pathology

There is no known true cause of GBS, but it is suspected that certain forms of bacteria or viruses could initiate the process. The commonly reported ones are *Campylobacter jejuni*, cytomegalovirus, *Haemophilus influenzae*, and Epstein-Barr.[15,24] The demyelination seen in GBS is theorized to be a result of an autoimmune reaction as it develops 2 to 4 weeks after a viral infection or mild flu-like respiratory infection or infrequently following immunizations.[17,21,25-28] The presence of GBS in immunosuppressed individuals after an organ transplant points to the fact that there could be another cause other than autoimmune in the pathogenesis of this disease.[21]

An inflammatory process involving antibody-mediated demyelination triggers the macrophages to release products that degrade the myelin at the node of Ranvier.[15] The Schwann cells of the axons are mainly attacked and destroyed, which leads to a reduction in electrical conduction along the nerve.[20] After 3 weeks of demyelination, the Schwann cells may start to regenerate and proliferate. With variations noted in each case, the inflammation may resolve, and there may be restoration of remyelination.[15] In some cases, recovery can take a long time, as there is axonal degeneration in addition to the demyelination.[16,20]

GBS is a lower motor neuron condition because all the nerves that are damaged are located outside of the CNS. The location and severity of impairments is determined by which nerves were demyelinated and to what degree. In GBS, the demyelination is seen in the peripheral and autonomic nerves. With GBS, 50% of cases have cranial nerve involvement, and 50% have autonomic nerve involvement.[15] The muscular weakness and sensory impairments result from demyelination of the axons in the peripheral nervous system.[25] The initial symptom of GBS is sensory loss that eventually progresses to ascending, symmetrical motor loss from distal to proximal affecting LEs, UEs, trunk, and face.[15,28] The motor loss can be isolated to only the skeletal muscles, or it can be more severe involving the respiratory and swallowing musculature in about 5% to 10% of individuals. If demyelination progresses to the respiratory and swallowing muscles, the patient is in a more life-threatening state requiring mechanical ventilation, which accounts for 10% to 20% of individuals diagnosed with GBS.[23,26,29] Of these patients, 20% will present with dysautonomia as the preganglionic fibers of the autonomic system are myelinated and susceptible to attack in GBS.[23,29]

Clinical Manifestations

Many patients will present first with paresthesia in the toes or sensory symptoms, followed by progressive symmetrical motor weakness.[21,26] The motor weakness may present as difficulty with bed mobility, transfers, balance, and gait. Patients may present with speech and swallowing disturbances too. Some GBS patients may present with autonomic dysfunction, sensory deficits, sleep disturbances, anxiety, and respiratory failure.[17,30] Patients may present with bowel and bladder symptoms such as constipation, urinary retention, and urge incontinence.[17]

Types

There are multiple types of GBS: acute inflammatory demyelinating polyradiculoneuropathy, acute motor axonal neuropathy, and acute motor sensory axonal neuropathy. The most common type in developed countries is the acute inflammatory demyelinating polyradiculopathy.[23] Despite GBS affecting the neurons and not the cerebral cortex, some patients do experience difficulties with language and cognition.[18,31] Miller-Fisher syndrome, a variant of GBS, primarily affects the cranial nerves, and patients present often with ocular disturbances.[16,17]

Medical Diagnosis

Medical diagnosis is often drawn from a person's clinical presentation and by ruling out other diagnoses. If a patient presents with progressive weakness in one or more than one extremity and exhibits loss of deep tendon reflexes, it can lead the physician to investigate further for GBS. Rapid development of symmetric weakness that ceases to progress after 4 weeks, mild sensory signs and symptoms, symmetric facial weakness, oral-bulbar weakness, and absence of fever support the diagnosis of GBS. A positive spinal tap of cerebrospinal fluid and the presence of antinuclear antibodies can support a diagnosis of GBS. Cerebrospinal fluid with elevated albumin protein levels is typically noted after the first week, and these levels continue to rise. The cerebrospinal fluid will exhibit low mononuclear leukocytes.[21] Slow nerve conduction velocities are noted on electrophysiological studies in nerves that are demyelinated.

Phases and Medical Managements

The course of progression is fairy predicable and can be separated into 3 phases: progression, plateau, and recovery.

- The *progression* phase lasts for 1 to 4 weeks and is characteristic of the individual losing sensory and motor function. During this phase, the main goal of the medical team is to reduce the progression and eliminate respiratory involvement. Once other diagnoses have been ruled out, the individual may undergo plasmapheresis and intravenous immunoglobin.
- Once the progression has been stabilized and the individual is no longer losing sensory and motor function, then the *plateau* stage has been reached. This is a period when the individual is neither declining nor improving.
- Once the individual begins to have any improvement of the sensory or motor impairments, the *recovery* phase begins.

Plasmapheresis, a process in which the circulating plasma is removed from the circulation, filtered, and diluted of the circulating antibodies, is commonly recommended within the first 4 weeks of onset of GBS for non-ambulatory patients and within the first 2 weeks for ambulatory patients. Patients undergoing plasmapheresis and intravenous immunoglobulin show more improvements and have a quicker recovery compared to those who are not treated with plasmapheresis or intravenous immunoglobin.[15,20,22,28,32] These medical interventions are implemented to slow the demyelination of the axons and preserve the peripheral nervous system integrity. Intravenous administration of immunoglobulin (intravenous Ig) is effective in treating GBS, as the body's immune system uses intravenous Ig protein to attack the invading foreign organisms.[15,28]

Examination and Evaluation of Clients With Guillain-Barré Syndrome: The Role of the Physical Therapist Assistant

Similar to the client with MS, a thorough evaluation must be completed prior to beginning treatment. The *Guide* must be used to ensure that proper information is obtained and measured so that an optimal treatment plan can be developed. Discussion with the supervising physical therapist throughout will facilitate patient outcomes and safety.

The setting will determine the standardized test that the supervising physical therapist will complete. In the acute stages, the focus will be on the client's ROM, strength, sensory testing, functional mobility, and assistance required for the activity. In the inpatient rehabilitation phase, the Functional Independence Measure is a common measure to assess functional mobility. It is a reliable tool to assess a person's level of disability and caregiver burden.[33]

Multiple other measures could also be used in the inpatient rehabilitation and outpatient settings, and the impairment needed to be tested and functional level of the client will guide which one is chosen. The Tinetti Performance Oriented Mobility Assessment has been shown to predict falls in the elderly population and assesses standing balance and gait.[34] Other measures that could be appropriate are the Berg Balance Scale, 10-meter walk test for velocity, Modified Clinical Test for Sensory Interaction in Balance, Functional Reach Test, and Timed Up and Go Test. As with the client who has MS, these outcome measures give information on balance and gait.

Therapeutic Interventions

Rehabilitation through a multidisciplinary approach (eg, psychological, social, speech, occupational therapy, and physical therapy) should be initiated as soon as the individual is medically stable to tolerate therapy.[17,19,29] Individuals with GBS have been shown to make substantial motor and cognitive gains through inpatient rehabilitation during the early phases of recovery.[17,18,19,26] After the medical team clears the patient for mobilization and the physical therapist completes an evaluation, then intervention can begin.

Early mobilization, if appropriate for the patient, helps with quicker recovery compared to patients who are on prolonged bed rest and develop further complications from being on bed rest.[35] Early introduction of physical therapy can prevent common complications such as deep vein thrombosis, dysautonomia, orthostatic hypotension, and respiratory muscle weakness seen in GBS patients.[26] The goals of therapy will change as the individual moves through the 3 phases. During the progression phase, the focus is on the medical management to obtain a quick diagnosis and begin treatment to reduce the severity of progression. During this time, therapy can be instrumental in patient and family education. Due to the loss of motor function, the individual will be confined to a sedentary position for an unknown period of time. It is crucial that the therapist educate the patient and caregivers about ROM exercises to preserve joint and tissue integrity needed for future mobilization.[36] Additionally, educating the patient and family on proper positioning and bed mobility techniques will decrease the risk of pressure spots and wounds. Gentle stretching and active or active assistive exercises are recommended, depending on the patient's strength. Massage and stretching help with managing pain, stimulating proprioceptive sensation, and improving circulation.[26,30] Caution must be exerted as overstretching and overexercising can result in muscle fatigue, further delaying recovery. Patients with respiratory involvement will benefit from deep breathing exercises, diaphragmatic breathing, and respiratory hygiene. As the individual enters the plateau and recovery phase, more challenging activities can be initiated, and goals progressed.

After the acute phase, the goal is to introduce therapeutic exercises to improve the tone of muscles and to recover from the motor and sensory deficits.[23,25] Nerves are not as vascular as muscles, and exercise increases blood flow to the muscle, thus providing nutrients to the surrounding nerve tissue, reducing nerve damage, and improving muscle plasticity.[16] Therapeutic exercises are an integral part of the second phase of rehabilitation and should incorporate isometrics, isotonic exercises with low resistances and progressive resisted exercises.[16,23] It may help to gradually progress from TheraBand (TheraBand) products to weights, depending on the degree of paresis.[26] During the plateau phase, patients benefit from neuromuscular facilitation techniques. Aquatic therapy may be beneficial in certain cases to initiate movement. Higher intensity exercises produce better functional improvements. When exercising the GBS patient, it is important to avoid rapid increases in intensity and overexercising the patient, as it results in relapses and reversal of strength.[25] It is ideal to terminate the therapy session before the patient reports fatigue.[26] Cycling seems to be the most effective exercise.[25] Patients with postural and balance issue benefit from exercises that incorporate weight-shift, retraining for static and dynamic balances, and gait training with eyes closed.[26] Yoga is shown to help GBS patients with management of sleep disturbances, pain, and breathing techniques.[30]

Even a year after the initial diagnosis, 20% of patients do not recover completely.[17,24] Safety with bed mobility, transfers, functional activities, and gait determine the appropriate discharge environment. Before discharging the patient, it is important to determine if the patient would benefit from orthosis, adaptive equipment, assistive devices, home modifications, and mobility devices such as wheelchairs or scooters.[17,29]

Physical therapist assistants should focus on low-intensity loads, few repetitions, with the treatment sessions split to short treatment sessions at different times of the day before progressing to increasing the time duration and intensity. After a patient is tolerating standing with an assistive device with minimum assistance, the physical therapist assistant should consult with the supervising physical therapist to progress to gait training.

Good predictors of poor outcomes include older age at onset, need for mechanical ventilation, reduced motor potential amplitudes, and prolonged time before recovery.[15,21,29]

Clinical Pearls

Focus 1: Multiple Sclerosis

- Educate the patient regarding the importance of achieving optimum health and well-being.[10] It is important to allow the patient to take the responsibility for health and well-being through engaging in daily exercise, ensuring appropriate nutrition and hydration, following the medical advice provided by the physician, and maintaining a positive and optimistic mental outlook. Patients need to learn not only to maintain a daily exercise routine but also to recognize when they have exercised too much and weakness overcomes them.
- Watch out for fatigue and overheating.[11] Precautions for patients and clients with MS include fatigue and decreased tolerance to heat. Always consider the environment where the treatment occurs. Regulate the temperature to minimize overheating, which will cause fatigue of the patient. Consideration of precooling therapy seems to be beneficial in these clients to help control body heating during exercise.[12] Timing and sequencing of the treatment are also important. Encourage the patient to perform the more difficult and potentially more fatiguing activities early in the day, and to conserve energy when possible. Many patients like to exercise in water, but they need to make sure the water is not too warm and does not cause fatigue.
- Improve balance and coordination. An optimal level of balance and coordination decreases the risk of falls and prevents the development of secondary complications that may be detrimental to the patient.[13]
- Compensate for impaired sensation by teaching the patient to do frequent skin checks for skin breakdown, use appropriate footwear when walking, and be cognizant of situations where lack of protective sensation may be dangerous (such as cooking, taking a bath, or walking on uneven surfaces).[14] Discourage people with MS from walking and standing without appropriate footwear even inside the home.
- Discuss with the supervising physical therapist the need to refer the patient to appropriate medical professionals as necessary. The patient may present with other signs and symptoms that can be better managed by other health care professionals. Referral to a neuropsychiatrist, speech therapist, or occupational therapist may assist the patient in improving function.

Focus 2: Guillain-Barré Syndrome

- Overwork fatigue presents risks.[37]
  - This is a reduction in muscular production and endurance because of excessive activity. As the nerves are recovering and remyelinating, there are fewer available motor units for force production. As a person is attempting to complete a functional activity or strengthening, overstressing the available motor units could lead to damage and delay recovery. Signs and symptoms of overwork fatigue are medical and physical in nature. An increase in creatine kinase levels can indicate the muscle fibers have been used too much. From a clinical perspective, the client will present with excessive muscle soreness that lasts 1 to 5 days after activity, or functional loss of strength. An example of functional loss would be if a client requires more assistance for bed mobility or transfers, or demonstrates a reduction in the ability to ambulate.
- Shorter and frequent bouts of activity are best.
  - To decrease the risk of overfatiguing the client, shorter bouts of activity are safest. While in the hospital, having the client perform upright sitting for a portion of the hour every hour would be an ideal plan for improving tolerance to upright positioning. As the client progresses and endurance increases, providing education on energy conservation techniques will facilitate safer completion of daily activities.
- Positioning is important in initial weeks.
  - In the initial weeks after diagnosis, the client will be declining in function and then transitioning to the plateau phase. During this period, each client will have various levels of function and mobility, but most will spend an extended time in bed. It is important to educate the client, family, and medical team on the importance of ROM exercises to reduce the risk of contractures and deep vein thrombosis. In addition, proper position in the bed and frequent pressure reliefs will decrease the risk of skin breakdown.
- Educate the client on the length of time to recover.
  - After the initial stage, the client may progress to the plateau phase, during which the client's signs and symptoms are neither worsening nor improving. The plateau phase is a temporary phase that later leads to the recovery phase. Client and family education during the plateau phase—with

emphasis on maintaining ROM and proper positioning protocol to prevent skin breakdown—is of great benefit to minimize complications. Caution should be exerted to not introduce intensive exercises prior to the recovery phase to minimize complications related to nerve and muscle damage. Low-intensity strengthening exercises are ideal for the recovery phase. The goal should be to increase sitting tolerance to 1 hour, 4 times/day. The physical therapist assistant should consult with the physical therapist to come up with an individualized sitting schedule that would be appropriate for the patient. Considering the patient and family's needs when setting up the schedule will promote success in adherence to the schedule.

- Discuss referral to other disciplines with the supervising physical therapist.
  - The patient may benefit from speech therapy to address swallowing problems, speech problems, and communication disorders. Patients who have been on a mechanical ventilation may have temporary speech issues related to the edema and trauma of the tubes placed in the pharynx.
  - Psychologist consultation may help the patients experiencing anxiety about the future and prevent onset of depression. The physical therapist assistant can discuss with the supervising physical therapist to establish a common time to work with a psychologist during the physical therapy treatment session to facilitate patient cooperation in those patients who are refusing therapy related to depression.
  - Respiratory therapy can be helpful in those patients who have needed ventilatory support. In settings where no respiratory therapists are available, the physical therapist assistant, after consulting with the physical therapist, can work on breathing techniques, diaphragmatic breathing, respiratory hygiene, and active cycles of breathing.
  - Discuss with the supervising physical therapist any changes noted in functional mobility, as the physical therapist can reassess the Functional Independence Measure score. Improvements and declines need to be reported to the physical therapist to initiate a reevaluation for the appropriate assistive devices and orthotics.

Case Studies

Case #1: Multiple Sclerosis

The client is a 45-year-old woman who was diagnosed with MS 5 years ago. She works part-time as a telemarketer and has a phone and computer setup that allow her to work at home. She reports progressive decline in functional ability in the past few years. Since the diagnosis, she has had several periods of exacerbations and remissions. She lives with her husband and teenage daughter, who both help her with her ADL. Her current complaints include weakness of the LEs, fatigue, and bouts of vision disturbances (eg, double vision). She reports lack of sleep at night due to leg cramps. She also mentions having fallen several times, usually during the night when she gets up to go to the bathroom.

The client is able to ambulate independently at home, holding onto walls and furniture for support as needed. In the community, she is able to ambulate short distances using a front-wheeled walker, but fatigues easily. She uses a w/c as her primary mode of locomotion when outside. ROM testing reveals tightness of bilateral hamstrings and calf muscles. Tone assessment using the Modified Ashworth Scale reveals a grade of 2 in the LEs. The patient demonstrates impaired UE and LE light touch and proprioception sensation, with the LEs more affected than the UEs.

Bed mobility, supine-to-sit, and transfers to the w/c are independent, but the patient performs these movements slowly. Sitting balance is good for static and fair+ to good for dynamic. Balance in standing is good for static and fair for dynamic. She scored a 16/28 on the Tinetti Performance Oriented Mobility Assessment and a 41/56 on the Berg Balance Scale. Both results indicate the patient's increased risk for falls.

Questions

1. When discussing the patient with the supervising physical therapist, what intervention areas could the physical therapist assistant suggest to the physical therapist as important to consider?
2. What would be important considerations must the physical therapist assistant note in providing interventions to this patient?

Case #2: Guillain-Barré Syndrome

The client is a 52-year-old man who was seen in the emergency room 8 weeks ago with complaints of sudden extremity numbness and weakness. Upon admission to the ER, he reported that he is an active and otherwise healthy individual. Through examination, it was determined that he had experienced a gastrointestinal bug 2 weeks prior to the symptom development.

Once other conditions had been ruled out, he was diagnosed with GBS. Over the course of 8 days, he progressed rapidly and required ventilator support. Additionally, he lost all motor movement of bilateral LEs and UEs over this time. He underwent 5 rounds of plasmapheresis and intravenous immunoglobin therapy. On day 9, he began to plateau with no further decline. His plateau phase lasted about 2 weeks, and then he became to gain strength, and his respiratory status began to stabilize. He was weaned from the ventilator after 21 days.

The client was recently discharged from acute care into an inpatient rehabilitation setting. He has significant weakness in all extremities, where he is able to move in a gravity eliminated position. Trunk weakness limits his ability to statically sit independently, requiring moderate assist, and he presents with extremely limited aerobic capacity and tolerance to upright supported sitting longer than 30 minutes. Currently, he needs moderate assistance for stand-pivot transfer and is non-ambulatory.

Questions

1. What are the signs and symptoms of overwork fatigue in this client?
2. What types of strengthening exercises would be appropriate in first week?
3. What types of exercises would be appropriate for improving cardiopulmonary status?

References

1. Widener G. Multiple sclerosis. In: Umphred D, Lazaro R, Roller M, Burton G, eds. *Umphred's Neurological Rehabilitation*. 6th ed. St. Louis, MO: Elsevier; 2012.
2. Confavreux C, Vukusic S, Moreau T, Adeleine P. Relapses and progression of disability in multiple sclerosis. *N Engl J Med.* 2000;343(20):1430-1438. doi:10.1056/NEJM200011163432001
3. What Causes MS? https://www.nationalmssociety.org/What-is-MS/What-Causes-MS. Accessed November 29, 2018.
4. *Guide to Physical Therapist Practice 3.0*. Alexandria, VA: American Physical Therapy Association; 2015.
5. MS-EDGE Outcome Measures for In and Out Patient Rehabilitation. http://www.neuropt.org/docs/default-source/ms-edge-documents/ms-edge-in-out-patient-rehab.pdf?sfvrsn=4a6f5543_0. Accessed November 29, 2018.
6. Khan F, Amatya B. Rehabilitation in Multiple Sclerosis: A Systematic Review of Systematic Reviews. *Arch Phys Med Rehabil.* 2017;98(2):353-367. doi:10.1016/j.apmr.2016.04.016
7. Jakowec MW, Wang Z, Holschneider D, Beeler J, Petzinger GM. Engaging cognitive circuits to promote motor recovery in degenerative disorders. exercise as a learning modality. *J Hum Kinet.* 2016;52(1):35-51. doi:10.1515/hukin-2015-0192
8. Braley TJ, Chervin RD. Fatigue in multiple sclerosis: mechanisms, evaluation, and treatment. *Sleep.* 2010;33(8):1061-1067. doi:10.1093/sleep/33.8.1061
9. Halabchi F, Alizadeh Z, Sahraian MA, Abolhasani M. Exercise prescription for patients with multiple sclerosis; potential benefits and practical recommendations. *BMC Neurol.* 2017;17(1):185. doi:10.1186/s12883-017-0960-9
10. Wellness for People with MS: What do we know about Diet, Exercise and Mood And what do we still need to learn? http://www.nationalmssociety.org/nationalmssociety/media/msnationalfiles/brochures/wellnessmssocietyforpeoplewms.pdf. Accessed December 8, 2019.
11. Storr LK, Sørensen PS, Ravnborg M. The efficacy of multidisciplinary rehabilitation in stable multiple sclerosis patients. *Mult Scler.* 2006;12(2):235-242. doi:10.1191/135248506ms1250oa
12. Kaltsatou A, Flouris AD. Impact of pre-cooling therapy on the physical performance and functional capacity of multiple sclerosis patients: A systematic review. *Mult Scler Relat Disord.* 2019;27:419-423. doi:10.1016/j.msard.2018.11.013
13. Jackson K, Mulcare JA, Donahoe-Fillmore B, Fritz HI, Rodgers MM. Home balance training intervention for people with multiple sclerosis. *Int J MS Care.* 2007;9(3):111-117. doi:10.7224/1537-2073-9.3.111
14. Managing Sensory Symptoms of Multiple Sclerosis. https://www.everydayhealth.com/multiple-sclerosis/symptoms/managing-sensory-symptoms-multiple-sclerosis/. Accessed December 8, 2019.
15. Fisher TB, Stevens JE. Rehabilitation of a marathon runner with Guillain-Barré syndrome. *J Neurol Phys Ther.* 2008;32(4):203-209. doi:10.1097/NPT.0b013e31818e0882
16. Dombale VV, Kumar S. A pilot study to compare between effectiveness of functional mobility and strengthening exercises and strengthening exercises alone in Guillain-Barré syndrome patients. *Indian J Physiother Occup Ther.* 2012;6(2):125-130.
17. Khan F, Amatya B. Rehabilitation interventions in patients with acute demyelinating inflammatory polyneuropathy: a systematic review. *Eur J Phys Rehabil Med.* 2012;48(3):507-522.
18. Alexandrescu R, Siegert RJ, Turner-Stokes L. Functional outcomes and efficiency of rehabilitation in a national cohort of patients with Guillain-Barré syndrome and other inflammatory polyneuropathies. *PLoS One.* 2014;9(11):e110532. doi:10.1371/journal.pone.0110532
19. Khan F, Pallant JF, Amatya B, Ng L, Gorelik A, Brand C. Outcomes of high- and low-intensity rehabilitation programme for persons in chronic phase after Guillain-Barré syndrome: a randomized controlled trial. *J Rehabil Med.* 2011;43(7):638-646. doi:10.2340/16501977-0826
20. Tomita MR, Buckner K, Saharan S, Persons K, Liao SH. Extended occupational therapy reintegration strategies for a woman with Guillain-Barré syndrome: case report. *Am J Occup Ther.* 2016;70(4):7004210010p1.
21. Gisbert R, Fuller K. The Peripheral Nervous System. In: Goodman CFK, ed. *Pathology: Implications for the Physical Therapist.* 4th ed. St. Louis, MO: Elsevier; 2015:1689-1691.

22. Gupta A, Patil M, Khanna M, Krishnan R, Taly AB. Guillain-Barre syndrome in postpartum period: rehabilitation issues and outcome - three case reports. *J Neurosci Rural Pract.* 2017;8(3):475-477. doi:10.4103/jnrp.jnrp_474_16
23. Albiol-Pérez S, Forcano-García M, Muñoz-Tomás MT, et al. A novel virtual motor rehabilitation system for Guillain-Barré syndrome. Two single case studies. *Methods Inf Med.* 2015;54(2):127-134. doi:10.3414/ME14-02-0002
24. Wada S, Kawate N, Morotomi N, Matsumiya T, Ono G, Mizuma M. Experience of rehabilitation for Guillain-Barré syndrome during and after pregnancy: a case study. *Disabil Rehabil.* 2010;32(24):2056-2059. doi:10.3109/09638281003797422
25. Simatos Arsenault N, Vincent PO, Yu BHS, Bastien R, Sweeney A. Influence of exercise on patients with Guillain-Barré syndrome: a systematic review. *Physiother Can.* 2016;68(4):367-376. doi:10.3138/ptc.2015-58
26. Dimitrova A, Izov N, Maznev I, Grigorova-Petrova K, Lubenova D, Vasileva D. Physical therapy and functional motor recovery in patient with Guillain-Barré syndrome—case report. *Eur Sci J.* 2017;13(33):11-19. doi:10.19044/esj.2017.v13n33p11
27. Damjanov I. *Pathology for Health Professions.* 4th ed. St. Louis, MO: Elsevier; 2012.
28. Reisner EG, Reisner HM, Crowley LV. *Crowley's An Introduction to Human Disease Pathology and Pathophysiology Correlations*. 10th ed. Burlington, MA: Jones and Bartlett Learning; 2017.
29. Gupta A, Taly AB, Srivastava A, Murali T. Guillain-Barre Syndrome—rehabilitation outcome, residual deficits and requirement of lower limb orthosis for locomotion at 1 year follow-up. *Disabil Rehabil.* 2010;32(23):1897-1902. doi:10.3109/09638281003734474
30. Sendhilkumar R, Gupta A, Nagarathna R, Taly AB. "Effect of pranayama and meditation as an add-on therapy in rehabilitation of patients with Guillain-Barré syndrome—a randomized control pilot study". *Disabil Rehabil.* 2013;35(1):57-62. doi:10.3109/09638288.2012.687031
31. Andrews AW, Middleton A. Improvement during inpatient rehabilitation among older adults with Guillain-Barré syndrome, multiple sclerosis, Parkinson disease, and stroke. *Am J Phys Med Rehabil.* 2018;97(12):879-884. doi:10.1097/PHM.0000000000000991
32. Inokuchi H, Yasunaga H, Nakahara Y, et al. Effect of rehabilitation on mortality of patients with Guillain-Barre Syndrome: a propensity-matched analysis using nationwide database. *Eur J Phys Rehabil Med.* 2014;50(4):439-446.
33. Hamilton BB, Laughlin JA, Fiedler RC, Granger CV. Interrater reliability of the 7-level functional independence measure (FIM). *Scand J Rehabil Med.* 1994;26(3):115-119.
34. Tinetti ME, Williams TF, Mayewski R. Fall risk index for elderly patients based on number of chronic disabilities. *Am J Med.* 1986;80(3):429-434. doi:10.1016/0002-9343(86)90717-5
35. Dennis D, Mullins R. Guillain-Barré syndrome patient's satisfaction with physiotherapy: A two-part observational study. *Physiother Theory Pract.* 2013;29(4):301-308. doi:10.3109/09593985.2012.732196
36. Jorge LL, de Brito AM, Marchi FH, Hara AC, Battistella LR, Riberto M. New rehabilitation models for neurologic inpatients in Brazil. *Disabil Rehabil.* 2015;37(3):268-273. doi:10.3109/09638288.2014.914585
37. Curtis CL, Weir JP. Overview of exercise responses in healthy and impaired states. *Neurol Rep.* 1996;20(2):13-19. doi:10.1097/01253086-199620020-00014

Please visit www.routledge.com/9781630915650 to access additional material.

Chapter 16

Cardiopulmonary Issues Associated With Patients Undergoing Neurorehabilitation

Ronald De Vera Barredo, PT, DPT, EdD, FAPTA

KEY WORDS Aerobic exercise | Breathing retraining | Cardiovascular system | Chronic obstructive pulmonary disease | Congestive heart failure | Dyspnea | Exercise intolerance | Progressive deconditioning | Pulmonary system | Restrictive lung disease

Chapter Objectives

- Describe the basic anatomy and physiology of the cardiovascular and pulmonary systems.
- Explain how neuromuscular pathologies can affect cardiovascular and pulmonary function.
- Discuss common cardiovascular and pulmonary comorbidities that may affect patients undergoing neurorehabilitation.
- Describe physical therapy examination procedures and common diagnostic tests used with individuals with primary or secondary cardiovascular and pulmonary problems.
- Describe procedural interventions that are used to manage patients with cardiovascular and pulmonary conditions.

Oxygen delivery and carbon dioxide elimination are important to sustaining life. Normal body functioning requires the presence of oxygen for cell metabolism and energy production. Without enough oxygen, the cells will not work properly, eventually impairing neuromuscular and musculoskeletal function. A byproduct of cell metabolism and energy production is carbon dioxide, which is transported to the lungs so that it may be eliminated from the body through the process of exhalation.

The entire process of oxygen delivery and carbon dioxide elimination is mediated through the cardiovascular and pulmonary systems. The cardiovascular and pulmonary systems are complementary systems that participate in gas exchange, oxygen transport, and carbon dioxide elimination. Problems with either or both systems may interfere with the rehabilitation process by limiting muscle performance, exercise tolerance, and functional capacity. Likewise, conditions of the neuromuscular and musculoskeletal systems that affect the cardiovascular and pulmonary systems can impair the latter's ability to deliver oxygen and eliminate carbon dioxide.

The purpose of this chapter is three-fold: first, to describe how impairments resulting from neuromuscular pathologies can alter cardiovascular and pulmonary function; second, to discuss how cardiovascular and pulmonary comorbidities affect neurorehabilitation; and third, to outline examination and intervention strategies appropriate for the physical therapist assistant to perform commensurate to his or her scope of practice. A sufficient understanding of the dynamics between the neuromuscular system and the cardiovascular and pulmonary systems will allow

Lazaro RT, Umphred DA, eds.
Umphred's Neurorehabilitation for the Physical Therapist Assistant, Third Edition (pp 373-385).

Table 16-1

Cardiovascular and Pulmonary Responses to Sympathetic and Parasympathetic Stimulation

System Component	Sympathetic Response	Parasympathetic Response
Heart	↑ Heart rate and contractility	↓ Heart rate and contractility
Peripheral vessels	Vasoconstriction	Vasodilation
Lungs	Bronchodilation	Bronchoconstriction

the physical therapist assistant to employ appropriate strategies within the established plan of care.

Review of Anatomy and Physiology of Cardiovascular and Pulmonary Systems

The pulmonary system is integral to gas exchange and carbon dioxide elimination. The cardiovascular system transports oxygenated blood from the lungs to cells, tissues, and organs. Waste products, including carbon dioxide from the cells, tissues, and organs, are transported back to the lungs for waste elimination. In supplying oxygen to and eliminating carbon dioxide from the body, the pulmonary system is able to regulate the body's pH balance.

The pulmonary system is composed of a network of airways that begins in the nose and mouth; proceeds inferiorly to the pharynx, larynx, trachea, and airways; and terminates into the alveoli, which are surrounded by capillaries. Inhaled air passes through these airways until it reaches the alveoli, where gas exchange occurs. Oxygen from the inhaled air diffuses through the alveoli into the arterial system, while carbon dioxide from the venous system diffuses into the alveoli and exits the body through the same network of airways during exhalation.

Essential in the mechanics of breathing is the integrity of the chest wall mechanics and respiratory muscle function. The chest wall should be able to expand and return to its resting position without compromise. The primary and accessory muscles of respiration should function appropriately to the needs of the person and the demands of the body. Consequently, neuromuscular and musculoskeletal pathologies and impairments that interfere with the normal functioning of the chest wall and the respiratory muscles may affect the mechanics of breathing, which would manifest itself in difficulty inhaling, exhaling, or both.

The cardiovascular system is composed of the heart and the blood vessels that not only supply oxygenated blood to the various parts of the body (*systemic circulation*), but also transport deoxygenated blood from the parts of the body to the lungs for oxygenation and waste elimination (*pulmonary circulation*). The heart is central to both systemic and pulmonary circulation. It is a 4-chambered organ consisting of 2 atria and 2 ventricles. The atria act as temporary storage chambers as the blood is transmitted to the ventricles. The ventricles function to eject the blood to either the lungs or the rest of the body. Between the atria and ventricles are valves that prevent the backflow of blood from one chamber to another.

The right side of the heart participates in pulmonary circulation. Deoxygenated blood coming from systemic circulation passes through the right atrium, the tricuspid valve, and the right ventricle, and is ejected to the lungs via the pulmonary arteries. The left side of the heart participates in systemic circulation. Oxygenated blood coming from the lungs is transported back to the heart via the pulmonary veins. The blood then passes through the left atrium, the mitral valve, and the left ventricle, and is ejected to the body via the aorta, systemic arteries, arterioles, and capillaries.

Both the parasympathetic and sympathetic nervous systems innervate the heart, lungs, and blood vessels. Parasympathetic innervation is effected primarily through the vagus nerve, while sympathetic innervation is effected through the pre- and post-ganglionic neurons that extend through the thoracolumbar regions of the spinal cord (Table 16-1). Consequently, neuromuscular pathologies and impairments that interfere with the normal functioning of the parasympathetic and sympathetic systems would affect the response of the cardiovascular and pulmonary systems.[1]

Neuromuscular Pathologies Affecting Cardiovascular and Pulmonary Function

Neuromuscular pathologies and impairments have the potential of affecting cardiovascular and pulmonary function. The physical therapist assistant needs to be aware of this potential to address issues of a cardiovascular or pulmonary nature when working with patients undergoing neurorehabilitation. For example, changes in muscle tone may affect muscle performance. Upper motor neuron lesions generally result in increased muscle tone, while lower motor neuron lesions generally result in decreased muscle tone. Such changes in muscle tone may not only

Table 16-2

Effects of Changes in Tone on the Mechanics of Breathing

Location of the Lesion	*Change in Muscle Tone*	*Musculoskeletal Effect*	*Cardiopulmonary Consequence*
Upper motor neuron lesion (eg, stroke, SCI, Parkinson's disease)	Increased	Decreased motor control	• Postural impairment due to weakness or increased tone • Altered chest movement • Difficulty recruiting accessory muscles • Inability to produce an effective cough
Lower motor neuron lesion (eg, poliomyelitis, neuropathy, muscle dystrophy)	Decreased	Muscular weakness	

affect motor performance, but may also contribute to impairments in posture. Consequently, impairments in muscle performance and postural control can affect the mechanics of breathing (Table 16-2).

Neuromuscular pathologies such as stroke and amyotrophic lateral sclerosis may also result in impairments of bulbar functions or cranial nerve involvement, which include chewing, swallowing, and speech. Paralysis of the muscles involved with bulbar function may result in the patient aspirating fluid and food particles to the lungs, resulting in aspiration pneumonia. The physical therapist assistant should recognize signs that point to problems with chewing, swallowing, or aspiration. These include excessive drooling, especially at mealtime; pocketing of food in the cheeks; choking or trouble swallowing certain foods or liquids; having a gurgling voice during or after a meal; coughing before or after swallowing; and frequent throat-clearing during or after a meal.

In addition to their impact on respiratory muscle function, breathing mechanics, and bulbar function, neuromuscular pathologies may also result in impairments of autonomic nervous system function. Patients with spinal cord injuries (SCIs), for example, may have problems regulating blood pressure (BP), but these tend to change with time following the injury. During the spinal shock stage (hours to days), there is massive dilation of the blood vessels, resulting in profound hypotension. As time progresses (days to weeks), spinal shock diminishes; however, patients experience frequent bouts with hypotensive episodes during changes in position or prolonged sitting, including lightheadedness, dizziness, and syncope. Conversely, instead of hypotensive episodes, patients with SCIs above T5 or T6 may experience bouts of hypertensive episodes brought about by noxious stimuli below the level of the lesion (*autonomic dysreflexia*), such as a distended bladder, a blocked catheter, or tight clothing. During these instances, the presence of noxious stimuli activates the sympathetic nervous system, resulting in increased BP, flushing of the face and upper body, and complaints of pounding headache. Current studies show that autonomic dysreflexia occurs more frequently during the early phases of SCI, while hypotensive episodes can persist for years after the injury.[2] The physical therapist assistant should recognize signs and symptoms of hypertension and hypotension with this population, especially during neurorehabilitation, to avert any untoward consequences to the patient, such as falls during hypotensive episodes and stroke during hypertensive episodes. Table 16-3 outlines signs and symptoms associated with hypotensive and hypertensive episodes that the physical therapist assistant needs to be familiar with.

Table 16-3

Signs and Symptoms Representative of Hypotensive and Hypertensive Episodes

Hypotensive	*Hypertensive*
• Lightheadedness • Dizziness • Syncope • Shortness of breath • Irregular heartbeat	• Pounding headache • Flushing of face • Sweating • Goose pimples • Nausea

Primary Cardiovascular and Pulmonary Pathologies Affecting Neurorehabilitation

Cardiovascular Pathologies

Patients undergoing neurorehabilitation may have cardiovascular comorbidities that require attention during the development and implementation of the plan of care. Some of these comorbidities may have been preexisting conditions that contributed to the development of the neurological condition. A classic example of this is the role of hypertension (systolic BP equal to or greater than 130 mm Hg; or diastolic BP equal to or greater than 80 mm Hg) in the development of stroke. Consistently high BP weakens the blood vessels and damages the flow to organs such as

Table 16-4
Ranges of Blood Pressure

Normal	Systolic less than 120 mm Hg; diastolic less than 80 mm Hg
Elevated	Systolic 120 to 129 mm Hg; diastolic less than 80 mm Hg
Hypertensive	Systolic equal to or greater than 130 mm Hg; diastolic equal to or greater than 80 mm Hg

the brain, thereby resulting in a stroke. Table 16-4 outlines the BP readings considered normal, elevated, and hypertensive.[3]

Physical therapist assistants working with patients who are hypertensive need to be familiar with the signs and symptoms of hypertension. Additionally, they should consider taking BP readings in the unaffected arm, since BP readings are unreliable if taken in the affected arm. Studies have shown that muscle tone in the affected arm can influence the BP reading in that extremity. Spastic extremities yield higher BP readings, while flaccid extremities yield lower BP readings.[4,5]

Atherosclerosis refers to the hardening of arteries usually caused by deposition of fat, cholesterol, and other substances that harden and form structures called *plaques*. The narrowing of the arteries results in decreased blood flow, starving cells, and tissues of oxygen-rich blood. Decreased blood flow to the cardiac muscles results in chest pain, also known as *angina*. Angina may feel like pressure or squeezing in the chest and can radiate to the shoulders, chest, jaw, or back. Sometimes, in the absence of chest pain, other symptoms are present, such as dyspnea, profuse sweating, extreme fatigue, and belching; these are known as *anginal equivalents* that also indicate decreased blood flow to the cardiac muscles. Stable angina occurs with activity or stress. This type of angina is predictable because symptoms are absent at rest or with mild activity. However, in the presence of increasing activity, decreased blood flow is unable to meet the oxygen demands of the heart, thereby eliciting angina. A decrease in activity or the administration of nitroglycerin may minimize the symptoms. On the other hand, unstable angina does not follow a predictable pattern. Angina may occur at rest and may not respond to medication. Therefore, unstable angina is a medical emergency. The physical therapist assistant should be able to recognize the signs and symptoms of angina. Should anginal onset occur during neurorehabilitation, the physical therapist assistant needs to cease the activity and notify the physical therapist immediately. Additionally, if nitroglycerin has been prescribed, the patient needs to be instructed to take the medication as prescribed by the physician.

Arrhythmias refer to problems with the rate and/or rhythm of the heart. Patients undergoing neurorehabilitation may report having palpitations, fluttering, or pounding in the chest. This may be accompanied by other symptoms, such as lightheadedness, dizziness, dyspnea, chest discomfort, or fatigue. In addition to recognizing the signs and symptoms of arrhythmias, the physical therapist assistant who works with a patient who has arrhythmia should continually monitor the patient's pulse and BP. Additionally, the physical therapist assistant should be trained not only in cardiopulmonary resuscitation, but also in the use of an automated external defibrillator.

Deep vein thrombosis (DVT) refers to a blood clot in the legs. The blockage causes pain, swelling, and warmth in the legs. DVT may be caused by prolonged bedrest or immobility, such as those caused by stroke or during the acute phase of a SCI. DVT is an important consideration, especially during the early phases of rehabilitation, because a medically unmanaged DVT may result in the release of an embolus from the site of the DVT, which eventually lodges itself in the lungs, causing a pulmonary embolism. Because Homan's sign is of no clinical use,[6] using the Wells Prediction Rule (Table 16-5) is a better alternative to determining the probability of a DVT. By determining the clinical presentation of the patient and assigning scores to the clinical features, the rule classifies patients as having either low, moderate, or high probability of having a DVT.[7]

The physical therapist assistant needs to be familiar with the risk factors for and the signs and symptoms of DVT. Additionally, the assistant should be familiar with the signs and symptoms of pulmonary embolism, should this occur during neurorehabilitation. Signs and symptoms include sudden and unexplained shortness of breath, difficulty with breathing, chest pain, tachypnea, palpitations, coughing, or coughing up blood. Individuals with DVT should not participate in physical therapy until cleared by the physician.

Like hypertension, congestive heart failure (CHF) has been recognized as a risk factor for stroke. CHF occurs when the heart is unable to pump adequately to meet the needs of the body. This can result from coronary artery disease, valvular diseases of the heart, and hypertension. Right-sided heart failure occurs when the right ventricle is unable to eject blood to the pulmonary circuit, which is involved with gas exchange. Left-sided heart failure occurs when the left ventricle is unable to eject blood to the systemic circuit, which is involved with supplying oxygenated blood to the body.

Regardless of which side of the heart is involved, the signs and symptoms of heart failure may be classified as the result of either *forward failure* (consequences resulting from blood not moving forward) or *backward failure* (consequences resulting from blood backing up from whence it came). In right-sided heart failure, for example, the right ventricle is unable to eject a sufficient amount of blood for gas exchange, thereby resulting in hypoxemia (forward failure). Concurrently, since the right ventricle is unable to fully eject blood from the right ventricle, blood is dammed back to the right atrium, then to the superior and inferior vena cava, and back to the venous system, thereby resulting in distended neck veins, dependent edema, and hepatomegaly (backward failure). On the other hand, in left-sided heart failure, the left ventricle is unable to eject a sufficient amount of blood for systemic circulation, which may result in lightheadedness and hypotension (forward failure). Additionally, since the left ventricle is unable to eject a sufficient amount of blood forward, blood is dammed back to the left atrium, then back to the lungs, thereby resulting in pulmonary edema, shortness of breath, and wheezing (backward failure). Table 16-6 outlines the representative signs and symptoms associated with right- and left-sided heart failure.

The physical therapist assistant needs to be familiar with the signs and symptoms of heart failure. Additionally, the physical therapist assistant should remember that patients undergoing neurorehabilitation who have CHF as a comorbidity may also report having dyspnea, fatigue, exercise intolerance, and weight gain. The assistant should report these findings to the physical therapist or to other appropriate personnel.

Table 16-5

Clinical Model for Predicting Pretest Probability for Deep Vein Thrombosis

Clinical Feature	*Score*
Active cancer (treatment ongoing or within previous 6 months or palliative)	1
Paralysis, paresis, or recent plaster immobilization of the lower extremities	1
Recently bedridden for more than 3 days or major surgery, within 4 weeks	1
Localized tenderness along the distribution of the deep venous system	1
Entire leg swollen	1
Calf swelling by more than 3 cm when compared with the asymptomatic leg (measured 10 cm below tibial tuberosity)	1
Pitting edema (greater in the symptomatic leg)	1
Collateral superficial veins (nonvaricose)	1
Alternative diagnosis as likely or greater than that of DVT	−2

Low probability, 0 or less; moderate probability, 1 to 2; high probability, 3 or more. Reprinted with permission from Wells PS, Anderson DR, Bormanis J, et al. Value of assessment of pretest probability of deep-vein thrombosis in clinical management. *Lancet*. Copyright 1997, with permission from Elsevier.

Pulmonary Pathologies

Patients with pulmonary comorbidities may exhibit exercise and activity limitations while undergoing neurorehabilitation. The physical therapist assistant needs to be familiar with the impairments resulting from these pathologies to implement strategies that will allow the patient to maximize the rehabilitation process while operating within his or her pulmonary limitations. Chronic obstructive pulmonary disease (COPD) and restrictive lung diseases represent 2 types of pulmonary pathologies. Obstructive lung conditions make it difficult for patients to expel air (*expiration*), while restrictive lung conditions make it difficult for patients to expand the lungs (*inspiration*). Despite these differences, obstructive and restrictive lung conditions result in patients having dyspnea or shortness of breath. During the early stages of obstruction or restriction, dyspnea would limit the performance of exercises and other activities and may limit the person's ability to participate in social interactions. As the condition progresses, dyspnea worsens to the point that it interferes with normal functioning and activities of daily living (ADL).

Patients with obstructive conditions experience dyspnea because they are unable to expire the air that is trapped in the lungs. Air-trapping can result from the destruction of the alveolar walls, such as seen in emphysema. When the lining of the alveolar walls is destroyed, the alveoli permanently expand, causing air to be trapped within it. The more chronic the condition, the more alveolar destruction is present, and the more air-trapping takes place, causing the patient to exhale slowly and longer in an effort to expel the air. Another cause of air-trapping is the narrowing of the airways. The presence of mucus, such as seen in chronic bronchitis, or a state of bronchoconstriction, such as seen in asthma, makes the diameter of the airways narrower. Because resistance to air movement is greater on expiration than inspiration, air can get in the lungs but has difficulty getting out. Like in emphysema, air-trapping takes place, causing the patient to exhale slowly and longer in an effort to expel air.

Patients with restrictive conditions experience dyspnea because they are unable to fully inspire air due to some type of pulmonary or extrapulmonary restriction. This restriction may be related to the inability of the lung tissue to fully expand, such as seen in *pneumothorax* (air in the intrapleural space) or *pleural effusion* (fluid in the intrapleural space); stiffness of the lung parenchyma, such as seen in interstitial lung disease; structural defects of the thoracic cage, such as seen in kyphoscoliosis; weakening of the respiratory muscles, such as seen in muscular dystrophy; increased tone of the muscles of the thorax, such as seen in hemiplegia; or damage to nerves that assist with breathing, such as in phrenic nerve compression.

Because of the increased respiratory effort and work associated with dyspnea, patients with obstructive and restrictive conditions may limit their food intake. Their use of accessory muscles contributes to higher energy expenditure. These 2 factors result in unintended weight loss. In addition to dyspnea and unintended weight loss, cough may also present among patients with pulmonary patholo-

Table 16-6

Signs and Symptoms Associated With Left- and Right-Sided Heart Failure

Left-Sided Heart Failure

• Forward failure
  ◦ Hypotension
  ◦ Lightheadedness
  ◦ Dizziness
  ◦ Cool extremities
• Backward failure
  ◦ Pulmonary edema
  ◦ Dyspnea
  ◦ Orthopnea

Right-Sided Heart Failure

• Forward failure
  ◦ Hypoxemia
• Backward failure
  ◦ Dependent edema
  ◦ Hepatomegaly
  ◦ Visible neck veins
  ◦ Ankle swelling

gies. For patients with obstructive conditions, cough is usually productive; for patients with restrictive conditions, cough is usually dry. Finally, for more chronic conditions, patients manifest with hypoxemia and may require supplemental oxygenation to meet the demands of the body. Hypoxemia may, in turn, cause restlessness, altered mental status, tachycardia, and diaphoresis.

Despite body system impairments caused by pulmonary comorbidities, patients undergoing neurorehabilitation need not stop exercising. Exercise can increase physical capacity, decrease anxiety, reduce fatigue, and improve independence. The physical therapist assistant needs to communicate closely with the physical therapist on the exercise parameters appropriate for the patient. Pacing and rest breaks are also important considerations during therapy. Finally, the physical therapist assistant should be able to recognize the signs and symptoms of respiratory distress and respond appropriately to the needs of the patient within the established plan of care.

Common Participation Restrictions, Functional Activity Limitations, and Body System Impairments of the Cardiopulmonary System

Participation limitations for patients with cardiopulmonary pathologies are largely a result of progressive deconditioning. Because dyspnea is central to most cardiopulmonary conditions, patients who experience this and other symptoms, such as leg fatigue and discomfort, minimize or avoid physical activity.[8,9] Patients become sedentary, and the resulting decrease in physical activity contributes to continued physical deconditioning, resulting in dyspnea on minimal exertion and eventual inability to participate in normal life activities and loss of function performing ADL. The loss of function in social participation and ADL also results in depression.[9] Figure 16-1 illustrates the role of dyspnea in deconditioning.

In addition to dyspnea, exercise intolerance is evident in patients with cardiopulmonary conditions, particularly those with CHF.[10] *Exercise intolerance* is defined as the reduced ability to perform activities that involve dynamic movement of large skeletal muscles because of symptoms of dyspnea, muscle weakness, or fatigue.[11] For a patient undergoing neurorehabilitation, exercise intolerance is a primary consideration. The physical therapist assistant should accommodate for dyspnea and muscle weakness or fatigue while implementing the established plan of care.

The physical therapist assistant should always be aware and cognizant of cardiac decompensation, which is indicative of the sudden worsening of symptoms related to heart failure. Symptoms may be manifested as increasing shortness of breath; onset of coughing and wheezing; worsening fatigue; and the development of hypotension, lightheadedness, cyanosis, angina, or arrhythmias.

Examination Tools, Tests, and Measures Used to Evaluate Cardiovascular and Pulmonary Function

Physical Examination

For patients undergoing neurorehabilitation, neurological assessment should include an examination of the cardiopulmonary system, especially since impairments in cardiovascular and pulmonary function may interfere with the rehabilitation process. While the physical therapist of record should perform the initial examination/evaluation, parts of the reexamination are often delegated to the physical therapist assistant. Similarly, a problem might develop during any intervention, and the physical therapist assistant needs to be aware of the signs and symptoms of a cardiopulmonary problem. For that reason, the physical therapist assistant needs to understand and be skilled at examining the cardiopulmonary system. If a problem develops and the physical therapist assistant does not feel comfortable with the reexamination, the physical therapist of record should be contacted immediately to prevent a delay in recognizing potential life-threatening dangers in the patient's cardiopulmonary system.

Physical therapy examination of the cardiovascular and pulmonary systems encompasses 4 areas: observation, palpation, percussion, and auscultation.[1,12,13] *Observation*

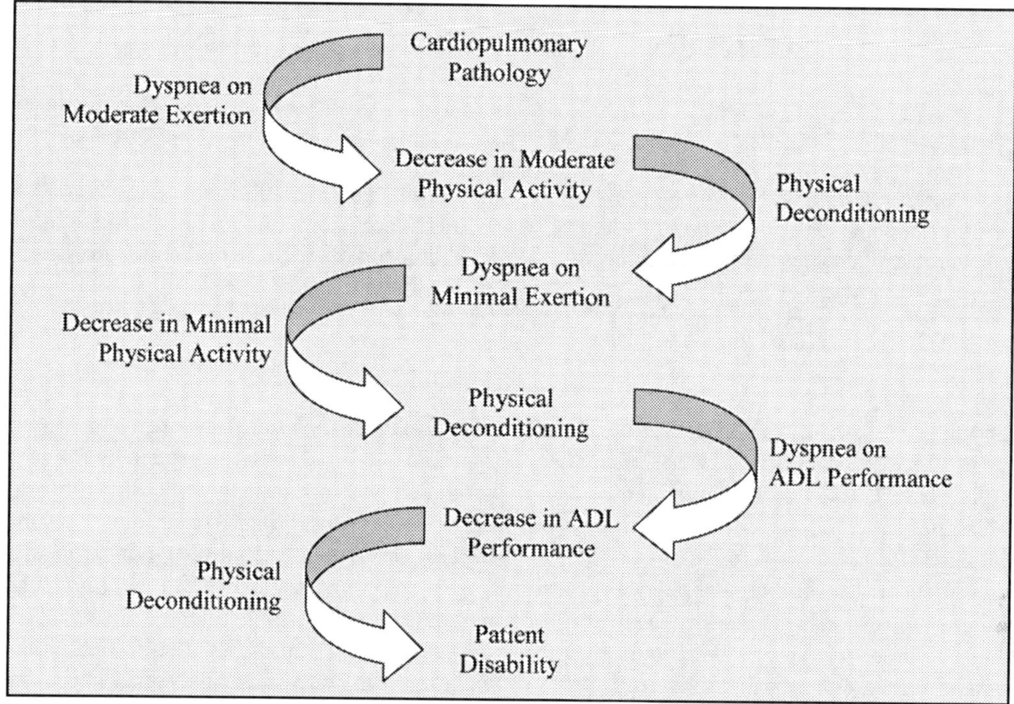

Figure 16-1. Dyspnea: deconditioning spiral.

refers to the visual inspection of the patient, which includes an assessment of the patient's general appearance, integumentary status, and breathing pattern. When observing the patient's general appearance, the physical therapist assistant should recognize signs of respiratory distress. The assumption of a tripod posture is characteristic of a patient having respiratory distress. In the tripod posture, a patient leans forward in sitting or standing and supports the upper body with the hands on the knees or on another surface. In this position, with the head and upper extremities fixed, the accessory muscles in the neck and chest are able to contract in reverse origin insertion to expand the chest when breathing. Another observable sign of respiratory distress is the increased work of breathing, manifested not only in the use of accessory muscles but also in the increased rate of breathing (*tachypnea*). Nasal flaring or the widening of the openings of the nose during breathing may also be observed.

When observing the patient's integumentary status, the physical therapist assistant should be aware of changes in the skin that may result from cardiovascular and pulmonary pathologies. Cyanosis or bluish discoloration of the skin occurs when the patient is not receiving adequate amounts of oxygen. This may occur centrally (eg, around the mouth and lips) or peripherally (eg, in the fingers). On the other hand, pallor or paleness of the skin occurs when there is decreased blood flow to the area, such as seen in arterial occlusion. Another observable skin condition is digital clubbing, characterized by changes in the base of the nails that result in the formation of convex distal phalanges. The condition may be seen among patients with lung neoplasms, chronic pulmonary infections, *corpulmonale* (right-sided heart failure), or chronic CHF.[14] For patients with CHF, edema may be observed in the lower extremities due to the damming of blood from the right ventricle to the peripheral venous circulation. Edema is usually manifested by swelling caused by fluid accumulating in the tissues. In prolonged upright postures, swelling accumulates in the lower extremities, causing dependent edema.

When observing the patient's breathing pattern, the physical therapist assistant should be aware of changes in the type, symmetry, rate, and depth of breathing. Patients in respiratory distress may manifest with tachypnea and accessory muscle use. Depending on the pulmonary condition, both the rate and depth of breathing may increase. An important consideration in observing the patient's breathing pattern may also include the neurological impairments that the patient has. In hemiplegia, for example, symmetry of breathing may be compromised because of changes in muscle tone and posture. Hemiparesis of the diaphragm causing involvement of one side of the diaphragm is almost always present following a middle cerebral artery stroke. Paradoxical breathing may be observed in patients whose SCI occurs at a high level. Paradoxical breathing occurs because of the loss of thoracic muscle tone and the paralysis of the thoracic muscles whose innervations come from the thoracic segments. The work of quiet breathing is borne solely by the diaphragm whose innervation comes from C3 to C5. When the patient inhales, the abdomen rises while the upper chest retracts. This type of paradoxical breathing is opposite that of patients in the latter stages of COPD. For these patients, the diaphragm has descended inferiorly

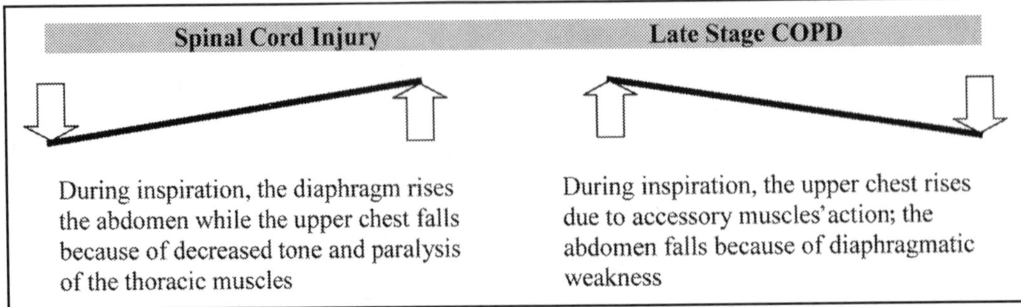

Figure 16-2. Differences in paradoxical breathing.

because of air-trapping, so the work of breathing is performed largely by the accessory muscles. When the patient inhales, the upper chest rises while the abdomen retracts. Figure 16-2 illustrates the difference between both types of paradoxical breathing.

Palpation represents the second area of physical examination. Palpation involves touching the patient to feel for and examine structures underneath. Palpation may be performed to determine the presence of tenderness. When patients report being short of breath, but it is not noticeable to anyone else, palpation may be used to feel for accessory muscle use. Edema may also be palpated to determine whether it is pitting or nonpitting. When pressure applied over an edematous area causes an indentation in the skin that persists after the pressure is released, then the edema is considered pitting. Conditions involving the heart and kidneys result in salt and fluid retention, usually leading to pitting edema. Additionally, skin turgor may also be assessed to determine the level of hydration. Skin that remains elevated after being pulled up and released indicates decreased turgor, which is indicative of decreased hydration.

Palpation is essential when taking the pulse. By palpating the pulse, the physical therapist assistant can determine not only the heart rate but also the rhythm and amplitude of the pulses. By determining the pattern of pulsations (rhythm), the physical therapist assistant can confirm the presence of arrhythmias and describe the pulses as regular, regularly irregular, or irregularly irregular. The amplitude or strength of the pulsations may be described as absent, faint, weak, strong, and bounding. Unfortunately, because a description of amplitude comes with subjectivity, determining amplitude should take into consideration the patient's condition, presentation, and comorbidities.[15] Outside of determining the heart rate, palpation can also be used to determine the presence of peripheral pulses. In the presence of peripheral vascular disease, the absence of peripheral pulses may indicate compromised blood flow.

Percussion represents the third area of physical examination. It involves the tapping of the thorax and abdomen to determine the condition of structures underneath it. Since thoracic and abdominal structures have different densities, the vibrations they generate during percussion vary. For example, air-filled structures, such as the lungs, normally produce resonance during percussion. However, when the lung tissue is consolidated (pneumonia), resonance changes to dullness on percussion. In the presence of increased air (ie, air-trapping), resonance changes to hyperresonance on percussion.

Auscultation represents the fourth area of physical examination. During auscultation, a stethoscope is used to listen to heart and lung sounds. Lung sounds are produced with the movement of air in and out of the lungs during each breath (*breath sounds*). Conditions that result in air trapping, such as emphysema, make it difficult for air to move in and out of the lungs; this results in decreased breath sounds. At other times, additional lung sounds are heard in addition to the breath sounds (*adventitious sounds*). These adventitious sounds indicate lung pathologies. Wheezing, for example, is an adventitious lung sound generated by air moving through narrowed airways, such as in asthma. Crackles (*rales*) is another example of an adventitious lung sound generated when air moves through pus, fluid, or mucus, such as in chronic bronchitis.

Heart sounds are produced by blood flow and valve closure. During cardiac auscultation, the closure of the atrioventricular valves produces the "lub" in the lub-dub sound of the heart, while the closure of the semilunar valves produces the "dub" sound. The former represents the S1 sound, while the latter represents the S2 sound. The presence of an S3 sound (heard immediately after S2) may be normal in children but may also indicate cardiac failure in adults. The presence of an S4 sound (prior to S1) may indicate a pathological condition such as myocardial infarct. In addition to the closure of the valves, a heart sound called *murmurs* may be produced by turbulent blood flow. Murmurs may be classified as innocent or abnormal. Innocent murmurs are not caused by heart conditions, but are nonetheless common in children. On the other hand, abnormal murmurs are caused by heart problems. They are generated when blood flows through either narrowed valves (*stenosis*) or incompetent valves (*regurgitation*).

Tests and Measures to Evaluate Cardiopulmonary Function

Diagnostic tests and outcomes measures are used to measure cardiovascular and pulmonary function. Although details on the administration of some of these tests and measures may be beyond the scope this text, the physical therapist assistant needs to be familiar with what these tests do and what type of information they provide to understand the test result found in the medical record and the effect those results may have on exercise or performance of ADL. The following tests will be covered in this section: pulmonary function tests, oximetry, arterial blood gases, activity and endurance evaluation, and stress testing.

Pulmonary function tests are used to determine how well the lungs function. More specifically, they measure the lungs' ability to hold air, move air in and out, and exchange oxygen and carbon dioxide from the blood. During testing, a patient breathes in and out of a mouthpiece into a recorder that measures the actual lung volumes and capacities and compares these values with predicted values that are based on the patient's age, sex, and height. Patients who undergo pulmonary function testing may be asked to breathe in and out normally and quietly. At other times, they may be asked to breathe in or out forcefully after taking a deep breath. An example of the latter is performed when measuring forced vital capacity (FVC). Since FVC involves maximum air exhalation after maximum air inhalation, the test reveals how fast and how much air patients can expire. Normally, a healthy individual can exhale between 75% and 80% of air during the first second of the FVC maneuver (FEV1). For patients with obstructive conditions, the value of FEV1/FVC is lower (ie, it takes longer for them to exhale). On the other hand, for patients with restrictive conditions, the value of FEV1/FVC is higher (ie, the patients are able to expire most of the air quickly). Another use of pulmonary function tests is to determine the efficacy of pulmonary medications in improving lung function. Baseline measures of lung function are taken and compared with values taken after administering pulmonary medications, such as bronchodilators. Should there be sufficient improvement in lung function, the medications become part of the patient's regimen, especially during functional activities that increase the demand on the pulmonary system.

Oximetry measures the concentration of oxygen in the blood by determining how saturated the hemoglobin is with oxygen molecules. The more saturated the hemoglobin is with oxygen molecules, the higher the oxygen saturation. Oxygen saturation can be measured using a pulse oximeter or through arterial blood gas analysis. When a pulse oximeter is used, oxygen saturation is labeled SpO_2; when arterial blood gas analysis is used, oxygen saturation is labeled SaO_2. Normal oxygen saturation is 97% to 99%, with 95% representing a clinically acceptable level of saturation for patients with a normal hemoglobin level. Generally speaking, activity should be stopped when oxygen saturation falls below 90%.[16,17] While working with a patient undergoing neurorehabilitation, the physical therapist assistant should ensure that the patient is above the clinical threshold determined by the physical therapist. When oxygen saturation falls below this threshold, the physical therapist assistant needs to cease the activity and consult with the physical therapist.

Arterial blood gas measurements determine not only the amount of oxygen and carbon dioxide in the blood, but also maintain the acid-base balance of the body through buffer mechanisms between the respiratory and renal systems. During instances of hypoventilation (such as in COPD), levels of carbon dioxide increase in the body and result in a condition known as *respiratory acidosis*. During instances of hyperventilation (such as in anxiety hyperventilation), carbon dioxide levels decrease in the body and result in a condition known as *respiratory alkalosis*.[18] When the underlying cause of either respiratory acidosis or alkalosis is untreated, the patient may manifest multisystemic signs and symptoms (Table 16-7).

For patients who have been bedridden or are just starting to get out of bed, an activity evaluation can be used to determine whether the patient is able to tolerate a variety of self-care activities performed first in supine, then progressed to sitting, and then to standing. During the performance of these self-care activities, the patients are monitored for symptoms including shortness of breath, lightheadedness, fatigue, fainting, and chest pain. Additionally, their heart rate and BP are monitored with each change in position. A drop of more than 20 mm Hg systolic BP and a drop of more than 10 mm Hg diastolic BP accompanied by a 10% to 20% increase in heart rate indicates postural hypotension.[14] Should postural hypotension be present, care should be taken for the patient to accommodate changes in position through gradual adaptation to changes in position. Once the patient is able to assume the standing position without any symptoms of or objective measures indicating hypotension, then the patient can proceed with progressive distance ambulation.

An endurance evaluation is used to determine whether the patient is able to perform an activity for a prolonged period of time. During an endurance evaluation, the patient walks a predetermined circuit for 2 to 3 minutes, after which vital signs are taken while the patient is marching in place. During this time, the patient is also monitored for symptoms such as shortness of breath, lightheadedness, fatigue, fainting, and chest pain. In the absence of physiological changes or subjective complaints that warrant termination of the test, the patient continues for a series of 2- to 3-minute intervals of walking and monitoring. The evaluation ends when the patient's perceived exertion is rated as "somewhat hard" (13/20) using the Borg Rating of Perceived Exertion Scale. At the conclusion of the test, the distance walked by the patient is recorded as a baseline measure.[19]

Table 16-7

Signs and Symptoms of Respiratory Acidosis and Respiratory Alkalosis

Respiratory Acidosis	*Respiratory Alkalosis*
• Confusion • Disorientation • Dyspnea • Headache • Hypercapnea • Respiratory distress • Restlessness • Shallow respirations	• Blurred vision • Dizziness • Hypocapnea • Inability to concentrate • Muscle cramps • Muscle twitching and weakness • Numbness and tingling • Palpitations

Whereas an endurance evaluation is a symptom-limited measure of exercise capacity, the use of the 6-minute walk test is a time-limited, submaximal exercise test that provides an objective measure of functional exercise capacity. The test measures the distance that a patient can quickly walk in 6 minutes. During the administration of the test, the patient is monitored for symptoms similar to those identified in the endurance test. At the conclusion of the test, the distance covered is recorded as a baseline measure.

Stress testing provides information on how the heart functions during conditions of physical stress. Patients who are able to perform exercise stress tests (graded exercise tests) usually walk on a treadmill or pedal a bicycle. As the heart contracts harder and beats faster, its demand for oxygenated blood increases. However, in the presence of coronary artery disease, the narrowed arteries are unable to supply the needs of the heart, thereby resulting in symptoms such as angina, shortness of breath, and changes in the heart's rate, contraction, and rhythm. Because of myriad physiological responses taking place in response to physical stress, the patient is monitored using equipment and devices including an electrocardiogram to record and monitor changes in cardiac activity; a spirometer to record and monitor changes in breathing and gas exchange; a pulse oximeter to record and monitor oxygen saturation; and a sphygmomanometer to record and monitor changes in BP.[20] Additionally, the patient may be asked to respond to the level of effort or exertion being expended during the stress test using a perceived exertion scale, such as the Borg Rating of Perceived Exertion Scale.[21]

The Borg Rating of Perceived Exertion Scale goes from 6 ("minimal exertion") to 20 ("maximal exertion") and has been shown to correlate linearly with oxygen uptake and heart rate.[17] Perceived exertion ratings of 12 to 14 (13 is "somewhat hard") usually indicate a moderate level of intensity. This table can be found on the Centers for Disease Control and Prevention website (https://www.cdc.gov/physicalactivity/basics/measuring/exertion.htm).

Interventions

Physical therapist assistants provide physical therapy services under the direction and supervision of a physical therapist. The physical therapist assistant implements selected interventions, obtains data related to the interventions provided, and makes modifications within the plan of care to progress the patient or to maintain patient safety and comfort. When working with patients who are undergoing neurorehabilitation, the physical therapist assistant may be directed to implement interventions specific to impairments in body structure and function and activity limitations resulting from cardiovascular and pulmonary comorbidities that may interfere with or have an impact on the neurorehabilitation process. These may include breathing exercises, coughing exercises, chest mobilization exercises, respiratory resistance training, bronchial hygiene techniques, and aerobic exercise training.[1,12,13]

Breathing exercises have numerous purposes. Deep breathing exercises help promote chest expansion and ventilate underventilated areas of the lung. This is especially important with patients who are bedridden. Patients who have recently had chest surgery are also encouraged to perform deep breathing exercises; oftentimes, an incentive spirometer is used to promote sustained inspiration. Diaphragmatic breathing exercises help promote the use of the diaphragm instead of accessory muscles to minimize energy expenditure. Patients who use accessory muscles when breathing are taught to use the diaphragm to minimize the work of breathing. Pursed-lip breathing exercises help create backpressure in the airways to prevent them from closing prematurely. By expiring through pursed lips (such as when blowing a candle or whistling), expiration is prolonged. Because patients with COPD use accessory muscles and have air-trapping in the lung, they are often instructed to perform diaphragmatic breathing with pursed-lip expiration. Segmental breathing exercises help promote ventilation to underventilated areas; facilitation strategies, such as the use of tactile stimuli over the area to be ventilated, usually precede instructions to breathe into or toward the area of the tactile stimulus.

Research indicates that breathing exercises and ventilatory training alter both the rate and depth of breathing. However, despite using these breathing techniques as interventions, they do not impact alveolar oxygenation or gas exchange.

Coughing exercises help promote expectoration of mucus from the lower airways. Patients who are bedridden benefit from coughing exercises as a prophylactic intervention against pneumonia. Patients with pulmonary conditions that result in excessive secretions, such as chronic bronchitis or cystic fibrosis, also benefit from coughing exercises because coughing helps remove the secretions that are accumulating in the lungs. Finally, patients who have a weak cough, such as those with neuromuscular weakness or those who recently had chest surgery, benefit from coughing exercises for their prophylactic and therapeutic effects.

To perform an effective cough, a person should be able to inhale deeply, hold his or her breath momentarily, and expel the air forcefully. Sometimes, however, patients are unable to perform any or all of this sequence of events. Therefore, patients need to learn techniques that compensate for or facilitate coughing. Huffing is performed by forcefully exhaling air through an open airway.

For patients who are unable to perform an effective cough, huffing may be the first step in training the patient to do so. Self-assisted coughing is performed when the UEs are thrust inward and upward on the upper abdomen in Heimlich-like fashion. Another method of self-assisted coughing is by having the patient flex the trunk forward during the expulsive phase of the cough. With hands behind the neck, the patient doubles down on him- or herself in either the short-sitting or long-sitting positions. Patients who have weak abdominals, for example, can benefit from these examples of self-assisted coughing. During instances when a patient is unable to perform self-assisted coughing, therapist-assisted coughing is used. The hand of the therapist is placed over the upper abdomen and pushed upward and inward during the expulsive phase of the cough. Splinting is a coughing technique used by patients who have had chest surgery. By placing a towel or pillow over the surgery site, the patient is able to support and relieve the pressure on the suture during the cough.

Chest mobilization exercises help improve chest mobility by incorporating chest wall, trunk, and/or arm movements with breathing. For example, a patient whose trunk muscles are tight on one side, such as those with hemiplegia, may not expand that side of the trunk during inspiration. Another patient who manifests with a kyphotic posture and pectoral muscle tightness, such as seen among patients with Parkinson's disease, may not be able to retract the shoulders and extend the trunk during inspiration. In the former example, the patient may be instructed to perform side-bending and rotation exercises away from the side of tightness during inspiration. In the latter example, the patient may be instructed to perform bilateral UE flexion or horizontal abduction with trunk extension during inspiration.

Care should be exercised when performing chest or trunk mobilization exercises. Sometimes the patient's spine is purposely being exposed to conditions that would cause the spine to tighten to maintain an upright posture. The physical therapist assistant should continually confer with the physical therapist regarding questions or concerns about the plan of care.

Respiratory resistance training is used to strengthen and improve the endurance of respiratory muscles of patients who have weak abdominal and chest wall musculature. Patients with an SCI, for example, may have reduced respiratory function because of the weakness of the respiratory muscles around the chest and abdomen. By using respiratory resistance training flow devices, patients are able to strengthen the respiratory muscles. Respiratory resistance training flow devices provide a training stimulus by decreasing the diameter through which air flows, thereby increasing the resistance to it. Inspiratory resistance loading provides resistance on inspiration, while concurrent flow devices provide resistance on inspiration and expiration. Over time, the muscles become stronger and more efficient when breathing.[22,23]

Bronchial hygiene techniques consist of noninvasive airway-clearance techniques designed to facilitate gas exchange by mobilizing and clearing secretions from the airways. Bronchial hygiene techniques include postural drainage and manual techniques such as chest percussion, vibration, and shaking. Postural drainage involves placing the patient in positions that would allow the affected lung segments to be placed in the most vertical position, thereby allowing gravity to mobilize the secretions. Patients are required to assume the position for several minutes, after which they are instructed to cough voluntarily to expel any secretions that have been drained. To facilitate the mobilization of secretions, manual techniques may also be applied to the chest while the patient is in a postural drainage position. Percussion is performed by tapping on the chest over the lung segment being drained. After 2 to 3 minutes of chest percussion, vibration is applied while the patient exhales. In so doing, secretions that have been drained by positioning and/or percussion are moved centrally and superiorly for expectoration.

Aerobic exercise training is a hallmark of any cardiac or pulmonary rehabilitation program. Aerobic exercise training involves the exercising of large muscle groups for an extended period of time. Initially, the program may start at a low level and progress to a longer duration as the patient's cardiopulmonary fitness improves. An aerobic exercise program begins with a warm-up phase, followed by the aerobic phase, and finally a cool-down phase. The aerobic phase may involve continuous training, interval training, circuit training, or circuit-interval training. Continuous training requires sustained effort until the exercise has been completed. Interval training involves alternating sessions of exercise and recovery. Circuit training allows for the training of specific muscle groups as the patient moves through the various stations in the circuit. Circuit-interval training involves the use of stations to train specific muscle groups and to provide recovery. In developing the exercise program, the physical therapist should consider the following principles of exercise training—specificity, progression, overload, rest/recovery, and tedium (Table 16-8)—and apply them to the specific needs of the patient.[24,25]

When a patient is participating in an aerobic exercise training program, the physical therapist should determine baseline measures and tailor an appropriate program for

Table 16-8

Principles of Exercise Training

Specificity	The type of exercise chosen should be appropriate for the type of improvement expected.
Progression	Because the body adapts to exercise intensity, the amount and intensity of exercise should be increased gradually.
Overload	Fitness improves when workloads are greater than those normally encountered in daily life.
Reversibility	Any gains in physical fitness due to exercise can be reversed when physical activity ceases.
Tedium	A variety of exercises must be incorporated in a training program to prevent the onset of tedium.

the patient, including the duration, intensity, and frequency of the program. The physical therapist needs to determine acceptable parameters of physiological response, including heart rate, BP, and oxygen saturation, and communicate these to the physical therapist assistant. Concurrently, the physical therapist assistant needs to continually communicate with the physical therapist regarding the status of the patient, including progress toward established goals. During the treatment session, the physical therapist assistant should be able to recognize signs and symptoms of respiratory failure and cardiac decompensation, including dyspnea, angina, exercise intolerance, and others, and terminate the session as needed.

Conclusion

Physical therapist assistants provide physical therapy services under the direction and supervision of a physical therapist. When working with patients who are undergoing neurorehabilitation, the physical therapist assistant may be directed to implement interventions specific to impairments in structure and function, activity limitation, and participation restriction resulting from cardiovascular and pulmonary comorbidities that may interfere with or have an impact on the neurorehabilitation process. Toward this end, the physical therapist assistant should be familiar with the anatomy and physiology of the cardiovascular and pulmonary systems and the impact of neuromuscular pathologies on the cardiovascular and pulmonary systems, and vice versa. Additionally, the physical therapist assistant should be familiar with examination procedures and diagnostic tests that measure cardiovascular and pulmonary function. Finally, the physical therapist assistant should be able to implement selected interventions, obtain data related to the interventions provided, and make modifications within the plan of care to progress the patient or to ensure that patient safety and comfort are maintained.

Case Studies

Case #1

A 74-year-old patient sustained a stroke 3 days ago and is in acute care. The patient has type 2 diabetes and has a history of coronary artery disease. The medical record indicates that the patient has *dysarthria* (slurred speech) and requires thickened liquids as part of the meal. For the past 3 days, the patient has been bedridden and is just now getting out of bed. Before doing so, however, the physical therapist directs the physical therapist assistant to take the vital signs of the patient in supine, then in sitting on the side of the bed, and finally in standing.

Questions

1. What cardiovascular and pulmonary complications should the physical therapist assistant expect?
2. What is the rationale for monitoring vital signs in supine, sitting, and standing?
3. Is the information gathered from taking vital signs sufficient to progress the patient from one position to another? Why or why not?
4. When taking the vital signs, what parameters would be indicative of orthostatic hypotension?
5. How would the physical therapist assistant determine the patient's tolerance for the activity?

Case #2

A patient sustained an SCI at the level of T4 6 weeks ago. The patient is in inpatient rehab undergoing intensive physical therapy and occupational therapy. While performing wheelchair/mat transfers in the gym, the patient reports having a pounding headache. This is accompanied by redness of the face and upper body along with hypertensive readings on the sphygmomanometer.

Questions

1. Is the patient's current condition a medical emergency? Why or why not?
2. What steps should the physical therapist assistant take initially to address the patient's current condition?
3. What relationship, if any, does the patient's SCI have to do with his current condition?
4. Is there anything that the physical therapist assistant can do in the future to minimize the likelihood of events such as this?
5. What other cardiovascular and pulmonary complications should the physical therapist assistant expect?

References

1. Hillegass E. *Essentials of Cardiopulmonary Physical Therapy.* 4th ed. St. Louis, MO: Elsevier; 2017.
2. Claydon VE, Steeves JD, Krassioukov A. Orthostatic hypotension following spinal cord injury: understanding clinical pathophysiology. *Spinal Cord.* 2006;44(6):341-351. doi:10.1038/sj.sc.3101855
3. Whelton PK, Carey RM, Aronow WS, et al. 2017 ACC/AHA/AAPA/ABC/ACPM/AGS/APhA/ASH/ASPC/NMA/PCNA guideline for the prevention, detection, evaluation, and management of high blood pressure in adults: a report of the American College of Cardiology/American Heart Association task force on clinical practice guidelines. *Hypertension.* 2018;71(6):1269-1324. doi:10.1161/HYP.0000000000000066
4. Dewar R, Sykes D, Mulkerrin E, Nicklason F, Thomas D, Seymour R. The effect of hemiplegia on blood pressure measurement in the elderly. *Postgrad Med J.* 1992;68(805):888-891. doi:10.1136/pgmj.68.805.888
5. Uijen AA, Hassink-Franke LJA. Blood pressure measurement in hemiparetic patients: which arm? *Fam Med.* 2008;40(8):540.
6. Tovey C, Wyatt S. Diagnosis, investigation, and management of deep vein thrombosis. *BMJ.* 2003;326(7400):1180-1184. doi:10.1136/bmj.326.7400.1180
7. Wells PS, Anderson DR, Bormanis J, et al. Value of assessment of pretest probability of deep-vein thrombosis in clinical management. *Lancet.* 1997;350(9094):1795-1798. doi:10.1016/S0140-6736(97)08140-3
8. Thomas M, Decramer M, O'Donnell DE. No room to breathe: the importance of lung hyperinflation in COPD. *Prim Care Respir J.* 2013;22(1):101-111. doi:10.4104/pcrj.2013.00025
9. Corbridge SJ, Nyenhuis SM. Promoting physical activity and exercise in patients with asthma and chronic obstructive pulmonary disease. *J Nurse Pract.* 2017;13(1):41-46. doi:10.1016/j.nurpra.2016.08.022
10. Fleg JL. Improving exercise tolerance in chronic heart failure: a tale of inspiration? *J Am Coll Cardiol.* 2008;51(17):1672-1674. doi:10.1016/j.jacc.2008.01.027
11. Piña IL, Apstein CS, Balady GJ, et al; American Heart Association Committee on exercise, rehabilitation, and prevention. Exercise and heart failure: A statement from the American Heart Association Committee on exercise, rehabilitation, and prevention. *Circulation.* 2003;107(8):1210-1225. doi:10.1161/01.CIR.0000055013.92097.40
12. O'Sullivan SB, Schmitz TJ, Fulk GD. *Physical Rehabilitation.* 6th ed. Philadelphia, PA: FA Davis; 2014.
13. Frownfelter D, Dean E. *Cardiovascular and Pulmonary Physical Therapy Evidence to Practice.* 5th ed. St. Louis, MO: Elsevier Mosby; 2012.
14. Karnath B. Digital clubbing: a sign of underlying disease. *Hosp Physician.* 2003;39:25-27.
15. Higgins D. Patient assessment part 5—measuring pulse. *Nurs Times.* 2008;104(11):24-25.
16. American Association of Critical Care Nurses. *Oxygen Saturation Monitoring by Pulse Oximetry.* 4th ed. Philadelphia, PA: Saunders; 2001.
17. Goodman CC, Fuller KS. *Pathology Implications for the Physical Therapist.* 4th ed. St. Louis, MO: Saunders; 2014.
18. Acid-Base Regulation and Disorders. Merck Manuals Professional Edition. https://www.merckmanuals.com/professional/endocrine-and-metabolic-disorders/acid-base-regulation-and-disorders. Accessed May 14, 2018.
19. Barredo R. Phase I cardiac rehabilitation. In: Jobst EE. *Physical Therapy Case Files Acute Care.* 1st ed. McGraw-Hill Education; 2013.
20. National Heart Lung and Blood Institute. Stress Test. https://www.nhlbi.nih.gov/health-topics/stress-testing. Accessed May 14, 2018.
21. Shirely Ryan AbilityLab. Rating of Percieved Exertion: Borg Scales. https://www.sralab.org/sites/default/files/2018-04/Rating_of_perceived_exertion_-_Borg_scale.pdf. Accessed March 17, 2020.
22. Piepoli MF, Conraads V, Corrà U, et al. Exercise training in heart failure: from theory to practice. A consensus document of the Heart Failure Association and the European Association for Cardiovascular Prevention and Rehabilitation. *Eur J Heart Fail.* 2011;13(4):347-357. doi:10.1093/eurjhf/hfr017
23. Litchke LG, Russian CJ, Lloyd LK, Schmidt EA, Price L, Walker JL. Effects of respiratory resistance training with a concurrent flow device on wheelchair athletes. *J Spinal Cord Med.* 2008;31(1):65-71. doi:10.1080/10790268.2008.11753983
24. Powers SK, Dodd SL, Jackson EM. *Total Fitness & Wellness.* 6th ed. San Francisco, CA: Pearson; 2013.
25. Kisner C, Colby LA. *Therapeutic Exercise Foundations and Techniques.* 6th ed. Philadelphia, PA: FA Davis; 2012.

Chapter 17

The Role of the Physical Therapist Assistant in the Management of Clients With Lifelong Impairments and Activity Limitations Secondary to Neurological Conditions

Hazel Anderson, PT, DPT, cert. MDT; Germaine Ferreira, PT, DPT, MSPT, BHMS; and Amy Walters, PT, DPT, SCS, GCS

KEY WORDS Aging | Cerebral palsy | Post-polio syndrome | Rehabilitation | Spinal cord injury | Traumatic brain injury

Chapter Objectives

- Identify how aging affects populations with acquired and developmental neurological diagnoses.
- Identify the typical concerns specific for aging adults with cerebral palsy (CP), spinal cord injury (SCI), traumatic brain injury (TBI), and post-polio syndrome (PPS).
- Analyze the role of the physical therapist assistant in helping optimize mobility and function in aging adults with neurological diagnoses.
- Discuss the importance of environmental modifications, psychological issues, and weight management in the care of aging adults with neurological diagnoses.

As the lifespan increases, we understand the importance of physical therapy in the management of many of the conditions that are common with aging. In addition to assessing the impact of multiple comorbidities and polypharmacy on an aging patient, we must also consider chronic movement impairments that result from neurological diagnosis at a younger age, or the effects of aging and movement limitations when met with a medical diagnosis from a neurological impairment. Improvements in health care have resulted in patients with neurological diagnoses living longer, which increases the need for physical therapists and physical therapist assistants to be aware of the impact of aging on these individuals.

This chapter will discuss aging in patients with non-progressive developmental conditions, such as CP, and with neurological conditions acquired during the lifespan, such as SCIs, TBIs, and PPS. Specific considerations for these populations will be investigated and a discussion of common impairments that go along with these conditions as these individuals age will be presented.

Lazaro RT, Umphred DA, eds.
Umphred's Neurorehabilitation for the Physical Therapist Assistant, Third Edition (pp 387-398).

Cerebral Palsy and Aging

Background and Prevalence

With a prevalence of 2 to 3 incidents in every 1000 live births, CP is the most common physical disability affecting children.[1] Children with CP typically present with problems with ambulation, posture, and balance. This often results in low physical activity, as well as decreased muscular and bone strength.[1] In addition to motor dysfunction, these children also struggle with cardiorespiratory impairment, altered sensation and cognition, communication difficulties, and other comorbid conditions such as epilepsy.[2] (Refer to Chapter 9 for additional information.)

As the lifespan of the entire population has increased, so has the population of adults and the elderly with CP. The prevalence of CP has remained stable, and the life expectancy of these individuals is only slightly decreased relative to the non-disabled population. With these individuals living longer, they also have developed age-related impairments on top of the original movement imitations and resulting activity limitations.[2]

Concerns and Clinical Manifestations

While the original insult that causes CP is not progressive, this population often struggles with pain, fatigue, weakness, falls, contractures, and spasticity.[3] This results in decreased physical activity throughout both childhood and adulthood, leading to conditions such as osteoporosis, cardiovascular deconditioning, and musculoskeletal joint problems earlier than their age-related peers.[2]

Therapeutic Interventions

Therapeutic intervention for older adults with CP should focus on managing pain, improving balance to prevent falls, managing spasticity, decreasing joint stiffness, and prescribing appropriate exercises to maintain cardiovascular function and mobility, as well as those activities the individual values and wants to participate in.

Pain Management

Pain is one of the most common complaints of older adults with CP. Almost 75% of adults with CP report chronic pain that tends to increase over time.[4] Pain most commonly affects the lower body, with the most common locations being the low back (71%), hips (58%), legs (58%), and feet (54%).[5] A lifetime of struggling with pelvic obliquity, scoliosis, ankle/knee/hip abnormalities, and contractures is likely to blame for much of the pain.[6] Medical providers often overlook and undertreat this pain.[7]

Initial medical treatment of pain typically consists of pharmacological management. Botox injections, baclofen pumps, opioids, anticholinergics, and nonsteroidal anti-inflammatory drugs are commonly used to manage pain in this population.[6] Many of the oral medications used to manage spasticity and pain, such as benzodiazepines, dantrolene sodium, and tizanidine, produce sedative side effects that may be detrimental to an aging population due to an increased risk of falls.[6] While physical therapist assistants cannot change a patient's medication or offer advice regarding a medication regimen, it is important to notify your supervising therapist if you believe that a medication is causing a patient to have falls.

Non-pharmacological management of pain may include massage techniques, relaxation exercises, movement exercise, positioning, and use of modalities such as heat and cold. In surveys assessing the most effective pain management techniques, most patients with CP cite a preference for heat over ice, but either is appropriate.[5] Additionally, one of the best methods for managing pain is exercise, so encouraging patients to stay active and moving in whatever manner they can is beneficial. Patients struggling with balance and gait on land may still benefit from exercise in the form of body weight–support treadmill training to increase endurance and strength, aquatic therapy for buoyance and support, or community swimming. In addition to aerobic exercise, range of motion and strengthening exercises have also been found to help with pain.[5] For those unable to participate in an exercise program, appropriate positioning in a wheelchair or when sleeping can help manage pain by improving joint alignment.

General Exercise Information

While exercise may be encouraged as a pain management technique, there are other benefits as well. Exercise is important to counter the negative effects of immobility and inactivity that many patients with CP struggle with throughout their lives. When exercising with these patients, as with any other clients, it is important to challenge them enough to stimulate change. This can be achieved by increasing distance, time, or resistance with exercise.[3]

Types of exercise that have found to be beneficial with this population are interactive gaming activities for balance and ambulation with rhythmic auditory stimulation, which can be done on dry land or in an aquatic environment.[8] Other interventions that may be beneficial include whole-body vibration, treadmill training with and without body weight–support, dynamic balance and gait activities, and progressive resistance training. However, there is not a lot of reliable research to support the use of many of these interventions due to the complexity of studying a population that presents across such a broad spectrum of function.[8] Of the research that does exist, most of it has been performed on young adults and adolescents, so guidelines may need to be altered if a patient is more deconditioned or struggling with many comorbidities.

Strengthening

Strengthening throughout the lifespan is essential for individuals with CP to help with cardiovascular fitness and to decrease functional decline. Strength training was previously avoided with this population due to a fear of increasing spasticity, but current research supports that strengthening is not detrimental to spasticity and may even improve it.[9] Strengthening should generally focus on the lower body with attention on the plantar flexors to aid balance.[10] Plantar flexor strength in patients with CP was found to be less than half of that of a traditionally developing adult.[10]

Strength training should ideally align with American College of Sports Medicine guidelines with a frequency of 2 to 3 times/week, with 2 to 4 sets of 10 to 12 reps, and a duration of 8 to 12 weeks.[11] However, a large number of these individuals may not be accustomed to strength training, so may need a more gradual transition with low-dosage training for several weeks and a longer duration of 12 to 16 weeks.[9]

Patients struggling with gripping weights may benefit from aids such as flexion mitts, straps or wrist and ankle weights with Velcro (Velcro) straps.[12] To avoid aggravating spasticity, it is better to start with less intense and longer duration exercise sessions.[12] Individuals with CP should be encouraged to develop a lifelong engagement in strengthening to improve or maintain mobility.

Stretching

Stretching should also be general but must address the lower extremities, specifically plantar flexors, to target ankle joint stiffness, gait, and balance.[10] Stretching and flexibility training is especially important for individuals with spastic CP. Full range of motion may not be possible, but individuals should still work within the range available. It is best to warm the muscles with aerobic activity before stretching, then hold stretches for 30 to 60 seconds.[12] Timing is important, as stretching during a cool-down may decrease the incidence of spasticity stimulated by the workout. Further techniques to avoid spasticity include focusing on slow and controlled movements to avoid activating a stretch reflex. If patients have difficulty stretching on land, stretching in a warm pool may be a better alternative.[12] Wheelchair-bound patients should pay particular attention to gaining flexibility in the chest and shoulders as well as the hip flexors due to being in a prolonged seated position. (Refer to Chapter 18 on complementary approaches for additional ideas of activities that will lead to strength and greater flexibility.)

Cardiorespiratory Endurance Training

Aerobic exercise is essential in increasing cardiorespiratory endurance in individuals with CP who are aging. If adults with CP are deconditioned, starting with 1 to 2 training sessions/week may be appropriate, with a goal of increasing to 2 to 4 sessions.[9] These sessions should last for at least 20 minutes and should ideally follow American College of Sports Medicine guidelines with an intensity of 64% to 95% of the maximum heart rate.[9] The exercise should be continuous and rhythmic, such as swimming, propelling a wheelchair, performing upper extremity ergometry, stair training, walking, or running.[9] In adults and especially older adults who use wheelchairs, swimming or aquatic therapy can be beneficial not only for the cardiovascular system, but also for the integumentary system, due to the change in position that it provides.[6]

Balance and Gait Training

Balance problems, postural imbalances, and gait dysfunction present from an early age in individuals with CP but will progress with the natural decline of the central nervous system and musculoskeletal system with aging, as occurs in the general population. This increased balance dysfunction may result in increased falls.[13] Preventing falls is paramount for any age individual with CP, but especially the elderly, as many of these patients have an earlier onset of osteoporosis from a lifetime of inactivity. It is crucial to implement static and dynamic exercises to improve both balance and gait. Also, stretching and strengthening of the plantar flexors may prove helpful in improving balance, but individuals with CP may ultimately need assistive devices such as a cane or walker if fall risk is high. Part of balance training and fall prevention with these patients should include education on how to get up off the floor in the event of a fall. Encouraging individuals to participate in community-based activities as adults that also tend to improve strength, flexibility, and endurance while encouraging social interactions should always be part of the physical therapist assistant's toolbox of recommendations for these individuals as they age.

Home Modifications

Home safety checklists allow a family member or caregiver to do a room-by-room assessment for potential safety concerns. These safety checks may need to be implemented earlier in individuals with CP due to earlier onset of osteoporosis and musculoskeletal problems. Inspections should include checking for grab bars in the shower and near toilets, putting fall monitoring systems in place for those that may not be able to get up off the floor after a fall, and checking for other risk factors such as poor lighting and loose throw rugs which may increase the occurrence of falls.

Conclusion

While there is not, to date, much research on physical therapy interventions for older adults with CP, many of these individuals will benefit from the same exercise and pain management techniques that physical therapist assistants employ to aid any aging population. However, the impact of aging may be seen earlier in this population due to a lifetime of reduced physical activity, movement limitations due to central nervous system damage, and musculoskeletal dysfunction. The pain and functional movement decline resulting from these conditions could be minimized by addressing the complications of CP not only in childhood but also throughout adulthood. Encouraging lifelong engagement with physical exercise might help these individuals stay active into their later years.

While there is not much evidence-based research on treating an older adult with CP, providers should consider the individual's knowledge and experience with their disability when developing a treatment program. Being respectful of and considering an individual's personal experience with their condition may be more important than the practitioner's knowledge of that condition.[2]

Spinal Cord Injury and Aging

Background and Prevalence

There are estimated to be 17,000 new cases of SCI every year in the United States.[14] Approximately 300,000 people with SCIs live in the United States currently. In the 1970s, an SCI was thought to commonly affect the healthy, active young adult males, with an average age of approximately 28.7 years at the time of injury. As the American population has aged, we have seen a shift in the average age at the time of injury from 37.1 years from 2005 to 2008, to 42 years in the 2010s.[14,15] Females too are affected, but it is predominantly a condition affecting males with approximately 80% new cases affecting men.[14]

Advancement in emergency medical care, acute care treatments, medical management, and rehabilitation have helped more individuals survive an SCI.[14,16] Mortality is the highest in the first year after an SCI, with fatalities being worst in individuals needing ventilator support.[14] No matter the level of the SCI, individuals are living with long-term disabilities.[16] The life expectancy of SCI patients has increased over the last decades. However, it is still less than the life expectancy of a normal healthy individual without an SCI. A 20-year-old healthy individual without SCI has a life expectancy of 78.6 years, compared to a 20-year SCI patient with an incomplete injury, who has a life expectancy of 72.6 years, or a 20-year-old SCI patient with complete paraplegia, who has a life expectancy of 65.2 years.[15]

The human body reaches its maximal function by age 25, following which there is a 1% decline in function every year.[14] As the SCI population starts to age, it has been noted that there is accelerated aging of an SCI individual. Immediately after an SCI, there is an increased functional and metabolic decline, which later stabilizes, allowing the aging process to continues normally.[14-16] The decreased secretion of human growth hormone following an SCI has been hypothesized to contribute to the premature aging noted in the SCI patient.[14] (Refer to Chapter 11 for a more thorough discussion.)

Common Disease Considerations

Cardiovascular diseases are commonly seen to be prematurely developing in the SCI population. Cardiovascular disease is the leading cause of death in these patients.[17] The common preventable risk factors such as smoking, sedentary lifestyle, and obesity need to be addressed in this population, especially since these individuals have an underlying neurologic disorder that amplifies metabolic changes related to inactivity.[14,16,17] Post-SCI patients commonly develop cardiometabolic syndrome, which presents with hypertension, obesity, insulin resistance, and a decrease in high-density lipoprotein.[18] Poor diet, decreased activity, and increased caloric intake further contribute to the aggravation of cardiovascular health.[14] C-reactive protein and homocysteine values that are good predictors of vascular disease are noted to be high in patients post-SCI.[14] Physical therapist assistants and the rehab team should educate patients with SCIs about these risk factors and encourage daily exercise and good heart-healthy nutrition. Many patients with SCIs desire to exercise but do not have access to a gym because of mobility issues, physical barriers, financial issues, and psychological concerns about the exercise being difficult.[14] Physical therapy can work with these patients to get them to be confident about the recommended exercise program to ensure compliance. Physical therapists working closely with social workers to address other barriers can help promote an active lifestyle with SCI patients. Regular cardiovascular fitness is a vital part of rehabilitation and should be tailored to be patient-specific depending on the level of injury.[15]

Patients with higher-level SCIs on ventilatory support have increased mortality within the first year.[17] Pulmonary problems are one of the leading causes of death both in the early years and later in the life of the aging SCI patient. A crucial part of physical therapy is reeducating and reminding these patients about proper breathing techniques and coughing techniques to prevent respiratory episodes that can be fatal at any age. As these patients age, it is important to revisit diaphragmatic breathing, self-assisted coughing to clear secretions, and respiratory muscle strengthening with inspiratory muscle devices.[15] The physical therapist assistant may be asked to work with an individual who has been hospitalized due to respiratory pathologies who also in the past suffered a SCI. In this case, the physical therapist assistant must again reemphasize the importance of diaphragmatic breathing and the importance of maintaining pulmonary function throughout the lifespan.

The aging SCI patients may report increased fatigue and decreased strength due to muscular changes such as atrophy, increased adipose tissue in the muscle, muscle imbalance, and the aging nervous system. These patients report shoulder complications from overuse injuries during transfers and wheelchair mobility.[15] Imbalance in the innervation of different shoulder muscles can contribute to the degeneration of the glenohumeral joint.[14] Physical therapy can address safety with transfers, mobility, use of devices to ensure maximal independence, and help protect joint integrity with the aging patient with a SCI.[14]

There is little research to show that there is an increase or decrease in the neuropathic pain related the SCI patients as they age. These patients will continue to have neuropathic pain following the SCI, and that needs to be addressed and managed. New treatment approaches will be developed throughout the individual's lifetime and keeping informed of current research and available adaptive devices that might enhance the quality of life of individuals with SCI should be part of both the physical therapist's and physical therapist assistant's role in educating patients.

Home Modifications

With increased age, there is often a decline in the independence of individual's daily life activities. This is no different with the SCI patient. As the SCI patient who already has limited independence ages, these functional limitations can further limit social interaction and impact the quality of life.[14] The premature aging seen in SCI patients may require early planning to consider home environment modifications before rushing to find nursing home placement.[14,15] Additional adaptive equipment to address the progression of dependence, safety features, the need for more nursing care and therapy should be discussed with all patients, their family, and the rehabilitation team. These patients often have a decline in renal function 4 to 5 years after the SCI injury, which may require long-term care placement.[15] When working with these patients, be vigilant and educate them to recognize early signs of urologic problems and minimize the risk factors that lead to system problems and additional health care issues.

Conclusion

Independence and employment affect the quality of life of the patient post-SCI, although the Americans With Disabilities Act has opened up many barriers. But the effects of premature aging in the SCI patient can impact when and if an individual needs to stop working. These potential problems need to be addressed early in the post-injury stages to help these patients cope.[14,15] It is important to have a holistic approach when dealing with an individual who is aging with a preexisting SCI. While physical therapy addresses the physical impairments and functional limitations related to aging, careful consideration should be paid to the social, psychological, and financial concerns that affect these patients as well.

Traumatic Brain Injury and Aging

Background and Prevalence

A TBI occurs when there is damage to the brain tissue from a force outside the cranium that results in disruption in brain function, loss of consciousness, and post-traumatic amnesia with or without changes in brain pathology.[19,20] Approximately 1.7 million people in the United States suffer a TBI annually.[19,21] We need to be able to treat and meet the rehabilitation needs of this growing TBI population. The TBI population comprises those who sustained a TBI as a child, those who suffered one as a young adult, and the growing number of elderly who succumb to a TBI. The younger population most affected by TBI are those between the age group of 0 and 5 years old and those between 15 and 25 years old.[19] The growing geriatric TBI population is due to the active elderly population.[20,21] The leading cause of TBI in those over 65 years of age is a fall.[6-8] A TBI in those over 65 results in higher rates of hospitalization.[19,20,22] The number of TBI cases rises significantly in individuals above the age of 85 years of age.[20] Individuals older than 55 years of age at the time of TBI typically have a more extended rehabilitation stay and a lower rate of change or function at discharge on the Functional Independence Measure score.[23] The impact of the TBI is not just felt by the patients and their families, but also impacts the economy as a whole.[19,21]

Following a TBI, a significant focus during acute care and rehabilitation is to prevent secondary complications associated with skin breakdown, immobilization, and development of contractures. With the older patient who suffers a TBI and with an aging patient who received the TBI as a younger person, the focus of rehabilitation has to shift towards comorbidities such as diabetes mellitus, osteoarthritis, cardiovascular issues, and visual deficits.[19,20,21] (Refer to Chapter 12 for an additional discussion.)

Management Considerations for People Aging With a Traumatic Brain Injury

A patient with a TBI, like any other person who ages, may start to have new movement problems related to the already compromised gait and transfers. The physical therapy team can work with these patients on gait modifications and the need for different assistive devices, and readdress gait training and transfer training.[23]

A longitudinal follow-up study on patients following a TBI showed that after 10 years post-TBI, these patients were reporting greater irritability, difficulty in motor planning, and fatigue upon movement. Some of these patients reported additional cognitive and emotional problems.[24] However, these cognitive and emotional problems were not attributed to aging, but rather to the fact that the TBI population with the time elapsed since the injury, were more aware of these problems they were experiencing.[24] As we work with the patients following TBI to address mobility and improve safety, therapists must become aware of signs of social isolation so the interdisciplinary team can address these issues. These problems can develop at any time throughout the lifespan, and will often result in reduced participation in leisure activities, which further culminates in social isolation.

Patients with a TBI can often present early with agitation, pain, insomnia, depression and behavioral issues for which they may be on psychotic medications.[19,21] These medications, and medications prescribed for comorbidities seen in the aging TBI patient, can affect the patient's ability to participate in therapy as well as future life participation.[19] There needs to be good communication among physical therapist assistants, the supervising therapist, and the rest of the interdisciplinary team to address the effects of polypharmacy on the patient's ability to optimize the physical therapy sessions, and how that might affect life activities as the individual ages. There should be good communication among the health care providers working with the patient and support system to determine if these symptoms are due to polypharmacy or a cognitive decline and will be expected to increase with general aging.

Head trauma, as seen in a TBI, can increase the risk for neurodegenerative diseases such as Parkinson's disease (see Chapter 14).[25] Patients with a TBI have elevated levels of amyloid beta plaques that are commonly seen in neurodegenerative diseases.[19,21] These patients have a higher risk of developing early-age-onset Alzheimer's disease.[19] After a TBI, the brain tissue undergoes progressive atrophy, which is further accelerated by the aging process.[21] Following a TBI, neuroendocrine disorders such as chronic growth hormone deficiency, hypothyroidism, and hypogonadism may follow, due to dysfunction of the hypothalamic-pituitary function.[21] The patient with a TBI may have comorbidities associated with aging such as diabetes, hypertension, and cardiovascular diseases. Diabetes mellitus may result in neuropathies affecting mobility in this already-compromised population.[21]

Older patients with a TBI often present with orthostatic hypotension.[19] Orthostatic hypotension is often a contributor to falls, which further increases the risk for these patients to suffer physical injuries as well as potential additional TBIs. The physical therapy team working with these patients should focus on slow transitioning of movement, use of compression stockings, use of abdominal binders, and interaction with the interdisciplinary team about these concerns. The medical team should address the overuse of medications, which may be contributing to orthostatic hypotension.[19]

Home Modifications

Patients following a TBI are at risk for falls, as are the elderly, so extra steps should be taken to educate the patient and caregivers on fall-prevention. Checking the room for unnecessary lines and tubes that may be an obstacle to safe mobility, use of low beds and padded floor mats, proper sleep hygiene routines to minimize waking up at night, and correct eyewear can help reduce the risk for falls.[21]

Like any other geriatric patient who may need assistive devices, patients following a TBI may be more dependent on assistive devices as they start to age. One needs to be aware of the sensitivity to loud noises that affect these patients.[24] Caution must be exerted when using tools such as bed alarms and chair alarms that produce a loud noise that can further aggravate the irritability of these patients or startle them as they move from one position to another.

These patients often experience visual disturbances such as difficulty with detecting low-contrast hazards, judging distance, and navigating spatial relationships.[21,24] As these symptoms can also be associated with aging, the patient and support systems need to be monitoring these behaviors. As this population ages, there is a need not to underplay the fact that these patients may have visual disturbances related to the TBI and to the aging process that can compromise safety with mobility. Patients with a TBI, no matter the age, may need more than visual cues to lock the brakes on their wheelchair or walker. Adequate room lighting and use of nightlights for patients who are independent of toileting can minimize falls from poor vision. Educating the caregiver of these concerns can decrease the irritability and behavioral issues these patients will experience.

Conclusion

Despite the shortage of studies available on the impact of aging on the TBI population, we must treat all patients holistically and recognize that patients with a history of TBI may report symptoms not typical of a geriatric patient.[22] Further research studies will help us understand if these clinical presentations are part of the aging process in these patients, or if they have nothing to do with the fact that they experienced a TBI. The long-term rehabilitation of patients with TBI should continue to address mobility, cognitive, psychological, and behavioral problems that this population will face.[24] Having them engage in social activities that encourage physical participation will help to maintain their functional skill as they age.

Post-Polio Syndrome and Aging

Background and Prevalence

Acute paralytic poliomyelitis (polio), caused by the polio virus, is a crippling and potentially deadly, infectious disease that selectively attacks lower motor neurons.[26,27] It can invade an infected person's brain and spinal cord, causing asymmetrical, flaccid muscular paralysis.[27-29] PPS, often occurring many years if not decades after the initial illness, is a specific neurological disorder characterized by progressive or new muscle weakness and lack of endurance, cold intolerance, profound fatigue, and pain at rest or during activities.[30] In 2016, 15 to 20 million polio survivors were estimated to be alive worldwide, with almost 573,000 of those residing in the United States.[30] The physiologic cause of PPS is not well understood; however, a widely accepted hypothesis is based on the deterioration of overused motor units that have accommodated orphaned muscle fibers since the initial recovery period from the infection.[31] Individuals in the acute phase of polio were taught to work hard, strengthen the system through exercise, and push themselves to functional movement even though they were weak and easily fatigued. So a behavior was taught that with weakness or fatigue, one should exercise more. Individuals with PPS experience a different time course than most others who age with neurological diagnoses, with early disability, a period of recovery or stability, and then a later onset of new weakness that needs to be addressed with energy conservation and not work hardening.[31] The effects of PPS are compounded by the fact that the population presenting with PPS is predominantly elderly, having acquired polio in their early years, and, consequently, have developed comorbidities and normal effects of aging that compound the functional problems and need to be considered.[32]

Concerns, Diagnosis, and Clinical Manifestations

Halstead and Gawne identified key symptoms of PPS as new or amplified muscle weakness, fatigue, and muscle/joint pain with neuropathic electromyographic changes in an individual with a previous positive diagnosis of polio.[32] Other symptoms may include difficulty breathing, voice changes, problems with swallowing, and sleep disorders and falls.[25,27,31] Due to the lack of certainty surrounding the cause of PPS and the overlap of normal aging processes, no conclusive test exists to diagnose the late effects of polio or PPS. Currently, it is a diagnosis of exclusion. The criteria most commonly used for establishing a medical diagnosis of PPS were developed by Halstead and Weicher,[33] and include a previous history of paralytic polio in childhood or teenage years; partial to complete muscle strength and functional recovery; a period of at least 15 years of neurological and functional recovery; slow onset of new muscle weakness, generalized whole-body and muscular fatigue, and muscle atrophy; and no other medical, orthopedic, or neurological conditions to explain these new health problems.[33]

Considerations, Treatment, and Management of Post-Polio Syndrome

Physical therapy examination and management for PPS is challenging due to the complex nature of the condition. Intervention design should take a multisystem, holistic approach and emphasize optimizing and maintaining activity and participation while protecting the residual motor units from additional degeneration.[34-36] Therapeutic interventions should focus on managing pain and fatigue, energy conservation, and pacing strategies, as well as a customized strengthening, stretching, and aerobic exercise program to promote optimal function and correct posture where possible.[37]

Cardiopulmonary assessment and interventions must be included in the management priorities. Functional mobility training and gait training using appropriate assistive devices and orthotics (with a reassessment of these as needed) will be necessary as part of the goal of conserving energy. To this end, fall consideration and education to avoid the risk of this should be incorporated.[30,35] By using energy conservation early the individual may stay functionally independent for a long time as they age.

Pain Management

Chronic muscle and joint pain of varying severity often affect PPS patients, with more than 65% of individuals with PPS reporting neck, shoulder, and back pain radiating to the hip and leg.[38,39] Interventions for pain are further complicated by osteoporosis, lack of compensatory substitutions to rest the injured part, and often, a modest response to exercise. Unsuccessful joint fusions, limb size differences, progressive scoliosis, poor posture, and abnormal mechanics may also contribute to pain.[40] The deep, aching pain described[37] is worsened by physical activity, stress, and cold temperature, and frequently interferes with sleep.[35,36,38,40] Interestingly, the pain normally occurs 1 to 2 days after the triggering event and is rarely associated with inflammation. Joint pain usually results primarily from long-term microtrauma from abnormal biomechanical forces. An example is an overuse of the shoulder girdle from years of Loftstrand (Lofstrand Labs) crutch use to compensate for lower-extremity impairments after polio. Pain due to progressive skeletal deformities such as scoliosis and joint deterioration is also common.

Medical interventions have been investigated for their effectiveness in alleviating signs and symptoms of PPS. Intravenous immunoglobulin therapy has shown promising results in reducing pain, improving quality of life, and possibly increasing strength.[27,41] Lamotrigine (an anticonvulsant drug) may improve quality of life, reduce pain, fatigue and muscle cramps in this population but larger trials are needed to validate these findings.[37,42] Amitriptyline is recommended to improve sleep.[34] Nonsteroidal anti-inflammatories and analgesics such as acetaminophen are most frequently prescribed when rest and rehabilitation do not provide enough relief.[37] Steroid injection and, rarely, surgery may also be indicated to improve joint stability and thus decrease pain.[34,36]

Non-pharmacological management of pain may include the use of physical agent modalities and electrotherapy as appropriate.[36] Transcutaneous electrical nerve stimulation may also assist in strengthening weakened muscles and reducing pain although overuse must be monitored. Magnet therapy (applied over trigger points) has also been found to alleviate symptoms, although more research is required in this area.[37] Other techniques to manage pain and maintain joint health may include the use of ergonomic equipment such as elevated chairs and bathtub/shower stools. Advice for alleviating pain in the neck and upper body include seating and workstation adaptations, headsets, rolling carts for carrying items, adjustable computer screens, wrist pads, and ergonomic keyboards.

Rehabilitation Strategies and Adaptive Equipment/Gait Aids

Education and training are important parts of the plan of care for patients with PPS. Patients need to be aware of pacing or grading activities, means of modifying their lifestyles, and how to employ possible energy-conserving techniques to reduce overall exhaustion and overuse injuries.[30,36] General lifestyle changes, including weight control, modification of daily activities, and elimination of unnecessary activities are encouraged to reduce fatigue. Specific recommendations for activities of daily living include scheduling regular rest periods during the day as well as taking frequent breaks during taxing activities, especially when (or ideally before) feeling fatigued. Rotating difficult chores and breaking tasks down into more manageable components has also been shown to be beneficial for decreasing fatigue and pain in PPS.[30] Furthermore, alternating activities requiring different muscular regions of the body and different energy requirements is another method of energy conservation, and this can be done in 15 to 30 minute periods (work-rest intervals) until all activities are completed.[30,43] Exploring more efficient ways of performing necessary occupational activities may also assist persons with PPS to manage their symptoms and optimize function.

Use of assistive devices and equipment in appropriate patients may allow better, safer functioning and an ability to ambulate at work or in the home. An occupational therapy examination is often helpful to this end. Incorporating the use of aids like stair glides, grab bars, raised toilet seats, adapted utensils, and other home modifications may also be suggested. A small study using bioceramic fabrics in clothes and mattresses for patients with PPS has also shown promising results (including relief from cold intolerance, pain relieving, and anti-inflammatory properties), but require further study.[44]

Gait and mobility aids, such as canes, walkers, wheelchairs (powered or manual), or scooters, may be handy for patients with PPS, by optimizing functioning and mobility, providing energy conservation, and pacing. As well, the use of these devices may reduce a PPS patient's self-reported level of fatigue.[45] Recommendation for the aid required is unique to each patient and dependent on their work/leisure needs and environment. A physical therapy assessment is required for gait aid trials and fitting a wheelchair to the patient.[46]

Recommendations for mobility aids can be emotionally upsetting to many individuals with PPS because they worked so hard during the acute phase of polio to prevent the need for such aids. Thus, the patient needs to be an active participant in this discussion and final decisions. Patients should never be pushed to fatigue no matter the motivation of the individual to work on function. After exercising, the patient should regain strength from an exercise quickly. Lingering fatigue is contraindicated and may cause more damage to the nervous system. Patients should be taught energy conservation whenever possible no matter if the individual is still working or is homebound. That is, if a patient has to walk from a parking lot to the office and then once at the office does not have the energy to walk the rest of the day, a therapist might recommend using a mobility aid such as a scooter to get from the car to the office, and then the patient can walk around the work place without fatigue. The patient should be making those decisions or choices as to what to participate in and where to conserve energy throughout the day.

Orthotic Intervention

Orthotic interventions, such as ankle-foot orthoses (AFOs) or knee-ankle-foot orthoses and even hip-knee-ankle-foot orthoses may be beneficial for patients to improve balance, mobility, and ambulation.[36] In patients who are at high fall risk, orthoses may be particularly helpful if the bracing can support the weak musculature causing the falls. A knee-ankle-foot orthosis may be recommended if the falls are due to knee-buckling or giving way of the knee secondary to quadriceps weakness. AFOs are excellent for falls as a result of foot drop, dorsiflexor weakness, or tripping over toes. In those with weak calf muscles, a dorsiflexion-restricting ankle-foot orthosis may be beneficial for enhancing gait biomechanics, speed, and patient's confidence with ambulation.[47] Use of light carbon fiber as compared with usual thermoplastic and metal materials reduces the weight by about a third, but is more costly.[48] Reducing the weight may reduce fatigue, overuse of muscle power and help to maintain function for a longer time. These carbon fiber knee-ankle-foot orthoses have demonstrated they improve gait efficiency, reduce oxygen consumption, and generally are much less energy-demanding for PPS survivors to use regularly when compared with no orthoses or conventional options.[49]

Exercise

The literature clearly documents the benefits of physical activity for those with PPS, and compliance with an appropriate individualized program must be emphasized.[35] There is concern that high-intensity exercises may cause overuse injury, but non-fatiguing exercises with adequate rest periods between sets for muscles with a fair plus grade (3+/5) or higher is reported to be safe and beneficial for improvement of overall functional performance and reduction in pain.[30,35,36] Weakness in PPS patients can occur in both previously affected and unaffected muscles; however, it is mainly observed in those muscles most affected by the initial infection.[50] According to the literature, the lower limbs and particularly the muscles supplied by the L4 and L5 spinal segments are the most commonly involved, and of these, the quadriceps, hip adductors and tibialis anterior are most often affected.[51] In the upper limb, the deltoid, followed by the elbow flexors and extensors, and opponents pollicis, will be affected most frequently.[52]

Strengthening

As far as strengthening exercise regimes, research on specific methods is varied. However, several 6- to 12-week supervised training programs (3 to 4 times/week) including isometric, isokinetic, and endurance muscle training have resulted in statistically significant increases in strength, improved fatigue and pain levels, and a better quality of life.[53,54] Furthermore, in comparison to healthy geriatric patients, those with PPS were weaker at the start, and their improvements in strength were better with no adverse effects on motor unit survival.[25,55] As far as more specific guidelines, subjects in a Canadian study performed 3 sets of 8 reps for 3 to 5 seconds of voluntary contractions. The training load was started at a low level of 50% maximal voluntary contraction to reduce the risk of overuse. As long as subjects made or exceeded the target load, repetitions were slowly progressed by 10% per week but limited to no more than 70% maximal voluntary contraction.[56] Another earlier study, focusing on dynamic knee extension exercises (aimed at strengthening the frequently affected quadriceps muscles), progressed the program based on the rating of perceived exertion after 12 reps. If the rating was less than 19 (corresponding to "very, very hard") at that point, the weight, used at the ankle in this case, was increased by 0.5 pound to 1 pound for the next visit. No problems or adverse effects were noted by subject or on the muscles affected.[57] Importantly, most studies agree that non-fatiguing strengthening exercises be interspersed with rest intervals, and that different muscle groups should be trained on alternate days to avoid overuse and decline in muscle function.[30,53,54,58]

Whole body vibration training has also been considered as an alternative to resistance training in these individuals and has shown in small studies to show improvement in walking speed and pain levels although no significant change has been noted in muscle strength.[59] Larger, randomized, controlled studies are required to determine this intervention's ability to benefit patients with PPS, but it is always recommended that the therapist pay close attention to the patient's level of fatigue and recognize when to stop prior to muscle power giving out.

Stretching and Range of Motion Exercises

While no high-quality research studies have been performed, use of rehabilitation principles for passive stretching and passive range of motion exercises that are similar to those used in other neuromuscular diseases seem sensible.[60] These methods, combined with splinting, may be beneficial for preventing and slowing the progression of milder contractures in PPS patients.[60] However, sometimes, compensatory contractures may develop and benefit patients by stabilizing joints with surrounding muscle weakness, and in these cases, stretching would not be indicated. A comprehensive physical therapist evaluation and ongoing examination are necessary before performing any stretching interventions in each muscle region.[30]

Cardiopulmonary Conditioning

Cardiovascular conditioning is an essential part of the management of individuals with PPS.[61,62] Aerobic exercise such as walking, use of a bicycle ergometer, or swimming are recommended, but the client must be interested in the activity to increase long-term compliance. Regarding specific parameters, the 20% rule has been recommended.[63] Once a patient's exercise capacity is determined, the patient performs the exercise at 20% of this level 3 to 4 times/week for 30 days, and gradually increases in 10% increments. An example may be cycling, where a patient could do it for 1 hour at max speed, and therefore is asked to do just 12 minutes 4 days/week for 1 month, and then increase by 6 minutes the following month.[36] As mentioned, aquatic therapy is also highly recommended. A Swedish study suggested that non-swimming dynamic exercise in warm water may be beneficial because it decreases the biomechanical stresses on the muscles and joints, and a subjective positive response was reported.[64] This same study recommended that any similar program is done more than twice a week to see objective improvement in aerobic capacity.[64] These individuals, similar to all aging individuals, will lose muscle power over time. Individuals with PPS loss will often seem quicker and more devastating than their aging counterparts. As is true with all elderly individuals, having a support system around them that helps them deal with these losses can help maintain dignity and a quality of life no matter their respective functional capabilities.

Clinical Pearls

- Ensure careful consultation with PPS patient and adhere to an individualized program.
- Avoid overuse of any muscle groups, especially those initially affected by poliomyelitis.
- Include adequate warm-up and cool-down periods.
- Guard patient appropriately while performing exercises to minimize the risk of falls.

- Encourage short periods of activity with adequate rest periods.
- Alternate days for full recovery of individual muscle groups.
- Educate patient on energy conservation and joint protection techniques.
- Encourage incorporating breathing, relaxation, mental imagery, and meditation into daily activities.

Other Considerations

Psychological (Coping)

The psychosocial issues challenging aging persons with PPS are often more disruptive than the physical problems due to an increasing loss of independence and an inability to perform previous personal and societal roles. There is no one specific method of addressing this, but individuals should be encouraged to become involved in PPS support groups and seek professional counseling when necessary.[35]

Weight Management

Obesity is a challenge in this population, especially with added effects of aging and comorbidities. Education on weight control/reduction is appropriate to help alleviate stress and strain on the muscles and joints that occur with heavier individuals.

At the moment, no cure exists for PPS, and the effects of aging along with PPS do impact these patients, although there is limited evidence on the exact experience of aging with PPS.[30,65] However, this population can be managed very successfully with the correct treatment strategies, adequate education and counseling, rehabilitative equipment and gait aids, orthotics, and most important, exercise recommendations. It is essential to take care in examining and working with these patients to develop individualized approaches to their care.

Conclusion

This chapter identifies the fact that aging causes physical changes that often lead to functional loss. Those losses occur regardless of insults that might have occurred over a lifetime. Individuals with prior central nervous system damage such as birth insults, trauma from head or spinal injuries, or development of PPS often find the aging experience more difficult and challenging. Empowering individuals to the function they have and can maintain will play a critical role in quality of life as those individuals age. These individuals need to decide what activities they want to participate in and how best to maintain their function. A physical therapy program with little carryover in the future by the individual will have little effect on maintaining function, so active participation and decision-making needs to place the patient at the center of the process.

References

1. Whitney DG, Hurvitz EA, Devlin MJ, et al. Age trajectories of musculoskeletal morbidities in adults with cerebral palsy. *Bone*. 2018;114:285-291. doi:10.1016/j.bone.2018.07.002
2. Mudge S, Rosie J, Stott S, Taylor D, Signal N, McPherson K. Ageing with cerebral palsy; what are the health experiences of adults with cerebral palsy? A qualitative study. *BMJ Open*. 2016;6(10):e012551. doi:10.1136/bmjopen-2016-012551
3. Turk MA. Health, mortality, and wellness issues in adults with cerebral palsy. *Dev Med Child Neurol*. 2009;51(suppl 4):24-29. doi:10.1111/j.1469-8749.2009.03429.x
4. Benner JL, Hilberink SR, Veenis T, Stam HJ, van der Slot WM, Roebroeck ME. Long-term deterioration of perceived health and functioning in adults with cerebral palsy. *Arch Phys Med Rehabil*. 2017;98(11):2196-2205.e1. doi:10.1016/j.apmr.2017.03.013
5. Hirsh AT, Kratz AL, Engel JM, Jensen MP. Survey results of pain treatments in adults with cerebral palsy. *Am J Phys Med Rehabil*. 2011;90(3):207-216. doi:10.1097/PHM.0b013e3182063bc9
6. Vogtle LK. Pain in adults with cerebral palsy: impact and solutions. *Dev Med Child Neurol*. 2009;51(suppl 4):113-121. doi:10.1111/j.1469-8749.2009.03423.x
7. American Academy for Cerebral Palsy and Developmental Medicine. Pain in adults with cerebral palsy. https://www.aacpdm.org/UserFiles/file/fact-sheet-pain-011516.pdf. Accessed November 20, 2018.
8. Lawrence H, Hills S, Kline N, Weems K, Doty A. Effectiveness of exercise on functional mobility in adults with cerebral palsy: a systematic review. *Physiother Can*. 2016;68(4):398-407. doi:10.3138/ptc.2015-38LHC
9. Verschuren O, Peterson MD, Balemans ACJ, Hurvitz EA. Exercise and physical activity recommendations for people with cerebral palsy. *Dev Med Child Neurol*. 2016;58(8):798-808. doi:10.1111/dmcn.13053
10. Gillett JG, Lichtwark GA, Boyd RN, Barber LA. Functional capacity in adults with cerebral palsy: lower limb muscle strength matters. *Arch Phys Med Rehabil*. 2018;99(5):900-906.e1. doi:10.1016/j.apmr.2018.01.020
11. Ross SM, MacDonald M, Bigouette JP. Effects of strength training on mobility in adults with cerebral palsy: A systematic review. *Disabil Health J*. 2016;9(3):375-384. doi:10.1016/j.dhjo.2016.04.005
12. Peter Harrison Centre for Disability Sport. Fit for life: a guide for adults with cerebral palsy. https://www.lboro.ac.uk/media/media/research/phc/downloads/Cerebral%20Palsy%20guide_Fit_for_Life.pdf. Accessed October 30, 2018.
13. Morgan PE, McGinley JL. Falls, fear of falling and falls risk in adults with cerebral palsy: a pilot observational study. *Eur J Physiother*. 2013;15(2):93-100. doi:10.3109/21679169.2013.795241
14. Frontera JE, Mollett P. Aging with spinal cord injury: an update. *Phys Med Rehabil Clin N Am*. 2017;28(4):821-828. doi:10.1016/j.pmr.2017.06.013
15. Fulk G, Behrman AST. Traumatic spinal cord injury. In: O'Sullivan S, Schmitz T, Fulk G, eds. *Physical Rehabilitation*. 6th ed. Philadelphia, PA: FA Davis Company; 2014.

16. Jörgensen S, Iwarsson S, Norin L, Lexell J. The Swedish aging with spinal cord injury study (SASCIS): methodology and initial results. *PM R.* 2016;8(7):667-677. doi:10.1016/j.pmrj.2015.10.014
17. Saunders LL, Clarke A, Tate DG, Forchheimer M, Krause JS. Lifetime prevalence of chronic health conditions among persons with spinal cord injury. *Arch Phys Med Rehabil.* 2015;96(4):673-679. doi:10.1016/j.apmr.2014.11.019
18. Upadhya B, Taffet GE, Cheng CP, Kitzman DW, Hospital HM. Heart failure with preserved ejection fraction in the elderly: scope of the problem. *J Mol Cell Cardiol.* 2015;83:73-87. doi:10.1016/j.yjmcc.2015.02.025
19. Mas MF, Mathews A, Gilbert-Baffoe E. Rehabilitation needs of the elder with traumatic brain injury. *Phys Med Rehabil Clin N Am.* 2017;28(4):829-842. doi:10.1016/j.pmr.2017.06.014
20. Dijkers M, Brandstater M, Horn S, Ryser D, Barrett R. Inpatient rehabilitation for traumatic brain injury: the influence of age on treatments and outcomes. *NeuroRehabilitation.* 2013;32(2):233-252. doi:10.3233/NRE-130841
21. Crownover J, Galang GNF, Wagner A. Rehabilitation considerations for traumatic brain injury in the geriatric population: epidemiology, neurobiology, prognosis, and management. *Curr Transl Geriatr Exp Gerontol Rep.* 2012;1(3):149-158. doi:10.1007/s13670-012-0021-6
22. Graham JE, Radice-Neumann DM, Reistetter TA, Hammond FM, Dijkers M, Granger CV. Influence of sex and age on inpatient rehabilitation outcomes among older adults with traumatic brain injury. *Arch Phys Med Rehabil.* 2010;91(1):43-50. doi:10.1016/j.apmr.2009.09.017
23. Pedersen AR, Severinsen K, Nielsen JF. The effect of age on rehabilitation outcome after traumatic brain injury assessed by the Functional Independence Measure (FIM). *Neurorehabil Neural Repair.* 2015;29(4):299-307. doi:10.1177/1545968314545171
24. Ponsford JL, Downing MG, Olver J, et al. Longitudinal follow-up of patients with traumatic brain injury: outcome at two, five, and ten years post-injury. *J Neurotrauma.* 2014;31(1):64-77. doi:10.1089/neu.2013.2997
25. Koopman FS, Beelen A, Gilhus NE, de Visser M, Nollet F. Treatment for postpolio syndrome. *Cochrane Database Syst Rev.* 2015;(5):CD007818.
26. Mayo Clinic. Post-polio syndrome. https://www.mayoclinic.org/diseases-conditions/post-polio-syndrome/symptoms-causes/syc-20355669. Published 2017. Accessed November 21, 2018.
27. Gonzalez H, Olsson T, Borg K. Management of postpolio syndrome. *Lancet Neurol.* 2010;9(6):634-642. doi:10.1016/S1474-4422(10)70095-8
28. World Health Organization. Poliomyelitis (polio). http://www.who.int/topics/poliomyelitis/en/. Published 2018. Accessed November 21, 2018.
29. Latham J, Foley G, Nolan R, et al. Post Polio Syndrome Management and Treatment in Primary Care. Dublin, Ireland: Post Polio Support Group; 2007, https://www.polio.dk/media/2195/management-of-post-polio-ireland.pdf. Accessed November 21, 2018.
30. Lo JK, Robinson LR. Post-polio syndrome and the late effects of poliomyelitis: Part 2. treatment, management, and prognosis. *Muscle Nerve.* 2018;58(6):760-769. doi:10.1002/mus.26167
31. McNalley TE, Yorkston KM, Jensen MP, et al. Review of secondary health conditions in postpolio syndrome: prevalence and effects of aging. *Am J Phys Med Rehabil.* 2015;94(2):139-145. doi:10.1097/PHM.0000000000000166
32. Halstead LS, Gawne AC, Pham BT. National rehabilitation hospital limb classification for exercise, research, and clinical trials in post-polio patients. *Ann N Y Acad Sci.* 1995;753(1):343-353. doi:10.1111/j.1749-6632.1995.tb27560.x
33. Halstead LS, Wiechers DO, eds. Research and Clinical Aspects of the Late Effects of Poliomyelitis. White Plains, NY: March of Dimes Birth Defects Foundation; 1987. http://www.polioplace.org/sites/default/files/files/Research-and-Clinical-Aspects-of-LEP-1987ocr.pdf. Accessed October 18, 2018.
34. Trojan DA, Finch L. Management of post-polio syndrome. *NeuroRehabilitation.* 1997;8(2):93-105. doi:10.3233/NRE-1997-8204
35. Umphred DA. *Umphred's Neurological Rehabilitation.* 6th ed. St. Louis, MO: Elsevier; 2013.
36. Burke-Doe A, ed. *Physical Therapy Case Files: Neurological Rehabilitation.* New York, NY: McGraw-Hill Education/Medical; 2014.
37. Gevirtz C. Managing postpolio syndrome pain. *Nursing.* 2006;36(12 Pt.1):17. doi:10.1097/00152193-200612000-00013
38. Stoelb BL, Carter GT, Abresch RT, Purekal S, McDonald CM, Jensen MP. Pain in persons with post-polio syndrome: frequency, intensity, and impact. *Arch Phys Med Rehabil.* 2008;89(10):1933-1940. doi:10.1016/j.apmr.2008.03.018
39. Smith LK, McDermott K. Pain in post-poliomyelitis—addressing causes versus treating effects. *Birth Defects Orig Artic Ser.* 1987;23(4):121-134.
40. Jubelt B, Agre JC. Characteristics and management of post-polio syndrome. *JAMA.* 2000;284(4):412-414. doi:10.1001/jama.284.4.412
41. Farbu E, Rekand T, Vik-Mo E, Lygren H, Gilhus NE, Aarli JA. Post-polio syndrome patients treated with intravenous immunoglobulin: a double-blinded randomized controlled pilot study. *Eur J Neurol.* 2007;14(1):60-65. doi:10.1111/j.1468-1331.2006.01552.x
42. National Institute of Neurological Disorders and Stroke. Post-Polio Syndrome Fact Sheet. https://www.ninds.nih.gov/Disorders/Patient-Caregiver-Education/Fact-Sheets/Post-Polio-Syndrome-Fact-Sheet. Published 2018. Accessed November 21, 2018.
43. Agre JC, Rodriquez AA. Intermittent isometric activity: its effect on muscle fatigue in postpolio subjects. *Arch Phys Med Rehabil.* 1991;72(12):971-975.
44. Vatansever F, Hamblin MR. Far infrared radiation (FIR): its biological effects and medical applications. *Photonics Lasers Med.* 2012;4(4):255-266. doi:10.1515/plm-2012-0034
45. Santos Tavares Silva I, Sunnerhagen KS, Willén C, Ottenvall Hammar I. The extent of using mobility assistive devices can partly explain fatigue among persons with late effects of polio - a retrospective registry study in Sweden. *BMC Neurol.* 2016;16(1):230. doi:10.1186/s12883-016-0753-6
46. Wise HH. Effective intervention strategies for management of impaired posture and fatigue with post-polio syndrome: a case report. *Physiother Theory Pract.* 2006;22(5):279-287. doi:10.1080/09593980600927831

47. Ploeger HE, Bus SA, Brehm MA, Nollet F. Ankle-foot orthoses that restrict dorsiflexion improve walking in polio survivors with calf muscle weakness. *Gait Posture.* 2014;40(3):391-398. doi:10.1016/j.gaitpost.2014.05.016
48. Hachisuka K, Makino K, Wada F, Saeki S, Yoshimoto N, Arai M. Clinical application of carbon fibre reinforced plastic leg orthosis for polio survivors and its advantages and disadvantages. *Prosthet Orthot Int.* 2006;30(2):129-135. doi:10.1080/03093640600574474
49. Hachisuka K, Makino K, Wada F, Saeki S, Yoshimoto N. Oxygen consumption, oxygen cost and physiological cost index in polio survivors: a comparison of walking without orthosis, with an ordinary or a carbon-fibre reinforced plastic knee-ankle-foot orthosis. *J Rehabil Med.* 2007;39(8):646-650. doi:10.2340/16501977-0105
50. Halstead LS. Assessment and differential diagnosis for post-polio syndrome. *Orthopedics.* 1991;14(11):1209-1217.
51. Sharma SC, Sangwam SS, Siwach RC, et al. The pattern of residual muscle paralysis in poliomyelitis. *Int Orthop.* 1994;18(2):122-125. doi:10.1007/BF02484424
52. Kumar K, Kapahtia NK. The pattern of muscle involvement in poliomyelitis of the upper limb. *Int Orthop.* 1986;10(1):11-15. doi:10.1007/BF00266267
53. Spector SA, Gordon PL, Feuerstein IM, Sivakumar K, Hurley BF, Dalakas MC. Strength gains without muscle injury after strength training in patients with postpolio muscular atrophy. *Muscle Nerve.* 1996;19(10):1282-1290. doi:10.1002/(SICI)1097-4598(199610)19:10<1282::AID-MUS5>3.0.CO;2-A
54. Fillyaw MJ, Badger GJ, Goodwin GD, Bradley WG, Fries TJ, Shukla A. The effects of long-term non-fatiguing resistance exercise in subjects with post-polio syndrome. *Orthopedics.* 1991;14(11):1253-1256.
55. Chan KM, Amirjani N, Sumrain M, Clarke A, Strohschein FJ. Randomized controlled trial of strength training in post-polio patients. *Muscle Nerve.* 2003;27(3):332-338. doi:10.1002/mus.10327
56. Chan KM, Amirjani N, Sumrain M, Clarke A, Strohschein FJ. Randomized controlled trial of strength training in post-polio patients. *Muscle & Nerve.* 2003;27(3):332-338. doi:10.1002/mus.10327
57. Agre JC, Rodriquez AA, Franke TM. Strength, endurance, and work capacity after muscle strengthening exercise in postpolio subjects. *Arch Phys Med Rehabil.* 1997;78(7):681-686. doi:10.1016/S0003-9993(97)90073-3
58. Einarsson G. Muscle conditioning in late poliomyelitis. *Arch Phys Med Rehabil.* 1991;72(1):11-14.
59. Brogårdh C, Flansbjer UB, Lexell J. No effects of whole-body vibration training on muscle strength and gait performance in persons with late effects of polio: a pilot study. *Arch Phys Med Rehabil.* 2010;91(9):1474-1477. doi:10.1016/j.apmr.2010.06.024
60. Skalsky AJ, McDonald CM. Prevention and management of limb contractures in neuromuscular diseases. *Phys Med Rehabil Clin N Am.* 2012;23(3):675-687. doi:10.1016/j.pmr.2012.06.009
61. Jones DR, Speier J, Canine K, Owen R, Stull GA. Cardiorespiratory responses to aerobic training by patients with postpoliomyelitis sequelae. *JAMA.* 1989;261(22):3255-3258. doi:10.1001/jama.1989.03420220069029
62. Kriz JL, Jones DR, Speier JL, Canine JK, Owen RR, Serfass RC. Cardiorespiratory responses to upper extremity aerobic training by postpolio subjects. *Arch Phys Med Rehabil.* 1992;73(1):49-54.
63. Yarnell SK. Non-fatiguing general conditioning exercise program (the 20% rule). *Post-Polio Heal.* 1991;7(3). http://www.post-polio.org/edu/pphnews/pph7-3a.html.
64. Willén C, Sunnerhagen KS, Grimby G. Dynamic water exercise in individuals with late poliomyelitis. *Arch Phys Med Rehabil.* 2001;82(1):66-72. doi:10.1053/apmr.2001.9626
65. Duncan A, Batliwalla Z. Growing older with post-polio syndrome: social and quality-of-life implications. *SAGE Open Med.* 2018;6:2050312118793563. doi:10.1177/2050312118793563

Chapter 18

Complementary Therapies or Integrative Health Care

Amy Broekemeier, PT, DPT, COMT, PMA-CPT; Darcy A. Umphred, PT, PhD, FAPTA; and Carol Davis, PT, DPT, EdD, FAPTA

KEY WORDS Body talk | Body work | Ch'i | Complementary therapies | Energy work | Holistic | Integrative medicine | Mind work

Chapter Objectives

- Identify types of complementary or integrative therapies.
- Differentiate traditional allopathic from holistic medicine.
- Identify complementary therapies integrated within a traditional physical therapy intervention program.
- Discuss appropriate roles of the physical therapist assistant when taught or asked to use complementary therapies as part of intervention within both traditional and alternative environments.

The 21st century has brought many changes to health care. Many individuals have advanced from knowing they have control over their health care (whether it is through their political choices or through their daily health habits) to actively owning the responsibility to change. The mentality of Americans has undergone a paradigm shift due to rising health care costs and has resulted in many people taking active steps to change not only how they take care of themselves but also how they view their health. Health care in the coming years will focus more on the personal responsibility of the individual to manage health. Whether it is through monitoring our bodies, eating right, avoiding stress as much as possible, or partaking in exercises such as yoga or Pilates that call for body awareness, individuals will no longer be passive participants in their health, but instead will hold the control to make changes.

The face of rehabilitation in health care has changed as well. The increasing prevalence of patients seeking complementary and alternative therapies for acute and chronic illness[1,2] and the increasing number of health care professionals practicing complementary and alternative therapies have influenced the practice of rehabilitation in a major way. Complementary and alternative therapies embrace the concept of self-responsibility and allow individuals control over their health. In a survey, 68% of respondents reported having tried at least one form of complementary therapy, and 4 out of 10 individuals are currently using some form of complementary or alternative therapy.[3,4] Even if physical therapist assistants are not practitioners of alternative and complementary therapies themselves, having a rudimentary understanding of the therapies that exist will enrich their practice and ability to connect with patients. Physical therapist assistants, along with other therapists, are able to use holistic therapies to augment their practice with patients. When integrating a complementary therapy with traditional intervention, the physical therapist and physical therapist assistant need to ask, "What factors make the

Lazaro RT, Umphred DA, eds.
Umphred's Neurorehabilitation for the Physical Therapist Assistant, Third Edition (pp 399-412).

administration of that therapy a part of rehabilitation?" rather than simply saying "yoga or tai chi." This chapter will answer that important question regarding justification of complementary therapies as part of physical therapy intervention.

Holistic Health

Complementary therapies are often termed *holistic*. What we mean by holistic therapies and holistic health is that the totality of a person can be seen to incorporate 4 areas of need and function: the physical (traditionally the body and movement), the intellectual (the brain and mind functions), the emotional (feelings and needs), and the spiritual (the eternal questions that help us organize meaning: Who am I? Why have I lived? Why am I ill? What am I to do?).[5,6] How these 4 areas function while interrelating in the world refers to the social aspect of need and function. This social aspect becomes the fifth area to consider.

In rehabilitation, the focus is on helping patients correct disorders of function that are primarily physical or movement-related, but physical therapists and physical therapist assistants are strongly influenced by patients' intellectual, emotional, and spiritual needs as well. The physical therapist and physical therapist assistant who practice holistically question the patient in such a way—most pointedly while taking the history—that illuminates problems and unmet needs in all 5 areas, and then advocate to see that all those needs are addressed.[5] Indeed, this is the ethical responsibility of all health care professionals.

Traditionally, fragmented care, in contrast to holistic care, is concerned only with the "part" of the person that falls under each professional's province. One result of this fragmentation is recognized when patients become labeled by their illness or disability, and not seen as a whole person.[6] Therapists may respond to the question "Who are you seeing next?" with "The low back at 1:30." In Eisenberg et al's[1,6] classic study from the early 1990s on the patterns of use of holistic therapies in the United States, the increasing frequency of use of holistic therapies was, in part, reportedly due to patients' objections to the fragmentation and impersonal aspects of traditional health care. Astin's[2] later study found that people were turning to holistic and complementary therapies primarily because these approaches seemed more consistent with their ideas of health and healing, and took into consideration their individual problems, needs, and quality of life issues.

Complementary Therapies: Integrative Health Care

In general, complementary and alternative therapies can be termed holistic and focus on using to advantage the inextricable link between mind and body. These therapies are administered in an effort to help a person regain health and stay healthy by facilitating the flow of that person's human energy or *ch'i*. Holistic theory posits that when human energy is balanced and flowing freely, it contributes to overall homeostasis, but when blocked, it interferes with health and renders the body and mind together vulnerable to pathogens and/or biochemical imbalance. The natural state of the human is to be in balance, to be healthy. Blocks to ch'i can occur from disruptions not just physically but in each of the 4 quadrants of function: physical, intellectual, emotional, and spiritual. Ideally, once a block to homeostasis of the ch'i occurs, a holistic practitioner would be able to detect that blockage and reverse it without the need for medications or major interventions. Evidence that people often heal themselves has made necessary the traditional double-blind, placebo-based clinical trial.[7]

Complementary and alternative therapies, once thought non-traditional interventions, can be administered either as a substitute to (alternative to) traditional allopathic therapies or in conjunction with (complementary with) traditional therapies. As they become more prominently used, they are commonly integrated seamlessly into rehab programs. They can be classified as systems, approaches, or techniques within approaches.[8] Examples of health care systems include chiropractic, Ayurveda, traditional Chinese medicine, homeopathy, and naturopathy. Within systems are approaches such as acupuncture, acupressure, and herbal therapies in traditional Chinese medicine. Even more basic is a technique within an approach, such as auricular acupuncture, found within the system of traditional Chinese medicine, and transcendental meditation and sesame seed oil massage, both found within the system of Ayurveda.[8] One of the first categorizations of holistic approaches was found in the Chantilly report of the National Institutes of Health,[8] which listed the following categories of alternative therapies.

Alternative Systems of Medical Practice

Ironically, 70% to 90% of all health care worldwide is considered an alternative system to Western medical allopathic practice. Popular health care, community-based care, professionalized health care, traditional Oriental medicine (including acupuncture and Ayurveda), homeopathy, anthroposophically extended medicine (elements of homeopathy and naturopathy), and naturopathic medicine[7] fall under the category of alternative medical practice.

Mind-Body Interventions

Psychotherapy, support groups, meditation, imagery, hypnosis, biofeedback, dance and music therapies, art therapy, prayer, mental healing, yoga, tai chi, Qigong, Alexander Technique, Feldenkrais Method, and Pilates are examples of mind-body interventions. Many interventions used by physical therapists and physical therapist assistants incorporate techniques drawn from the philosophies and techniques of these approaches.[9,10] Although the body of literature with regard to complementary and alternative therapies with neurological populations is small, patients with neurological dysfunctions are seeking complementary and alternative therapies more than individuals without neurological disorders.[11] Some of the most beneficial aspects of mind-body interventions are reductions in stress, anxiety, depression, and pain.[12]

Bioelectromagnetics Application to Medicine

Thermal applications of nonionizing radiation, radio-frequency hyperthermia, laser and radio-frequency surgery, low-energy laser, radio-frequency diathermy, nonthermal applications of pulsed electromagnetic field stimulation for bone repair, magnets, and nerve stimulation fall within this classification.[9,10,13,14]

Manual Healing Methods

Among this group are touch, manipulation, osteopathy, chiropractic, massage therapy, Rolfing, soma therapy, neuromuscular therapy, and biofield or bioenergy therapeutics, which include healing touch, noncontact therapeutic touch, myofascial release, both osteopathic and sustained release or Barnes Method, craniosacral therapy, Reiki, Jin Shin Do, and manual lymph drainage. Specific Human Energy Nexus therapy, a biofield method of treating psychosomatic disorders by releasing repressed and suppressed debilitation emotions, would also be classified here.[9]

Pharmacological and Biological Treatments

Certain pharmacological and biological treatments can be classified as alternative medications and are not accepted by allopathic medicine. These therapies are not regulated by the U.S. Food and Drug Administration. As a physical therapist assistant, it is important to make sure that the patient knows the possible interactions of alternative therapies while taking medication prescribed by their physician, and they should be informed to notify the physician of any additional medication or treatments. The following list includes some of those alternative medications:

- Chondroitin sulfate derived from shark cartilage has been shown to have a protective effect within joints.[15]
- Marijuana is legally prescribed in certain states for pain control and is being studied to evaluate its effectiveness on spasticity in patients with neurological dysfunctions.[16]
- Linoleic acid found in evening primrose oil, sunflower seeds, and safflower oil is used to relieve some symptoms of multiple sclerosis (MS).[17]
- Biologically guided chemotherapy takes into consideration individual differences of the patient.[9]
- St John's Wort has been shown to assist with depression and anxiety.[18]
- Ginkgo biloba is said to improve circulation and prevent ischemia in the central nervous system, leading to a neuroprotective effect. It is also known for improving memory.[19]

Diet and Nutrition

For the prevention of chronic disease, Dean Ornish's program, the Pritikin program, Junger's detox plan,[20] and the Atkins plan are based on the philosophy that nutritional intake and, thus, diet are critical for not only maintaining health but also preventing common diseases such as diabetes, cardiovascular disease, cancer, and Alzheimer's.[9,10,21] A small research pilot study, involving a multimodal intervention including a Paleolithic diet (Wahl's), demonstrated significant improvement in fatigue for patients with secondary progressive MS.[22] Although the specific diet that optimizes the healing component of the human body has not yet be identified in research, and may never be given the number of variables under consideration, diet and nutrition certainly play an important role in not only maintaining health of all bodily systems but also in regaining quality of life following any nervous system trauma. Dolan has identified the need to analyze nutrition as a critical aspect of body function that plays a key role not only in maintaining health, but also in healing.[23]

Complementary Therapies Commonly Integrated in Neurorehabilitation

Energy medicine is another term given to holistic therapies integrated within traditional rehabilitation therapies such as neuromuscular facilitation, exercise, work hardening and, neurological rehabilitation.[24] All medicine and all health care, traditional and holistic, can be seen as energetically based because we are influencing the flows of energy within our own bodies, and also in each of our interventions, whether that flow of energy is found in blood flow, nerve flow, lymph flow, neurotransmitter flow, neuropeptide flow, steroid flow, hormone flow, or the flow of thoughts.[9] The goal of clinicians as facilitators of healing integrating complementary or holistic therapies is to help restore normal function, balance, and rhythm to the body systems so that the body can once again be in homeostasis and a state of healing or self-regulation. As practitioners, therapists become transmitters of a healing energy that surrounds the patient as well as the clinician. By way of intention, the energy is focused through the clinician into patients so that resonance is achieved.[25]

The fourth edition of *Complementary Therapies in Rehabilitation: Evidence for Efficacy in Therapy, Prevention, and Wellness*[8] lists the following as approaches commonly used by therapists in rehabilitation settings. Physical therapist assistants can study and practice these techniques to add to their repertoire of treatment options.

Body Work

Therapeutic Massage

Therapeutic massage is an array of ancient healing practices of manual therapies that include stroking, tapping, stretching, shaking, vibrating, rolling, rubbing, using friction, clapping, gliding, kneading, applying percussion, and manipulating tissue. This is practiced with the intent of altering the structure of the tissue and the consciousness of the recipient. It engages the musculoskeletal, neurological, lymphatic, and circulatory systems.[26] According to Juhan, without adequate tactile input, the human organism will die. Touch is one of the principal elements necessary for the successful development and functional organization of the central nervous system, and is as vital to our existence as food, water, and breath. All of the body's tissues are a great deal more plastic and responsive to change and improvement throughout our lifetimes than we normally assume. Far from being fixed and determined by our biological inheritance, we are all still "works in progress."[27]

This premise supports the necessity of touch therapies to be included in treatment protocols for individuals with neurological compromise over their lifespans. Many traditional physical therapy techniques, although described according to neuromusculoskeletal research and science, could also be considered body work.

Craniosacral Therapy

This holistic manual therapy that energetically manipulates the flow of the cerebrospinal fluid within the craniosacral system promotes self-correction and healing throughout the entire body. The practitioner restricts and then allows movement of cerebrospinal fluid according to the rhythm of breath and pulse of the flow of the cerebrospinal fluid. This technique has been found to improve pain, sleeping habits, and overall well-being.[28,29]

Myofascial Release (Barnes Method)

Myofascial release is a holistic manual therapy that focuses on releasing inappropriate fascial restrictions that distort tissue and the shape of the body. These restrictions can be found within the macrolevel of muscles and fascial layers down to the cellular level in such a way that flow or normal fascial and muscle gliding is restricted. Fascial tightness causes the body to lose its physiological adaptive capacity, and homeostasis is disrupted because fascia encapsulates muscle, bone, and organs. Recent probe-based technology allowed examination of live tissue at a microscopic level inside the body and in real time. Researchers describe the anatomy and histology of a previously unrecognized, though widespread, macroscopic, fluid-filled space within and between tissues, a novel expansion and specification of the concept of the human interstitium.[30] Dr. Jean-Claude Guimberteau has documented this phenomena for the past 20 years and has created a brilliant video called *Strolling Under the Skin* and co-authored the book *Architecture of the Human Living Fascia: The Extracellular Matrix and Cells Revealed Through Endoscopy*.[31,32] Another researcher and orthopedic surgeon, Stecco, in her paper on "The Fascia: The Forgotten Structure," discusses the three-dimensional continuity of the myofascial.[33] Although scientific research in the area of fascia has most recently been documented, rehabilitation clinicians including Barnes, Barral, and others have been using and teaching fascial techniques for decades with empirical data to support its use clinically.[34,35]

It is believed that sustained myofascial release facilitates the release of electrons through a piezoelectric effect to restore the length of the fascia by releasing primarily the ground substance of the fascia so that soft tissue is restored to its original shape.[36] This release is not only able to be felt by the clinician and patient as a tightness that "melts" or gives way, but it is able to be seen using dynamic ultrasound and is correlated with pain reduction.[37] Individuals with spinal cord injury could benefit from myofascial release due to restrictions secondary to cervical and lumbar fusions and tissue trauma sustained at the initial insult. Broekemeier has experienced individuals with MS, Parkinson's disease, cerebral palsy, and post-stroke and brain injury benefitting from the effectiveness of myofascial techniques to reduce spasticity and encourage efficient tissue length tension relationships for improved function.

Complete Decongestive Therapy (Manual Lymphatic Drainage)

Manual lymphatic drainage (MLD) is one component of a comprehensive lymphedema management program termed *complete decongestive therapy*. In many European countries, this approach is considered traditional physical therapy intervention. In the United States, lymph drainage is generally used with post-surgical cancer patients. Molecular and energetic flows are affected. Complete decongestive therapy consists of skin care, lymphatic massage, and bandaging of the swollen limb, followed by active exercises.[38] Individuals who undergo MLD can experience decreases in limb girth and volume that significantly affect the gait and lead to increased quality of life and the ability to perform activities of daily living.[39]

Rolfing or Structural Integration

Developed by Ida Rolf, this is a manual body-based therapy that mechanically and energetically changes the tissues of the body. The myofascial system is aligned so that gravity flows through the body tissues and supports upright posture and movement. In this way, structure and function are realigned to promote health and homeostasis. Structural integration can increase the ability to process sensory information and make a patient more receptive, reduce anxiety, and improve neuromotor organization and overall well-being.[40] Deviations in posture and tissue restrictions serve to locate dysfunction. The therapy consists of 10 systematic and prescribed sessions of both structural integration and intense deep connective tissue manipulation to restore appropriate tissue length and upright posture.[41] The patient takes an active part in the session by moving the body part while pressure is applied as tissue gives way.

Mind and Body Work

Tai Chi

Tai chi is described as choreography of body and mind. Originally a martial art, tai chi movements are a response to an attacker. That attacker's own movement and, thus, energy, are used against that person by moving in such a way as to sidestep and throw the attacker off balance. There are numerous forms of tai chi containing as many as 108 postures and movements. Family names are associated with different forms, such as Wu, Ch'en, Ch'uan, and Chih. Each is distinctive but follows classic tai chi principles that are based on integrating the mind and body to facilitate the flow of energy in the movements.[16] Tai chi is a low-impact form of movement exercise that has been shown by well-documented research studies to improve respiratory status, functional balance, and aerobic control.[42,43] Tai chi has grown in use with the neurological populations, such as individuals with Parkinson's disease, chronic migraines, and MS.[43-45] Also important are the psychological aspects of tai chi, such as stress and anxiety reduction.[46-48]

Biofeedback

Biofeedback is a process of electronically using information from the patient's body to teach that person to recognize processes taking place inside his or her body, brain, nervous system, and muscles. Instruments reveal conscious and unconscious actions that are occurring, and patients or clients are then instructed to use this sensory feedback information to change unwanted activity. In this way, people are able to learn how to control unwanted activity, such as muscle tension, blood pressure, and congestion of blood in the vessels of the brain that cause migraine headaches.[49] Biofeedback is also important with individuals who might have a decreased sense of self and awareness of surroundings, such as people who have had a stroke or have Parkinson's disease. Therapists use verbal, visual, and kinesthetic biofeedback through voice, demonstration, and manual contacts every day, but may not recognize when one system is contradicting the other. With the advent of interactive video gaming, such as the Wii (Nintendo), the therapist can integrate this software into the therapy session to give real-time feedback to patients.[50] This type of biofeedback is effective, inexpensive, and easy for physical therapists and physical therapist assistants to access. The use of game-oriented training sessions as biofeedback can easily be used to augment home programs in outpatient rehabilitation. The key to success of this type of intervention is that the patient enjoys the activity and practices often between therapy sessions, and that the feedback can change with improvement in skill and is appropriate to the ability of the person.[51] (Refer to Chapter 17 for additional information and ideas on biofeedback techniques.)

Yoga

Yoga is derived from a Sanskrit verb meaning to unite, as in uniting the body, mind, and spirit. Classic yoga practice includes more than body movements and positions, or *asanas*, performed with mindfulness and attention, especially to breathing. It is a broad philosophical model of health based on human experience.

There are many forms or approaches to yoga. The most commonly used in rehabilitation is hatha yoga. Hatha yoga is especially useful in rehabilitation to facilitate patients' attention to the importance of breathing and moving mindfully through a full range of motion. Bringing attention to the breath unites body and mind, and the meditative movement facilitates the spirit to be "in the now."[52] Integrating movement with body awareness, as practiced in yoga, reduces stress, depression, and anxiety.[53]

Yoga has been shown to be an effective treatment for neurological movement dysfunctions and pain management, as well as for the community-dwelling elderly.[54-56] A meta-analysis of the effectiveness of yoga based on the International Classification of Functioning, Disability and Health model for use in MS, stroke, and children with cerebral palsy was conducted, resulting in the conclusion that yoga was no better or worse than other exercise modalities, but the positive social and emotional benefits may contribute to improved quality of life.[57] A protocol for a randomized control study comparing yoga to stretch and resistance training exercises on psychological distress in clients with Parkinson's disease has been proposed.[58] It is clear that yoga has a benefit to clients with neurological compromise and is sought for physical, intellectual, emotional, spiritual, and social benefits; however, further research in this area is needed.

Alexander Technique

Based on the study of his own habits of movement that interfered with function, Frederick Matthias Alexander developed a technique whereby the teacher helps the student organize the position of the head to the neck and back, redistributing muscle tone and opening up consciousness. Poor habits of movement are identified to the patient by way of touch and direction, and the patient is directed to change in ways that facilitate conscious control of movement, overriding poor habits of motion. Choice is thus given to the patient to move in ways that reinforce an "extended field of consciousness."[59] The Alexander Technique can influence control of voluntary movement and balance and was shown to improve the ability of individuals with Parkinson's disease to conduct activities of daily living.[60]

Feldenkrais Method

Each person develops patterns of movement to maximize basic needs when growing to maturity. Many of these highly individual patterns of movement are limited in skill, flexibility, and practice. Mental and physical aspects are incorporated into these habitual patterns. Some movements optimize physical performance, while others are inefficient ways of moving. Moshe Feldenkrais developed a method of movement that would assist people in functioning at a higher level. Efficient postural patterns and movements away from and back toward those postures are taught. Those patterns are performed with a minimal amount of effort accompanied by a well-developed kinesthetic sense of awareness. In this way, a person should easily recover from any movement or postural challenge or trauma. Functional integration is a one-on-one, hands-on approach, and awareness through movement is a verbally directed movement process that can be performed in groups.[61] The Feldenkrais Method can translate to improvements in level of perceived pain, in the ability to perform activities of daily living, and most important, in patients' quality of life.[62] Applying movement principles coupled with self-awareness takes patients beyond their limitations and opens up new possibilities of fluid, pain-free movement for all individuals.[63,64]

Pilates

Joseph Pilates overcame his physical frailties by developing this exercise method that is performed on mats and on several types of apparatus that use springs to assist an injured individual in successfully completing movements that would be otherwise restricted. By altering spring tension or increasing the challenge of gravity, an individual can be assisted in strengthening toward efficient functional movement. The Pilates environment consists of appliances such as the reformer, trapeze table, chair, ladder barrel, and mat. The focus of exercise is on strengthening the core or trunk so that the extremities can be supported in movement. Attention is given to the breath, alignment, and smoothness of movement.[65] Symmetry can be emphasized using the reformer, on which both lower extremities can go through a motion at the same time with graduated springs to assist or resist the movement. Pilates-evolved methods have taken Joseph Pilates' original work further by incorporating current theories and recent knowledge in areas such as neurorehabilitation, orthopedic manual therapy, training progressions, fascial slings and tensegrity, eccentric loading, biomechanics, functional-relational anatomy, imagery, and mind/body systems.[66-68] Pilates has most recently been used in many physical therapy practices as a useful tool in the rehabilitation of clients with neurological compromise particularly adults with MS, and children with cerebral palsy. In a randomized controlled study comparing Pilates with traditional physical therapy for clients with MS, walking speed and step length significantly improved in both groups.[69] Clients with MS participating in mat and reformer Pilates programs made significant gains in balance, functional mobility, core stability, fatigue severity, and quality of life.[70] When comparing aerobic exercise and Pilates for clients with MS, improvements were shown in physical performance and cognitive tests in the Pilates group.[71] A 10-week Pilates program was found effective to improve sensory integration and to decrease fatigue in clients with MS.[72] Pilates may be an important rehabilitation technique for children with CP who present mild deficits in motor structures and high functional level, especially when the aims are to improve muscle strength and postural control during quiet standing.[73] Empirically, practitioners see the benefits of Pilates for use with clients who have neurological compromise including after stroke, brain injury, and spinal cord injury. However, more formal research is required to demonstrate the total effectiveness of the Pilates method.

Body Talk

Body talk is the active experience of observing and analyzing the posture, appearance, and movements of an individual to evaluate factors involved in the patient's health state. Body talk combines concepts and research from Western medicine with techniques of traditional Chinese medicine, yoga, and acupuncture.[74] Body talk works on the premise that the body can be thrown out of homeostasis where internal energy is disrupted, which leads to disease and dysfunction in the body. Along with other complementary therapies, body talk views the patient as an active participant who is capable of directing and channeling energy to encourage healing. The body talk philosophy uses techniques such as breathing, rearranging energy, hands-on analysis of energy blockages, and visualization techniques.[75,76]

Energy Work

Reiki

Reiki is a Japanese word meaning universal life force that animates all living things. The meaning of Reiki is similar to that of *ch'i, prana, pneuma,* or *ruah.* Reiki is a healing system that channels the universal life force surrounding all of us through the practitioner's hands into the mind and body of the recipient, promoting energy balance, healing, and a state of well-being within the physical, mental, emotional, social, and spiritual domains. Anyone can learn Reiki, but it must be transferred from a Reiki master to the student during the induction process called *attunement.* The learner opens up to channel the energy to another. Intentionality is critical to this process. Reiki practitioners focus attention of thought or concentration in a specific way to bring about a healing or balance by way of energy flow.[77] Evidence for the use of Reiki for improving function in neurological illnesses is weak, but in one study, Reiki therapy led to improved pain and anxiety associated with chronic illness.[78] Reiki certainly has been shown to have a positive effect on individuals who are going through traumatic medical interventions as well as reducing stress levels and relaxation.[79,80]

Qigong

Qigong is the foundational energy that underlies all energy techniques, including tai chi. This ancient Chinese medicine philosophy states that health and healing depend on a balance of vital energy, a still mind, and controlled emotions. Physical dysfunction results from disordered patterns of long-standing energy. To balance and restore energy flow, Qigong uses exercises that include slow, controlled, nonimpact-type movements and postures that gain control over the center of gravity. Qigong integrates deep breathing, movement, and postures while stressing expansion of the base of support, trunk control, and improving rotation of the trunk and coordination of isolated extremity motions. The meditative component serves to make an individual more aware of the body, enhancing the ability to control muscle tension, posture, and movement and facilitating a peace of mind that leads to an overall sense of well-being.[81] A bounty of literature exists showing improvements in quality of life and balance and a decrease in falls. Studies promote Qigong and tai chi as effective additions to traditional physical therapy practice.[82]

Magnets

Often grouped with crystals, magnets are thought to be worthless in health and healing by most allopathic health practitioners. The research, as limited as it is, indicates that there may indeed be a healing effect of magnetic energy on the body and mind. Magnets exert their influence by way of a magnetic field emanating from them. *Unipolar* and *bipolar* refer to the presence of which poles (ie, north, south, or both) face the surface. Manufacturers claim one or the other is more therapeutically beneficial. In the literature, many claims are made that are not substantiated with good research. However, some studies with patients who are medically diagnosed with pain, wounds, and fibromyalgia indicate that magnets seem to offer a therapeutic effect.[83] The literature must be studied with a careful eye to ascertain the true benefits of which strength of magnet and which polarity seemed to be most beneficial.[83] The therapeutic community needs to be aware of this research to advise patients who are seeking relief. Although there is benefit to magnetic therapy, the quality of magnets and their use (which are shown to have benefit, especially in wound healing), are not widely available to the general population.[84]

Acupuncture

Having been in existence as a therapeutic modality for more than 2000 years, acupuncture is one part of the system of traditional Chinese medicine. Its theory is based on the concept that the flow of ch'i can be influenced by mechanically and energetically stimulating acupuncture points that lie along pathways (or *meridians*) to restore balance and flow. Disease results in and from a deficiency of flow of ch'i. Acupuncture physicians study the signs that indicate an imbalance in one or both forms of ch'i, the yin and yang energy. These clinicians learn how to facilitate flow through needling the acupuncture points, direct stairways to the pathways of flow (or meridians).[85] A study by Hsing et al using electroacupuncture, not traditional acupuncture, on stroke patients found significant improvements in functional ability as measured by the National Institutes of Health Stroke Scale.[86] Like any intervention, the location and application of treatment were extremely important, because the sham electroacupuncture group showed no improvement as compared with the treatment group.[86] In a recent retrospective review of Chinese medicine techniques used for clients with Parkinson's disease, a positive correlation was noted using acupuncture, musical/rhythmic therapy, and deep brain stimulation.[87]

Therapeutic Touch

A manual therapy developed by Delores Kreiger, RN, PhD, and Dora Kunz, therapeutic touch is considered a nursing intervention in which the patient/client is not touched by the practitioner, but the electromagnetic energy field of that person is manually manipulated in such a way as to remove blocks and disturbances in it.[88] In this way, noncontact therapeutic touch facilitates an improvement in energy flow in the environment around the patient so the natural healing powers of the patient can be maximized. Because of Kreiger's position as an academic, this holistic therapy is one of the few that have been taught in college curricula for credit.[88] This approach has been found to be beneficial in preterm newborn children to help develop a protective response to abnormal autoregulation of blood flow.[89,90]

The Role of the Physical Therapist Assistant in the Integration of Complementary Integrative Therapies in Neurorehabilitation

Each of these (and other) complementary therapies carries a learning process requiring that the person performing the therapy be schooled in the theory and practice of the technique. Some require extensive coursework followed by examination and certification. Others require learning of the technique but do not require official certification. When offered in a rehabilitation setting, the physical therapist assistant, acting within the scope of practice of an assistant to the physical therapist, must work with the physical therapist in instituting complementary therapies. For a physical therapist assistant to be delegated the total responsibility of interventions using the following therapies, that physical therapist assistant must be licensed or certified by agencies providing education in this modality: acupuncture, biofeedback, yoga, Pilates, Reiki, MLD, Alexander Technique, Feldenkrais Method, or Rolfing.

When offering modalities that require certification without the supervision of a physical therapist, the physical therapist assistant should step outside the boundaries of practice as a physical therapist assistant and practice according to the stipulations of the license or certification that the complementary therapy offers. In other words, the physical therapist assistant should perform as a certified or licensed complementary therapy practitioner, but not as a physical therapist assistant. And, for risk management purposes, a physical therapist assistant should provide these therapies outside of traditional allopathic health care environments. Within an acute care, rehabilitation, or long-term care environment, the physical therapist assistant will provide interventions delegated by the physical therapist. For that reason, autonomy of practice by the physical therapist assistant using any of these approaches would not be appropriate and would place the physical therapist assistant's certification or license at risk. If the physical therapist is licensed or certified to offer the above therapies, then the physical therapist assistant can assist the physical therapist according to the instructions of the physical therapist in the rehabilitation setting. This is true of all of the complementary therapies described.

There is risk associated with the use of complementary therapies in traditional Western medical management settings. For example, if a physical therapist decides that a patient would benefit from yoga exercises and the physical therapist assistant has been educated in the application of yoga as exercise, then the physical therapist assistant is still required to work under the overall supervision of the physical therapist even if the physical therapist assistant knows more about yoga than the physical therapist does. Once a complementary therapy becomes part of the physical therapy program administered within the practice environment of the physical therapist, the physical therapist is still responsible for the process of patient care.

The Importance of a Good Communicating Relationship Between the Physical Therapist and Physical Therapist Assistant

The optimal relationship between the physical therapist and the physical therapist assistant requires ongoing communication and decision-making for the benefit of the patient/client. This does not change with the integration of complementary and alternative therapies. The application of these energy-based techniques requires special education and development of the intention of the physical therapist and physical therapist assistant to be successful in using them with patients and clients. Ideally, the physical therapist and physical therapist assistant will learn, for example, myofascial release or Pilates or craniosacral therapy together and, thus, both will be able to benefit patients with these holistic methods as complementary to their rehabilitation process. Communication is critical to the effective partnership of the physical therapist and physical therapist assistant. However, in the rehabilitation setting when complementary therapies are offered to patients, whether it is magnets, myofascial release, therapeutic touch, or MLD, the physical therapist assistant must work under the specific supervision of the physical therapist, no matter how skilled the physical therapist assistant is in the application of these complementary therapies.

Conclusion

Holistic therapies have a great deal to offer in helping patients regain a higher quality of life and empowerment toward better health. Although best used immediately upon onset of symptoms or as a preventative measure to support consistent homeostasis of the system, at the least, these approaches offer energy-based methods that are often helpful when all traditional therapies have failed. At the most, holistic therapies require an interaction with patients that restores therapeutic presence to the application of physical therapy; they move both the physical therapist and the physical therapist assistant out of the business mode of the managed care administration of therapy and back into an emphasis on the whole person and empowerment. Research now has shown physiological evidence regarding how and why some of these techniques seem to be effective. For example, water molecules can be affected by words and music that surround the individual,[91] and the body is made up of 80% water. Our thoughts and feelings about our bodies have the ability to heal tissues, and human beliefs can assist cells to obtain optimal function.[92,93] Therapist have seen that fear of movements that previously created pain can impede the body's ability to perform a task or function even after the physiological healing of injured tissue occurs.[94] An accepted fact is that our brain has neuroplasticity and plays a direct role in healing of movement problems seen in the body.[92,93,95]

Evidence that all matter existed in a vast web of connection, or life force, which has been proposed in ancient myth and religion since the beginning of time,[96-98] has shown that every action in the human body is a unique array of fibrils under load in an irregular, chaotic, fractal, nonlinear organization that is irregular but not random. This supports Laplace's 1795 theory that order is created by random events and deterministic chaotic behavior, and is one of nature's potential dynamic capabilities. These concepts broaden the field of possible solutions or treatment outcomes that allow treatment to be explored more efficiently, and permit greater complexity.[32] In essence, the search for equilibrium or balance in life is constant and ever-changing, not only for the body, but also for all systems in nature. If Guimberteau's conclusion is correct that matter is the key to everything, then it should be at the center of scientific debate. In the future, a clinician's intention and presence, along with technical skill and knowledge, will very likely be shown to significantly influence healing on a totality of levels; physical, intellectual, emotional, spiritual, and social. Complementary research today certainly has illustrated that a physical therapist's or physical therapist assistant's thoughts and intentions play a larger variable in how a patient responds to intervention than what can be identified in the scientific literature.

Sacrosanct in this process of administering complementary therapies is the mandated supervisory relationship of the physical therapist and physical therapist assistant. No matter how knowledgeable the physical therapist assistant is in the administration of holistic therapies, the physical therapist maintains supervisory control of the patient care process when practiced within Western medical environments. As the physical therapist assistant is delegated additional responsibilities for the intervention of patients receiving physical therapy, having training in complementary approaches should provide an environment that leads to a feeling of wellness and empowerment within the patient. Hopefully, empathic communication among the physical therapist, the physical therapist assistant, and the patient will round out the treatment so that the experience is fulfilling for each person.

Case Studies

Case #1

Mrs. J was referred to Dr. Hagen, DPT for examination and evaluation of balance problems. Dr. Hagen was a staff physical therapist in an outpatient neurorehabilitation center of a large teaching hospital. Upon examination, Dr. Hagen determined that Mrs. J, who was in good health overall, had developed her unsteady gait after moving from her 2-story home to an apartment where she no longer had any stairs to climb. As a result of using the elevator and only walking on flat surfaces, her balance problems began from increasing weakness in her hips and knees. Examination using the Berg Balance Scale, including the forward reach and manual muscle testing, revealed that her problem was muscle weakness. She scored 3(-) in hip extensors, knee extensors, and ankle dorsiflexors bilaterally. No inner-ear problems were noted, but she was experiencing some difficulty with her vision and her hearing.

Dr. Hagen consulted with PD, a physical therapist assistant who worked with her in the neurorehabilitation setting. Together, they devised an exercise program that included systematic strengthening of her pelvis and lower extremities and suggested participation in a group tai chi class taught by PD on Mondays, Wednesdays, and Fridays from 10:30 am to noon.

PD had studied tai chi with a tai chi master and had gained skill to the extent that she was able to teach tai chi at the rehabilitation center, as a physical therapist assistant under the supervision of the director of physical therapy. The state in which they practiced allowed her to practice out of line of sight of the supervising physical therapist, and her group met in a quiet common area near the main rehab gym. PD employed the assistance of several aids and family members as "spotters" for her patients during the group session.

Mrs. J recovered her strength very rapidly with exercises and tai chi. PD did a follow-up assessment of her balance and reported that Mrs. J was functioning safely, and she felt she was ready for the supervising physical therapist to do a final discharge evaluation. Mrs. J liked the tai chi group exercises so much that she enrolled in a wellness center group and continued with tai chi for several months.

Questions

1. Was an appropriate protocol used by both the physical therapist and physical therapist assistant with the delegation to the physical therapist assistant of a group class that included the complementary approach referred to as tai chi?
2. Once Mrs. J met the objectives of the traditional interventions as well as the functional balance activities of the tai chi, was it appropriate for the physical therapist assistant to recommend that Mrs. J go back to the supervising physical therapist for final examination and discharge, or could the physical therapist assistant, as a tai chi instructor, do this independently?

Case #2

Physical therapist Connie W evaluated Mr. K, a 65-year-old executive at a local bank, for beginning Parkinson's symptoms that were limiting his participation. Upon examination, Mr. K showed no involvement in his handwriting and moderate rigidity in his back and shoulders. He held his left arm in slightly more flexion at the elbow, and the fingers of his left hand were straight with slight metacarpophalangeal flexion. His head flexed forward 6 inches; his left arm showed diminished swing with gait, and his steps were shortened to a 12-inch stride. His turn-around time to the left was slower than the right, taking several more steps to complete. No shuffling gait was noted. No detectable tremor was found, but Mr. K reported that a slight tremor of his left hand was present upon awakening some mornings. He had full animation of his face, no seborrhea; his speech was clear and easily understood, but quiet. He reported no difficulty in self-care. He was quite concerned about how this diagnosis would affect his career at the bank, which included interaction with many powerful people who trusted him with their money. He was most anxious that he not show any sign of weakness or pathology.

Muscle strength was normal throughout. Range of motion in left shoulder flexion was slightly diminished to 150 degrees. Trunk rotation and cervical rotation were limited to two-thirds normal. With regard to balance, one-legged stance time was less than 10 seconds on either foot. He was able to stand from a chair 10 times in 30 seconds without using his arms to assist. He was able to pick up a pencil off the floor, but was unable to tandem stand. Connie

W devised a therapeutic program composed of myofascial release, which she performed focusing on releasing deep fascial restrictions on the psoas area bilaterally, opening up the occipital ridge, the thoracic inlet, and pectoral areas and working to improve fascial length for trunk rotation and shoulder flexion. Exercises were designed to emphasize deep breathing and increasing fluidity of spine rotation and gait. In addition, she had Mr. K practicing one-legged stance and tandem stance at the sink at home, and wanted him to start practicing yoga on a regular basis.

Estelle F, a physical therapist assistant working with Connie W in the rehabilitation center, was also a certified yoga instructor and had a part-time evening and weekend yoga practice in a small storefront location quite near the rehabilitation center. Connie W knew that Estelle F was also an excellent yoga instructor who specialized in assisting people with disabilities in assuming postures with supporting towels, and who emphasized therapeutic breathing. She suggested to Mr. K that he enroll in Estelle F's yoga classes on Tuesday and Thursday evenings. Thus, Connie W would see Mr. K as an outpatient in the rehabilitation center on Mondays and Fridays, and Mr. K would take yoga on Tuesday and Thursday evenings. This plan appealed to Mr. K, who sensed that he really must not be "all that disabled" if he could take yoga as part of his physical therapy.

Estelle F spoke with Connie W about Mr. K when he enrolled in her evening yoga class. Connie W was able to share her examination and evaluation information on Mr. K and suggested an emphasis on trunk rotation and upper extremity range in addition to yoga breathing exercises. Estelle F was able to supplement Mr. K's rehabilitation by implementing these suggestions in Mr. K's yoga practice with much success.

Questions

1. Would the myofascial release techniques and the traditional exercises be considered physical therapy?
2. Would recommending yoga as a life activity be considered physical therapy, and should the physical therapist assistant consider her class as part of the physical therapy interventions designed by the physical therapist? If so, how would the physical therapist and physical therapist assistant deal with the concept of supervision? If not, why would the physical therapist recommend the individual enroll in the yoga class?
3. Once the individual completed the intervention aspect of the traditional physical therapist program and continued with the yoga, would it still be considered physical therapy?

Case #3

Candace is a 40-year-old patient who, 25 years ago, was in a motor vehicle accident in which her sister died and she suffered a mild head injury, C5/6 incomplete cervical fracture with fixation, and other soft tissue injury. She received 12 months of traditional inpatient and outpatient neurorehabilitation. At the time of discharge from rehabilitation, she used a wheelchair and returned to independent living. For the last 10 years, she has sought weekly treatment from a trainer to improve strength and endurance. The trainer referred her to an outpatient, non-traditional, physical therapy center using manual therapy, Barnes myofascial release, Pilates, and other movement modalities. Upon evaluation, Candace complained of constant thoracic spine pain while seated and while propelling her wheelchair, raspy vocalization, decreased rib expansion, and intermittent spasticity in bilateral lower extremities. She was able to stand and walk short distances with hand-held assist, transfer independently, and participate independently in all activities of daily living, including driving. Upon orthopedic assessment, Candace had a functional scoliosis convex left thoracic with the inability to rest on her left ischial tuberosity when seated in her wheelchair. Rib expansion during breathing was 1-inch gain in diameter when measured from full expiration to full inspiration. She had limited use overhead of the left upper extremity secondary to severe right rotation of the thoracic spine and rib cage. The severe curve of her spine followed a direct physical line from an anterior abdominal feeding tube insertion scar that Candace had acquired directly following the accident while in acute neurorehab. It also appeared that the scoliotic curve progressed rapidly while Candace had been required to sit in her wheelchair and propel it independently over the last 25 years. Candace has been participating in Barnes myofascial release and manual therapy treatments weekly for 1 year with a physical therapist. She was referred to a Pilates instructor certified in Pilates and the Gyrotonic Method for whole body movement and retraining once a week. The instructor was practicing within the same non-traditional physical therapy practice as the physical therapist, but was not certified as a physical therapist assistant. After working with the physical therapist and Pilates instructor, Candace now has no thoracic spine pain, can sit on her ischial tuberosity while seated in her chair upright and symmetrical, has full use of her left upper extremity, and can stand and ambulate distances in her home unassisted. Her inspiration diameter of her ribs has doubled in volume since beginning her sessions, and voice difficulties have dissipated since participating in myofascial release of scar tissue in the anterior cervical spine.

Questions

1. Would any of the interventions used by the physical therapist and the Pilates instructor be considered physical therapy services? When physical therapy services are rendered at an outpatient non-traditional physical therapy center that is cash-based, are the services physical therapy?
2. If the Pilates instructor was also licensed as a physical therapist assistant, would the services be deemed physical therapy?

3. Is it appropriate to continue the services to this client indefinitely if improvement continues to be made? And are these services still considered physical therapy services? What about the Pilates and Gyrotonic instruction provided under the supervision of the physical therapist also certified in these modalities?

Case #4

Mark is a 46-year-old patient who, while visiting family 2 years ago, suffered a severe full occlusion stroke in the left hemisphere with resultant right hemiplegia. The medical system predicted that, due to the severity of the stroke, he would not recover any function in either his right upper or lower extremity, but today he is functioning independently with minimal support. Prior to his injury, Mark was an avid outdoorsman and ice climber with no fear of heights or limitations in his physical and mental performance.

Upon evaluation by Broekemeier, a physical therapist, Mark was ambulating independently with cane use in the left hand and an ankle-foot orthosis on the right lower extremity. His right upper extremity was severely spastic and at the time deemed unusable with a deteriorated axillae skin condition, severely restricted glenohumeral joint, tightened finger flexors, and severe upper extremity myofascial and neural restriction associated with the internally rotated and adducted positioning of the upper extremity. Mark could articulate short sentences, but had a very difficult time with specific word retrieval. His memory seemed fully intact, and cognition was close to normal as recognized by his close friends who assisted him on a daily basis. Mark had received 2 years of inpatient and outpatient physical, occupational, and speech therapies, but insurance coverage had run out by the time Mark was referred to a cash-based, non-traditional, outpatient physical therapy center at Pinnacle Performance. While the previous therapies had addressed Mark's gait, activities of daily living, and speech, no intervention had addressed the right upper extremity spasticity, myofascial restrictions or lack of use.

Broekemeier used Barnes myofascial release techniques, proprioceptive neuromuscular facilitation-based contract relax, neural mobilization, and assisted neuromuscular retraining in efficient postures to obtain improved right upper extremity use for Mark. Mark was treated weekly for 4 weeks, then periodically over 6 months when the therapist could get Mark into her very busy schedule on a pro bono basis. At the current status, Mark is able to open his hand upon request, mildly grasp and hold objects, elevate his right upper extremity to 100 degrees shoulder flexion, and lie supine with his hand placed behind his head comfortably. He has started to participate in paddle boarding with balance assist using a brace to open and attach the paddle to his right hand. He also participates independently in a daily home exercise program to keep range of motion in the right shoulder, elbow, wrist, and hand. Mark demonstrates improved skin health in his axillary tissue with increased neural and fascial mobility throughout the right upper extremity. The plan is to continue with pro bono services when available. The physical therapist is curious and open to whatever functional improvements can be made in Mark's use of the right upper extremity. Mark is eager to return to outdoor activity and recreation, which the physical therapist would encourage him to participate in as long as these movements remain easy to perform. He feels encouraged and continues to practice what he enjoys, and he is motivated as part of his life choices.

Questions

1. Is it appropriate to call the services provided by the physical therapist "physical therapy" when Barnes myofascial release does not have scientific research to prove its effectiveness?
2. Can the physical therapist legally instruct a physical therapist assistant in the use of the above skill sets, turn the treatment intervention over to the physical therapist assistant in order to practice all these functional skills, and continue to call the services physical therapy services?
3. How long can the above services be ethically provided by the physical therapist and physical therapist assistant?

References

1. Eisenberg DM, Kessler RC, Foster C, Norlock FE, Calkins DR, Delbanco TL. Unconventional medicine in the United States. Prevalence, costs, and patterns of use. *N Engl J Med.* 1993;328(4):246-252. doi:10.1056/NEJM199301283280406
2. Astin JA. Why patients use alternative medicine: results of a national study. *JAMA.* 1998;279(19):1548-1553.
3. Kessler RC, Davis RB, Foster DF, et al. Long-term trends in the use of complementary and alternative medical therapies in the United States. *Ann Intern Med.* 2001;135(4):262-268. doi:10.7326/0003-4819-135-4-200108210-00011
4. Barnes PM, Powell-Griner E, McFann K, Nahin RL. Complementary and alternative medicine use among adults: united States, 2002. *Adv Data.* 2004;2(343):1-19. doi:10.1016/j.sigm.2004.07.003
5. Davis CM. *Patient Practitioner Interaction: An Experiential Manual for Developing the Art of Health Care.* 5th ed. Thorofare, NJ: SLACK Incorporated; 2011.
6. Koloroutis M, Trout M. *See Me as a Person: Creating therapeutic relationships with patients and their families.* Minneapolis, MN: Creative Health Care Management Inc; 2016.
7. Davis CM. Complementary therapies in rehabilitation. In: Gonzalez EG, Myers SM, Edelstein JE, Lieberman J, Downey JA, eds. *Downey and Darling's Physiological Basis of Rehabilitation Medicine.* 3rd ed. Boston, MA: Butterworth-Heinemann; 2001.
8. Davis CM. *Integrative Therapies in Rehabilitation; Evidence for Efficacy in Therapy, Prevention, and Wellness.* 4th ed. Thorofare, NJ: SLACK Incorporated; 2016.

9. Alternative Medicine: Expanding Medical Horizons. The Chantilly, Virginia, workshop report on alternative medical systems and practices in the United States to the National Institutes of Health. Pittsburgh, PA: Superintendent of Documents; 1992.
10. Spencer JW, Jacobs JJ. *Complementary/Alternative Medicine: An Evidence-Based Approach*. 2nd ed. St. Louis, MO: Mosby; 2002.
11. Erwin Wells R, Phillips RS, McCarthy EP. Patterns of mind-body therapies in adults with common neurological conditions. *Neuroepidemiology*. 2011;36(1):46-51. doi:10.1159/000322949
12. Wahbeh H, Elsas SM, Oken BS. Mind-body interventions: applications in neurology. *Neurology*. 2008;70(24):2321-2328. doi:10.1212/01.wnl.0000314667.16386.5e
13. Shen WW, Zhao JH. Pulsed electromagnetic fields stimulation affects BMD and local factor production of rats with disuse osteoporosis. *Bioelectromagnetics*. 2010;31(2):113-119.
14. Becker RO, Selden G. *The Body Electric: Electromagnetism and the Foundation of Life*. New York, NY: Morrow; 1985.
15. Imada K, Oka H, Kawasaki D, Miura N, Sato T, Ito A. Anti-arthritic action mechanisms of natural chondroitin sulfate in human articular chondrocytes and synovial fibroblasts. *Biol Pharm Bull*. 2010;33(3):410-414. doi:10.1248/bpb.33.410
16. Husseini L, Leussink VI, Warnke C, Hartung HP, Kieseier BC. [Cannabinoids for symptomatic therapy of multiple sclerosis] [in German]. *Nervenarzt*. 2012;83(6):695-704. doi:10.1007/s00115-011-3401-9
17. Namazi MR. The beneficial and detrimental effects of linoleic acid on autoimmune disorders. *Autoimmunity*. 2004;37(1):73-75. doi:10.1080/08916930310001637968
18. Benzie IFF, Wachtel-Galor S. *Herbal Medicine: Biomolecular and Clinical Aspects*. 2nd ed. Boca Raton, FL: CRC Press; 2011. doi:10.1201/b10787
19. Mdzinarishvili A, Sumbria R, Lang D, Klein J. Ginkgo extract EGb761 confers neuroprotection by reduction of glutamate release in ischemic brain. *J Pharm Pharm Sci*. 2012;15(1):94-102. doi:10.18433/J3PS37
20. Junger A. *Clean: The Revolutionary Program to Restore the Body's Natural Ability to Heal Itself*. New York, NY: Harper Collins; 2009.
21. Accardi G, Caruso C, Colonna-Romano G, Camarda C, Monastero R, Candore G. Can Alzheimer disease be a form of type 3 diabetes? *Rejuvenation Res*. 2012;15(2):217-221. doi:10.1089/rej.2011.1289
22. Bisht B, Darling WG, Grossmann RE, et al. A multimodal intervention for patients with secondary progressive multiple sclerosis: feasibility and effect on fatigue. *J Altern Complement Med*. 2014;20(5):347-355. doi:10.1089/acm.2013.0188
23. Byl N, Barbe M, Dolan C, Glass G. Repetitive Strain Injuries. In: McGee DJ, Zachazewski JE, Quillen WS, Maske RC. *Pathology and Intervention Musculoskeletal Rehabilitation*. New York, NY: Elsevier Health Science; 2015.
24. Lazaro R, Reina-Guerra S, Quiben M. *Umphred's Neurological Rehabilitation*. 7th ed. St. Louis, MO: Elsevier; 2019.
25. Oschman JL. *Energy Medicine: The Scientific Basis*. 2nd ed. St. Louis, MO: Elsevier; 2016.
26. Kahn J. Therapeutic massage and rehabilitation. In: Davis CM, ed. *Integrative Therapies in Rehabilitation; Evidence for Efficacy in Therapy, Prevention, and Wellness*. 4th ed. Thorofare, NJ: SLACK Incorporated; 2016.
27. Juhan D. *Job's Body: A Handbook for Bodywork*. Barrytown, NY: Station Hill Press; 2003.
28. Jäkel A, von Hauenschild P. Therapeutic effects of cranial osteopathic manipulative medicine: a systematic review. *J Am Osteopath Assoc*. 2011;111(12):685-693.
29. Giaquinto-Wahl DA. Craniosacral therapy. In: Davis CM, ed. *Integrative Therapies in Rehabilitation: Evidence for Efficacy in Therapy, Prevention, and Wellness*. 4th ed. Thorofare, NJ: SLACK Incorporated; 2016.
30. Benias PC, Wells RG, Sackey-Aboagye B, et al. Structure and distribution of an unrecognized interstitium in human tissues. *Sci Rep*. 2018;8(1):4947. doi:10.1038/s41598-018-23062-6
31. Guimberteau JC. *Strolling Under the Skin* [Video]. SFRS Service du Film de Recherche Scientifique; 2005.
32. Guimberteau JC, Armstrong C. *Architecture of Human Living Fascia: The Extracellular Matrix and Cells Revealed Through Endoscopy*. Edinburgh, UK: Handspring Publishing Limited; 2015.
33. Stecco C, Macchi V, Porzionato A, Duparc F, De Caro R. The fascia: the forgotten structure. *Ital J Anat Embryol*. 2011;116(3):127-138.
34. Barnes JF. *Myofascial Release: the search for excellence, a comprehensive evaluator and treatment approach*. MFR Seminars; 1990.
35. Barral JP, Mercier P. *Visceral Manipulation*. Seattle, WA: Eastland Press, Inc; 2005.
36. Barnes JF. Myofascial release: the missing link in traditional treatment. In: Davis CM, ed. *Integrative Therapies in Rehabilitation: Evidence for Efficacy in Therapy, Prevention, and Wellness*. 4th ed. Thorofare, NJ: SLACK Incorporated; 2016.
37. Tozzi P, Bongiorno D, Vitturini C. Fascial release effects on patients with non-specific cervical or lumbar pain. *J Bodyw Mov Ther*. 2011;15(4):405-416. doi:10.1016/j.jbmt.2010.11.003
38. Funk B, Kunlel KR. Complete decongestive therapy. In: Davis CM, ed. *Integrative Therapies in Rehabilitation: Evidence for Efficacy in Therapy, Prevention, and Wellness*. 4th ed. Thorofare, NJ: SLACK Incorporated; 2016.
39. Cohen MD. Complete decongestive physical therapy in a patient with secondary lymphedema due to orthopedic trauma and surgery of the lower extremity. *Phys Ther*. 2011;91(11):1618-1626. doi:10.2522/ptj.20100101
40. Jacobson E. Structural integration, an alternative method of manual therapy and sensorimotor education. *J Altern Complement Med*. 2011;17(10):891-899. doi:10.1089/acm.2010.0258
41. Deutsch J. The Ida Rolf method of structural integration. In: Davis CM, ed. *Integrative Therapies in Rehabilitation: Evidence for Efficacy in Therapy, Prevention, and Wellness*. 4th ed. Thorofare, NJ: SLACK Incorporated; 2016.
42. Bottomley JM. T'ai chi: choreography of body and mind. In: Davis CM, ed. *Integrative Therapies in Rehabilitation: Evidence for Efficacy in Therapy, Prevention, and Wellness*. 4th ed. Thorofare, NJ: SLACK Incorporated; 2016.
43. Li F, Harmer P, Liu Y, et al. A randomized controlled trial of patient-reported outcomes with tai chi exercise in Parkinson's disease. *Mov Disord*. 2014;29(4):539-545. doi:10.1002/mds.25787

44. Vergara-Diaz G, Osypiuk K, Hausdorff JM, et al. Tai chi for reducing dual-task gait variability, a potential mediator of fall risk in Parkinson's disease: a pilot randomized controlled trial. *Glob Adv Health Med.* 2018;7:2164956118775385. doi:10.1177/2164956118775385
45. Winser SJ, Tsang WW, Krishnamurthy K, Kannan P. Does Tai Chi improve balance and reduce falls incidence in neurological disorders? A systematic review and meta-analysis. *Clin Rehabil.* 2018;32(9):1157-1168. doi:10.1177/0269215518773442
46. Li F, Harmer P, Fitzgerald K, et al. Tai chi and postural stability in patients with Parkinson's disease. *N Engl J Med.* 2012;366(6):511-519. doi:10.1056/NEJMoa1107911
47. Field T. Tai Chi research review. *Complement Ther Clin Pract.* 2011;17(3):141-146. doi:10.1016/j.ctcp.2010.10.002
48. Wahbeh H, Elsas SM, Oken BS. Mind-body interventions: applications in neurology. *Neurology.* 2008;70(24):2321-2328. doi:10.1212/01.wnl.0000314667.16386.5e
49. Bottomley JM. Biofeedback: connecting the body and mind. In: Davis CM, ed. *Integrative Therapies in Rehabilitation: Evidence for Efficacy in Therapy, Prevention, and Wellness.* 4th ed. Thorofare, NJ: SLACK Incorporated; 2016.
50. Esculier JF, Vaudrin J, Bériault P, Gagnon K, Tremblay LE. Home-based balance training programme using Wii Fit with balance board for Parkinsons's disease: a pilot study. *J Rehabil Med.* 2012;44(2):144-150. doi:10.2340/16501977-0922
51. Byl K, Byl N, Byl M. Integrating technology into clinical practice in neurological rehabilitation. In: Umphred DA, Lazaro R, Roller M, Burton G, eds. *Umphred's Neurological Rehabilitation.* 6th ed. St. Louis, MO: Elsevier; 2013. doi:10.1016/B978-0-323-07586-2.00047-9
52. Taylor MJ. Yoga therapeutics: an ancient practice in a 21st century setting. In: Davis CM, ed. *Integrative Therapies in Rehabilitation: Evidence for Efficacy in Therapy, Prevention, and Wellness.* 4th ed. Thorofare, NJ: SLACK Incorporated; 2016.
53. Smith JA, Greer T, Sheets T, Watson S. Is there more to yoga than exercise? *Altern Ther Health Med.* 2011;17(3):22-29.
54. Guner S, Inanici F. Yoga therapy and ambulatory multiple sclerosis Assessment of gait analysis parameters, fatigue and balance. *J Bodyw Mov Ther.* 2015;19(1):72-81. doi:10.1016/j.jbmt.2014.04.004
55. Martins RF, Pinto e Silva JL. Treatment of pregnancy-related lumbar and pelvic girdle pain by the yoga method: a randomized controlled study. *J Altern Complement Med.* 2014;20(1):24-31. doi:10.1089/acm.2012.0715
56. Tiedemann A, O'Rourke S, Sherrington C. Is a yoga-based program with potential to decrease falls perceived to be acceptable to community-dwelling people older than 60? *Public Health Res Pract.* 2018;28(2):28011801. doi:10.17061/phrp28011801
57. Veneri D, Gannotti M, Bertucco M, Fournier Hillman SE. Using the International Classification of Functioning, Disability and Health model to gain perspective of the benefits of yoga in stroke, multiple sclerosis, and children to inform practice for children with cerebral palsy: a meta-analysis. *J Altern Complement Med.* 2018;24(5):439-457. doi:10.1089/acm.2017.0030
58. Kwok JYY, Kwan JCY, Auyeung M, Mok VCT, Chan HYL. The effects of yoga versus stretching and resistance training exercises on psychological distress for people with mild-to-moderate Parkinson's disease: study prxotocol for a randomized controlled trial. *Trials.* 2017;18(1):509. doi:10.1186/s13063-017-2223-x
59. Zuck D. The Alexander technique. In: Davis CM, ed. *Integrative Therapies in Rehabilitation: Evidence for Efficacy in Therapy, Prevention, and Wellness.* 3rd ed. Thorofare, NJ: SLACK Incorporated; 2009:207-224.
60. Woodman JP, Moore NR. Evidence for the effectiveness of Alexander Technique lessons in medical and health-related conditions: a systematic review. *Int J Clin Pract.* 2012;66(1):98-112. doi:10.1111/j.1742-1241.2011.02817.x
61. Stephens J, Miller TM. Feldenkrais method in rehabilitation: using functional integration and awareness through movement to explore new possibilities. In: Davis CM, ed. *Integrative Therapies in Rehabilitation: Evidence for Efficacy in Therapy, Prevention, and Wellness.* 4th ed. Thorofare, NJ: SLACK Incorporated; 2016:203-225.
62. Connors KA, Pile C, Nichols ME. Does the Feldenkrais Method make a difference? An investigation into the use of outcome measurement tools for evaluating changes in clients. *J Bodyw Mov Ther.* 2011;15(4):446-452. doi:10.1016/j.jbmt.2010.09.001
63. Teixeira-Machado L, Araújo FM, Cunha FA, Menezes M, Menezes T, Melo DeSantana J. Feldenkrais method-based exercise improves quality of life in individuals with Parkinson's disease: a controlled, randomized clinical trial. *Altern Ther Health Med.* 2015;21(1):8-14.
64. Torres-Unda J, Polo V, Dunabeitia I, et al. The Feldenkrais Method improves functioning and body balance in people with intellectual disability in supported employment: A randomized clinical trial. *Res Dev Disabil.* 2017;70:104-112. doi:10.1016/j.ridd.2017.08.012
65. Anderson B. Pilates rehabilitation. In: Davis CM, ed. *Integrative Therapies in Rehabilitation: Evidence for Efficacy in Therapy, Prevention, and Wellness.* 4th ed. Thorofare, NJ: SLACK Incorporated; 2016.
66. Myers TW. *Anatomy Trains: Myofascial Meridians for Manual and Movement Therapists.* Edinburgh, UK: Elsevier; 2009.
67. Vleeming A, Mooney V, Stoeckart R. *Movement, Stability & Lumbopelvic Pain: Integration of research and therapy.* 2nd ed. Edinburgh, UK: Elsevier; 2007.
68. Franklin E. *Dynamic Alignment Through Imagery.* Leeds, UK: Human Kinetics; 1996.
69. Kalron A, Rosenblum U, Frid L, Achiron A. Pilates exercise training vs. physical therapy for improving walking and balance in people with multiple sclerosis: a randomized controlled trial. *Clin Rehabil.* 2017;31(3):319-328. doi:10.1177/0269215516637202
70. Bulguroglu I, Guclu-Gunduz A, Yazici G, et al. The effects of Mat Pilates and Reformer Pilates in patients with Multiple Sclerosis: A randomized controlled study. *NeuroRehabilitation.* 2017;41(2):413-422.
71. Kara B, Küçük F, Poyraz EC, Tomruk MS, İdıman E. Different types of exercise in Multiple Sclerosis: aerobic exercise or Pilates, a single-blind clinical study. *J Back Musculoskeletal Rehabil.* 2017;30(3):565-573. doi:10.3233/BMR-150515

72. Soysal Tomruk M, Uz MZ, Kara B, İdiman E. Effects of Pilates exercises on sensory interaction, postural control and fatigue in patients with multiple sclerosis. *Mult Scler Relat Disord*. 2016;7:70-73. doi:10.1016/j.msard.2016.03.008
73. Dos Santos AN, Serikawa SS, Rocha NA. Pilates improves lower limbs strength and postural control during quite standing in a child with hemiparetic cerebral palsy: A case report study. *Dev Neurorehabil*. 2016;19(4):226-230.
74. Gale NK. From body-talk to body-stories: body work in complementary and alternative medicine. *Sociol Health Illn*. 2011;33(2):237-251. doi:10.1111/j.1467-9566.2010.01291.x
75. International Body Talk Global Healing. International Body Talk Association Body Talk Principles, Knowledge, Applications. https://www.bodytalksystem.com/learn/bodytalk/research/journal_articles.cfm. Accessed June 28, 2018.
76. Fiery MF, Martz DM, Webb RM, Curtin L. A preliminary investigation of racial differences in body talk in age-diverse U.S. adults. *Eat Behav*. 2016;21:232-235. doi:10.1016/j.eatbeh.2016.03.004
77. Singg S. Reiki: an alternative and complementary healing therapy. In: Davis CM, ed. *Integrative Therapies in Rehabilitation: Evidence for Efficacy in Therapy, Prevention, and Wellness*. 4th ed. Thorofare, NJ: SLACK Incorporated; 2016.
78. Lee MS, Pittler MH, Ernst E. Effects of reiki in clinical practice: a systematic review of randomised clinical trials. *Int J Clin Pract*. 2008;62(6):947-954. doi:10.1111/j.1742-1241.2008.01729.x
79. Bukowski EL. The use of self-Reiki for stress reduction and relaxation. *J Integr Med*. 2015;13(5):336-340. doi:10.1016/S2095-4964(15)60190-X
80. Orsak G, Stevens AM, Brufsky A, Kajumba M, Dougall AL. The effects of Reiki therapy and companionship on quality of life, mood, and symptom distress during chemotherapy. *J Evid Based Complementary Altern Med*. 2015;20(1):20-27. doi:10.1177/2156587214556313
81. Bottomley JM. Qi gong for health and healing. In: Davis CM, ed. *Integrative Therapies in Rehabilitation: Evidence for Efficacy in Therapy, Prevention, and Wellness*. 4th ed. Thorofare, NJ: SLACK Incorporated; 2016.
82. Jahnke R, Larkey L, Rogers C, Etnier J, Lin F. A comprehensive review of health benefits of qigong and tai chi. *Am J Health Promot*. 2010;24(6):e1-e25. doi:10.4278/ajhp.081013-LIT-248
83. Spielholz NI. Magnets: what is the evidence of efficacy? In: Davis CM, ed. *Integrative Therapies in Rehabilitation: Evidence for Efficacy in Therapy, Prevention, and Wellness*. 3rd ed. Thorofare, NJ: SLACK Incorporated; 2009.
84. Song BW, Hong H, Jung YJ, Lee JH, Kim BS, Lee HB. Combination therapy comprising a static magnetic field with contractility improves skin wounds. *Tissue Eng Part A*. 2018;24(17-18):1354-1363. doi:10.1089/ten.tea.2017.0470
85. LaRiccia PJ, Sowers K, Littman LB, Galantino ML. Acupuncture theory and acupuncture-like therapeutics in physical therapy. In: Davis CM, ed. *Integrative Therapies in Rehabilitation: Evidence for Efficacy in Therapy, Prevention, and Wellness*. 4th ed. Thorofare, NJ: SLACK Incorporated; 2016.
86. Hsing WT, Imamura M, Weaver K, Fregni F, Azevedo Neto RS. Clinical effects of scalp electrical acupuncture in stroke: a sham-controlled randomized clinical trial. *J Altern Complement Med*. 2012;18(4):341-346. doi:10.1089/acm.2011.0131
87. Han L, Xie YH, Wu R, Chen C, Zhang Y, Wang XP. Traditional Chinese medicine for modern treatment of Parkinson's disease. *Chin J Integr Med*. 2017;23(8):635-640. doi:10.1007/s11655-016-2537-7
88. Anderson EZ. Therapeutic touch. In: Davis CM, ed. *Integrative Therapies in Rehabilitation: Evidence for Efficacy in Therapy, Prevention, and Wellness*. 4th ed. Thorofare, NJ: SLACK Incorporated; 2016.
89. Honda N, Ohgi S, Wada N, Loo KK, Higashimoto Y, Fukuda K. Effect of therapeutic touch on brain activation of preterm infants in response to sensory punctate stimulus: a near-infrared spectroscopy-based study. *Arch Dis Child Fetal Neonatal Ed*. 2013;98(3):F244-F248. doi:10.1136/archdischild-2011-301469
90. Vanaki Z, Matourypour P, Gholami R, Zare Z, Mehrzad V, Dehghan M. Therapeutic touch for nausea in breast cancer patients receiving chemotherapy: composing a treatment. *Complement Ther Clin Pract*. 2016;22:64-68. doi:10.1016/j.ctcp.2015.12.004
91. Emoto M. *Water Knows the Answer*. Tokyo, Japan: Sunmark Publishing; 2001.
92. Pert CB. *Molecules of Emotion: The Science Behind Mind-Body Medicine*. Simon & Schuster; 1997.
93. Lipton BH. *The Biology of Belief: Unleashing the Power of Consciousness, Matter, & Miracles*. Carlsbad, CA: Hay House Inc; 2008.
94. Schultz RL, Feitis R. *The Endless Web: Fascial Anatomy and Physical Reality*. Berkeley, CA: North Atlantic Books; 1996.
95. Doidge N. *The Brain's Way of Healing. Remarkable Discoveries and Recoveries from the Frontiers of Neuroplasticity*. New York, NY: Penguin Books; 2016.
96. McTaggart L. *The Field: The Quest for the Secret Force of the Universe*. New York, NY: Harper; 2008.
97. Talbot M. *The Holographic Universe*. New York, NY: Harper Perennial; 2011.
98. Laszlo E. *Science and the Akashic Field: An Integral Theory of Everything*. Rochester, VT: Inner Traditions; 2007.

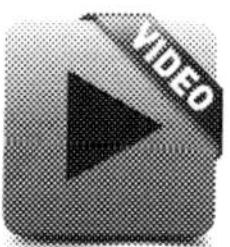

Chapter 19

Technologies in Neurorehabilitation

Arvie Vitente, PT, DPT, MPH, GCS, CDP, CCI, PhD(c)

KEY WORDS Activity tracking devices | Body weight–supported treadmill training | Cell phone applications | Exoskeletons | Gaming programs | Neurorehabilitation | Neurorobot | Neurorobotic training | Regenerative rehabilitation | Virtual reality environment

Chapter Objectives

- Discuss the use of body weight–supported treadmill training (BWSTT), exoskeletons, and robotic training in neurorehabilitation.
- Discuss the use of virtual reality (VR) environment in strength, balance and coordination, and cognitive training in patients with neurological conditions.
- Explain the use of common technologies found in the household such as the Wii (Nintendo), PlayStation (Sony), and Kinect (Microsoft) as part of neurorehabilitation.
- Explain the use of activity tracking devices and cell phone applications in neurorehabilitation.
- Explain the role of a physical therapist and physical therapist assistant in regenerative rehabilitation.

The third edition of *The Guide to Physical Therapist Practice* (the *Guide*) explains[1] in detail the steps in the patient/client management that the physical therapist and physical therapist assistant must follow. These steps include the examination, evaluation, diagnosis, prognosis, interventions, and outcomes. The principal element in which the physical therapist or the physical therapist assistant has both an interaction with the patient/client is the *intervention* portion.[2] Physical therapy interventions related to neurological rehabilitation delegated to a physical therapist assistant can be grouped into 5 categories: functional activity training, impairment training, hands-on guidance by the therapist, somatosensory retraining, and participation training.

This chapter discusses accepted interventions in neurorehabilitation that focus on the integration of technology into clinical practice. This includes BWSTT, exoskeletons, robotics, and the use of the VR environment for strength, balance coordination, and cognitive training. The chapter will also discuss the common technologies found in the household that patients can use to continue their neurorehabilitation once leaving the facility, including the Wii, PlayStation, and Kinect, and activity tracking devices and cell phone applications (apps). A discussion about the future of regenerative medicine as related to neurorehabilitation will also be briefly covered.

Goals of Neurorehabilitation

The goals of the interventions in neurologic rehabilitation may be classified into therapeutic, assistance, or substitution for neurological deficits.[3] The use of appropriate technology can help achieve those goals. An entry-level physical therapist assistant is expected to provide safe and effective interventions and to discuss with the supervising physical therapist any concerns regarding safe administration of any interventions.

Lazaro RT, Umphred DA, eds.
Umphred's Neurorehabilitation for the Physical Therapist Assistant, Third Edition (pp 413-422).

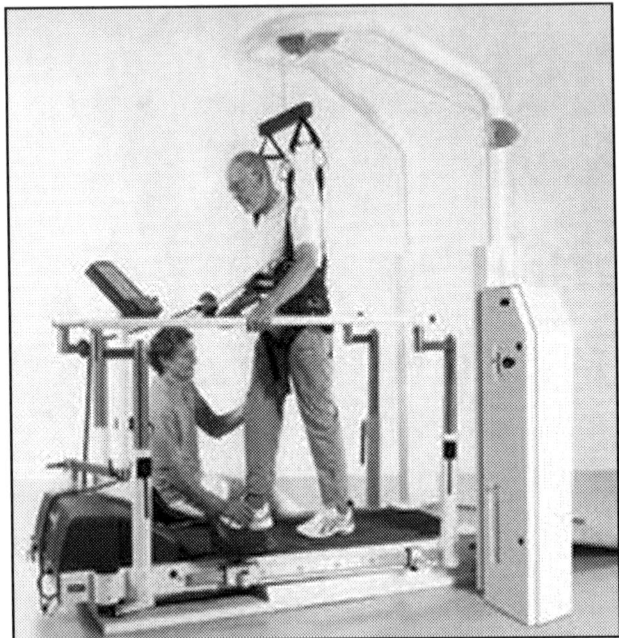

Figure 19-1. An example of BWSTT. (Picture: Hocoma, Switzerland.)

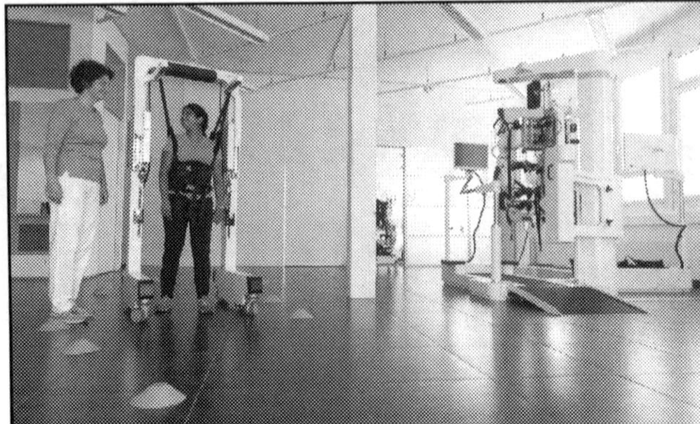

Figure 19-2. Body weight–supported overground training. (Picture: Hocoma, Switzerland.)

Advanced Clinical Technology

The integration of advanced clinical technology to help achieve the goals of the interventions in neurorehabilitation are gaining popularity and acceptance. Rehabilitation robotics is being seen as a safe and effective adjunct to physical therapy treatment. These novel intervention approaches show promising outcomes in maximizing independence and improving quality of life in people with neurological insults. Results of studies on neuroplasticity and motor relearning associated with stroke and other neurologic conditions are now being used to support the use of these technologies in rehabilitation practice (see Chapters 4 and 5).[4] These technologies can assist the clinician in providing early mobilization, optimal repetition, saliency, and safety that can improve patient outcomes through the enhancement of functional mobility. Evidence also shows that these innovative therapies could facilitate improvement in cognitive abilities, motor skills, and movement quality in patients.[5]

Body Weight–Support Systems

Body weight–support systems can help in the therapeutic process by providing stability, support, and unweighting of the body to allow more normal movements to occur and be practiced repeatedly by the patient with the assistance of a clinician. Body weight–support systems could be overground or with the use of a treadmill (eg, BWSTT; Figure 19-1). A brief description of this intervention in patients with stroke can be found in Chapter 13; additional information and applications of this technology in other conditions can be found in Chapters 5, 9, 11, and 12. Body weight–support systems can also be configured in a therapeutic pool as part of an aquatic therapy program. This set up incorporates buoyancy to help further unweight the joints, and also gives the option of exercising using water as resistance. Whether overground (Figure 19-2) or using a treadmill, the patient is placed on a harness and attached to a suspension system that allows unweighting of the body. The amount of body weight supported by the device will be set at a level that will appropriately facilitate bilateral limb loading while preventing knee buckling, which is defined as premature knee flexion during weight-bearing. The environment enhances patient safety and confidence because the risk for falling is removed via the suspension system. It requires less demand on the patient to use his or her upper extremity for support while training. It also affords less physical strain on the therapist, who would otherwise need to provide more support and assistance to facilitate movements while keeping the patient safe. Because of the safe and supported environment, repetitions—and therefore the opportunity to practice in a task-specific environment of walking—are optimized, potentially leading to better outcomes than conventional therapy alone.[6]

The usual progression of the intervention using this device includes pre-gait training, then treadmill training, and then overground gait training. The important pre-gait activities that can be facilitated by using this device include weight-shifting, stepping in place, and sit-to-stand squat. Weight-shifting activities during pre-gait training could be helpful in improving stance symmetry by allowing increased load acceptance in the patient's paretic lower extremity.[7]

During treadmill training, assistance to move the lower extremities can be done unilaterally or bilaterally as appropriate. Increased repetitions allow the patient to practice the task over and over. Treadmill speed can be adjusted; slowing the speed focuses on the movement pattern and weight-bearing components, while increasing the speed allows for a more intense training that supports functional speeds for walking. Repetition, salience, and intensity can be focused with the training.

Overground training prepares the patient to walk on real environments and focuses on transference of skill from walking on treadmill to overground.

Another benefit of using body weight–support systems is early mobility. Using the equipment provides a safe system to move the patient to vertical, thereby facilitating early standing and weight-bearing. Early mobilization is associated with fewer complications and better long-term outcomes in people with stroke.[8]

Body weight–support can also be done through lower-body positive pressure systems, where a person's lower body is contained in an airtight chamber that also contains a treadmill, then inflated to create a force that unweights a person. Commercially available lower-body positive pressure devices such as the AlterG treadmill (AlterG) can unweight up to 80% of the person's body weight. The advantage of this method of body weight–support is the ability of the person to perform upper extremity functional and dual-task activities while walking or running on a treadmill with body weight–support. These units have been used to rehabilitate after total hip or knee replacements and to help in returning to sports. Neurological applications include training to improve mobility in persons with stroke, Parkinson's disease, and other neuromuscular conditions.[9]

Rehabilitation Robotics in Neurorehabilitation

The Robot Institute of America defines a robot as "a programmable, multi-functional manipulator designed to move material, parts or specialized devices through variable programmed motions for the performance of a variety of tasks."[10] In the field of neurorehabilitation, the type of robot that is being used is called a *neurorobot*—defined as an electromechanical device programmed with an artificial intelligence that can perform a variation of humanoid functions. These robots were first developed in the 1980s,[11] and in the early 2000s[12] robotic exoskeletons—such as the Lokomat (Hocoma), Armeo (Hocoma), Anklebot (MIT), EksoGT (Ekso Bionics)—became available in the market. Most of the barriers associated with the use of neurorobots include fear of use, risks for bodily harm, and ethical issues.[13]

Isamov[13] discussed the 3 laws related to robotic technology that may be applied to neurorobots as follows:

1. A neurorobot may not allow a patient to be injured or to come to harm.
2. A neurorobot must follow the orders given by clinicians, except where such orders would conflict with the first law.
3. A neurorobot must adapt its behavior to the patient's abilities in a visible manner as long as it does not conflict with the first or second laws.

The main types emerging therapies using neurorobots that include verticalization robots such as the Erigo (Hocoma), body weight–supported treadmill systems with robotics (eg, Lokomat), wearable assistive robotic device (eg, Armeo for upper extremities and EksoGT for lower extremities), and body weight–supported mobile walking aids such as the Andago (Hocoma).

Verticalization Robots

These robots are primarily used to get an acutely impaired patient progressively in the upright position for early mobilization. Patients with severe neurological diseases could be at risk for secondary complications due to the damaging effects of immobilization such as weakness, decreased endurance, skin breakdown, and impairments in mobility. Verticalization robots such as Erigo have 2 main therapeutic goals: to prevent joint stiffness through early passive range of motion of bilateral lower extremities by the device, and improvement of muscle strength through passive range of motion of bilateral lower extremities by the device, which the therapist ultimately progresses to progressive resistive exercises. Through verticalization, the clinician could also help the patient perform object manipulation with the use of bilateral upper extremities. Moreover, this intervention can be used to manage orthostatic hypotension, similar to the use of a tilt-table (Figure 19-3).

Verticalization using robotic devices can start as early as the first day in an intensive care unit to allow the patient to increase awareness of their surroundings. Preliminary evidence supports that the system is safe for early mobilization.[12,14] Erigo can permit tilt-table functionality in combination with the stepping movement with or without functional electrical stimulation (FES; Figure 19-4).[15] Evidence suggests that robotic tilt-table training such as Erigo could be more effective as compared to tilt-table training alone.[15] Furthermore, if started during the acute stage, an intensive stepping verticalization protocol in patients with severe acquired brain injury has been found to improve the short- and long-term functional and neurological outcomes of patients with disorders of consciousness.[16] Therefore, early mobility using robotic technology is recommended, provided that there is hemodynamic, respiratory, and intracranial stability.[16]

Body Weight–Supported Treadmill Systems With Robotics

Robotic technology can be incorporated with treadmill gait training to allow optimal intensity and repetition while still maintaining a safe environment for both the patient and clinician. This is achieved through the use of *exoskeletons*, which are robotic devices that provide an external support to the patient. Lokomat, a robotic device that is essentially a computerized gait orthosis (Figure 19-5), can

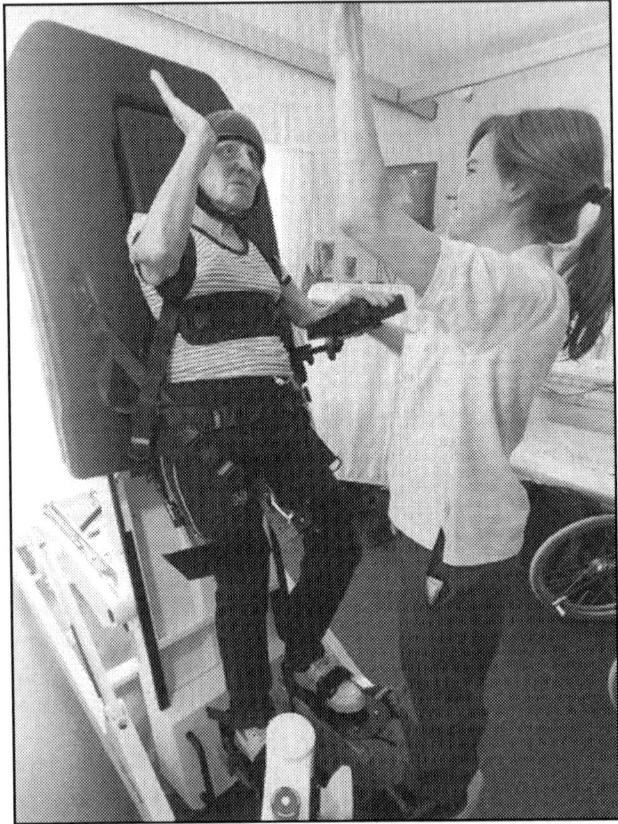

Figure 19-3. Example of a verticalization robot. (Picture: Hocoma, Switzerland.)

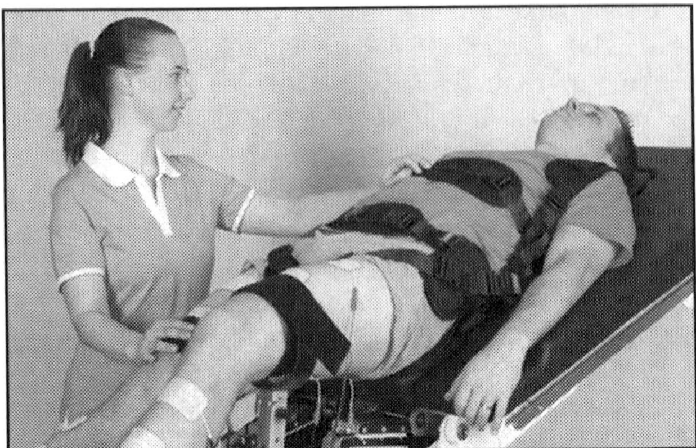

Figure 19-4. Verticalization robots can facilitate stepping movements with the incorporation of FES. (Picture: Hocoma, Switzerland.)

be used in conjunction with BWSTT.[17] Evidence suggests that robotic training, like ones that can be done using the Lokomat combined with conventional physical therapy, can produce a better improvement in gait, balance, functional status, cognitive function, and quality of life in patients post-stroke.[18] Evidence also suggests positive effects of conventional gait training and BWSTT on gait and clinical manifestations in patients with idiopathic Parkinson's disease. The advantages of BWSTT with robotics over conventional therapy include the following:

- Therapists are not exposed to increased physical strain, decreasing therapist burnout.
- Staffing becomes more efficient because a single therapist can provide therapy.
- The patient will have longer training duration and higher intensity, repetition, and feedback.
- The therapy will help the patient perform a gait pattern that is highly reproducible and more physiological.

A more physiological gait pattern can be done by adjusting the exoskeleton to the individualized needs of patients. The Lokomat permits the following characteristics of a good gait pattern in a complete gait cycle: natural plantar pressure distribution, sensory feedback, and physiological vertical displacement. This device provides a task-specific performance feedback that will augment the patient's motivation.

Wearable Assistive Robotic Devices for the Upper Extremity

Impairments of arm and hand functions are common in patients with neurological conditions. Robotic devices are available to assist in regaining upper extremity function. The Armeo Power therapy is a fixed, upper-extremity service robotic device that facilitates highly repetitive and intensive early arm rehabilitation (Figure 19-6). The device supports the weight of the patient's arm and guides the movement of the arm. Game-like exercises, which are highly challenging and motivating to the patients, can be programmed. These types of exercises are examples of an augmented performance feedback and are designed to train functional movement patterns used to perform activities of daily living. The exercises are individualized based on the patient's motor and cognitive capabilities and can be progressed based on the stage of the patient's motor recovery. It can also be programmed for fine motor control training, and upper limb dysfunctions (Figure 19-7). This is also a wearable exoskeleton device with an integrated spring mechanism allowing variable upper limb gravity support. Evidence suggests that this is an effective intervention for enhancing upper limb functions in patients with multiple sclerosis.[19]

Wearable Assistive Robotic Devices for the Lower Extremity

The wearable overground robotic exoskeletons can assist weight-bearing and ambulation in patients with a spinal cord injury. The EksoGT is intended to facilitate ambulation in patients with stroke and spinal cord injury patients (Figure 19-8). The devices are designed as adjuncts to neurorehabilitation to facilitate relearning of physiological step patterns, weight-shifting, and lessening compensatory patterns during sit-to-stand transfers and ambulation. Evidence states that supervised locomotor training program using a wearable overground robotic exoskeleton such as the EksoGT is feasible and relatively safe.[20]

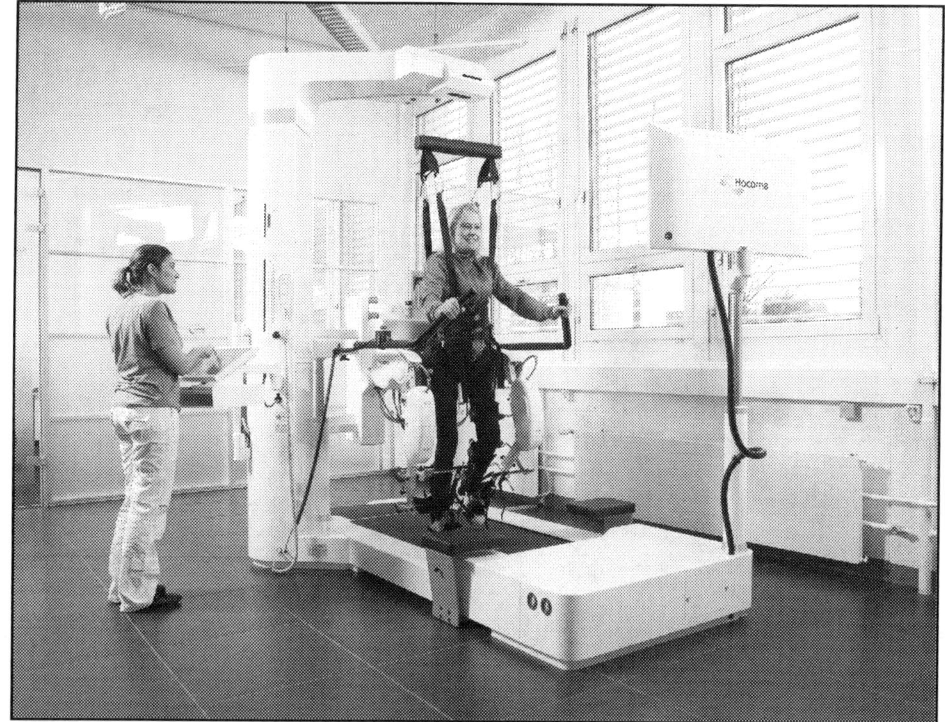

Figure 19-5. Example of a robotic device that is essentially a computerized gait orthotic. (Picture: Hocoma, Switzerland.)

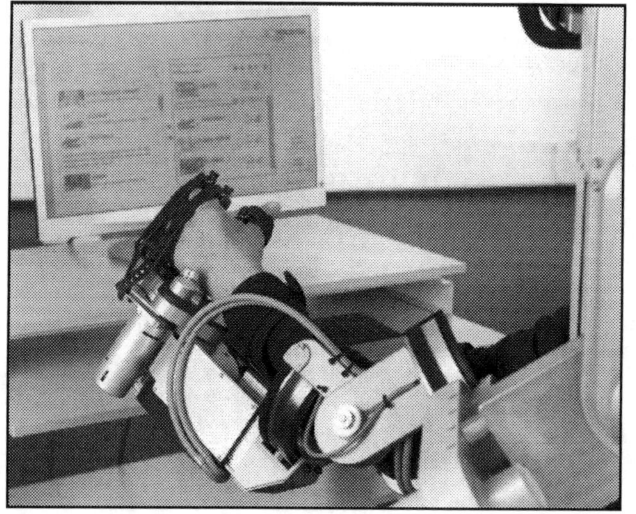

Figure 19-6. Example of an upper extremity robotic device. (Picture: Hocoma, Switzerland.)

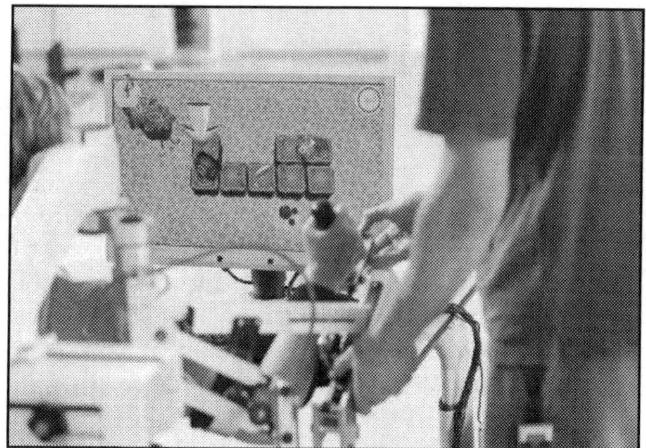

Figure 19-7. The upper extremity robotic device can be paired with a game-like device with a monitor to allow purposeful arm movements. (Picture: Hocoma, Switzerland.)

It is important to note that the physical therapist must evaluate, and the physical therapist or physical therapist assistant must complete a training program prior to the use of this neurorobot. Presently, the devices are not recommended for use in sports activities or stair-climbing functions.

Neuroprosthesis

It is also important to briefly discuss the use of neuroprosthesis in neurorehabilitation as a wearable assistive non-robotic device. A neuroprosthesis uses FES for therapeutic gain or functional assistance to both upper and lower extremities. This intervention uses surface, percutaneous, and implanted electrodes to enable muscle contraction. For example, available neuroprostheses enable grasp-and-release

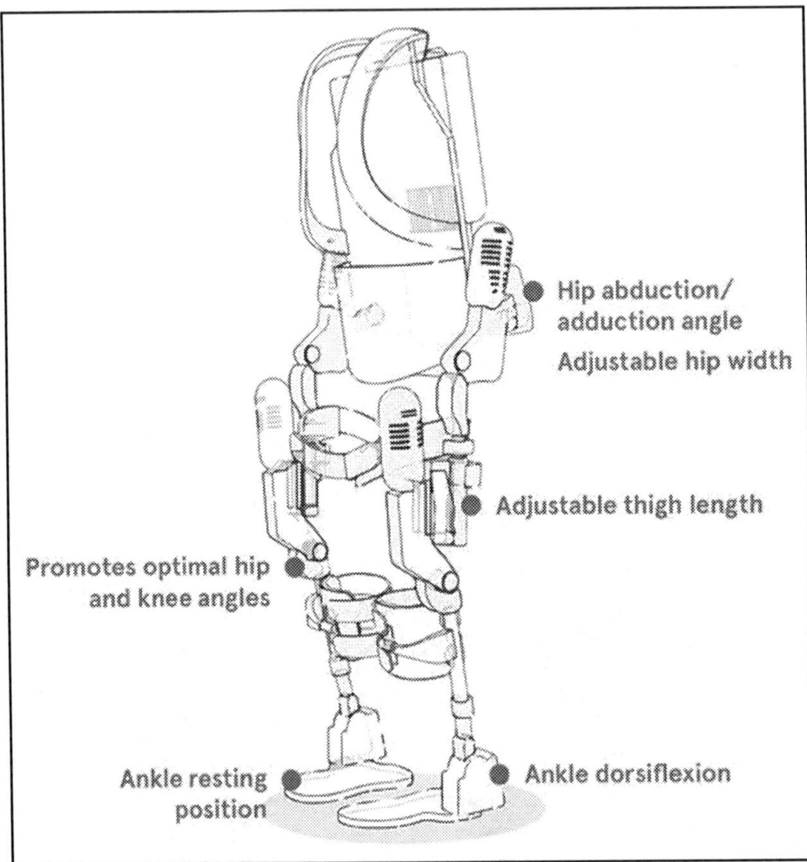

Figure 19-8. EksoGT is a wearable overground robotic exoskeleton. (Reprinted with permission from Ekso Bionics.)

to be used in performing tasks such as eating, personal hygiene, writing, and completing office tasks.[21,22] The NESS H200 Hand Rehabilitation System (Bioness) can be used to allow synchronized muscle activity of the flexors and extensors of the wrist and hand following stroke or a spinal cord injury to reduce muscle spasm, improve local blood circulation, retard disuse atrophy, and prevent joint contractures.[23]

Body Weight–Supported Mobile Walking Aids

Body weight–supported mobile walking aids allow the patient to perform self-directed gait activities while on a body weight–support system. This neurorobot actively follows the patient and permits the patient to explore locations in the clinic and at home. Andago is an example that transitions the patient from treadmill-based gait training such as BWSTT or with the use of the Lokomat, and overground free ambulation (Figure 19-9). This neurorobot has a dynamic body weight–support that helps the patient perform normal walking. Therapists will be able to focus on giving the patients the cues they need during the gait training because patients are secure. It also decreases physical strain on the therapists.

Virtual Reality

VR is a type of interaction between an individual and a computer-generated environment that can stimulate sensory modalities including visual, auditory, or haptic (ie, tactile and proprioceptive) experiences.[24,25] This application describes a virtual, computer-generated world scenario in which the user can interact in three dimensions to feel part of it.[26] VR offers clinicians the opportunity to bring the patient into a contrived environment, but with the complexity of the physical world. This can facilitate the patient's balance and postural control in the environment with different physical variables that can influence the patient's behavior toward these variables. At the same time, this intervention allows the therapist to record the patient's physiological and kinematic responses.[27]

Studies show that VR interventions were clinically effective and well-tolerated by patients, but a systematic review in 2017 suggested the need for larger, well-controlled studies to indicate clinical and cost-effectiveness of the use of VR in medical inpatient settings.[24]

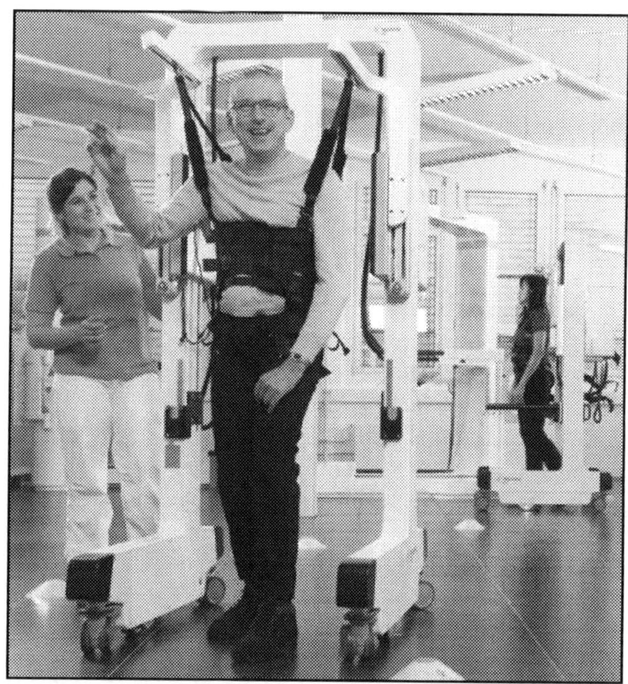

Figure 19-9. Overground walking with body weight–support. (Picture: Hocoma, Switzerland.)

Body Weight–Supported Treadmill Training With Virtual Reality Technology

Newer technologies combine BSWTT and VR technology for balance and postural control training. C-Mill by Motek (Hocoma) enables the therapist to perform balance assessments and training exercises. This makes it easier to establish the baseline balance level of the patient and the effect of the balance training. Early intervention is possible with the device. Safe balance assessment methods and training can be provided because of the support from the device (Figure 19-10).

Virtual Reality Technology to Improve Impairments and Activity Limitations

Evidence suggests that rehabilitation using VR to provide intensive and repetitive training sessions can increase strength that improves lower limb motor function in patients with incomplete spinal cord injury. It was suggested that initial training to the patient and/or caregivers is needed to ensure proper execution of the program at home. This home-based training could be beneficial to patients with neurological conditions in terms of reducing transportation cost and effort. Through this rehabilitation technique, patient adherence and outcome could be enhanced.[28]

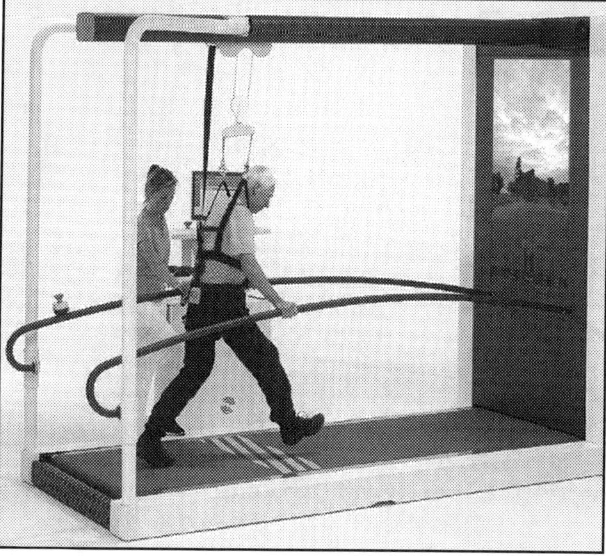

Figure 19-10. Example of gait training in a VR environment. (Picture: Hocoma, Switzerland.)

VR has also been used to improve functional outcomes of patients with Parkinson's disease who demonstrate freezing of gait. In one study, a physical rehabilitation program using a customized video game within the Kinect was used as an intervention for Parkinson's disease patients with gait and balance disorders. Results revealed decreased freezing of gait episodes, increased balance confidence, and improved kinematic gait parameters. Though larger studies are needed, the results show the potential of this technology to assist in optimizing function in people with neurological disorders.[29] However, these data serve as preliminary evidence for further larger and controlled studies to propose this intervention at home.

Virtual Reality and Computerized Cognitive Training

Patients with cognitive impairments may benefit from VR training. Computerized cognitive training on an individual electronic device (eg, computer, laptop, or tablet/iPad) that requires a physical response such as a button press is an example of a complex mental activity being used to enhance cognitive function in the aging population.[30] Multi-domain computerized cognitive training has been found to increase hippocampal functional connectivity that may lead to better memory and cognitive functions.[31]

Gaming Programs for Home-Based Exercises

VR-based gaming programs are cost-effective rehabilitation interventions. The Wii, PlayStation, and Kinect are examples of gaming devices that can be easily adapted for patient use while undergoing rehabilitation, and also as part of their home exercise program. Evidence suggests that these gaming program-based exercises may be an effective alternative to more conventional forms of exercise in improving balance control.[32] A television set or a liquid crystal display projector, gaming console, and game program are the basic equipment needed for the therapeutic intervention. Using gaming programs such as bowling, golf, and tennis can challenge weight-shifting, stepping, and static and dynamic balance. It is helpful to train the patients and their caregivers prior to discharge from the facility to ensure correct use and progression of the training programs. Many of these devices can track the patient's performance over time, so improvements can be documented. Therapists can use these logs to provide feedback to the patient to progress or regress the activity as needed so that the patient is able to exercise at an appropriate intensity. Another alternative is the use of a video recorder to document the session. Therapists can use the playback of the recorded video as a form of augmented performance feedback. Additionally, computer-assisted technologies may give reminders to patients to exercise, summarize the completed programs, and even provide positive reinforcement as appropriate to optimize adherence to the home program.

Activity Tracking Devices and Cell Phone Applications

Adherence to home exercise programs is a significant factor that contributes to the improvement of the patient. Activity tracking devices use behavior change techniques to enhance motivation, goal-setting, self-monitoring, and augmented performance feedback.[33] Examples of consumer physical activity monitors include, BodyMedia Fit (Jawbone), DirectLife (Philips), Fitbit (Fitbit), Vivofit (Garmin), Shine (MisFit), and FuelBand (Nike). Most monitors use accelerometry, which is considered as an objective method of monitoring physical activity and energy expenditure.[34] Many of these devices are worn on the wrist for step-counting; however, evidence suggests that placing these monitors on the hip provides the most accurate reading.[35] The Shine, which can also be worn as a pendant, placed in a pocket, or clipped onto shoe. offers some flexibility, but could be easily misplaced or forgotten, especially in patients who have cognitive deficits. Some consumer technologies such as the Fitbit have algorithms that can differentiate walking from other activities such as running, riding a bike, performing aerobic workouts, or swimming.[36]

There are mobile applications that provide health coaching. Vida Health (Vida Health) is a mobile application that gives personalized health coaching that can be used in combination with the Fitbit to provide feedback and motivation. Other behavioral intervention applications available in similar devices include alarms and texting. Another emerging application in the field of neurorehabilitation is Concussion Tracker. Concussion Tracker (Complete Concussion Management) is an application that provides seamless communication between sport teams, schools, parents, and the local medical team when concussions happen. This application can track physical activity, heart rate patterns, and cognitive function for 6 weeks after a head trauma.[36]

Regenerative Rehabilitation

Regenerative medicine is the "process of creating living, functional tissues to repair or replace tissue or organ function lost due to age, disease, damage, or congenital defects."[37] This collaboration between the fields of regenerative medicine and rehabilitation is termed *regenerative rehabilitation*. The American Physical Therapy Association defines regenerative rehabilitation as the "integration of principles and approaches from rehabilitation and regenerative medicine with the ultimate goal of developing innovative and effective methods that promote the restoration of function through tissue regeneration and repair."[38]

Numerous organisms have a natural process of tissue regeneration to repair themselves following injuries.[39] Technological advances take the process forward by using technology to restore injured, diseased, or degraded tissues such as bone, muscle, cartilage, ligaments, and nerves to a more functional state. Physical therapy then plays an important role in optimizing the patient's functional capacity that could lead to improved quality of life.

The following are examples of physical therapy involvement in this developing area of medicine. Patients who opt for regenerative procedures as an alternative to joint replacement surgery may be referred for physical therapy to improve mobility and function. Regenerative interventions such as autologous bone marrow aspirate concentrate combined with platelet-rich plasma or stem cell injections could decrease pain and improve mobility in the hips and knees that have been lost due to osteoarthritis.[40] With physical therapy, the patient can then optimize movement patterns and potentially regain mobility and ambulation.

Another application involving the rehabilitation team includes patients who will be receiving *autologous* (from the patient, taken before chemotherapy and radiation) or *allogenic* (from a healthy donor) stem cell therapy to treat leukemia, lymphoma, and myeloma. These patients are seen as soon as possible prior to the procedure by the rehab team, which could include physical therapist assistants for exercises as tolerated. After the procedures, the patients continue with physical therapy to optimize mobility and function.[40]

In terms of neurological rehabilitation, there is beginning evidence that a combination of stem cell therapy and exercise interventions involving physical therapy is beneficial to neuroregeneration and recovery from conditions such a cerebrovascular accidents and traumatic brain injuries.[41] The role of physical therapists and physical therapist assistants in this emerging field will continue to increase as we better understand the mechanisms behind neuroregeneration.

Many of the technologies presented in this chapter are part of the mainstream rehabilitation interventions that can be provided by the physical therapist/physical therapist assistant team. Regenerative rehabilitation is an emerging field that is anticipated to involve the rehabilitation team to ensure optimal functional outcomes that can improve the patient's quality of life. In either case, the physical therapist assistant must expect and therefore be prepared for higher practice expectations because of the nature of the practice area. Many of the concepts presented in this text, particularly those related to motor control, motor learning, and neuroplasticity, should be applicable to the patient population.

Case Studies

Case #1

The patient is a 75-year-old African-American man who was fairly active until approximately 3 months ago when his diabetic neuropathy progressed, resulting in numerous ground-level falls with minor injuries in the past few weeks. The patient has a history of hypertension controlled by medications. The patient has no history of blood clots, heart disease, or lung disease. He reports that his wife once tried to break one of his falls, resulting in both of them falling to the ground. He states that, since that incident, he has lost his confidence in his balance, and that he is very afraid that he will hurt his wife again. He is motivated in improving his balance and would like to learn about things that he can do at home.

Questions

1. Which gaming system mentioned previously could be used for strength and balance training by the physical therapist/physical therapist assistant?
2. How would the physical therapist assistant progress the strength and balance training mentioned in question #1?

Case #2

The patient is a 45-year-old Caucasian man who was admitted to the emergency department 3 weeks ago with chief complaints of weakness in all extremities. He reports progressive weakness starting about 3 weeks ago, with initial complaints of difficulty hammering as part of his job as a carpenter. This problem quickly progressed, leading to bilateral partial paralysis of the upper and lower extremities, in addition to complaints of developed difficulty breathing. He was diagnosed with Guillain-Barré syndrome. He is beginning to regain strength of the trunk and extremities but still requires maximum assistance of 2 people to stand up and transfer to the chair.

Questions

1. What is the advantage of using a verticalization robot with stepping movement compared to the traditional tilt-table during the early stage of his recovery?
2. What are some of the advantages of using a body weight–supported mobile walking aid in the rehabilitation process as the patient starts ambulating?

References

1. American Physical Therapy Association. Guide to Physical Therapist Practice 3.0. http://guidetoptpractice.apta.org/. Accessed May 5, 2018.
2. Clynch HM. *Role of the Physical Therapist Assistant: Regulations and Responsibilities*. Philadelphia, PA: FA Davis; 2012.
3. Sheffler LR, Chae J. Technological advances in interventions to enhance poststroke gait. *Phys Med Rehabil Clin N Am*. 2013;24(2):305-323. doi:10.1016/j.pmr.2012.11.005
4. Dimyan MA, Cohen LG. Neuroplasticity in the context of motor rehabilitation after stroke. *Nat Rev Neurol*. 2011;7(2):76-85. doi:10.1038/nrneurol.2010.200
5. Aminov A, Rogers JM, Middleton S, Caeyenberghs K, Wilson PH. What do randomized controlled trials say about virtual rehabilitation in stroke? A systematic literature review and meta-analysis of upper-limb and cognitive outcomes. *J Neuroeng Rehabil*. 2018;15(1):29. doi:10.1186/s12984-018-0370-2
6. Park BS, Kim MY, Lee LK, et al. Effects of conventional overground gait training and a gait trainer with partial body weight support on spatiotemporal gait parameters of patients after stroke. *J Phys Ther Sci*. 2015;27(5):1603-1607. doi:10.1589/jpts.27.1603
7. Horak FB, Henry SM, Shumway-Cook A. Postural perturbations: new insights for treatment of balance disorders. *Phys Ther*. 1997;77(5):517-533. doi:10.1093/ptj/77.5.517
8. Auriel E. Early Mobilisation Following Stroke. https://www.touchneurology.com/articles/early-mobilisation-following-stroke. Published January 27, 2013. Accessed October 15, 2018.
9. Alter-G. Clinical Summary, Resources & Case Studies. https://www.alterg.com/clinical-information?gclid=CjwKCAjw3-bzBRBhEiwAgnnLCpH4U9O10sFZy1kZourK67YiDP699ZfoOed5xJaQ-kPuyAYFoo9ImBoCyH0QAvD_BwE. Accessed December 10, 2018.
10. Morone G, Paolucci S, Cherubini A, et al. Robot-assisted gait training for stroke patients: current state of the art and perspectives of robotics. *Neuropsychiatr Dis Treat*. 2017;13:1303-1311. doi:10.2147/NDT.S114102
11. Krebs HI, Hogan N, Aisen ML, Volpe BT. Robot-aided neurorehabilitation. *IEEE Trans Rehabil Eng*. 1998;6(1):75-87. doi:10.1109/86.662623
12. Preising B, Hsia TC, Mittelstadt B. A literature review: robots in medicine. *IEEE Eng Med Biol Mag*. 1991;10(2):13-22. doi:10.1109/51.82001
13. Iosa M, Morone G, Cherubini A, Paolucci S. The three laws of neurorobotics: a review on what neurorehabilitation robots should do for patients and clinicians. *J Med Biol Eng*. 2016;36(1):1-11. doi:10.1007/s40846-016-0115-2

14. Rocca A, Pignat JM, Berney L, et al. Sympathetic activity and early mobilization in patients in intensive and intermediate care with severe brain injuries: a preliminary prospective randomized study. *BMC Neurol.* 2016;16(1):169. doi:10.1186/s12883-016-0684-2
15. Kuznetsov AN, Rybalko NV, Daminov VD, Luft AR. Early poststroke rehabilitation using a robotic tilt-table stepper and functional electrical stimulation. *Stroke Res Treat.* 2013;2013:946056. doi:10.1155/2013/946056
16. Frazzitta G, Zivi I, Valsecchi R, et al. Effectiveness of a very early stepping verticalization protocol in severe acquired brain injured patients: a randomized pilot study in ICU. *PLoS One.* 2016;11(7):e0158030. doi:10.1371/journal.pone.0158030
17. Colombo G, Joerg M, Schreier R, Dietz V. Treadmill training of paraplegic patients using a robotic orthosis. *J Rehabil Res Dev.* 2000;37(6):693-700.
18. Dundar U, Toktas H, Solak O, Ulasli AM, Eroglu S. A comparative study of conventional physiotherapy versus robotic training combined with physiotherapy in patients with stroke. *Top Stroke Rehabil.* 2014;21(6):453-461. doi:10.1310/tsr2106-453
19. Gijbels D, Lamers I, Kerkhofs L, Alders G, Knippenberg E, Feys P. The Armeo Spring as training tool to improve upper limb functionality in multiple sclerosis: a pilot study. *J Neuroeng Rehabil.* 2011;8(1):5. doi:10.1186/1743-0003-8-5
20. Gagnon DH, Escalona MJ, Vermette M, et al. Locomotor training using an overground robotic exoskeleton in long-term manual wheelchair users with a chronic spinal cord injury living in the community: lessons learned from a feasibility study in terms of recruitment, attendance, learnability, performance and safety. *J Neuroeng Rehabil.* 2018;15(1):12. doi:10.1186/s12984-018-0354-2
21. Ho CH, Triolo RJ, Elias AL, et al. Functional electrical stimulation and spinal cord injury. *Phys Med Rehabil Clin N Am.* 2014;25(3):631-654, ix. doi:10.1016/j.pmr.2014.05.001
22. Anderson KD. Targeting recovery: priorities of the spinal cord-injured population. *J Neurotrauma.* 2004;21(10):1371-1383. doi:10.1089/neu.2004.21.1371
23. Nathan RH. Functional electrical stimulation of the upper limb: charting the forearm surface. *Med Biol Eng Comput.* 1979;17(6):729-736. doi:10.1007/BF02441554
24. Dascal J, Reid M, IsHak WW, et al. Virtual Reality and Medical Inpatients: A Systematic Review of Randomized, Controlled Trials. *Innov Clin Neurosci.* 2017;14(1-2):14-21.
25. Gibo TL, Mugge W, Abbink DA. Trust in haptic assistance: weighting visual and haptic cues based on error history. *Exp Brain Res.* 2017;235(8):2533-2546. doi:10.1007/s00221-017-4986-4
26. Sherman WR, Craig AB. *Understanding Virtual Reality: Interface, Application, and Design.* San Francisco, CA: Morgan Kaufmann; 2002.
27. Carrozzo M, Lacquaniti F. Virtual reality: a tutorial. *Electroencephalogr Clin Neurophysiol.* 1998;109(1):1-9. doi:10.1016/S0924-980X(97)00086-6
28. Villiger M, Liviero J, Awai L, et al. Home-based virtual reality-augmented training improves lower limb muscle strength, balance, and functional mobility following chronic incomplete spinal cord injury. *Front Neurol.* 2017;8:635. doi:10.3389/fneur.2017.00635
29. Nuic D, Vinti M, Karachi C, Foulon P, Van Hamme A, Welter ML. The feasibility and positive effects of a customised videogame rehabilitation programme for freezing of gait and falls in Parkinson's disease patients: a pilot study. *J Neuroeng Rehabil.* 2018;15(1):31. doi:10.1186/s12984-018-0375-x
30. Ten Brinke LF, Davis JC, Barha CK, Liu-Ambrose T. Effects of computerized cognitive training on neuroimaging outcomes in older adults: a systematic review. *BMC Geriatr.* 2017;17(1):139. doi:10.1186/s12877-017-0529-x
31. Sheldon S, Levine B. The role of the hippocampus in memory and mental construction. *Ann N Y Acad Sci.* 2016;1369(1):76-92. doi:10.1111/nyas.13006
32. Laufer Y, Dar G, Kodesh E. Does a Wii-based exercise program enhance balance control of independently functioning older adults? A systematic review. *Clin Interv Aging.* 2014;9:1803-1813. doi:10.2147/CIA.S69673
33. Lyons EJ, Lewis ZH, Mayrsohn BG, Rowland JL. Behavior change techniques implemented in electronic lifestyle activity monitors: a systematic content analysis. *J Med Internet Res.* 2014;16(8):e192. doi:10.2196/jmir.3469
34. Plasqui G, Westerterp KR. Physical activity assessment with accelerometers: an evaluation against doubly labeled water. *Obesity (Silver Spring).* 2007;15(10):2371-2379. doi:10.1038/oby.2007.281
35. Swartz AM, Strath SJ, Bassett DR Jr, O'Brien WL, King GA, Ainsworth BE. Estimation of energy expenditure using CSA accelerometers at hip and wrist sites. *Med Sci Sports Exerc.* 2000;32(9)(suppl):S450-S456. doi:10.1097/00005768-200009001-00003
36. Wright SP, Hall Brown TS, Collier SR, Sandberg K. How consumer physical activity monitors could transform human physiology research. *Am J Physiol Regul Integr Comp Physiol.* 2017;312(3):R358-R367. doi:10.1152/ajpregu.00349.2016
37. National Institutes of Health. Regenerative Medicine. https://archives.nih.gov/asites/report/09-09-2019/report.nih.gov/nihfactsheets/ViewFactSheetc0d0.html?csid=62&key=R#R. Accessed May 30, 2018.
38. Bellamy J. Regenerative Rehabilitation. APTA. http://www.apta.org/RegenerativeRehab/. Accessed May 30, 2018.
39. Mason C, Dunnill P. A brief definition of regenerative medicine. *Regen Med.* 2008;3(1):1-5. doi:10.2217/17460751.3.1.1
40. Hayhurst C. The Role of PTs in Regenerative Medicine. APTA. http://www.apta.org/PTinMotion/2016/3/Feature/RegenerativeMedicine/. Accessed October 23, 2019.
41. Portis SM, Sanberg PR. Regenerative rehabilitation: an innovative and multifactorial approach to recovery from stroke and brain injury. *Cell Med.* 2017;9(3):67-71. doi:10.3727/215517917X693393

Please visit www.routledge.com/9781630915650 to access additional material.

Financial Disclosures

Dr. Hazel Anderson has no financial or proprietary interest in the materials presented herein.

Dr. Fritzie Arce-McShane has no financial or proprietary interest in the materials presented herein.

Dr. Rodiel Kirby Baloy has no financial or proprietary interest in the materials presented herein.

Dr. Ronald De Vera Barredo has no financial or proprietary interest in the materials presented herein.

Dr. Kristen Barta has no financial or proprietary interest in the materials presented herein.

Jan Black has no financial or proprietary interest in the materials presented herein.

Dr. Amy Broekemeier has no financial or proprietary interest in the materials presented herein.

Dr. Gordon U. Burton has no financial or proprietary interest in the materials presented herein.

Dr. Elizabeth Ching has no financial or proprietary interest in the materials presented herein.

Dr. Barbara H. Connolly has no financial or proprietary interest in the materials presented herein.

Dr. Kristine N. Corn has no financial or proprietary interest in the materials presented herein.

Dr. Carol Davis has no financial or proprietary interest in the materials presented herein.

Dr. Lauren Eberhardt has no financial or proprietary interest in the materials presented herein.

Dr. Germaine Ferreira has no financial or proprietary interest in the materials presented herein.

Lisa Ferrin has not disclosed any relevant financial relationships.

Dr. Amanda A. Forster has no financial or proprietary interest in the materials presented herein.

Patricia Harris has not disclosed any relevant financial relationships.

Dr. Brian Hickman has no financial or proprietary interest in the materials presented herein.

Dr. Bret Kennedy has no financial or proprietary interest in the materials presented herein.

Dr. Dennis Klima has no financial or proprietary interest in the materials presented herein.

Dr. Rolando T. Lazaro has no financial or proprietary interest in the materials presented herein.

Dr. Tony Lema has no financial or proprietary interest in the materials presented herein.

Dr. Nelson Marquez has no financial or proprietary interest in the materials presented herein.

Becky S. McKnight has no financial or proprietary interest in the materials presented herein.

Dr. Esmerita Roceles Rotor has no financial or proprietary interest in the materials presented herein.

Dr. Kelly Ryujin has not disclosed any relevant financial relationships.

Dr. Dale Scalise-Smith has not disclosed any relevant financial relationships.

Dr. Eunice Shen has no financial or proprietary interest in the materials presented herein.

Dr. James M. Smith has no financial or proprietary interest in the materials presented herein.

Dr. Irwin S. Thompson has no financial or proprietary interest in the materials presented herein.

Dr. Darcy A. Umphred has no financial or proprietary interest in the materials presented herein.

Dr. Arvie Vitente has no financial or proprietary interest in the materials presented herein.

Dr. Amy Walters has no financial or proprietary interest in the materials presented herein.

Index

Printed in the United States
by Baker & Taylor Publisher Services